Medical Keyboarding, Typing, and Transcribing

TECHNIQUES AND PROCEDURES

Medical Keyboarding, Typing, and Transcribing

TECHNIQUES AND PROCEDURES

4th Edition

Marcy Otis Diehl, BVE, CMA-A, CMT
Professor
Medical Transcription Specialist Curriculum
Grossmont Community College
El Cajon, California

Marilyn Takahashi Fordney, CMA-AC, CMT
Formerly Instructor of Medical Insurance,
Medical Terminology, Medical Machine Transcription,
and Medical Office Procedures
Ventura College, Ventura, California

W.B. SAUNDERS COMPANY
A Division of Harcourt Brace & Company
Philadelphia ▪ London ▪ Toronto ▪ Montreal ▪ Sydney ▪ Tokyo

W.B. SAUNDERS COMPANY
A Division of Harcourt Brace & Company

The Curtis Center
Independence Square West
Philadelphia, Pennsylvania 19106

Library of Congress Cataloging-in-Publication Data

Diehl, Marcy Otis.

Medical keyboarding, typing, and transcribing : techniques and procedures / Marcy Otis Diehl, Marilyn Takahashi Fordney.—4th ed.

p. cm.

Rev. ed. of: Medical typing and transcribing. 3rd ed. 1991.

ISBN 0-7216-6858-5

1. Medical secretaries. 2. Typewriting. 3. Dictation (Office practice) 4. Medical writing. I. Fordney, Marilyn Takahashi. II. Diehl, Marcy Otis. Medical typing and transcribing. III. Title. [DNLM: 1. Medical Secretaries—problems. 2. Medical Records—problems. 3. Medical Records—terminology. 4. Vocational Guidance. W 18.2 D559m 1997]

R728.8.D47 1997 652.3'26—dc20

DNLM/DLC 96-41729

MEDICAL KEYBOARDING, TYPING, AND TRANSCRIBING: TECHNIQUES AND PROCEDURES, 4th Edition ISBN 0-7216-6858-5

Printed in the United States of America.

Last digit is the print number: 9 8 7 6 5 4 3 2

To my new students and former students,
whose excitement about this challenging field
has inspired and delighted me.

MOD

To my sister Toni,
whose dedication to helping the deaf communicate
has been an inspiration.

MTF

Preface

This is the fourth edition of a book that has had a wonderful transformation each time it has been updated—and, of course, we feel that this time it is particularly enhanced and special. It is our hope that if you are picking up this text for the first time as a student or an instructor, you will be as pleased with it as we are. If you have used previous editions of the book, we hope you will find this edition more exciting and even easier to work with. The general format of the book is the same so that both student and instructor can utilize it in ways that are most convenient to them. Objectives introduce each chapter to let the student and instructor know exactly what will be taught. The instructor may test with these objectives in mind to see how well they have been met. The major change has been the addition of a computer component, in the form of a diskette, so that students can gain additional practice working on the screen—mainly editing—and enter the work force better prepared. Challenging medical transcripts will further prepare the student for the actual work place. Text narrative and examples assume that students are using computers in the classroom since nearly all medical transcription done today is on computers. A major change was made to Chapter 2, which describes various pieces of equipment currently being used in transcription, with the introduction of some exciting new applications that make transcribing easier and faster. Since medical transcriptionists work in a variety of settings, we have tried to address the responsibilities of the private office–based transcriptionist, the home-based entrepreneur, the hospital professional, and those employed in transcription services. Because of their difficulty, Chapters 3, 4, and 5 have a complete synopsis of rules at the end of the chapters, facilitating quick referencing. We have also incorporated handy hints that we have learned over the years, as well as information shared by students and colleagues.

A new reference section, Appendix B, consists of tear sheets (perforated pages) that may be used in each student's personal transcriptionist's notebook. This consists of additional new data, some tables appearing within chapters, and popular reference information found in several appendices in past editions. Having all of this information in one location makes it possible to access reference data easily and quickly. This enhancement gives students a good start for their collections and encourages use of reference materials.

This text is designed for the secretarial student who plans to major in medical transcription, seeking eventual employment in a private physician's office, clinic, or hospital or to be self-employed and freelance. There continues to be a serious shortage of well-trained medical transcriptionists resulting from the problems of training, the increase in the quantity of dictation due to longer reports and a larger number of diagnostic studies, the fact that documentation must show medical necessity and correspond to reimbursement, and the demand by hospitals for quality reports. It is an appropriate text for a first-semester medical typing class after completion of a medical terminology course. The legal secretary and court reporting student will also find it a useful introduction to medical terms and practices.

We have designed the book so that it may be used in the community college or vocational-technical institute, for in-service training in the hospital or private medical office, or in extension programs. It may also be used for independent home study if no formal classes are available in the community. The textbook may also be used by practicing medical or legal assistants who want to upgrade their skills but are unable to attend class. Finally, the book serves as a reference for the working medical or legal transcriptionist.

All the material included in the exercises is authentic medical dictation or writing. The facts in the examples have been altered only to the extent necessary to prevent identification of the cases or parties involved. No evaluation of medical practice, nor medical advice, nor recommendations for treatment are to be inferred from our selections. Actual medical documents illustrating format and content are used liberally throughout the major chapters.

Basic English rule books and style manuals form the backbone of the rules and guidelines with our own experience, that of our reviewers and colleagues, and field research determining which methods are most frequently and consistently utilized when there are a variety of choices. Changes in the way professionals do things are reflected in modification in rules and format.

Three audiotapes designed to provide the student with practice in medical transcription are available. The tapes consist of 60 medical reports, letters, and chart notes using a variety of voices to simulate how various physicians might dictate. Transcription may be attempted after completing Chapters 1 through 7. Initially, the letters are dictated slowly, indicating some punctuation and paragraphing. Later in the program, reports are dictated at a more natural dictating speed, and students are asked to employ their own skills in punctuation and paragraphing. These tapes are excellent for a beginning student and may be obtained from the publisher of this textbook. As the student advances, "live" dictation by local physicians is important before the student attempts to obtain employment.

An instructor's guide, available for use with this text, assists in the establishment of a transcription course and gives the teacher some ideas about how to use the text as an adjunct to an existing class. It provides a complete syllabus, features answers to each chapter's review exercises, and gives additional exercises that have no answers provided in the text. Performance evaluation sheets for review tests are included for those who wish to use them. The second half of the guide provides a key of the audiotapes.

As a result of this textbook, we have coauthored a handy reference book that has been well received by the working transcriptionist. It is entitled *Medical Transcription Guide: Do's and Don'ts.* In fact, we have discovered that many students seem to enjoy having this book for reference as well as *Saunders Manual of Medical Transcription, Dorland's Illustrated Medical Dictionary,* and a variety of word books. All of these publications may be obtained from the publisher of this book.

Marcy O. Diehl
San Diego, California

Marilyn T. Fordney
Oxnard, California

Acknowledgments

Credit for the production of this text is owed to many persons, including our husbands, families, and friends, who gave encouragement, advice, and understanding of the priority it had on our time.

We are thankful to the reviewers of each of the chapters who gave us concrete suggestions and extremely helpful criticisms:

Jerri Adler, BA, AA, CMA, CMT
Lane Community College, Eugene, Oregon

Sandie Baillargeon, CMS
Career Canada, Hamilton, Ontario, Canada

Janice E. Bennett
Guthrie Healthcare System, Waverly, New York

Jane L. Bragg
Whitewater, Wisconsin

Martha Garrel, MSA, MT(ASCP), CMA-C
Ivy Technical State College, South Bend, Indiana

Carolyn K. Grimes, RRA, CMT
Miami–Dade Community College, Miami, Florida

Cecilia M. Miller, RN, BSN, CMA
South College, Savannah, Georgia

Ruth Ott
Formerly of Stautzenberger College, Toledo, Ohio

Marsha Schultz, CMT
GateWay Community College, Phoenix, Arizona

Frances P. Steiner
Southeast Regional Occupational Program, Cerritos, California

We gratefully acknowledge the members of our local chapters of the American Association for Medical Transcription and the members of the California Association of Medical Assistant Instructors (CAMAI) who contributed suggestions over the years for improving the text and have been supportive in this project from its outset in 1979.

We are most indebted to many individuals on the staff of the W.B. Saunders Company for their participation in making this text a reality. We wish to express particular appreciation to Margaret Biblis, Senior Acquisitions Editor, and Developmental Editors, Linda C. Wood of The Woods Publishing Group and Dr. Barbara L. Halliburton. Our thanks also go to Agnes Byrne, Project Supervisor, and Shelley Hampton, Production Manager, both of the W.B. Saunders Company.

Special acknowledgment is given to Rita Naughton and Paul Fry, who designed the book.

We are grateful to the Staff of the Transcription Department at Camarillo State Hospital; Joan Marie Griffin, Psychiatric Counselor; and Dr. Hal Forman for their assistance in preparing the psychiatric report section of this textbook.

We wish to acknowledge the Joint Commission on Accreditation of Healthcare Organizations for always being there to answer our many questions so promptly.

In addition, we received many valuable suggestions and much help from the following people: Hazel Tank, CMT, Quality Assurance Manager, AlphaScribe Express, San Diego, California; George Morton, CMT, Instructor, Grossmont Community College, El Cajon, California; Eve Lafond, Transcriptionist; Gail E. Graham, Risk Control Consultant, St. John's Regional Medical Center, Oxnard, California; Danielle LaFrance; Joanne Kennedy, MSLS, Library Manager, Mercy Healthcare Ventura County, Biomedical Research Services, St. John's Regional Medical Center, Oxnard, California; Ofer Nadler, Sales Representative, Dictaphone, Ventura, California; Dr. Dominic Tedesco and staff, who graciously helped with additional research for the spelling of drug names; and Marlene M. DeMers, Clinical Laboratory Scientist, Medical Technologist (American Society of Clinical Pathologists), who reviewed and enhanced the laboratory section.

We appreciate the help from many students, whose questions and criticism while working with the material have been very constructive.

Numerous equipment and supply companies were kind enough to cooperate by supplying descriptive literature and photographs of their products. Their names are credited throughout the text.

MARCY O. DIEHL
MARILYN T. FORDNEY

Contents

CAREER ROLE AND RESPONSIBILITIES

TOOLS OF TRANSCRIPTION

TRANSCRIPTION GUIDELINES

Career Role and Responsibilities

CHAPTER

1

The Medical Transcriptionist's Career, Including Ethical and Legal Responsibilities

OBJECTIVES

After reading this chapter and working the exercises, you should be able to

1. Identify the background and importance of medical records.
2. Explain the skills a transcriptionist must possess and know why terminology is so vital.
3. Identify opportunities for the physically challenged transcriptionist.
4. Define and explain the purpose of a medical report or record.
5. Define privileged and nonprivileged information.
6. Enumerate the guidelines for release of information from both the private medical office and the hospital.
7. Explain the importance of subpoenas for patient records.
8. Assemble a reference notebook.

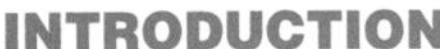

INTRODUCTION

Welcome to an exciting and vitally important career field. We hope that this text will assist you in maintaining an eager interest and excitement about the course of study you are undertaking as well as provide you with a strong foundation as a medical transcriptionist. This text has been designed to speed the beginner transcriptionist (who already knows how to type) on his or her way to proficiency. The more skills you bring with you, the faster you will progress. At the same time, we hope you will begin to experience the fascination and appreciation for medicine that working medical transcriptionists have come to enjoy.

MEDICAL COMMUNICATION

The recording of diseases and injuries goes back many centuries, as shown by hieroglyphics on the walls of the Egyptian tombs. Our first medical terms depicted treatments or remedies in the form of prescriptions. As shown in Figure 1–1, the picture of the bone looks perhaps like a tree with branches, and the heart is depicted as a vessel of some type. This communication has helped bridge the gap between ancient and modern civilizations. Part of the joy of being a transcriptionist is in knowing that you are the modern communicator in the medical field.

JOB OPPORTUNITIES

Health care reform across the United States and the development of a variety of managed care systems have made a significant impact on documentation for inpatient and outpatient settings, requiring increased detailed documentation to back up what is billed. Advances in computer and telecommunications technology have caused changes in how documentation is transmitted, increasing the cost of generating reports. To remain cost efficient, smaller facilities are merging with larger ones to remain a part of the medical industry. Many national organizations are involved in setting standards to determine how business is carried out in the future. It is important to take all this information into account when thinking about job opportunities in the region in which you wish to work.

When you have completed your course of study, you will be prepared to seek employment in a variety of medical settings or become a self-employed transcriptionist (independent contractor) or telecommunicator. The private physician's office, the hospital, and transcription agencies are exciting and interesting work environments, and the duties and responsibilities of an employee in these settings offer a real challenge for the modern career transcriptionist. Although transcribing correspondence, reports, and other medical documents will be your prime responsibility, you may find that there are other interesting business duties.

As more tasks are affected by computerization, career specialists have predicted that workers will become multiskilled. With a broad background in terminology, it is possible to enhance knowledge and skills by enrolling in classes on how to complete insurance claims or how to become proficient in procedural and diagnostic coding. In the physician's office, you may be responsible for processing insurance claims or assisting in patient care. In the hospital, you may work in the medical records department as a full-time transcriptionist or as a part-time transcriptionist with some records management duties. Other hospital departments that require the skills of medical transcriptionists are radiology, pathology, outpatient surgery, emergency, admissions, business, and executive.

Public health clinics, school health facilities, private insurance agencies, specialized computer and transcription agencies, large legal firms, military medical departments, and governmental agencies also offer challenging opportunities for the professional transcriptionist. Medical research is conducted in many settings, and as a medical transcriptionist, you may have the opportunity to participate in this forum. You might decide to work for a private transcribing service. In this setting, you could be working on several different accounts, and each may have different criteria.

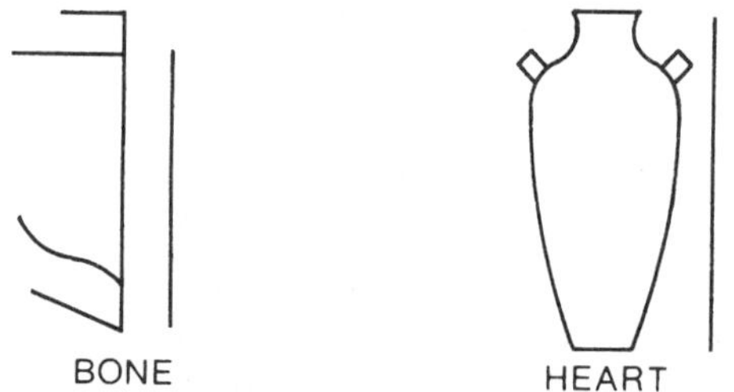

Figure 1–1. Hieroglyphics from the walls of Egyptian tombs depicting some of the first medical terms.

JOB DESCRIPTIONS

You will always be working with others who have chosen the field of medicine in some similar way, and you will find that you are a vital part of the team wherever you are employed; therefore, it is important that you also learn to respect and appreciate the duties of the other personnel with whom you work. To avoid confusion, the differences in duties of the medical typist, medical transcriptionist, and medical secretary are presented.

1. A *medical typist* is a professional who
   a. sets up medical records and accounting forms.
   b. prepares letters from drafts using proper mechanics.

c. does "light" transcribing of letters and chart notes.
d. completes workers' compensation and state disability forms.
e. writes letters to follow up insurance claims, order supplies, collect monies, and so forth.
f. responds to requests for data from life insurance companies.

2. A *medical transcriptionist* is a professional who
   a. possesses excellent typing and word processing skills.
   b. is highly skilled and knowledgeable about human anatomy, physiology, and pathophysiology.
   c. has excellent spelling, editing, and proofreading skills.
   d. has a good command of English grammar, structure, and style.
   e. has a thorough knowledge of medical terminology used in medical and surgical procedures, drugs, instruments, and laboratory tests.
   f. is an indispensable assistant to physicians, surgeons, dentists, and other medical professionals in producing medical reports, which become permanent records of medical, scientific, and legal value.
3. A *medical secretary* is a professional who
   a. possesses a mastery of all medical business office skills (appointment making, telephone procedures, accounting, insurance claim completion, collection of accounts, banking, payroll, mail processing, filing, patient records, office maintenance).
   b. has knowledge of medical terminology as well as excellent grammar skills.
   c. demonstrates the ability to assume responsibility without direct supervision.
   d. exercises initiative and judgment.
   e. makes decisions within the scope of assigned authority.
   f. writes letters over own signature or that of his or her employer.
   g. abstracts medical records and reports.
   h. edits and revises documents for the employer.

Because the role of a transcriptionist requires knowledge, skills, and performance standards, the American Association for Medical Transcription (AAMT) developed a model job description in 1990 (Fig. 1–2). This is not a complete list of duties and responsibilities but may assist as a guideline in the development of a job description by an employer. The subsequent chapters will help you develop the skills outlined in this job description and will illustrate how it ties in with the transcriptionist's job duties.

Because medicine is ever changing and because people and their problems are interesting, we can assure you that you will never get bored. Because of the heavy load of paperwork in the medical field that must be completed on a personal basis, you know that you will never be replaced by a machine. In fact, the demand for medical business personnel is increasing.* There is no age limit, provided that you work proficiently and maintain an acceptable standard of performance. The salary for high-quality professionals is excellent, depending on your experience and locality, of course.

You can be your own boss if you wish: many successful transcriptionists work out of their own homes, at night, or part-time or do freelance work to suit the hours they want. However, this involves more responsibility, because you will have to learn to set up your own business, obtain accounts, advertise and market your service, and so forth.

As you are embarking on this vocational field, you may be interested in where this career may lead. You can further your education and obtain a liberal arts degree or enroll in courses such as English, communications, journalism, professional writing, editing, or education. With experience and background, it is possible to find work as a medical writer, editor, or publications coordinator.

TRANSCRIPTION SKILLS

Medical transcription is both an exacting science and an artistic accomplishment. It is important to have a combination of skills, including the formatting of medical documents; spelling; proofreading; knowledge of medical terminology, disease processes, drugs, and typing or keyboarding; and a firm background in English grammar, structure, and style. The successful medical transcriptionist has accuracy and speed; a broad knowledge of anatomy; and a thorough knowledge of medical, surgical, drug, and laboratory terms; as well as knowing how to use all the standard reference materials, including the medical dictionary, word books, abbreviation reference books, specialty reference books, a standard English dictionary, and drug reference books.

As you proceed through the exercises in this text, you will become more aware of terms that

* The U.S. Department of Labor projects a faster than average employment growth in the health services classification from 1992 employment of 9613 to more than 13,789 by the year 2005, a 43.4% change.

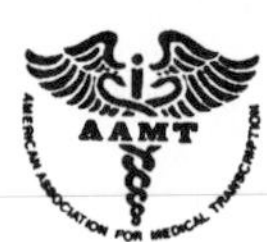

AMERICAN ASSOCIATION
FOR MEDICAL TRANSCRIPTION

AAMT Model Job Description:

MEDICAL TRANSCRIPTIONIST

The *AAMT Model Job Description* is a practical, useful compilation of the basic job responsibilities of a medical transcriptionist. It is designed to assist human resource managers, department managers, supervisors, and others in recruiting, supervising, and evaluating individuals in medical transcription positions.

The *AAMT Model Job Description* is not intended as a complete list of specific duties and responsibilities. Nor is it intended to limit or modify the right of any supervisor to assign, direct, and control the work of employees under supervision. The use of a particular expression or illustration describing duties shall not be held to exclude other duties not mentioned that are of a similar kind or level of difficulty.

Position Summary: Medical language specialist who interprets and transcribes dictation by physicians and other healthcare professionals regarding patient assessment, workup, therapeutic procedures, clinical course, diagnosis, prognosis, etc., in order to document patient care and facilitate delivery of healthcare services.

Knowledge, skills, and abilities:

1. Minimum education level of associate degree or equivalent in work experience and continuing education.
2. Knowledge of medical terminology, anatomy and physiology, clinical medicine, surgery, diagnostic tests, radiology, pathology, pharmacology, and the various medical specialties as required in areas of responsibility.
3. Knowledge of medical transcription guidelines and practices.
4. Excellent written and oral communication skills, including English usage, grammar, punctuation, and style.
5. Ability to understand diverse accents and dialects and varying dictation styles.
6. Ability to use designated reference materials.
7. Ability to operate designated word processing, dictation, and transcription equipment, and other equipment as specified.
8. Ability to work independently with minimal supervision.
9. Ability to work under pressure with time constraints.
10. Ability to concentrate.
11. Excellent listening skills.
12. Excellent eye, hand, and auditory coordination.
13. Certified medical transcriptionist (CMT) status preferred.

Working conditions:
General office environment. Quiet surroundings. Adequate lighting.

Physical demands:
Primarily sedentary work, with continuous use of earphones, keyboard, foot control, and where applicable, video display terminal.

AAMT gratefully acknowledges Lanier Voice Products, Atlanta, Georgia, for funding the development of the *AAMT Model Job Description: Medical Transcriptionist.*

For additional information, contact AAMT, P.O. Box 576187, Modesto, CA 95357-6187. Telephone 209-551-0883 or 800-982-2182. FAX 209-551-9317.

Figure 1–2. The American Association for Medical Transcription Model Job Description: Medical Transcriptionist. This is a practical, useful compilation of the basic job responsibilities of a medical transcriptionist. It is designed to assist human resource managers, department managers, supervisors, and others in recruiting, supervising, and evaluating individuals in medical transcription positions.

AAMT Model Job Description: Medical Transcriptionist

Job responsibilities:	*Performance standards:*
1. Transcribes medical dictation to provide a permanent record of patient care.	1.1 Applies knowledge of medical terminology, anatomy and physiology, and English language rules to the transcription and proofreading of medical dictation from originators with various accents, dialects, and dictation styles. 1.2 Recognizes, interprets, and evaluates inconsistencies, discrepancies, and inaccuracies in medical dictation, and appropriately edits, revises, and clarifies them without altering the meaning of the dictation or changing the dictator's style. 1.3 Clarifies dictation which is unclear or incomplete, seeking assistance as necessary. 1.4 Flags reports requiring the attention of the supervisor or dictator. 1.5 Uses reference materials appropriately and efficiently to facilitate the accuracy, clarity, and completeness of reports. 1.6 Meets quality and productivity standards and deadlines established by employer. 1.7 Verifies patient information for accuracy and completeness. 1.8 Formats reports according to established guidelines.
2. Demonstrates an understanding of the medicolegal implications and responsibilities related to the transcription of patient records to protect the patient and the business/institution.	2.1 Understands and complies with policies and procedures related to medicolegal matters, including confidentiality, amendment of medical records, release of information, patients' rights, medical records as legal evidence, informed consent, etc. 2.2 Meets standards of professional and ethical conduct. 2.3 Recognizes and reports unusual circumstances and/or information with possible risk factors to appropriate risk management personnel. 2.4 Recognizes and reports problems, errors, and discrepancies in dictation and patient records to appropriate manager. 2.5 Consults appropriate personnel regarding dictation which may be regarded as unprofessional, frivolous, insulting, inflammatory, or inappropriate.
3. Operates designated word processing, dictation, and transcription equipment as directed to complete assignments.	3.1 Uses designated equipment effectively, skillfully, and efficiently. 3.2 Maintains equipment and work area as directed. 3.3 Assesses condition of equipment and furnishings, and reports need for replacement or repair.
4. Follows policies and procedures to contribute to the efficiency of the medical transcription department.	4.1 Demonstrates an understanding of policies, procedures, and priorities, seeking clarification as needed. 4.2 Reports to work on time, as scheduled, and is dependable and cooperative. 4.3 Organizes and prioritizes assigned work, and schedules time to accommodate work demands, turnaround-time requirements, and commitments. 4.4 Maintains required records, providing reports as scheduled and upon request. 4.5 Participates in quality assurance programs. 4.6 Participates in evaluation and selection of equipment and furnishings. 4.7 Provides administrative/clerical/technical support as needed and as assigned.
5. Expands job-related knowledge and skills to improve performance and adjust to change.	5.1 Participates in inservice and continuing education activities. 5.2 Provides documentation of inservice and continuing education activities. 5.3 Reviews trends and developments in medicine, English usage, technology, and transcription practices, and shares knowledge with colleagues. 5.4 Documents new and revised terminology, definitions, styles, and practices for reference and application. 5.5 Participates in the evaluation and selection of books, publications, and other reference materials.
6. Uses interpersonal skills effectively to build and maintain cooperative working relationships.	6.1 Works and communicates in a positive and cooperative manner with management and supervisory staff, medical staff, co-workers and other healthcare personnel, and patients and their families when providing information and services, seeking assistance and clarification, and resolving problems. 6.2 Contributes to team efforts. 6.3 Carries out assignments responsibly. 6.4 Participates in a positive and cooperative manner during staff meetings. 6.5 Handles difficult and sensitive situations tactfully. 6.6 Responds well to supervision. 6.7 Shares information with co-workers. 6.8 Assists with training of new employees as needed.

Figure 1–2 *Continued* This is not intended as a complete list of specific duties and responsibilities, nor is it intended to limit or modify the right of any supervisor to assign, direct, and control the work of employees under supervision. The use of a particular expression or illustration describing duties shall not be held to exclude other duties not mentioned that are of a similar kind or level of difficulty. (From the American Association for Medical Transcription, Modesto, California, Copyright 1990.)

may sound alike but are spelled differently because they specify areas located in different parts of the body. For English-speaking persons, Greek terms are sometimes more difficult to spell than Latin terms. You will learn how to pluralize Greek and Latin words. In Chapter 8, you will find exercises that will help you to use the medical dictionary effectively. Other practice sets will develop your skills in punctuating and capitalizing, in using abbreviations, and in typing symbols. Your profession will become more rewarding as your understanding of medical terminology grows.

In Chapter 2, you will be introduced to the equipment used by the transcriptionist, such as computers, stenotype machines, transcribing machines, word processors, voice synthesizers, modems, facsimile equipment, and photocopiers.

It is also important for the medical transcriptionist and medical secretary to understand the ethical implications of handling medical records. Experience in medical transcription brings with it the ability to interpret, translate, and edit medical dictation for content and clarity as well as the ability to use deductive reasoning and detect medical inconsistencies in dictation.

MEDICAL RECORDS

In today's world, medical records are a vital key in patient care and medical research. If the records are kept neatly, thoroughly, and accurately, and if one is prompt in recording the data, they help the physician in the treatment of the patient as well as aid in future research on diseases and their management. As you will learn later in this chapter, properly kept records can eliminate medicolegal problems. Occasionally, records are seen by attorneys, employers, other physicians, insurance companies, and courts, so we cannot overemphasize the importance of keeping them correctly. An efficient system of keeping records can even allow the physician more time for patients. Therefore, the medical transcriptionist becomes an important figure in recordkeeping.

The professional transcriptionist types material that makes sense to him or her or asks the dictator to clean up inconsistencies by flagging the section for clarification. That is why it is important for you to understand medical terminology. Learning the component parts of medical terms (prefixes, suffixes, and roots) enables the transcriptionist to spell and pronounce words he or she may never have encountered.

TRANSCRIPTION SPEED

Unless copy is perfect, speed is worthless. You should always strive for accuracy. At the same time, your pay often will be based on the number of pages, characters, or lines typed, so speed also becomes a skill to work toward. However, some employers pay by the hour or provide a monthly salary. Opinions vary in regard to how many lines per hour a superior secretary should transcribe. A production norm in one situation cannot be applied to another because of a wide range of variables, such as type of hospital (local community, large metropolitan, university teaching medical center); type of dictators (medical students, residents, foreign-speaking, regional accent); type of equipment (word processors, computer-linked equipment, off-site printing); use of macros and alphabetical expanders; additional duties besides transcription; resource materials available; definition of a "line" or other measure of production (words, keystrokes by page, characters typed per day); and standards of quality. One suggested goal is 100 lines per hour, using a 6-inch line as the average. A 15-minute tape averages approximately 150 lines, and a 30-minute tape averages from 300 to 400 lines, depending on the speed of the dictator. As all experienced transcriptionists know, speed and accuracy come together only with constant practice.

If you do not know your typing speed at the beginning of the course and wish to take a timed typing test, ask the instructor for assistance. Your instructor may wish to time you with familiar and unfamiliar work.

THE PHYSICALLY CHALLENGED TRANSCRIPTIONIST

Wheelchair-bound and blind typists have done office work since the invention of the typewriter. When transcribing equipment came into use, many new career paths developed for the blind, making it possible for them to be promoted from corresponding secretary up to and including positions in management. Typists with limited dexterity use special equipment, e.g., a stenotype machine interfaced with a word processor or computer with voice technology or enlarged print. Typists with one hand can be as productive as those typing with both hands. With the need for professional medical transcriptionists and the shortage that is always apparent in most communities, training of the physically challenged has been started in private and community colleges across the nation. Many medical terminology textbooks have been put into braille and onto cassettes to make learning easier and faster.

If a person has a physical impairment and needs training or assistive devices, he or she should contact the appropriate state department of vocational rehabilitation. In addition to the Braille Institute, there are many other sources of help, such as the AAMT, the American Heart Association, the United Way, and the Easter Seal program. See Chapter 8 for materials developed specifically for the physically challenged.

There are a number of machines available to assist the physically challenged transcriptionist. See Chapter 2 for detailed discussion of some of this equipment.

Because listening and typing are the two most important skills in medical transcription, this field usually is not suitable for a person who has a significant hearing impairment.

CERTIFICATION FOR MEDICAL TRANSCRIPTIONISTS

After at least two years of experience in performing medical transcription in a variety of medical and surgical specialties, a qualified medical transcriptionist may wish to take the certification examination offered by the AAMT. The examination consists of two parts: written (multiple choice questionnaire) and practical (transcription of documents). The written examination must be passed to be eligible to take the practical examination. The practical examination must be passed within two years of passing the written examination, or the written examination must be passed again before taking the practical. No credential is given for passing only the written examination. Those passing the examination become certified medical transcriptionists (CMTs). A CMT is recognized as a professional medical transcriptionist who participates in an ongoing program of continuing medical education to increase knowledge of medicine and improve skills in medical transcription. CMTs are required to accrue 30 continuing education credits (CECs) in a three-year period after certification.

There are a number of other benefits of belonging to a professional association besides certification. As a student member, you will get to meet others in the field and learn how they cope with certain on-the-job problems. When attending local meetings, you receive further education from guest speakers on pertinent topics of current interest. From the professional publications you receive, you will learn about what is currently happening in the field. Sometimes part-time or full-time job opportunities are mentioned in the publications as well as at meetings, and this can lead to employment. Most importantly, you will become friends with those in your chosen profession and will feel more professional by belonging to a group.

For more information regarding membership, certification, recertification, and self-assessment products, contact

American Association for Medical Transcription
P.O. Box 576187
Modesto, California 95357
Telephone: 800-982-2182
Fax: 209-551-9317

ETHICAL AND LEGAL RESPONSIBILITIES

Before beginning work as a medical transcriptionist, it is wise to have some basic knowledge of ethical and legal responsibilities as they pertain to the medical profession and the medical transcriptionist. Ethics are not laws but are standards of conduct. AAMT adopted a Code of Ethics on July 10, 1995 (see Appendix B). If you become employed by a transcription service, you also should adhere to the code of ethics developed by the Health Professions Institute in Modesto, California (Fig. 1–3).

This section mentions those medicolegal aspects that concern medical records and how they relate to the medical transcriptionist or typist. These standards vary from state to state, so only commonly accepted practices and procedures are discussed. If you are employed by a health facility that has a policy manual or office procedure manual, familiarize yourself with its rules for the release of information. However, if a situation arises for which you do not have the answer, consult your supervisor or risk management department regarding hospital regulations. The AAMT explains risk management as follows: "Healthcare institution activities that identify, evaluate, reduce, and prevent the risk of injury and loss to patients, visitors, staff, and the institution itself. Medical transcriptionists play an important role in risk management through their commitment to quality in medical transcription and through their alertness to dictated information that indicates potential risk to the patient or the institution, including its personnel. When identified, such information should be brought to the attention of the appro-

Medical Transcription Industry Alliance Code of Ethics and Standards

The goal of the members of the Medical Transcription Industry Alliance (MTIA) is to promote superior performance standards for medical transcription companies and to provide a forum for industry representatives to exchange information. Members of MTIA subscribe to the following Code of Ethics and Standards:

1. We pledge to provide medical transcription service of the highest professional standards to our clients in order to contribute to the quality and efficiency of the healthcare industry.
2. We pledge to conduct ourselves and our businesses in such a way as to bring dignity and honor to the medical transcription profession and industry.
3. We pledge to deal with our clients with the highest standards for integrity and honesty, and to communicate clearly our standards for protection of confidentiality, quality of transcription, turnaround time, and billing practices which include definable and verifiable units of measurement.
4. We pledge to protect and promote the dignity of our employees, to show respect for them as individuals, to honor their right to privacy, to encourage and reward continuing education, to uphold the highest professional standards for confidentiality and quality work, and to respect their employment rights as reflected in federal, state, and local laws.
5. We pledge to follow the highest ethical principles and procedures in relationships with colleagues in the medical transcription industry.
6. We pledge to achieve and maintain the highest attainable levels of professional competence in medical transcription businesses.

Adopted May 2, 1992, Chicago, Illinois

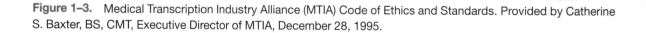

Figure 1–3. Medical Transcription Industry Alliance (MTIA) Code of Ethics and Standards. Provided by Catherine S. Baxter, BS, CMT, Executive Director of MTIA, December 28, 1995.

priate institutional personnel, identified in the institution's program policies."* If you are working in a private medical office, consult the local medical society or your employer's attorney if an unusual problem arises, since you fall under the jurisdiction of *respondeat superior*, or "let the master answer." This means that the physician/dictator is liable in certain cases for the wrongful acts of assistants or employees.

As we discuss the ethical and legal implications in regard to medical records, refer to the following vocabulary list to assist you in better understanding some of the difficult legal terms.

Vocabulary

Breach of confidential communication: In a medical setting, this means the unauthorized release of information about the patient.

Confidentiality: Treatment of the patient's medical information as private and not for publication.

Custodian of records: A person put in charge of medical records.

Defamation: A common tort; injury to reputation, i.e., slander or libel.

Documentation: The supplying of written or printed official information that can be used for evidence.

Ethics: Moral principles and standards in the ideal relationships between the physician and patient and also between physicians.

Etiquette: Customs, rules of conduct, courtesy, and manners of the medical profession.

Invasion of right of privacy: Unwarranted exploitation of another's personality or personal affairs with which one has no legitimate concern in such a way as to cause mental anguish or humiliation. Publication of a patient's medical record or photograph without the knowledge and authorization of the patient.

Libel: A false written or graphic statement to a third person that damages the reputation or subjects a patient to ridicule.

Medical record: Written or computer-stored information (medical reports), tissue samples, log books, or x-ray films are considered medical records and may be used as evidence in legal issues.

Medical report: Written or computer-stored information about the patient's medical history. It is part of the medical record.

Nonprivileged information: The patient's authorization is not needed to disclose the information unless the record is in a specialty hospital or in a special service of a general hospital, e.g., the Psychiatric Unit. Examples: dates of treatment, dates of admission and discharge, number of times the physician attended the patient, name and address of the patient, name of relative or friend given at the time the patient was seen in the hospital or in the physician's office.

Privileged communication: A confidential communication that may be disclosed only with the patient's permission.

Privileged information: Information related to the treatment and progress of the patient that can be given out only on the written authorization of the patient or guardian.

Release of information: Medical information given out to a third party with the written authority of the patient.

Respondeat superior: "Let the master answer." A physician is liable in certain cases for the wrongful acts of his or her assistants or employees.

Risk manager: Coordinates and manages claims and settlements in conjunction with administrative and legal hospital personnel, receives legal documents related to hospital liability, acts as liaison to hospital and medical staff for hospital policy and state and federal legislative requirements, reviews managed care contracts, and assesses losses in hospital activities and future ventures. A risk management department is also established to prevent situations leading to liability.

Slander: A false spoken statement in the presence of others that damages reputation or subjects a person to ridicule.

Subpoena duces tecum: "Under penalty you shall bring with you." A subpoena that requires the appearance of a witness with his or her records. Sometimes the judge permits the mailing of records, and the physician or medical record custodian is not required to appear in court.

Verbatim: word for word.

* From Tessier, Claudia: The AAMT Book of Style for Medical Transcription. American Association for Medical Transcription, Modesto, California, 1995, p 295.

Medical Reports and Records

Joint Commission on Accreditation of Healthcare Organizations

The Joint Commission on Accreditation of Healthcare Organizations (JCAHO) is a commission formed to improve the quality of care and services provided in organized health care settings via a voluntary accreditation process. Accreditation standards are continually updated and published in the *Accreditation Manual for Hospitals* (AMH). JCAHO conducts surveys of hospitals to measure and encourage compliance with the standards. When these standards are met, JCAHO awards accreditation to the health care facility. The Joint Commission's AMH does not address any legal aspects of the medical record as it applies to the transcriptionist. However, their chapter on "Medical Record Services" contains standards that require certain entries, information, and signatures to be entered into the medical record as determined by a prescribed format. A *medical record* is information set down in writing to authenticate evidence of facts and events and is a legal document in all cases of litigation. The transcriptionist is responsible only for the accuracy of the transcribed medical report and for seeing that it remains confidential. A *medical report* is a permanent legal document that formally states the results of an investigation.

Three main purposes of medical records are to

1. Assist in the diagnosis and treatment of a patient by communicating with the attending physician and other medical personnel working with the patient.
2. Aid and advance the science of medicine.
3. Comply with laws and serve in support of a claim.

The Joint Commission's AMH states requirements for medical report completeness, signatures, abbreviations, deadlines, and dates of documents; details of this information are mentioned here.

Authentication of Documents

Manual Signatures

All medical reports dictated by a physician must be signed by the physician responsible for the dictated material. In a case in which an intern does the physical examination of the patient and the attending physician dictates the history and physical, the attending physician may be the one signing the report. In regard to rubber signature stamps on medical reports, careful consideration of state regulations and statutes, system security, and system reliability must be made before such policies are adopted. Rubber signature stamps may be used by the individual whose signature the stamp represents, and there must be a signed statement placed in the hospital administration office attesting that only the physician responsible for the dictated material will use the stamp. Rubber signature stamps are not preferred to an original signature. In regard to pathology and laboratory reports, a laboratory technician must sign, initial, or stamp those reports he or she completes. A pathologist's signature is required only on work he or she performs or provides such as tissue, cytology, necropsy, and consultation reports. In regard to radiology reports, the radiologist must authenticate the examinations he or she interprets in transcribed reports. If the physician is away from the office after dictating a letter or report and the correspondence is urgent, the medical transcriptionist has two choices: he or she can either sign the physician's name with his or her own initials after it, or the medical transcriptionist can send a photocopy of the letter stating that the physician will sign and forward the original upon his or her return.

Electronic Signatures

Many facilities have reports generated via computer and an electronic signature is possible. This means that an individual has computer access and uses an identification system, such as a series of letters or numbers (alphanumeric computer key entries), electronic writing, voice, or fingerprint transmissions (biometric system) to authenticate portions of the medical record. For transcribed medical reports, JCAHO and the Medicare guidelines require that signatures, electronic or other, be written or entered by the physician and not be delegated. The legal requirements for electronic signature can be found in federal law, state law, and the accreditation standards of the JCAHO.

Medicare Signature Requirements

Federal law requires physician signatures in a medical record for hospital compliance with Medicare Conditions of Participation and to qualify for reimbursement under the Prospective Payment System (PPS). A handwritten signature, initials, or computer entry is allowed. However, a computer key signature system is permitted if the hospital keeps a list of computer codes and written signatures that are readily available to surveyors, adequately safeguards the codes against unauthorized access and use, and establishes sanctions for misuse. In regard to Medicare reimbursement, an electronic signature is permitted when the physician attests to the patient's diagnosis only if the fiscal intermediary has approved the system. If the attestation is transmitted by facsimile machines, the physician must keep in the files the hard copy of the original signature.

State laws vary, so it is important for you to know the legal requirements in your state so that you can comply with those laws.

JCAHO Signature Requirements

The JCAHO accreditation standards for hospitals require that all entries into a medical record be authenticated and dated. A method must be established to identify the authors of entries in the medical record. This identification may be a written signature, initials, or computer key. A rubber stamp is allowed if the physician has executed a statement of exclusive possession and use of the stamp. Always consult with JCAHO before implementing any other electronic signature systems.

Abbreviations. The JCAHO requires that the medical staff of each hospital approve abbreviations and symbols that may be used in its medical records, and each abbreviation must have a definition. In regard to the diagnosis section of a report, "Diagnoses and procedures should be written in full, without the use of symbols or abbreviations." Each health care facility's list of abbreviations and symbols will vary, and it is important for the medical transcriptionist to review these before beginning work as well as to refer to the approved list when necessary in performing medical transcription. Since physicians tend to dictate their own preferred abbreviations, it is the medical transcriptionist's responsibility to use only those approved by the medical institution whenever possible. Abbreviations dictated by the physician and approved by the medical facility may be transcribed as abbreviations or transcribed in full, depending on the physician's preference, the medical facility's policies, or the transcriptionist's style. Abbreviations dictated by the physician but not approved by the institution must be transcribed in full. A transcriptionist may not invent abbreviations for words and phrases by the physician. Each health care facility updates the approved abbreviation and symbol list from time to time, so it is important to make sure you have the current list for reference.

Deadlines for Medical Reports. The JCAHO states the following in regard to deadlines for medical reports.

Physical Examination. "The physical assessment shall be completed within the first 24 hours of admission to inpatient services." This document has priority when several items are pending.

Discharge Summaries. "The records of discharged patients shall be completed within a period of time that will in no event exceed 30 days following discharge; the period of time shall be specified in the medical staff rules and regulations."

Operative Reports. Operative reports "should be dictated or written in the medical record immediately after surgery."

Diagnostic or Therapeutic Procedures. "Reports of pathology and clinical laboratory examinations, radiology and nuclear medicine examinations or treatment, anesthesia records, and any other diagnostic or therapeutic procedures should be completed promptly and filed in the record, within 24 hours of completion if possible."

Autopsy Reports. "When a necropsy is performed, provisional anatomic diagnoses should be recorded in the medical record within three days, and the complete protocol should be made part of the record within 60 days."

Dates of Documents. When the date is given for a letter or medical report, the date used is the day the material was dictated and *not* the day it was transcribed. A dictator might ask the typist to date a report other than the actual date of dictation to make it appear that the report was completed in a timely fashion. The date *should not* be changed. This is very important for a number of reasons. Comments made in the document could reflect on this date. If the document should be entered as evidence in a court proceeding, it may be discovered that the date was changed, and the physician's credibility might be questioned and accusations of concealment, tampering, fabricating, and so forth could be made.

Completeness of Medical Reports. It cannot be overemphasized that if medical records are completed promptly after the physician sees the patient, there is less chance of an omission. In a physician's office, it is the office assistant's job to ensure that an entry is made in the chart each time a patient is seen and that all procedures are documented according to the reimbursement codes used for that service. In a hospital setting, it is the medical records personnel that alert the physician to complete a medical record.

A medical record is complete "when the required contents are assembled and authenticated, including any required clinical resume or final progress note; and when all final diagnoses and any complications are recorded, without use of symbols or abbreviations. Completeness implies the transcription of any dictated record content and its insertion into the medical record." All medical information must be entered into the record and all signatures entered within 30 days after the patient's discharge for the record to be considered complete.

Hospitals and physicians have been held liable because the handwritten notes in the charts were unclear. It is, therefore, important that the transcriptionist enter material that is accurate into the record.

Medicare Documentation Guidelines

Guidelines, not laws or rules, have been developed by the American Medical Association (AMA) and the Health Care Financing Administration to make physicians aware of the criteria that a Medicare fiscal intermediary or carrier uses to evaluate records if and when a Medicare audit is conducted. These guidelines affect evaluation and management services that are assigned code numbers from the *Current Procedural Terminology* code book annually published by the AMA. These are discussed in Chapter 11, Medical Chart Notes and Progress Notes.

Ownership

Medical records are the property of the physician, corporation, or institution, and, as such, the owner is legally and ethically obligated to protect them. The Code of Hospital Ethics adopted by the American Hospital Association and the American College of Surgeons states, "It is the responsibility of the hospital and its personnel to safeguard the clinical records of the patients and to see that such records are available only to properly authorized individuals or bodies." This also applies to physicians. Information received from other hospitals and physicians regarding past history or treatment is for informational use and is not considered the property of the hospital that receives it. Correspondence or social service information, which also may be filed in the hospital medical record, is not considered part of the medical record. When a patient is referred to a radiologist for x-ray films, the films belong to the radiologist and not to the referring physician.

Corrections

Medicolegal problems might arise, so it is important to know how to correct medical reports and chart notes. If a patient's medical record is presented in court as evidence in a professional liability case and the records have been sloppily corrected, a prosecuting attorney might win a case if it is proved that the records have been intentionally altered.

See Chapters 7 and 11 for detailed information on correction materials and how to make corrections. Some offices remove all regular pens from their supply and use only legal copy pens, since this eliminates alteration of records when a correction has been inserted. When self-adhesive typing strips are used, the strip should never be obliterated. Instead, place a new strip below it with the correction. If a typist in a hospital transcription pool makes so many errors on a report that it has to be sent back for retyping, insert the omitted words, correct erroneous ones, and initial each correction on the original transcript. If that produces a messy copy, retype it. Write "corrected for typing errors" on the second draft. The physician should sign both the second draft and the original and staple the two copies together. In court, the original will confirm that the report was made as soon as possible after treatment.

CONFIDENTIALITY

When transcribing for a hospital, at home, or in an office or a clinic, the transcriptionist has an obligation to protect the privacy of patients' medical information. Some employers require transcriptionists to sign a confidentiality agreement (Figs. 1–4 and 1–5). To obtain a comprehensive monograph addressing confidentiality, privacy, and security of patient care documentation through the process of medical dictation and transcription, contact the AAMT in Modesto, California.

Right of Privacy

The invasion of the right of privacy is the "unwarranted exploitation of another's personality or personal affairs with which one has no legitimate concern—particularly, intrusions into an other's affairs in such a way as to cause mental anguish or humiliation." An example of invasion of privacy is the publication of a patient's medical record without his or her knowledge or consent. Another example would be the publishing of a

STATEMENT OF CONFIDENTIALITY

TRANSCRIPTION COMPANY understands and agrees that in the performance of our duties as a contractor to COMMUNITY HOSPITAL, we must hold medical information in confidence.

Further, we understand that violation of our contractor's confidentiality may result in legal remedies being sought by COMMUNITY HOSPITAL.

Additionally, TRANSCRIPTION COMPANY's service facilities located at 1234 Main Street, Smalltown, USA, are secure under lock and key.

Security measures to insure confidentiality include, but are not restricted to, shredding of all disposable confidential material not returned, and a statement of confidentiality signed by all employees.

The confidentiality statement signed by all employees reads as follows:

> I understand that the services that TRANSCRIPTION COMPANY performs for its clients are confidential, and to enable TRANSCRIPTION COMPANY to perform those services, its clients furnish to TRANSCRIPTION COMPANY confidential information concerning their affairs. The legal responsibilities and good will of the clients and the people they serve depends, among other things, upon our keeping such services and information confidential.
>
> The Employee recognizes that the disclosure of information by the Employee may give rise to irreparable injury to TRANSCRIPTION COMPANY, the owner, or the subject of such information, and that accordingly, TRANSCRIPTION COMPANY, the owner, or the subject of such information may seek any legal remedies against the Employee which may be available.

__________ ______________________________

Date TRANSCRIPTION COMPANY
President

Figure 1–4. Example of a statement of confidentiality that may be used by a transcription service company when hiring a new employee. It was developed by the Health Professions Institute, Modesto, California.

CONFIDENTIALITY AGREEMENT

Agreement is entered into by ______________ (herein known as EMPLOYEE) and ______________ (herein known as FACILITY).

EMPLOYEE understands that, in the performance of duties as a medical transcriptionist, all patient and client information is to be held in strictest confidence, including but not limited to the transcription of medical documents. EMPLOYEE recognizes that the disclosure of such information shall result in immediate dismissal from FACILITY. EMPLOYEE also acknowledges that any such violation may give rise to irreparable damage to FACILITY, and that FACILITY and any injured party may seek legal remedies against EMPLOYEE.

This AGREEMENT is entered into on (date).

____
Employee signature

____
Witness signature

Figure 1–5. Example of a confidentiality agreement that may be used by a facility when hiring a new employee. It was developed by the Health Professions Institute, Modesto, California.

patient's photograph (from which the patient could be easily identified) without the consent of the patient.

Privileged Communication

Privileged communication is a confidential communication that may be disclosed only with the patient's permission. The right to the protection of the confidentiality of information in medical records belongs to the patient, not the physician. The transcriptionist should never mention the name of a patient away from the office or discuss a patient's condition within hearing distance of others. Everything he or she sees, hears, or reads about patients should remain confidential and should not leave the place of employment *under any circumstances.* Records, appointment books, charts, and ledgers should not be left where unauthorized people can see them. There are a few exceptions to the right of privacy and privileged communication. These include the records of physicians employed by insurance companies (especially for industrial cases) and reports of communicable diseases, child abuse, gunshot wounds and stabbings resulting from criminal actions, and diseases and ailments of newborns and infants.

Release of Medical Records

Information in medical records falls into two classifications, nonprivileged information and privileged information. They can be defined as follows:

1. *Nonprivileged information* is unrelated to the treatment of the patient. The patient's authorization is not needed to disclose these facts to anyone unless the record is in a specialty hospital or in a special service of a general hospital, such as the psychiatric unit. Even so, discretion must be used at all times, and care must be taken to make certain that the inquiry is a proper one that protects the best interests of the patient. Examples of nonprivileged information are as follows:
   a. Dates of treatment.
   b. Dates of admission and discharge.
   c. Number of times and dates when the physician attended the patient.
   d. Fact that the patient was ill or operated on.
   e. Complete name of the patient.
   f. Patient's address at the time the physician saw the patient or at the time the patient was admitted to the hospital.
   g. Name of relative or friend given at the time patient was first seen in the physician's office or at the time of admission to the hospital.
2. *Privileged information* is related to the treatment and progress of the patient and can be given out only on the written authorization of the patient or guardian (Fig. 1–6). A patient can sign an authorization to "release" only selected facts and not the entire record.

Guidelines for Release of Information

Following are guidelines for release of information.

1. The medical transcriptionist should become thoroughly familiar with state laws and with the ethics concerning release of medical information.
2. Whenever a patient fails to keep an appointment or to follow the physician's advice, a letter should be sent to the patient, since documentation is necessary in the medical record.
3. Requests from physicians concerned with patient care are honored with the written consent of the patient.
4. Requests from insurance companies, attorneys, and others concerned from a financial point of view are honored *only* with the written consent of the patient. (If the attorney cannot read the physician's handwriting, an appointment is made with the physician. The attorney should pay for the office call.) The medical transcriptionist should not attempt to interpret a medical record. Exception: See number 18.
5. When litigation is involved, information should *not* be released in the absence of a subpoena unless the patient has authorized it. Remember never to accept a subpoena or give records to anyone without the physician's prior authorization. In the case of a subpoena or interrogatories (questions directed to a physician who is being sued), the medical transcriptionist should not release records without first verifying them with the physician and having him or her correct any inaccuracies. Usually there is time to review such records, and any problems should be referred to the physician's lawyer before release.
6. Government and state agencies may have access to records pertaining to federal government-sponsored and state-sponsored programs, but these records should not be released without explicit consent of the patient.

AUTHORIZATION FOR DISCLOSURE OF CONFIDENTIAL INFORMATION

I hereby authorize and request Dr. ________________ to furnish

information or copy of my medical records to:

____

____

____

about medical findings and treatment about my illness and/or treatment

during the period from ______________to_________________

I understand that this is a required consent and I must voluntarily and knowingly sign this authorization before any records may be released, and that I may refuse to sign, but in that event the records will not be released.

I further release my physician from any liability arising from the release of information to the individual(s)/agency designated herein.

Signed________________________ Witness___________________

Address________________________ Date_____________________

____

Optional statements may include:
I agree that a photocopy of this form may be used in lieu of the original.

This authorization will automatically expire one year from the date signed or is effective until________________________.

Figure 1–6. Example of authorization for disclosure of confidential information.

7. Information of a psychiatric nature may present special or delicate problems. Generally the psychiatrist or another attending physician concerned with the case should be consulted before any data are released.

8. Special care should be exercised in the release of any information to an employer, even with the consent of the patient. See number 18 for additional information regarding industrial injuries.

9. It is preferable not to allow lay persons to examine records. In this way misunderstandings of technical terms are avoided. However, according to the Privacy Act of 1974, certain patients, such as those receiving Medicare and CHAMPUS benefits, have a right to their records, since federal agencies are bound by its provisions. If the physician determines that the release may not be in the patient's best interests, most states allow for release to a representative of the patient. The only way a physician can prevent patients from gaining access to privileged information in their own medical records is by noting on the charts that he or she believes knowledge of the contents would be detrimental to the patient's best interests. This entry, however, must be made before the patient makes his or her request. Usually the courts will uphold a physician's judgment under these instances. In many states it is consid-

ered risky to allow a patient to hand-carry his or her records to a consultant, since the patient may misinterpret what has been entered in the record and may become frightened or angered. If there is a time factor involved and sending the records with the patient is the best solution to get them there on time, seal them in an envelope and send copies, not the originals. It is also a good idea to have the patient sign a receipt for any x-ray films. Consultation reports from other physicians, even those stamped "confidential," as well as billing or accounting records may also be released to the patient. Only the paper they are typed on is the physician's.

10. Care must be exercised in the release of any information for publication, since this also constitutes an invasion of the patient's right to privacy and can result in legal action against the physician or health facility releasing such information.
11. When in doubt about the release of any information, obtain the patient's authorization in writing.
12. If the signed authorization form is a photocopy, it is necessary to state that the photocopy is approved by the patient or to write to the patient and obtain an original signed document.
13. Any transfer of records from hospital to hospital, physician to physician, or hospital to nursing home should be authorized in writing by the patient. If the patient is physically or mentally incapacitated, the next of kin or legal guardian may approve the transfer.
14. You cannot justifiably refuse to provide information to another physician just because a patient has a large outstanding bill with your office or institution.
15. If a legal photocopier comes to the office to copy the record, number the pages released or observe the record while it is copied. You may do it yourself and charge the attorney a fee for this service.
16. When working in a hospital, medical transcriptionists should check with the supervisor or risk manager at all times to make sure their actions conform with hospital policy in regard to release of medical information. Whether working in a hospital or for a physician, do not hesitate to ask for clarification of matters that are unclear. If you are employed by a health care facility that has a policy manual or office procedure manual, familiarize yourself with its rules regarding the release of information.
17. Oral requests can be handled in two ways. Either ask the caller to put the request in writing and include the patient's signature for release of information, or obtain the name and telephone number of the caller and relationship to the patient and have the physician return the call.
18. In an industrial injury (workers' compensation) case, the contract exists between the physician and the insurance carrier. When an insurance adjuster requests information in such a case by telephone, verify to whom you are speaking before giving out medical information. Such cases do not require a patient to have a signed release of information form on file.
19. If working in a physician's office, seek legal counsel if a patient who has a positive human immunodeficiency virus (HIV) test for acquired immune deficiency syndrome (AIDS) applies for life or health insurance and requests that the physician or hospital send medical records to the insurance company. Some state laws allow AIDS information to be given only to the patient's spouse. In a hospital setting, patients infected with HIV must sign an informed written consent before any medical information is released. The release of information from records of persons who have HIV infection or those tested for HIV must be handled very carefully, especially in states with restricted access, because information about test results may appear in many sections of the health record. If state law says test results may be placed separate from the patient's medical record, a file for cases (e.g., HIV or alcohol or substance abuse) that require special release of information forms may be established. The use of ICD-9-CM code 795.8 reflects a positive HIV test, so this information must be considered confidential. The American Health Information Management Association (AHIMA) has suggested the use of a consent for release of information form (Fig. 1–7). Besides completing the blanks, it is important to list the extent or nature of the information to be released, e.g., HIV test results of diagnosis and treatment with inclusive dates of treatment. Following authorized release of patient information, the signed authorization should be retained in the health record with notation of the specific information released, the date of release, and the signature of the individual who released the information. All information released on the request of a patient with a diagnosis of HIV infection should be clearly stamped with a

NAME OF FACILITY
Consent for Release of Information

DATE________________

1. I hereby authorize__________________to release the
Name of Institution
following information from the health record(s) of

____
Patient Name

____
Address
covering the period(s) of hospitalization from:
Date of Admission______________________________
Date of Discharge______________________________
Hospital #__________________Birthdate______________

2. Information to be released:
[ ] Copy of (complete) health record(s) [ ] Discharge Summary
[ ] History and Physical [ ] Operative Report
[ ] Other______________________________________

3. Information is to be released to_______________________

____

4. Purpose of disclosure_________________________________

____

5. I understand this consent can be revoked at any time except to the extent that disclosure made in good faith has already occurred in reliance on this consent.

6. Specification of the date, event, or condition upon which this consent expires.

____

7. The facility, its employees and officers and attending physician are released from legal responsibility or liability for the release of the above information to the extent indicated and authorized herein.
Signed____
(Patient or Representative)

____
(Relationship to Patient)

____
(Date of Signature)

Figure 1–7. Consent for release of information form. (Reprinted with permission from the American Health Information Management Association [AHIMA], formerly known as the American Medical Record Association [AMRA], Chicago, Illinois.)

statement prohibiting redisclosure of the information to another party without the prior consent of the patient. The party receiving the information should also be requested to destroy the information after the stated need is fulfilled.

Special Guidelines for Release of Hospital Information

Generally speaking, certain information is not available from the hospital medical record for release to third parties. This includes detailed psychiatric examination information, personal history of the patient or family, and information controlled by state law. If there is a question regarding the content of the medical information to be released, the attending physician should be consulted regarding its accuracy or interpretation. Hospitals prefer to release information by the use of summaries or abstracts or on standard forms recommended by the American Hospital Association or local hospital groups. Duplicating an entire record is expensive; furthermore, control of the record by the hospital would be lost, and the copy might be misused. If the attending physician wishes information from the hospital record, an abstract or a copy can be given without the patient's written permission, as long as it is for the physician's own use.

Retention of Records

State and local laws govern the retention of records, and many states set a minimum of 7 to 10 years for keeping records in their original form. Generally, most physicians retain medical records on their patients for an indefinite period of time for research or for historical significance. In the case of minors, records should be retained three to four years beyond the age of majority.

Subpoena Duces Tecum

Subpoena duces tecum requires the witness to appear and to bring certain records to the deposition, trial, or other legal proceeding. Usually, the records are mailed by certified mail, and the physician or custodian of the records is not required to appear in court. A subpoena is a legal document signed by the clerk of the court (Fig. 1–8). In cases in which a "pretrial of evidence" or deposition is set up, the subpoena may be issued by a notary public, in which event it is called a notary subpoena. If an attorney signs it, he or she must validate it in the name of a judge, the court clerk, or other proper officer.

A *subpoena duces tecum* must be served to the prospective witness in person. If the subpoena is accepted by someone authorized to receive it, it is the equivalent to personal service. The subpoena cannot be left on a desk. It must be served with the subpoena (witness) fee and mileage fee, if requested by the witness. In some states, provision is made for substitute service by mail or through newspaper publication if all reasonable efforts to effect personal service have failed. In certain states, such as California, it is illegal for the physician to tell the custodian of the records not to release medical records when a written authorization has been signed by an adult patient.

Here are nine points to remember if a subpoena is served and you are given permission to receive it for the physician.

1. Be courteous to the deputy who is serving the subpoena. Ask for the fee when the subpoena is served because in the absence of the fee the subpoena is not legally valid and may be refused.
2. Find out from the deputy to which physician the subpoena is addressed. Get the name of the custodian of records for that particular physician if you are not the custodian. Ask to see the subpoena so that you know what action to take.
3. If the physician is on vacation, explain that you cannot accept a subpoena in the physician's absence. Suggest that the deputy contact the physician's attorney and relay this information to the attorney. Discuss the subpoena in question with one of the other physicians in the office for advice or management.
4. After receiving the witness fee and the subpoena, obtain the patient's chart and place the medical record and the subpoena on the physician's desk for review. Willful disregard of a subpoena is punishable as contempt of court. After receiving a subpoena for a trial, verify with the court that the case is on the calendar. If the subpoena is for a deposition, verify the date and place to appear with the attorney.
5. You will have a prescribed time in which to produce the records. It is not necessary to show them at the time of service of the subpoena unless the court order so states. Telephone the attorney who ordered the subpoena and request permission to mail the record or a copy of the record. If the attorney agrees, send it by certified mail with return receipt requested. If the subpoena is for a trial, the witness or custodian of the records will have to appear in court unless there is permission to mail. If you do not appear, you may be in contempt of court and subject to fine or imprisonment.
6. Never give records to anyone without the physician's prior permission. When a subpoena is served, an authorization form for release of records signed by the patient is not required. Read the record to see that it is complete and that signatures and initials are identifiable.
7. Remove the records to a safe place so that they cannot be stolen or tampered with before the legal proceeding. Make photostatic copies of the records if you are in doubt about their safety. This may be expensive, but it can prevent total loss of the records and facilitate discovery of any altering while they are outside your custody. It also provides you with the record in case the patient is treated before the original is returned.
8. If you must appear in court with the records, comply with all instructions given by the court. *Do not* give up possession of the records unless

Name, Address and Telephone No. of Attorney(s)	Space Below for Use of Court Clerk Only
Mitchell & Green 210 W. "A" Street Los Angeles, California 90014 (213) 232-7461 Attorney(s) for Defendants	

SUPERIOR COURT OF CALIFORNIA, COUNTY OF LOS ANGELES

ALBERT OTTO — Plaintiff(s) vs. ROY M. LEDFORD, RALPH WALLACE, et al., — Defendant(s) (Abbreviated Title)	CASE NUMBER 353 957 **SUBPENA DUCES TECUM (Civil)**

THE PEOPLE OF THE STATE OF CALIFORNIA, to Dr. J. Brown,

You are ordered to appear in this court, located at 111 No. Hill Street, Los Angeles, Ca. (Street Address of Court and City),

on Feb. 8,199x (Date) at 9 a.m., (Time) Department 1 (Department, Division or Room No., if any), to testify as a witness in this action,

You must appear at that time unless you make a special agreement to appear another time, etc., with:

R. Mitchell, esq. (Name of Attorney or Party Requesting This Subpena Duces Tecum) at 232-7461 (Telephone Number)

You are also ordered to bring with you the books, papers and documents or other things in your possession or under your control, described in the attached declaration or affidavit, which is incorporated herein by reference.

Disobedience of this subpena may be punished as contempt by this court. You will also be liable for the sum of one hundred dollars and all damages to such party resulting from your failure to attend or bring the books, etc., described above.

Dated Jan. 31, 199x

SUPERIOR COURT, LOS ANGELES COUNTY, CALIFORNIA

Clarence E Cabell

CLARENCE E. CABELL, County Clerk and Clerk of the Superior Court of California, County of Los Angeles.

(To be completed when the subpena is directed to a California highway patrolman, sheriff, marshal or policeman, etc.)

This subpena is directed to a member of ____________ (Name of Employing Agency)

I certify that the fees required by law are deposited with this court.

Receipt No.____________ Amount Deposited $____________

CLARENCE E. CABELL, County Clerk By ____________, Deputy

NOTE: The original declaration or affidavit must be filed with the court clerk and a copy served with this subpena duces tecum.

(See reverse side for Proof of Service)

SUBPENA DUCES TECUM (Civil)

C.C.P. §§1985-1997; Evid. C. §§1560-1566; Gov. C. §§68097.1–68097.4; 35c.

Figure 1–8. Subpoena duces tecum (civil).

instructed to do so by the judge. *Do not* permit examination of the records by anyone who has not been identified in court. When you leave the records in the court in the possession of the judge or jury, obtain a receipt for them.

9. If you have additional questions, call the patient's attorney or the physician's attorney.

TRANSCRIPTIONIST'S NOTEBOOK OR FILE

As you prepare for your future career as a transcriptionist, you should organize two notebooks. One should be an alphabetical pocket-sized notebook and the other a standard-size three-ring binder with or without index tabs. These notebooks can become valuable tools. The alphabetical notebook is for writing down any new or unfamiliar words or phrases heard while listening to transcription tapes (Fig. 1–9). Make it a rule to add any word that you had to research because of spelling, capitalization, or usage. In this way, when you hear the word again, you will be able to find it with ease. It is always easier to locate a word in your own guide, even when you know the word is in the dictionary. Do not make this a chore or you will not be consistent. Write in the word, no definitions, with a few hints from time to time such as the following:

- An (a) or (n) after an adjective or noun term

  EXAMPLE

  mucous (a)   mucus (n)

- An (s) or (p) after a singular or plural word

  EXAMPLE

  bronchus (s)   bronchi (p)

- An extra word to complete a complicated pair

  EXAMPLE

  pleural poudrage   poudrage, pleural

B

babermycins (generic)

Berke ptosis forceps (Oph)

bleed (n)

bombe, iris (Dr. J.J.)

bougie (surg instr)

bruits (p)

BUS (Ob–Gyn) Bartholin's, urethral, Skene's glands

Figure 1–9. Page B from an alphabetical pocket-sized transcriptionist's notebook showing the following entries: a generic drug word, an ophthalmology term, a noun, a word dictated by Dr. John Jones, a surgical instrument, a plural word, and an obstetric and gynecologic abbreviation.

- A line under a capital letter so you will not wonder later if it is correct

EXAMPLE

pH

- A source clue that could help you to determine later that you have the correct word

EXAMPLE

CABG (cardio)

When working for a group of physicians, some transcriptionists prefer to indicate which physician dictated the word by placing his or her initials after the word. Any other individual hints you can think of to help you may certainly be incorporated because this is your reference book. As your material accumulates, be sure you carefully recopy it in strict alphabetical sequence. An alternative reference method is to prepare an index file of 3 × 5 inch cards with alphabetical dividers and to use the cards in the way mentioned previously.

A standard-size binder can be used for storing commonly needed information for quick reference while transcribing dictation, such as state abbreviations, proofreading marks, and so forth. Throughout this text/workbook, notations appear that give you instructions to insert special data sheets into your standard notebook. Your instructors may provide additional lists and data sheets as you progress. When you are employed, you will often come across articles or lists in journals or other publications that serve as excellent reference guides.

Now you are ready to begin Self-Study 1–1, on your way to becoming a medical transcriptionist.

1–1: SELF-STUDY

Directions: Let's start on the right foot by beginning a pocket-sized notebook and a standard three-ring notebook. Obtain an easy-to-handle, ½-inch thick, three-hole ring binder with 25 sheets of lined paper and A-Z index guides. If it is difficult to locate a set of 26 alphabetical index tabs, obtain the 2-letter combined alphabetical index tabs. As you come to words in the text that you have difficulty spelling or that you want to be able to refer to quickly, place them under the correct alphabet letter for easy reference. Beginning with Chapter 3, look for some words to place in your notebook. Write in any unusual words or abbreviations that appear in your examples or exercises.

1–2: REVIEW TEST

Directions: Complete the following statements by filling in the blanks.

1. According to standards of the Joint Commission on Accreditation of Healthcare Organizations, what is the deadline for completion of a physical examination report on an inpatient?

____

____

2. Explain briefly why it is important for the transcriptionist to understand medical terminology.

____

____

____

3. State at least four skills a good transcriptionist should have.

a. ______________ c. ______________

b. ______________ d. ______________

4. In transcribing, what is even more important than speed?

____

5. A permanent legal document that formally states the results of an investigation is a/an

____.

6. Written or typed information set down for the purpose of preserving memory that authenticates evidence of facts and events is a/an

____.

7. Briefly list three main purposes of medical records.

   a. ____

   b. ____

   c. ____

8. Who owns the patient's medical records? ____

9. Confidential communication that may be disclosed only with the patient's permission is also known as ____.

10. Name two classifications of information contained in medical records.

   a. ____

   b. ____

11. Name three places legal requirements for electronic signatures can be found.

   a. ____

   b. ____

   c. ____

12. Miss Freda Findley was in an automobile accident. Her attorney, James Burr, called and asked that a report of her condition be sent to him. What should the transcriptionist do?

____

____

13. Mr. Henry Waxman, an employer, calls the physician's office to inquire about the condition of one of his employees who had become ill while on vacation. The medical transcriptionist taking the call should do what?

____

____

____

14. Mrs. Jane Avers had plastic surgery done on her ears. Dr. Jeffers submitted an article to the *Medical World,* which was subsequently published, including the patient's photograph. No consent form was signed by the patient. What ethical and legal infringement would this be classified as?

____

15. The transcriptionist recognized the name of a patient as being the son of a friend of hers. The report indicated a good prognosis for the child. Since the mother had been depressed and uneasy for her child, the transcriptionist felt it was all right to telephone her and reassure her. Was this action correct? __________ Why? ____

____

Tools of Transcription

CHAPTER

2

Equipment

OBJECTIVES

After reading this chapter and working the exercises, you should be able to

1. State how dictation and transcription evolved over decades.
2. Describe the operation of different types of dictation and transcription equipment.
3. Identify components of a computer system.
4. Explain the capabilities of word processing computer software.
5. Name speed typing systems available.
6. Explain various methods to manage and store computer data.
7. Identify types and features of computer printers.
8. State the purpose of a modem.
9. Identify ergonomic factors that affect the transcriptionist's work environment.
10. Name two categories of voice recognition systems.
11. List some of the indication features used in dictation machines.
12. Define the hand/foot control of transcription equipment.
13. Demonstrate proper computer and transcriber equipment maintenance.
14. Perform the steps of transcription preparation.
15. Identify equipment for physically challenged individuals.
16. Explain how photocopying and facsimile machines may be used in the transcription process.
17. Define vocabulary terms related to office equipment.

2

HISTORY

Dictation

Initially, physicians made handwritten chart entries or dictated chart notes and medical reports in person to secretaries who wrote in shorthand. It was necessary for two people to be simultaneously engaged, a condition that was often difficult in a busy office. The clerk also had to convert his or her notes quickly because a certain amount of memory was involved. It was nearly impossible for someone other than the person who took the notes to transcribe them. Then, dictation machines, which have been traced back to Thomas Edison, made their appearance. The physician dictated reports directly and at any time, freeing the transcriptionist for other tasks during dictation and making it possible for others with skills to transcribe the reports. These machines had cylinders made of material that would easily chip, crack, or break into pieces if dropped. Sound was of poor quality. By the 1960s, Mylar tape was used, which substantially improved the sound quality of standard cassettes. Eventually, microcassettes and picocassettes were introduced. Still popular are *desk-top machines,* which are used by the physician and medical transcriptionist. The most common units available include the following:

- *Dictation unit,* for dictation only
- *Transcription unit,* designed for the transcriptionist who will transcribe the dictation (Fig. 2–1)
- *Combination unit,* which can be used for both dictation and transcription

Some transcriptionists use a *cassette-changer central recorder.* This holds 15 to 25 cassettes that can be programmed to change automatically, either according to the number of dictators having access to the recorders or according to the percentage of tape used. It can be set up so that each person who dictates is recorded on a separate cassette. Dictators can access the equipment from any telephone, at work or at home.

Physicians carry *portable dictating machines* to conventions or meetings or for use in an automobile or at home (Fig. 2–2). These are battery operated or can be used with AC current and a wall plug. Microcassettes can be played back at the office if the transcription equipment is fitted with an adaptor.

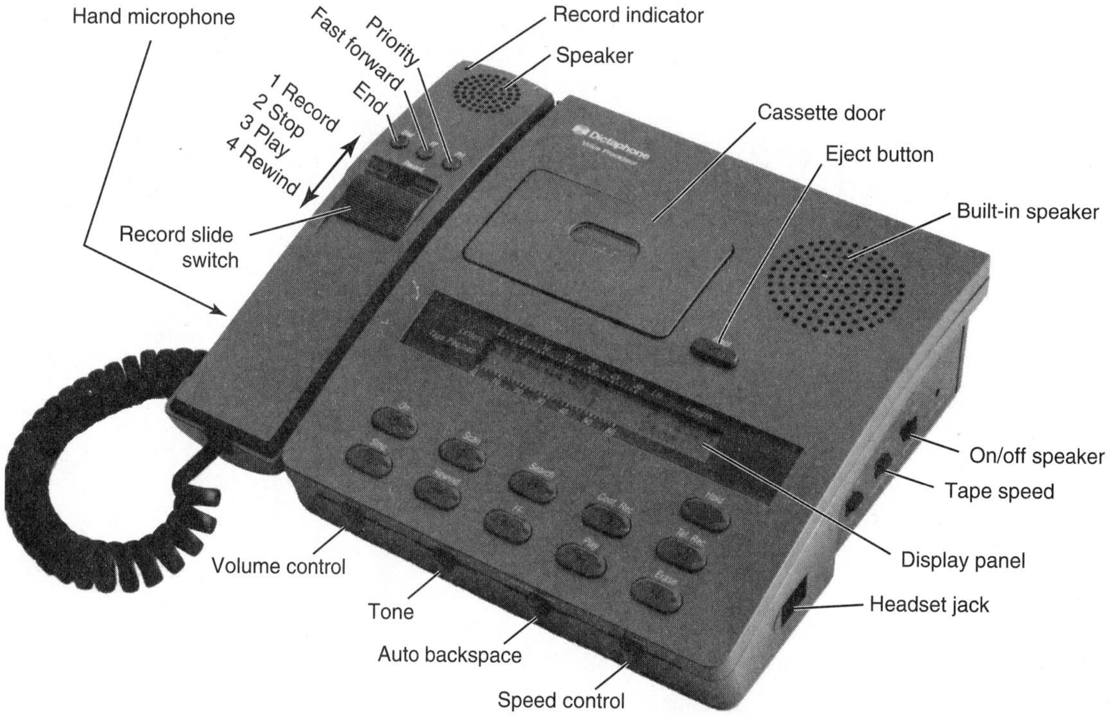

Figure 2–1. Dictaphone's Express Writer Plus voice processing system, a fully programmable compact desktop system, features advanced dictation and transcription capabilities. Light-emitting diode (LED) display shows various functions on the control panel for recording or transcribing a document. (Courtesy of Dictaphone Corporation, Stratford, Connecticut.)

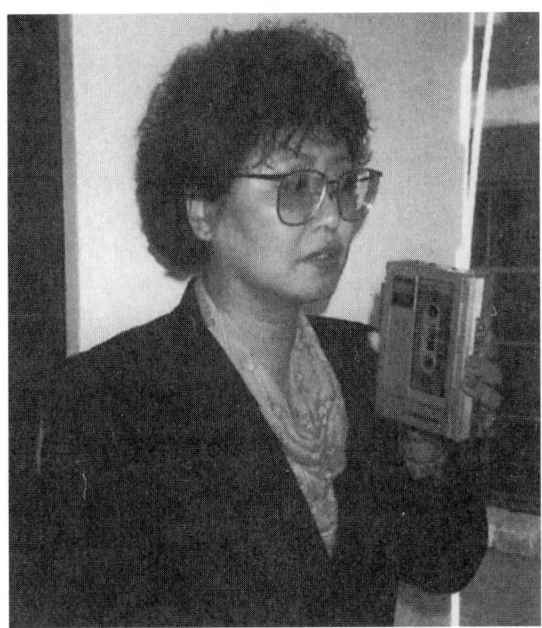

Figure 2–2. A physician using a portable dictating machine.

Digital Dictation

Digital dictation is used in many offices and hospital facilities, eliminating the use of Mylar tape. The dictated voice is digitized (converted to a string of 0s and 1s, representing the audio waveform) and stored as data on a computer disk with identifying information (patient and dictator identification and work type). Data are instantly and selectively accessible before, during, or after transcription. When accessed (from a dictation/transcription station or connections telephone), the binary digits are converted back to analog waveform to sound the same as the original dictation (Fig. 2–3). Therefore, sound quality is superior because there is no background noise, hiss, or other extraneous sounds. The dictator can insert or delete material for error-free dictation. Most transcriptionists in hospitals that are on digital systems use a connections telephone and a password to access dictation of an individual physician or a group of physicians, depending on how the system is set up. The connections telephone has buttons that are used to make the speed of the dictation slower or faster, volume louder or softer, and tone bass or treble. The backup feature of the foot control makes it easy to relisten to a short phrase or a long sentence.

Typewriter

To accomplish their work, medical transcriptionists must have tools, like everyone else in business. In the early 1800s, the tool was a manual typewriter with carriage and keys that hit onto a cylindrical platen. In 1872, Christopher Sholes along with

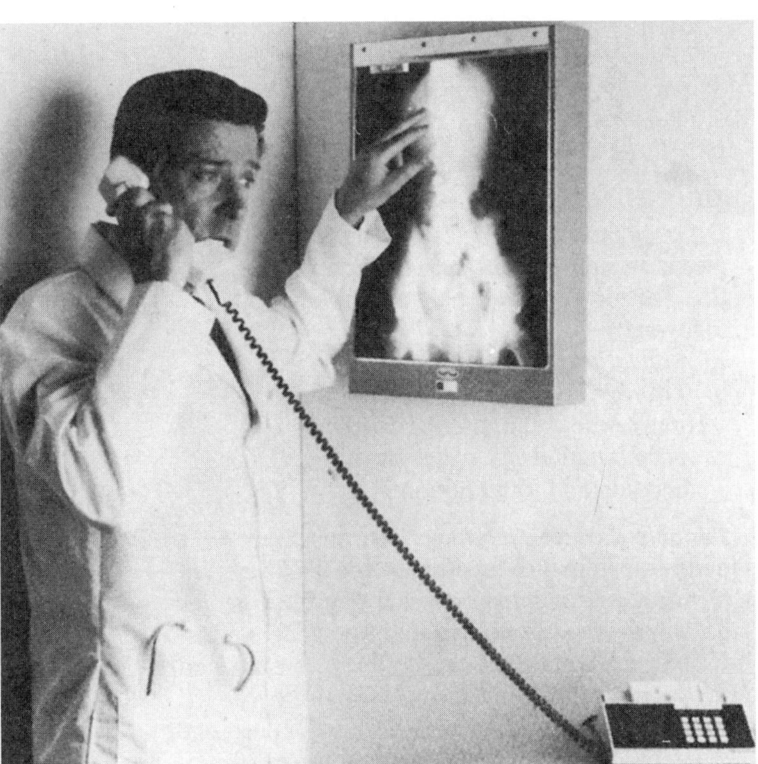

Figure 2–3. The physician's voice is digitized while using a dictation station (connections telephone–like device) to dictate medical reports from the hospital or office to the transcription department or outside service. (Courtesy of Dictaphone Corporation, Stratford, Connecticut.)

friends developed the QWERTY typewriter keyboard (named for the six keys above the home row of the left hand). In 1936, August Dvorak created the DVORAK arrangement of keys, increasing accuracy by 50% and speed by 15 to 20%. However, this keyboard arrangement never caught on. The first electric typewriter was manufactured by Remington and Sons in 1925. In the 1960s, the IBM Selectric typewriter was the next step in technology. Individual keys were replaced by a ball or spherical element containing all the letters and numbers in the standard pica and elite type in addition to a variety of other type styles. The element moved across the page, eliminating the movement of the carriage. In the late 1970s, the electronic typewriter was introduced, which was a forerunner to word processors. It had a small memory, and mistakes could be corrected on a small screen before a document was typed or printed. Then, word processors and computers were competitively marketed, making it possible to input entire pages, check for errors, and print error-free pages in one or more of hundreds of available fonts. The use of carbon paper was virtually eliminated.

COMPUTER SYSTEMS

In the 1990s, personal computers (PCs) that perform with a variety of word processing software packages are used in most offices. Computers perform a multitude of functions: telecommunication, filing, word processing, graphics, accounting and financial management, and so forth. Therefore, many hospital facilities, medical clinics, and physicians' offices are equipped with PCs.

Hardware

The physical components of a computer system (electronic, magnetic, and mechanical devices) are known as the *hardware* (Fig. 2–4). A computer has a *keyboard* in either the QWERTY or the DVORAK typewriter configuration plus function keys, also known as control keys, or *command keys.* A program instruction may be given by depressing certain keys or combinations of keys to enter a particular command into the software program. *Response time* is the time it takes the system to react to a command; it varies depending on the sophistication of the equipment. Computers are equipped with a *monitor* (video screen). Data are keyboarded *(input),* and the typist may electronically rearrange the material, revise it, and then put it into a variety of final formats for "error-free" copy *(output).* Computers allow the typist to rewrite or eliminate words or complete paragraphs within seconds.

In addition to keying in data, it is possible with some sophisticated equipment to handwrite or say special words to create data automatically. It is possible to point to a picture on a touch-sensitive video screen or computer pad to perform certain functions. Similar equipment is used in shopping malls to locate stores or make gift selections at a bridal registry. Computer accessories, such as a *mouse* or a light pen, are hand-maneuvered devices that enable the operator to draw images, mark choices, and add or delete text on the monitor. Light pens are used in some facilities to scan the patient's admitting information so that the operator does not have to type the patient's name and other identifying data.

Data are stored temporarily in the *memory,* the material is proofread from the screen, revisions and corrections are made, and it is printed as *hard copy.* Data in memory can be stored on floppy or hard disks or onto a CD-ROM rewriteable diskette for permanent or backup storage. Final output may be sent via telecommunication satellite, telephone lines, or facsimile machine with the use of a modem to be read by the receiver onscreen or printed out. It may be sent to a micrographic center for production directly into microfilm or be transmitted directly to phototypesetting equipment for in-house printing.

Software

The programs and instructions for a computer are known as the *software.* For word processing, some features of computer software are as follows:

1. *Cut and paste:* provides extensive *editing* and revising capabilities to *insert, delete,* and move copy *(cut and paste)* easily by using *command keys* on the keyboard and moving the *cursor* to the proper location on the monitor.
2. *Right margin justification:* justifies right margin (Fig. 2–5); however, some employers prefer *ragged text,* where the right margin does not align flush .
3. *Decimal tab alignment:* allows columns of figures with decimals to align automatically. (Fig. 2–5).
4. *Global search and replace:* allows the operator to use one instruction to search for a word or group of words everywhere in the text and automatically replace them with other words.

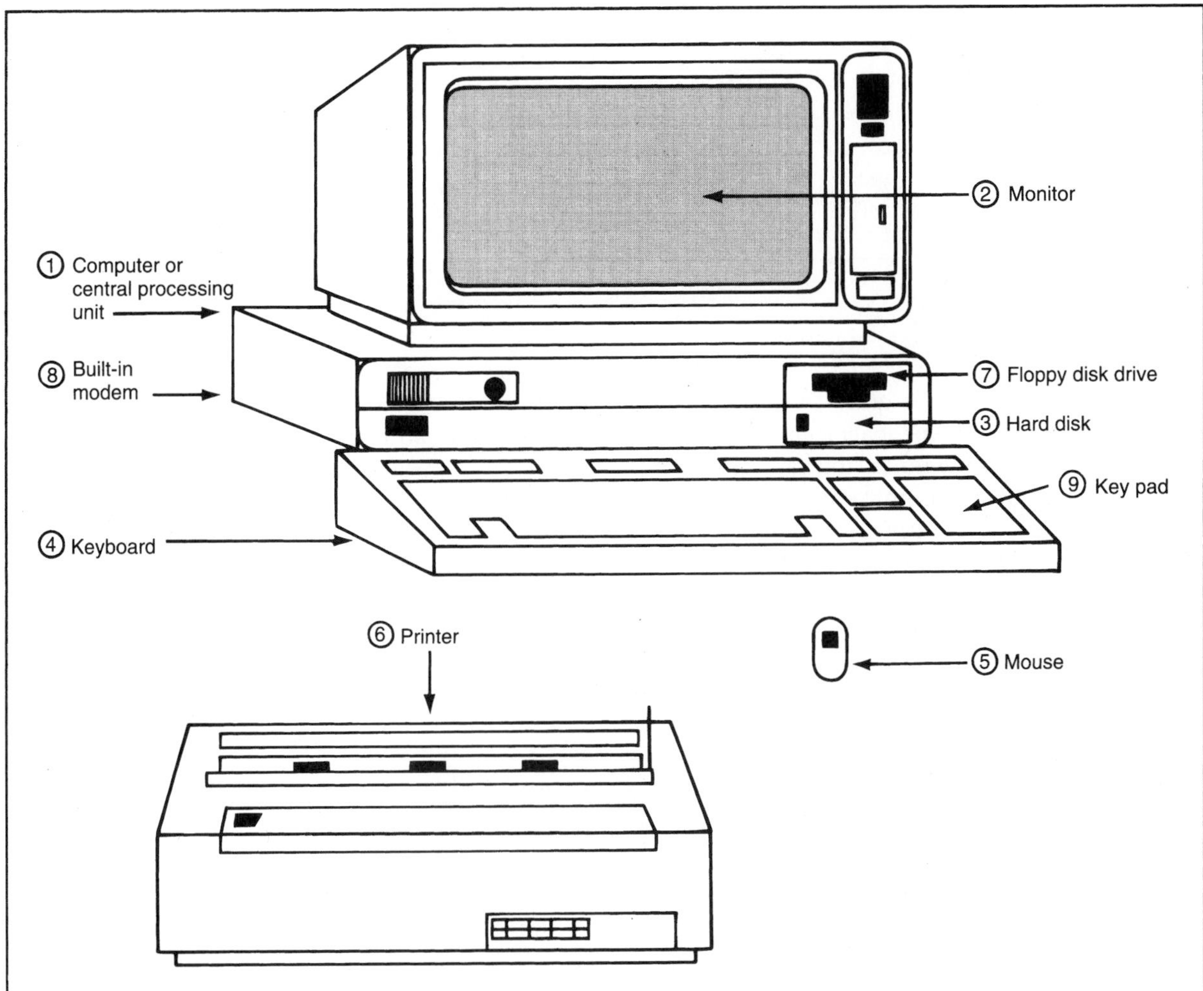

Figure 2–4. Illustration of the hardware components of a computer system. The system consists of input devices (keyboard [4], key pad [9], and mouse [5]), a central processing device (inside system unit [1]), output devices (monitor [2] and printer [6]), auxiliary storage devices (disk drives [3 and 7], also located within the system unit), and a transmission device or modem (inside the system unit [8]). (From Fordney MT: Insurance Handbook for the Medical Office, 4th edition. W. B. Saunders Company, Philadelphia, 1995.)

5. *Pagination:* instructs the text editor to determine the ends of pages of a document and number the pages in sequence.
6. *Menu:* aid the operator in making revisions and performing machine manipulations.
7. *Automatic hyphenation:* hyphenates a word that is too long to fit within the right margin and moves part of the word to the next line.
8. *Word wrap:* moves the last word of a line to the next line if the word goes outside the predetermined right margin.
9. *Document assembly:* allows combining prerecorded text with keyboarded text, combining selections from prerecorded text to form a new document, and inserting names and addresses to create a number of nearly identical documents. Also called *merge.*
10. *Reverse index:* allows for superscript and subscript.
11. *Scrolling:* allows moving the text vertically and horizontally as well as flipping pages of a document on the monitor.
12. *Indenting, underlining, centering, automatic tabulation to decimal points, and so forth:* allows these functions to be carried out (Fig. 2–5).
13. Dictionary: assists as a spell checker for English or medical terms in a sentence, paragraph, page, or document and can be expanded.

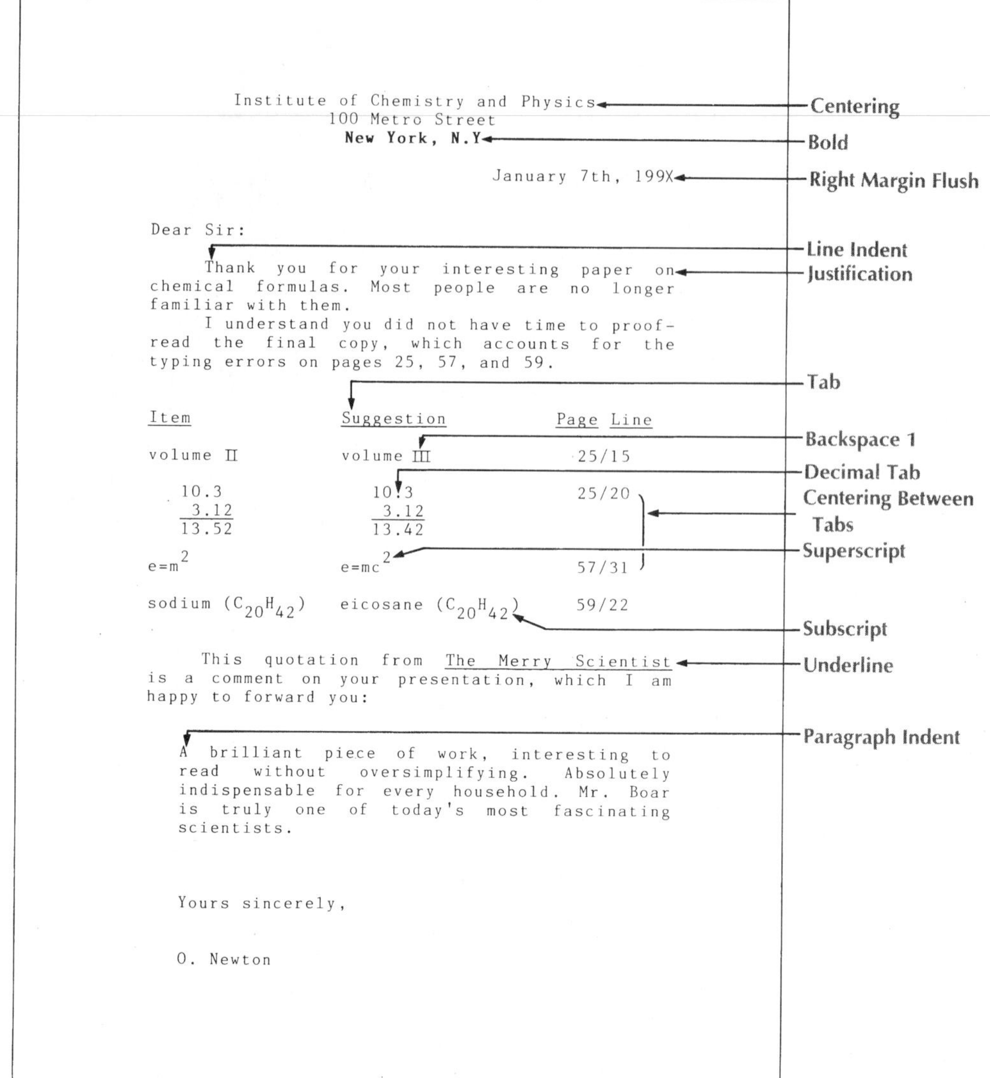

Institute of Chemistry and Physics
100 Metro Street
New York, N.Y

January 7th, 199X

Dear Sir:

Thank you for your interesting paper on chemical formulas. Most people are no longer familiar with them.

I understand you did not have time to proofread the final copy, which accounts for the typing errors on pages 25, 57, and 59.

Item	Suggestion	Page Line
volume II	volume III	25/15
10.3 + 3.12 = 13.52	10.3 + 3.12 = 13.42	25/20
$e=m^2$	$e=mc^2$	57/31
sodium ($C_{20}H_{42}$)	eicosane ($C_{20}H_{42}$)	59/22

This quotation from <u>The Merry Scientist</u> is a comment on your presentation, which I am happy to forward you:

A brilliant piece of work, interesting to read without oversimplifying. Absolutely indispensable for every household. Mr. Boar is truly one of today's most fascinating scientists.

Yours sincerely,

O. Newton

Figure 2–5. Illustration of some features when keyboarding word-processed documents using a computer. (Reproduced by permission of Brother International Corporation, Somerset, New Jersey.)

14. Thesaurus: assists in composition when trying to find a substitution for a word since it is a categorized index of synonyms and antonyms.
15. *Counter:* counts words and gives the number of words or characters per page and/or per document.
16. *Grammar checker:* checks grammar for common errors. A document can be scanned for violation of standard grammar rules.
17. *Forms processing:* completes insurance claims.
18. *Windows and split screens:* allows spread sheets to complete billing reports and incorporate totals into past due letters and allows graphics to be pasted into medical reports.

Computers have a disk operating system (DOS), which controls the loading and storage of files from and to the memory of the computer and onto a magnetic disk. Operating systems in the PC environment are MS/DOS (MicroSoft Disk Operating System), PC-DOS (the IBM PC operating system), Macintosh OS (Apple Computer operating system), and the UNIX system developed by Bell Laboratories. Word processing on a computer is accomplished with the use of sophisticated word processing software. To help you work efficiently, English, medical, and pharmaceutical dictionaries as well as word spellers for almost all medical specialties are available on diskette or CD-ROM. Some word processing software has preset alphabetical expanders or macro capabilities, or you can purchase software with a modified keyboard to allow the use of macros, or *chording,* by simultaneously depressing multiple keys (see "Macros and Alphabetical Expanders"). This feature is for frequently used words and phrases. For example, keying in "PE" would appear as "physical examination" on the computer screen. Integrated software packages have *windows* that let you see various functions simultaneously. As mentioned previously, a number of computer programs can be activated by voice instead of by keyboarding command keys. *Utility programs* are general-purpose software programs that perform activities that are not specific to an application, e.g., spell checkers, line count, macro makers, installation of fonts (size and style of type), initialization of a disk (to prepare the magnetic surface of a blank diskette so it will accept data), and so forth. Sometimes, word processing software programs incorporate these utility features. If data are to be stored, a blank disk is initialized and the information is given a file name so it can be retrieved from the system.

Speed Typing Systems

Shorthand Equipment

With this system, a computer is linked to electronic shorthand equipment similar to that used in court reporting, where transcription speeds of 225 words per minute and higher are attained. Instead of entering text by one keyboard stroke (one character at a time), one stroke (which can be one, two, or three keys hit simultaneously) is used to enter entire words, phrases, and sentences. The shorthand is instantly converted into correctly spelled words, phrases, and sentences. By producing multiple characters with each keyboard stroke, text is entered much faster and more efficiently than is possible with a one-stroke, one-character keyboard. It is possible to build extensive medical dictionaries that are unique to each medical specialty. The text is sent to remote systems via facsimile (fax) or modem so that the report does not have to be printed and delivered. Electronic signatures are used in some facilities when such high-tech systems are installed.

Macros and Alphabetical Expanders

Popular methods of more quickly keyboarding data into the computer memory are use of alphabetical expanders and macros. A *macro* can be created by the transcriptionist with the word processing software program by entering special abbreviations so that one key or a series of keystrokes, preferably two or three, will generate a phrase, a paragraph, or an entire report. These special abbreviations are saved to the program to access as needed. For example, PERRLA may be put into a single-key macro to generate "pupils are equal, round, and reactive to light and accommodation." A *keyboard macro* is when a keyboard key is reprogrammed; for example, every time you press Control E, "esophagogastroduodenoscopy" would appear in the document. Often, keyboard macros are used for foreign letters or symbols, e.g., μ, c, °, §, $\frac{1}{2}$, and $\frac{1}{4}$. A *temporary macro* can be made while you are working within a document and remains in effect until you exit the program.

Alphabetical expanders are preset in word processing software programs with letters that expand into words when proper keystrokes are made. For example, "e"/space could generate the word "examination," "uga"/space could generate "under general anesthesia" and "catx"/space could generate an entire cataract extraction operative note with fill-ins.

Data Forms

Because of the need for more documentation, reduced resources to pay for it, and speed in obtaining it, some hospital facilities use a simplified system of data forms and software. For an operative report, the surgeon completes the data forms after the operation and gives the forms to clerical staff, who manually enter the data with a computer or insert the forms into a scanning device. Data forms are available for history and physical examination and for each type of surgery and consist of boxes to check and a place to handwrite the diagnoses. Once completed and authenticated by the surgeon, a comprehensive, well-organized operative report is generated that contains a description of the surgical findings, the surgical treatment performed, the protocol used, any specimens removed, the name of the surgeon and assistant surgeon, and any details pertinent to the case. This system is used in a variety of settings, especially in orthopedic practices for those handling a large volume of industrial injury cases.

On-line Processing System

In large companies, computers may be linked to other systems, or *peripherals,* such as data processors, electronic mail, optical character readers (OCRs), and so forth. An *on-line processing system* is composed of a central processing unit (CPU), a communications linkage, a terminal, and a user,

2

which interact to carry out a task. The CPU is the brain of the computer and is where data are added, subtracted, multiplied, divided, and sorted; it coordinates the random access memory (RAM) and read-only memory (ROM). The software programs that give the computer the electronic instructions to do the work are executed in the CPU. Computers communicate and operate by using binary logic to process information. This binary number system is composed of 1s and 0s, which are called *bits* (*bi*nary dig*its*). A group of eight bits is called a *byte.* One byte is equal to one alphanumeric character and represents the amount of space a character takes up in the memory of the computer. A megabyte (meg) is almost 1 million bytes, approximately the number of characters in a novel. A gigabyte (gig), nearly 1 billion bytes, is comparable to 1000 novels. A *character* is anything that takes up a cursor position on the screen (letter, tab, header command, margin command, space between letters). If you type a three-letter word and then backspace and erase the word, you have added six bytes to the document even though nothing appears on the screen. Computers have RAM and ROM. RAM is used to describe machine memory that can be stored in any order, accessed immediately, and modified; it operates the software. ROM refers to computer memory that can be addressed but not modified. This is the primary area where operating (software) information is stored. Computers may be hooked up to the telephone line to assist in transmitting and receiving faxes or electronic mail.

Data Storage

Hard Disk Drive

A hard disk drive, magnetic media (tape drives and diskettes), or CD-ROM rewriteable disks may be used to store data. A *hard disk* may be inside (internal) or outside (external) the computer case. It is used when you need a fast device for access and to store large amounts of data (several million bytes of information).

Floppy Disk

A magnetic media *diskette* is a 3.5-inch, thin, circular piece of magnetically coated plastic that is contained in a protective cover to shield its surface from contamination by dust and fingerprints (Fig. 2–6). Storage capacity is determined by whether the diskette is single or dual sided and single or double tracked.

Computer software is sold on diskettes or CD-ROM disks, so it is always wise to make a *backup* of expensive software programs after their purchase. If a *crash* or a problem develops with the backup/working diskette, you will have the original. If the system does not automatically back up the data that are input, you should make backup copies of the data onto disks on a daily basis.

Because you will have important information stored on computer disks, it is wise to take care of them. The information is magnetically recorded. Therefore, any magnetic or electromagnetic field can scramble or destroy data recorded onto a disk. Your telephone, printer, and video terminal contain magnetic fields, so do not place a disk on top of this equipment. Disks should be properly stored in boxes. The container should be kept away from extreme heat (100°F or above) and out of direct sunlight, because valuable information could be destroyed or the disk could melt. Never attach rubberbands to disks, because these could bend or damage the disks.

Always label each disk before filing it in the storage box. Do not stack labels on a disk. Too many labels could cause an imbalance in the weight of the surface of the disk and may make it difficult for the computer head to read the data. Keep disks clean and out of the way of possible spills or stains. Never drink, eat, or smoke around the computer area. If a disk case must be cleaned, use a damp cloth to wipe it off.

Printer

Computers have a printer as a separate component. The most popular in use are nonimpact (ink jet, thermal transfer, laser) or impact (dot matrix). A tractor guides continuous-form stationery on sprockets or individual sheets may be fed manually or automatically by a sheet feeder. While data are keyboarded into a computer, the program instructions (commands or functions) signal the printer. For example, a stop code embedded in a document signals the printer to stop. There is a wide range of printing quality and speeds. Output from the printer is called *hard copy.* In many transcription departments, printing may be done off site. It is common for documents to print in another room in the building or across town or be transmitted via modem to a hospital floor for accessibility. Therefore, it cannot be overemphasized that you must read data on the screen while transcribing because you may not get another opportunity.

Cartridge ribbons for dot matrix printers may look identical, but they vary considerably in their construction, ink, fabric specifications, print quali-

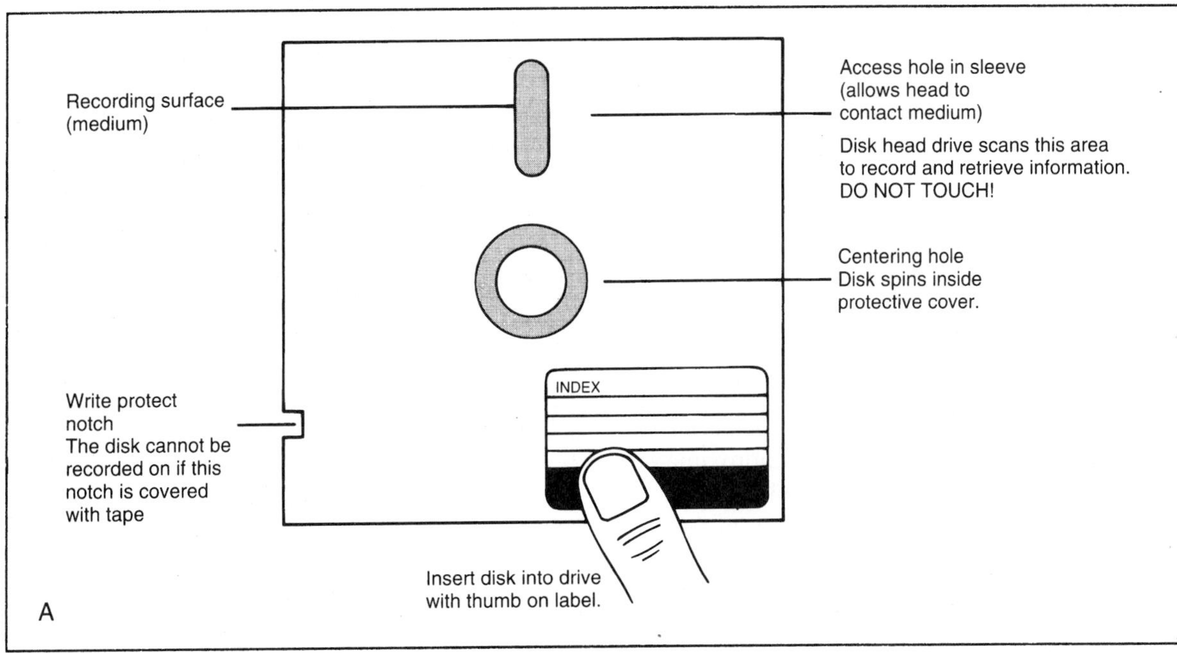

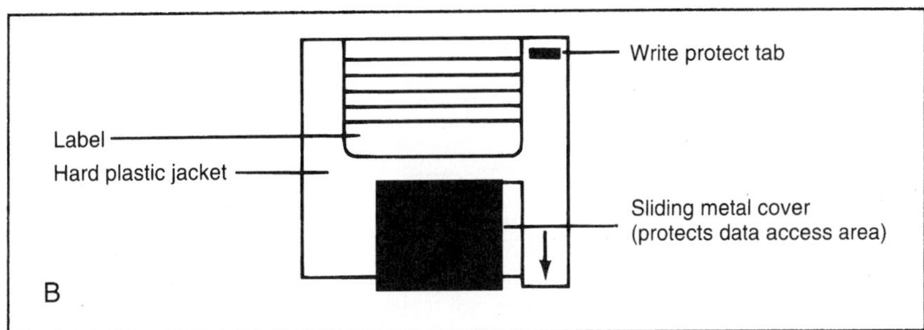

Figure 2–6. *A*, Illustration of the components of a 5.25-inch floppy disk and information on how to insert it into the disk drive. *B*, The components of a 3.5-inch disk. (From Fordney MT: Insurance Handbook for the Medical Office, 4th edition. W. B. Saunders Company, Philadelphia, 1995.)

ity, and print durability. The price of a ribbon is not always a good measure of product quality. Generic-brand ribbons are less expensive and may be acceptable. However, they may be of poor quality and possibly cause printer damage. Brand-name ribbons are usually of high quality but are also the most expensive. Some features to look for in a good-quality ribbon are crisp characters that do not smear, durable packaging so the ribbon does not dry out, and a guarantee by the dealer to replace or give a credit for defective ribbons.

Laser printers are fitted with cartridges. Some companies sell recycled refilled cartridges, which are less expensive than a new cartridge. However, check for high-quality rather than mediocre-quality refill powder and ask whether the company replaces the drum in each cartridge before it is refilled. This guarantees crisp clean printouts.

Modem

The word *modem* is an acronym for *mo*dulator *dem*odulator unit and is a device that sends and receives information over telephone lines. Some transcription services offer this type of telecommunication by hooking up their computer equipment to the telephone lines. Then, they can transmit correspondence or reports to an office, a clinic, or a hospital facility many miles away. Documents transmitted in this way can be revised and edited at the receiving office before they are printed out into a hard copy. Some modems include speaker-phone and voice mail capabilities called telephony. Major cities may have fiberoptic telephone lines, which speed up transmission from 14.4 to 28.8 kilobytes per second (kbps).

2

ERGONOMICS

Real problems exist for medical transcriptionists because they work in one position hour after hour and perform repetitive movements. These are known as cumulative trauma disorders (CTDs) or repetitive stress injuries (RSIs). Other factors that can contribute to on-the-job injuries are indoor air pollution, electromagnetic radiation, and stress. Therefore, steps must be taken to avoid these disorders or injuries.

The height of the surface on which the word processor or computer sits is very important (Fig. 2–7). Improper height can cause early fatigue and will reduce productivity. A high-quality chair is equally important and should be adjusted to the individual's height and build. A well-adjusted and properly designed chair can reduce fatigue and tension. Features to look for are foldaway arms, contoured seat pads, vertical adjustments, and built-in supports. Do not sit on keys, billfolds, or note pads because these may block circulation. Sometimes a small footstool will help the short typist to avoid back problems.

When retyping or doing copy work and to prevent fatigue, neck aches, backaches, eyestrain, or duplicating or leaving out a sentence, use an electronic copyholder with a foot pedal control and magnifying cursor so that proper posture can be maintained and material can be easily read. To prevent frozen shoulders and carpal tunnel syndrome, a split keyboard (one for each hand), keyboards on the arms of chairs, and keyboards that adjust for your comfort are available. The keyboard should be placed sufficiently low so the arms are relaxing comfortably in a neutral or downward position on the keys.

Match the overall brightness of your computer screen to its surroundings to protect your eyes from too much transient adaptation. Another con-

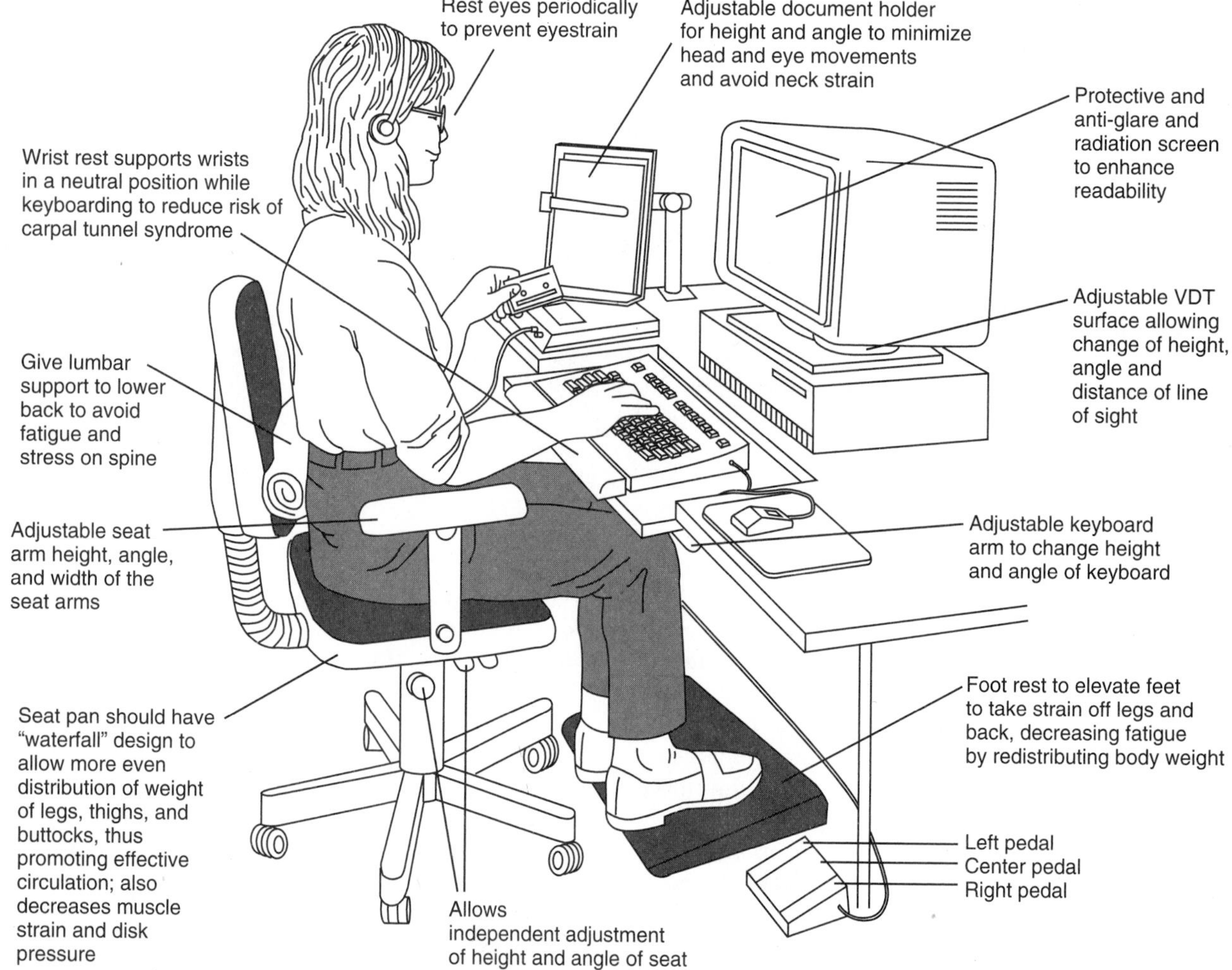
Rest eyes periodically to prevent eyestrain
Adjustable document holder for height and angle to minimize head and eye movements and avoid neck strain
Protective and anti-glare and radiation screen to enhance readability
Wrist rest supports wrists in a neutral position while keyboarding to reduce risk of carpal tunnel syndrome
Adjustable VDT surface allowing change of height, angle and distance of line of sight
Give lumbar support to lower back to avoid fatigue and stress on spine
Adjustable seat arm height, angle, and width of the seat arms
Adjustable keyboard arm to change height and angle of keyboard
Foot rest to elevate feet to take strain off legs and back, decreasing fatigue by redistributing body weight
Seat pan should have "waterfall" design to allow more even distribution of weight of legs, thighs, and buttocks, thus promoting effective circulation; also decreases muscle strain and disk pressure
Left pedal
Center pedal
Right pedal
Allows independent adjustment of height and angle of seat

Figure 2–7. Adjustments that may be made at a work station to improve the system ergonomically. (Modified from Sloane SB, Fordney MT: Saunders Manual of Medical Transcription. W. B. Saunders Company, Philadelphia, 1994.)

cern is the rate of flicker on the screen, which may be seen less if the screen background is dark. If you have a white background, lower the brightness to make the flicker less noticeable. Take frequent breaks and periodically do body and wrist stretches and focus the eyes on distant objects to eliminate eye strain, blurred vision, headaches, dry eyes, and lowered productivity. Diminish exposure to low-frequency radiation and prevent glare and light reflection by installing a Polaroid-type antireflection screen or radiation-blocking filter over the monitor screen. A seal of acceptance by the American Optometric Association means that the filter has met its high standards. Some filters also act as a privacy protection so that people viewing a screen from either side see nothing but a blank screen. An operator seated in front of the computer terminal has a completely unobstructed view. Some software programs are designed to signal the user to stop and exercise at preferred intervals and may even give exercise hints. If you begin to feel joint pain, apply ice to the area after work and on break to prevent inflammation.

DICTATION EQUIPMENT

Voice Recognition Systems

There are two basic categories of computerized voice recognition products: navigation and dictation. *Navigation* (or command control) software allows you to launch and operate software applications with spoken directions; *dictation* software is used in some departments (within hospitals and physicians' offices) to create medical reports, enter numbers into spreadsheets, and conduct on-line sessions. The physician trains the system to understand his or her speech patterns, and the system translates the tones of the human voice into computer commands and text on the screen. However, the report must be formatted, proofread, and edited for grammar and punctuation before it is printed and ready for signature. Persons who have repetitive-strain injuries or congenital deformities or lack full hand function have found voice-recognition systems to be of great help. Full dictation systems are available from the following:

Dragon Systems, Inc.
320 Nevada Street
Newton, MA 02160

IBM National Support Center for Persons with Disabilities
P.O. Box 2150
Atlanta, GA 30301-2150

Kurzweil Applied Intelligence, Inc.
411 Waverley Oak Road
Waltham, MA 02154-8414

Media

The media used in dictating machines are of a variety of types. No medium is involved when digital dictation is used. Media may be in the form of magnetic tapes, such as microcassettes or standard cassettes. It makes little difference what medium is used, because the transcribing process is the same; however, fidelity does vary considerably. Some instruments actually enhance the speaker's voice. Be sure to check carefully for good voice fidelity when purchasing new equipment.

Magnetic tapes, disks, or cassettes allow the dictator to correct his or her own errors so that the medical transcriptionist does not have to listen ahead for corrections. Microcassettes and standard cassettes are most popular and can record from 15 to 90 minutes on each side. They are easily erased and reused. Some machines have an adaptor so that you can use standard cassettes and smaller sizes.

Most machines emit a warning tone when approaching the end of a tape, and some machines warn you if the tape is broken.

Indication Features

Some machines use cue-tone indexing, which allows the dictator to insert this information magnetically onto the medium while dictating. Another method of indication involves a display window that electronically shows the type and number of documents recorded on the tape (letter, priority, special instructions), status and warning information about the job you are working on, how much time is left as you are typing the dictated material, the total time of all recordings, how many pieces of work you have completed, an average indication of the total time and quarter pages for each job, and which side of the tape is in use.

Indication features help you plan your day more efficiently, because you can judge the length of a document before transcribing it and can scan for special instructions.

HAND/FOOT CONTROL

Transcription machines have a foot pedal that will start the machine. Pressure on the pedal causes the machine to play; as soon as you release the pedal, the machine stops (see Fig. 2–7). You have complete control over how much of the dictation you hear. The control is so sensitive that you can stop and restart in the middle of a word. The machine also has a backup pedal that permits you to relisten to a few words or as much as you need to hear again before you transcribe. Some machines can be adjusted to replay a phrase or a word automatically every time you restart. This is also called auto rewind. In addition, the control may have a *fast forward* feature.

Initially, you will listen to as much of a sentence as you can retain by memory, and you will type it before listening to the next phrase. Eventually, you will learn to type as you listen, ceasing to listen only long enough to catch up to the dictation; then, just before you type the last of what you heard, start to listen again so that there is as little time as possible during which you are not typing at all. If the foot pedal of the transcription machine constantly or frequently slips out of reach, glue two strips of the looped side of some Velcro tape to the bottom of the pedal. Velcro sticks to a carpeted floor just as it would to the soft-side Velcro. If the floor is not carpeted, glue two matching strips of soft-side Velcro to the floor at the place where the pedal is most comfortable.

Dictation equipment has a speed control that should be adjusted to a natural voice sound, neither too fast nor too slow. The voice should not sound distorted. If the transcriptionist has difficulty understanding a word or phrase, the speed control can be adjusted to slow down the voice to see if this makes it audible or clear. However, the speed control should not be left in the slow mode; it should always be adjusted to a natural-sounding voice quality. In digitized dictation, no sound distortion occurs when the speed of the voice is changed.

Some manufacturers make a hand control available to the physically challenged as an alternative accessory. The operation of the control plays a vital role in developing the essential skill of typing steadily and quickly.

Table 2–1 will help you avoid some of the pitfalls and take advantage of some of the benefits when operating a transcriber.

DICTATION

Dictating is a communications skill, and there are good and poor dictators. Transcribing is definitely improved by good dictation. Sometimes the transcriptionist can aid his or her employer by talking about the problems encountered to see if there is some solution. If that does not work, try watching the dictator dictate. You might find the following problem-causing areas: eating while dictating, speaking directly into the mike and not across the mike as one should, having an "intimate conversation" with the mike (resulting in a low-pitched, quiet, sultry, and inaudible voice), stretching arms out with microphone in one of them (resulting in fade-in and fade-out). A little lecture from the salesperson who gave the original presentation on the equipment is often very helpful. There might be some features of the equipment that the dictator has forgotten existed or has never used or perhaps did not know were there in the first place. Many dictators neglect to use cuing and indication, and the transcriptionist should explain how important this is and why. Some dictators do not understand how to dictate and think they have to keep up with the machine or leave it on while thinking of what to say. This results in poor copy. Some dictators mislead the transcriptionist by dropping their voices as if they were finished and then going on with an "and" or a "but." You may help the dictator by tactfully letting him or her know about such problems. In a hospital setting where one does not have an opportunity to interact with the dictator, the supervisor and medical transcriptionists might prepare a check sheet for the dictator or an orientation packet for the new dictator giving hints, suggestions, policies, procedures, and so forth.

The transcriptionist should be sure that the dictator's equipment is always prepared for use. It should be plugged in, and the medium, such as tape, belt, disk, or cassette, should be properly installed. One should remove the medium as soon as the dictator completes recording and insert a new medium immediately, so the dictator can work if he or she wishes. In order to avoid misplaced patient's charts and to make dictating easier, a flow sheet can be designed for the physician's specialty. After a patient is seen, the sheet is removed from the patient's chart and placed inside a plastic sleeve. At the end of the day, place the accumulated pile of sheets into the physician's briefcase along with the portable dictation equipment. Thus, the physician can dictate at the hospital, at home, or wherever he or she may be and will not have to remove the patient's chart from the office. Another problem is the confusion of dictated tapes with transcribed tapes, which often results in tapes being transcribed again. The physician can be asked to apply a small, removable colored dot to media that are ready for transcription. After the

2

TABLE 2–1. GENERAL FEATURES OF THE TRANSCRIBER

Part Name		What They Do, What They Don't Do, and Handy Hints To Remember
Audio speaker control	*Does:*	Clarify words Disrupt room environment Maintain confidentiality when not in use Remember: Operate briefly when using
Cassette media	*Does:*	Have adaptors available on standard-size cassette Have transcriber for smaller size cassettes
	Does not:	Allow for prolonged use of media since this results in worn tape and poor sound reproduction
Foot pedal	*Does:*	Allow hands to remain on keyboard Have a setting adjustment so words are not backspace missed. This adjustment should be changed as the transcriptionist becomes more experienced. A zero adjustment (slight rewind of tape when stopped and then restarted) should be aimed for before obtaining a job
	Does not:	Have standardized pedal parts on machines, and location of function features can be easily confused
Erase button	*Does:*	Allow for clean erasure of tape
	Does not:	Have a safety feature, so accidental erasures can occur
Headset	*Does:*	Enhance sound quality biaurally Shut out office sounds Preserve confidentiality
	Does not:	Have loan out properties since earpiece fits inside ear canal, and infections can be transmitted unless the earpiece is thoroughly cleaned. Note: Clean earpieces from time to time
Indication feature	*Does:*	Locate special instructions or comments Indicate length of documents
	Does not:	Consistently line up accurately with the beginning of each report
Insert control	*Does:*	Allow insertion of dictation without rerecording or erasing dictation
Scanning	*Does:*	Allow for quick location and identification of all dictation on tape
Sensor for voice-activation	*Does not:*	Require the dictator to hold the microphone
	Does:	Provide gag-free dictation
Speed control	*Does:*	Distort speech when speed is decreased too much Slow down the fast dictator Increase a naturally slow dictator Match dictation speed with transcription speed
Tone control	*Does:*	Mute consonants when too much bass is used Accentuate consonants and clarify dictation when put in treble pitch Cause static when too much treble pitch is used
Volume control	*Does:*	Distort sound when the volume is too high. It is important to adjust the volume for each transcription

tape has been transcribed, the transcriptionist removes the dot. Thus, it becomes easy to distinguish the media that have been transcribed from those that have not.

Let your employer know if the dictation is good. Do not just scold—praise good dictation and show that you appreciate the punctuation, the clearly enunciated words, the nicely modulated voice, the paragraph indications, and so forth.

The following are some hints to aid the person dictating:

1. Prioritize and organize material.
2. Identify yourself.
3. Indicate what is being transcribed (such as a letter, memo, report, rough draft, or form letter) and on what kind of paper it should be typed (letterhead, personal stationery, or colored paper).
4. Indicate the number of copies needed and enclosures.

2

TABLE 2–2. DICTATION PROBLEM SOLVING

Problem	Solution
Fast dictation	Decrease the speed of the dictation if words and phrases are running together Write out slurred phrases phonetically and separate the syllables to try to form words
Foreign accent	Get a copy of a report by the same physician dictated and transcribed previously and compare words and phrases Distinguish the accent and substitute the correct sound to identify the word
Garbled word	Increase or decrease dictation speed and relisten Relisten on audio speaker Ask someone else to listen Leave a blank, continue transcribing, and listen for the word to be dictated again within the transcript
Mumbled dictation	Increase the tone control Clean the recording head with a cleaning cassette tape
Static obscures dictation	Decrease the tone control
Unfamiliar word	Look up the word in a medical or English dictionary Use the Sound and Word Finder Table in Appendix B

5. Give the names of the patient and the person for whom the item is intended, and spell out the names if they are difficult to ascertain.
6. Dictate the street address, city, state, and zip code to which the correspondence is being sent when this is not readily available to the transcriptionist.
7. Separate the ideas into paragraphs. Spell a word that you think the typist might have difficulty understanding.
8. Indicate the beginning of new paragraphs by stating after the first paragraph, "period paragraph."
9. Remember to say *comma* specifically where you want the reader to pause.
10. Indicate when a word is a plural, or needs quotes, parentheses ("paren open and paren close"), indentations, columns, or subparagraphs.
11. Keep a blank copy of the form in front of you while dictating information that is to be inserted into the form.
12. Eliminate extraneous sounds such as "ugh," "um," "eh," "and," "that." Remember to speak slowly and clearly. Do not slur word endings. Add a personal touch to the end of the tape by saying "thank you" to the transcriptionist. This will certainly make the transcriptionist feel he or she is a valuable part of the team.
13. Use the pause button or key when it is necessary to stop and think.
14. Mark each cassette with the date and other identification.

Table 2–2 presents information that will assist you in solving problem dictation.

MAINTENANCE

Computer

Because you want to have professional-looking reports and letters, it is essential that your equipment be maintained in good working condition. In a dusty environment, cover your equipment when you leave at the end of a work day. Periodically, the keyboard and body should be cleaned by using a vacuum and a slightly dampened cloth. Plastic keyboard skins are available to eliminate having to vacuum the keys. From time to time, the computer box should be opened and cleared of dust particles by using a series of short blasts from special pressurized cans (e.g., Dust-Off). Avoid using abrasive cleaners on any parts of your equipment. After the warranty time has expired, an annual service contract for computer and printer is essential. Know whom to call to make repairs. If the computer is producing erratic functions, locate the section in the manual dealing with the software you are using and find and read through the troubleshooting section. Save any printed material that demonstrates the problem so a sample is available to show the service person.

Before making a service repair call, be sure that you are not making an "idiot call," which may be quite costly. Check to see that all computer cables are properly connected. See whether the problem will clear itself by turning the terminal or printer off and then on again. Check to see whether the equipment is plugged in and has not been unplugged by cleaning personnel. Make sure the outlet is in working order by plugging another piece of equipment in and turning it on and off. Determine whether the equipment has been turned on. Make sure the screen brightness has not been turned down. Check to make sure that another electric device is not interfering with the computer. Check the equipment manual and locate the section on troubleshooting information. Check to see whether technical assistance is available over the telephone before calling a technician to the equipment location. Many companies have their own help department for resolving and tracking computer and/or software problems. Search out the machine's serial number, model, purchase date, warranty information, version of software in use, and so forth before telephoning for assistance. Keep a log of the service calls, noting the technician's name, time of call, time of arrival of technician, and resolution of the problem.

Transcriber

Use the following checklist when your transcriber is not working properly:

1. Is the equipment plugged in?
2. Is the outlet in working order?
3. Is the equipment turned on?
4. Is the "play" button pushed down, preventing you from hearing through the headset?
5. Is the foot pedal attached to the machine?

If you have decided that your equipment needs repairs, type a note explaining the problems your machine is giving you, then tape the note to the side of your machine. This way the repairperson will know what to look for even if you are not present. This also should be done in a classroom setting.

TRANSCRIPTION PREPARATION

Here are some suggestions to help you organize and plan your work before you begin to transcribe and to help you increase your efficiency and production.

1. Gather all necessary information and materials at your desk.
2. Make sure the headset, earphones (or amplifier), and foot control are attached to the unit and comfortably positioned.
3. Verify that the unit is operating properly, plugged in, and turned on.
4. Insert the medium. Priority (STAT) reports are transcribed immediately. Then the oldest dictation is transcribed, and the most recent dictation is typed last.
5. Use indication features and estimate the length of the report or letter. Listen for special instructions or comments.
6. Listen to the instructions or cue in to see if there are corrections by scanning the media.
7. Adjust the volume, *tone,* and speed controls to your taste. Remember too slow a speed will only distort the sound.
8. Make sure the format for margins and tabulation stops is proper before beginning a document.
9. Mark any problems with editing codes so the dictated report can be scanned and necessary corrections can be made.
10. Select the paper, and note how many copies are necessary.

Remember: Listen to *all* instructions *before* beginning to transcribe, since failure to do so may result in redoing the work. Punctuate as you go and leave a blank space for words that you do not understand. Attach notes to your transcript for any unclear phrases or sentences. See Chapter 7 for help in flagging unfamiliar copy. The more transcribing you do, the more you will retain in memory when coordinating listening and typing. Save the dictation until after the physician reads and signs the report in case a problem or question arises.

EQUIPMENT FOR THE PHYSICALLY CHALLENGED

Several methods have been developed to make it easier for the blind or visually handicapped transcriptionist or those with little or no hand/arm movement to type and transcribe.

A blind person who wishes to take notes can use a mechanical brailler known as the Perkins' Brailler. This uses six keys to emboss the proper configuration of the six dots in the braille cell (raised-dot) system that represent letters and punctuation. A correction is made by rubbing out the incorrect cell dots.

Computer equipment consists of several types, such as screen readers that use voice recognition systems, screen magnifiers, braille printers, Kurzweil reader, and book scanners.

A *screen reader* converts all text on the screen to spoken characters or words by using voice recognition technology. In order to eliminate the need to have other employees proofread text produced by a blind typist on a computer, voice synthesizers have been developed. A blind terminal user can hear the information that is displayed on the screen and can learn how to operate the machine by listening to cassette-recorded instructions or by braille writing. Usually, the audio output formats available on such systems include the following:

- *Pronounce* format. The contents of the screen are read in the same way as you would read a book, with each word pronounced separately but without incorporating punctuation. Numbers are announced individually, so that 132 would be announced "one, three, two."
- *Punctuate* format. This is similar to the pronounce format. In addition, single or double spaces are identified by a sound (the number of spaces are given if more than two), and punctuation marks are also announced.
- *Spell* format. All words are spelled out, spaces and capital letters are identified, number of spaces or repeated characters are given, and punctuation marks are announced. In cases of similar-sounding letters, the operator may select spelling by using the international alphabet, such as L for Lima, I for India, and so forth.

Speech can be slowed to aid transcription or sped up for casual scanning of data. Words can be spoken in monotone or with intonation on some systems. Some machines use a keypad to control the audio output, or when the operator's hands are busy, an external foot switch may be used. The cursor is positioned on the screen, and then the machine reads out the row number and column number. It will read the word at, before, or after the cursor; it may read the entire row on which the cursor is located, the row before it, or the row after it; or the complete screen may be read out. It is easy to go back and verify something not understood by backspacing and then changing the output format from pronounce to punctuate or spell.

A partially sighted typist can produce perfect letters and reports by using a *screen magnifier,* which may consist of software or hardware that enlarges the characters on a computer screen, such as that manufactured by V-Tek, 1625 Olympic Boulevard, Santa Monica, CA 90404, 800-345-2256.

A *braille printer* is a computer printer that prints computer documents in braille with raised dots and is available from International Business Machines, Inc.

A *Kurzweil reader* is a machine that reads a printed page and converts it to speech. This may run in tandem with a computer.

A *book scanner* easily scans books or other bound materials (e.g., magazines, photocopies, documents with multiple columns). It recognizes text, converts it into synthesized speech, and then reads the materials aloud.

The Optacon, or *op*tical to *ta*ctile *con*verter, is a device that allows a blind person to read any printed material. It consists of a small portable case with a removable electronic eye. The case is designed to allow a person's hand to be inside, with the index finger resting on a transmitter plate, so that the person can feel the images. With experience, an 8½ × 11–inch page of single-spaced copy can be read in minutes. A model is available for those working with a word processor or computer that enables the blind typist to read the luminous display of the screen. A portable module (hand or automatic scanning version) can be added to an Optacon to convert the output into natural-sounding synthetic speech and an automatic scanning system with voice output.

Braille-Edit is a sophisticated word processing program that enables blind and sighted people to work together in using the power of microcomputers. This program is used by a number of medical transcriptionists and works with voice or braille devices. A user can hear material entered by letter, word, phrase, or section, and material can be entered on a braille device, such as the VersaBraille (a paperless brailler). This program provides a broad range of translation, formatting, and printing operations. It can set up "transformation chapters" in which certain characters can be removed and replaced by other characters. For example, "qqra" could be replaced by a long medical phrase. The transformation chapters can be prestored and invoked by name. Thus, you can enter some medical phrases by using a personal abbreviation and obtain a printout of regular text. Braille-Edit has many additional features for blind, partially sighted, or sighted persons too numerous to mention here.

Another aid for medical transcriptionists who are blind or visually impaired is the series of ridges located in the upper right corner when side one of a Norelco minicassette or "ultra"-minicassette is facing the user. This allows quick determination of the cassette side being used.

Photocopy equipment has also been developed to produce raised copy images, such as raised-relief maps, drawings, and braille writing. Illustrations enhance the learning process, and such equipment decreases the cost and time involved in producing documents for the vision-impaired.

For persons with limited hand/arm movement or slight head movement, a Magic Wand Keyboard with a built-in mouse is available. To begin work, one simply unplugs the existing computer keyboard, plugs in the Magic Wand Keyboard, and uses a hand or mouthstick to touch the keys. No strength or dexterity is required. This device is manufactured by In Touch Systems, 11 Westview Road, Spring Valley, NY 10977, 800-332-MAGIC.

FACSIMILE MACHINES

Facsimile (fax) machines are used by clinics and physician's offices to send and/or obtain charts, electrocardiogram (ECG) tracings, laboratory reports, referral authorizations, letters, medical reports, and insurance claims; to order supplies; and so forth. Hospitals use them to transmit within the facility, such as medical records, laboratory and pathology reports, prescriptions to the hospital pharmacy, surgical scheduling, patient admissions, patient room scheduling, ECGs, face sheets, medical staff committee meetings, and so forth. Pharmacies send physicians requests and confirm orders, and physicians send prescription orders. Information can also be sent and received from medical libraries, attorneys, accountants, financial advisors, and vendors of medical and office supplies. Transcription services offer fax as a benefit for fast turnaround of medical reports. Documents can be faxed from the service to different floors within a hospital facility, from physician's office to the hospital across town, or around the world within a few minutes.

A fax machine is connected to a telephone line. A document is scanned, and this process converts the image to electronic impulses for transmitting over telephone lines. The receiving fax machine converts the impulses back to an identical hard copy of the original, and a printed copy is generated. Fax machines print on plain paper or thermally treated paper, but because thermal paper fades on exposure to sunlight, it is wise to photocopy important documents by using bond paper. Thermal paper also has a tendency to curl at the edges, so if the appearance of a document is crucial, you may prefer to use an overnight-delivery service instead of fax. Many fax machines generate open document communications, so someone must be assigned to secure incoming documents to provide for confidentiality. Some personal computer–based fax boards solve the security problem for sending and receiving documents because these boards give personal computers the ability to function like stand-alone fax machines. Thus, the documents are printed on quality bond paper and have very good image quality.

Many features are available for fax machines. The most useful are user and receiver confidentiality, automatic dialer, automatic document cutter, document feeder, 9600, 14,400, or 28,800 baud or bits per second (bps) transmission speed, half-tone or gray-scale mode, full-size (328 feet) paper roll, plain paper printing, autodialers, and delayed broadcasting for sending documents when telephone tolls are low.

When sending confidential material such as medical or legal records, telephone the recipient before faxing the information so that he or she can stand by. Incoming documents may be available for inspection by anyone at the receiving end, and the fax may be unstaffed. Begin every transmission with a cover sheet (a half-sheet size is sufficient) detailing the sender (name, telephone number, and fax number), the number of pages being sent, who is to receive the transmission (name and address), and any other information that will help get the fax to the proper person (Fig. 2–8). Include a telephone number to call in case there is a problem with the transmission, such as a lost page or dropped line. A handy hint is to make up a standard cover sheet letter on the employer's stationery and enclose it in a clear plastic sleeve (one that will allow you to fax a cover sheet within it). Fill in the information on the plastic sleeve with a dry erasable marker, using the cover sheet inside as your guide. After completing it, check to make sure the markings are dry, then fax. When the fax is complete, erase the cover information from the plastic sleeve with a blackboard eraser and put it aside for the next fax transmission. If you are concerned about clarity, test your material by making a copy on your fax machine before you send that important document. Perhaps you may have to make a photocopy of the document or enlarge the document on your copy machine and transmit the copied page. If the document contains numbers, type the numbers in words to avoid misinterpretation. Do not use color on fax documents without making a test copy. Dark colors can block copy and sometimes slow transmission. Do not use correction tape or fluid on

2

FAX TRANSMITTAL SHEET

To: ____________________ Date ____________

Fax Number: ____________________ Time ____________

Number of Pages (including this one): ____________________

From: ____________________ Phone ____________

Note: This transmittal is intended only for the use of the individual or entity to which it is addressed, and may contain information that is privileged, confidential, and exempt from disclosure under applicable law. If you are not the intended recipient, any dissemination, distribution, or photocopying of this communication is strictly prohibited. If you have received this communication in error, please notify this office immediately by telephone and return the original FAX to us at the address below by U. S. Postal Service. Thank you.

Remarks: ____________________

____

____

If you cannot read this FAX or if pages are missing, please contact:

PRACTON MEDICAL GROUP, INC.
4567 Broad Avenue
Woodland Hills, XY 12345-4700
Tel. 013/486-9002
Fax No. 013/488-7815

INSTRUCTIONS TO THE AUTHORIZED RECEIVER: PLEASE COMPLETE THIS STATEMENT OF RECEIPT AND RETURN TO SENDER VIA THE ABOVE FAX NUMBER.

I, ____________________**, verify that I have received** ____________
(no. of pages including cover sheet)

from ____________________
(sending facility's name)

Figure 2–8. Example of a facsimile cover sheet for medical document transmission illustrating a confidentiality statement with appropriate wording. (From Fordney MT: Insurance Handbook for the Medical Office, 4th edition. W. B. Saunders Company, Philadelphia, 1995.)

documents to be faxed. Always remove paper clips and staples to prevent damaging the fax machine. If the original document has copy near the left or right edges of the page, position the paper in such a way that the entire image will reproduce. Learn your fax's error messages and how to correct the problems that caused them. Noise or interference from telephone lines can garble your message, requiring you to resend or slow down the transmission rate. Be sure the transmission has been completed before you leave the fax machine.

PHOTOCOPYING MACHINES

Every office should have some type of copying equipment. Most equipment uses plain bond paper. Some machines copy only single sheets, whereas others copy pages from magazines or books as well as single sheets. It is important to make sure you invest wisely and purchase the equipment that will fit your particular needs. The copies are representative of you and your office, and a machine should be selected that produces the copies that most closely look like your original. Speed of copying may be another essential factor to consider. Before purchasing new equipment, you should discuss upkeep, ease of operation, and rate of breakdown with other owners. Special opaquing fluid specifically formulated for correcting copies can be obtained from your local stationers.

VOCABULARY

Audio device: Any computer device that produces sound. See *Voice synthesizer.*

Backup: A copy of a file that is kept in case the original file is destroyed.

Bit (binary digit): The smallest unit of information recognized by a computer.

Byte: A given number of bits considered as a unit of computer storage. (A byte is to a bit what a word is to a single letter.)

Cassette: A magnetic tape wound on two reels encased in a plastic or metal container that can be mounted on or inserted in a tape recording or playback device.

Character: Usually synonymous with byte. Also, a letter, symbol, or number contained in a text.

Command key: A key that enters a particular command into a word processing system. Also called control or function key.

Continuous form stationery: Forms, letterhead, or envelopes joined in a series of accordion-pleated folds and used in printers.

Copy: Text material in typed or printed form.

Crash: Sudden and complete failure of all or a substantial part of a system. See also *Head crash.*

Cue tone indexing: Inserting information magnetically onto a medium for the purpose of making corrections, deletions, or pertinent notes.

Cursor: A lighted indicator on a monitor that shows the place for entering new text or making editing changes.

Cut and paste: A term that means moving a piece of your copy to another place in your document or to another document.

Data: Information that can be processed or produced by a computer.

Default: A standard setting, preset for convenience, that may be changed when necessary. In word processing software, defaults define margins, tabs, page length, spacing, and so forth.

Delete: A command in word processing that removes a specific section of text from the recording medium.

Digital dictation: The process whereby the dictated voice is digitized (converted to a string of 0s and 1s representing the audio waveform) and stored as data on a computer disk. When instantly and selectively assessed from a dictation/transcription station or telephone, the binary digits are converted back to analog waveform sound.

Disk: A magnetic storage device made of rigid material (hard disk) or flexible plastic (floppy disk).

Disk drive: A device that holds the disk, retrieves information from it, and saves information on it.

Disk operating system (DOS): A program that controls the loading and storage of files from and to a computer's memory and to a magnetic disk.

Display: 1. Text appearing on the screen. 2. The act of commanding the computer to produce a document or specified text on the screen.

Document assembly: Device that allows combining of prerecorded text with keyboarded text, combining of selections from prerecorded text to form a new document, and inserting of names and addresses to create a number of nearly identical documents.

Dot matrix printer: An impact printer that prints characters composed of many dots.

Editing: Revision and correction of text (read back, scan, delete, insert, reformat) before final document printout.

Electronic mail system (EMS): Transmission of letters and reports from one computer to another via telephone lines.

Equipment service contract: Routine maintenance and emergency repair services provided for a set fee per year.

Ergonomics: The science of adapting working environment, conditions, and equipment to suit workers.

Error-free: A characteristic of recording on magnetic media that allows correction of errors by recording over unwanted material; in word processing, a term used when printing a document with no mistakes.

2

Facsimile machine: A machine connected to a telephone line and electric wall outlet that scans a document's image, transmits and/or receives it, and prints an exact facsimile. Also called fax.

Fast forward: A tape recorder feature that permits the tape to be run rapidly in normal-play direction for search purposes.

Fidelity: The degree of accuracy with which sound is reproduced.

File: A single stored unit of information that is given a file name so it can be accessed.

Floppy disk: See *Disk.*

Font: The size and style of type.

Global search and replace: The ability of a word processing system to change a word or other text element everywhere it appears in a document, with one instruction. Also called *global change.*

Hard copy: Written or printed document.

Hardware: The physical components (electric, electronic, magnetic, and mechanical devices) of a computer system, which, combined with software (programs, instruction, and so forth), create a system.

Head crash: When the read/write head of a disk drive flies above the disk and strikes the surface, severely damaging it. See *Crash.*

Initialize: To prepare the magnetic surface of a blank diskette so that it can accept data. This is sometimes referred to as formatting the disk.

Input: Information entered into a system to be processed.

Insert: A word processing function allowing introduction of new material within previously recorded text.

Justification: Alignment of text between fixed right and left margins by the addition of spacing between the words in a line of text; alignment of text margins on both right and left sides, i.e., flush left and flush right.

K (kilobyte): A symbol that refers to 1024 bytes or units of memory, i.e., 64 K means 64 times 1024 bytes or 65,536 bytes, not 64,000.

Keyboarding: Like typing, but including the extra instruction keys of a computer.

Light pen: A computer input device that looks like a pen on a string. It allows an operator to "draw" images on the screen of a video display terminal (VDT), mark choices on a displayed menu, add or delete displayed text, and so forth.

Medium (plural: media): Material on which information can be recorded.

Memory: The section of the computer where instructions, data, and information are stored; also called *storage* and *internal* or *main memory.*

Menu: Series of program options or commands displayed in a list on the computer screen that acts as an aid in using the word processing software. A menu may be referred to as main, mini, pull-down, or popup.

Merge: Document assembly, such as combining prerecorded text with keyboarded text, combining selections from prerecorded text to form a new document, and inserting names and addresses to create a number of nearly identical documents.

Modem: Acronym for *MO*dulator *DEM*odulator unit. A modem is a device that converts data into signals for telephone transmission and then (at the receiving end) back again into data.

Monitor: A screen attached to computer equipment; also known as video display or cathode ray tube (CRT).

Mouse: A hand-held computer input device, separate from a keyboard, used to control cursor position on a monitor.

Output: The final results after recorded information is processed, revised, and printed out.

Pagination: The automatic numbering of pages in a document.

Patching: A method of transferring recorded material from one tape or card to another.

Peripheral: Any input, output, or storage device (hardware) connected to the computer, such as hard disks, modems, or printers.

Playback: Listening to recorded dictation.

Power typing: A system that allows the typist to type at maximum or "rough draft" speed without concern for errors. These are corrected by backspacing and typing over to produce a perfect recording from which an error-free document is automatically printed out.

Program: See *Software.*

RAM: Random access memory. Memory that can be stored in any order and can be accessed immediately.

Response time: The time a computer takes to react to a given input.

Retrieve: Finding stored information from the archive.

ROM: Read-only memory. Memory that can be accessed but not modified.

Scanner: A machine or hand-held device that converts text or a printed image into a format readable by the computer and printer. Also referred to as optical character reader (OCR).

Scanning: To locate quickly, listening to a specific part of a recorded dictation by moving the sound head across a magnetic belt.

Scrolling: The ability to move the text vertically and horizontally and to flip pages of a document on the monitor.

Software: Programs or instructions used to support a piece of equipment, as opposed to the equipment itself or hardware.

Stop code: A code embedded in a document that signals the printer to stop.

Telecommunications: The transmission of information between widely separated locations by means of electric or electromagnetic systems such as telephone or telegraph.

Tone control: A feature on transcribing equipment used to vary treble and bass response during playback.

Touch-sensitive video screen: The user gives instructions to a computer by touching a picture on the screen instead of keyboarding.

Transcription: Conversion of recorded dictation to hard copy.

Tuning: Alignment of a sound head with the track on the recording medium.

Type: Refers to pressing the keys of a keyboard to input characters and symbols that when assembled become computer data.

Utility program: A general-purpose software program that performs activities (e.g., initializing a disk) that are not specific to an application.

Voice activation: Ability of a machine to recognize and respond to spoken words.

Voice recognition: The ability of a computer system (equipped with sound sensors) to translate the tones of the human voice into computer commands.

Voice synthesizer: A device that allows the computer to respond orally. It is used by visually impaired medical transcriptionists. Also called *Audio device.*

Warranty: A written statement from the manufacturer regarding responsibility for replacement and repair of a piece of equipment over a specified period of time.

Window: A graphics-based operating environment that provides a part of the video display area dedicated to a specific purpose. Multiple windows on the screen allow the user to treat the computer display screen like a desktop where various files may remain open simultaneously.

Word processing (WP): A combination of people, procedures, and equipment that transforms ideas into printed communications and helps facilitate the flow of related office work.

Word Processing Center: The room with equipment and personnel for processing written communications.

Word wrap: A feature in which a word that has more characters than will fit at the end of a line is moved to the beginning of the next line.

2-1: REVIEW TEST

Directions: Complete the following statements by filling in the blanks.

1. The first method used to make medical notes in charts was ____________________.
2. Initially, medical secretaries took dictation via ____________________.
3. The dictation method that has superior sound quality with no distortion, even when slowing down the voice, is called ____________________.

4. Physical parts of a computer system are called ____________, and programs that are used to support a piece of equipment are called ____________.
5. Computer function keys are also known as ____________ or ____________.
6. A screen attached to computer equipment is known as a/an ____________, ____________, or ____________.
7. Name four systems that speed up entering data via the computer.
   a. ____________
   b. ____________
   c. ____________
   d. ____________
8. A magnetic storage device made of flexible plastic is called a/an ____________.
9. Name four types of computer printers.
   a. ____________
   b. ____________
   c. ____________
   d. ____________
10. State why a transcriptionist would use a computer modem.
    ____
11. Name seven working characteristics to reduce computer fatigue and tension and increase productivity.
    a. ____________
    b. ____________
    c. ____________
    d. ____________
    e. ____________
    f. ____________
    g. ____________
12. Two categories of voice recognition products are ____________ and ____________.
13. Name two indication features that promote efficiency when transcribing a document.
    a. ____________
    b. ____________
14. List three features of the hand/foot control device used with transcribers.
    a. ____________
    b. ____________
    c. ____________
15. In regard to transcription preparation, what is the most important thing to do to prevent retyping a report or letter? ____________
    ____

16. Match the definitions in the first column with their correct terms in the second column. Place letters on blanks.

____ Printout of material recorded from a computer.

____ Alignment of the sound head with the track on the recording medium.

____ Information entered into a system to be processed.

____ Degree of accuracy with which sound is reproduced.

____ Materials on which information may be recorded.

____ Written statement from manufacturer stating responsibility for equipment replacement and repair.

____ Magnetic tape wound on two reels and encased, which is inserted in a dictation and/or transcription device.

____ Final results after recorded information is processed, revised, or printed out.

____ Standard setting preset for convenience that can be changed when necessary.

____ Program options listed on the computer screen as an aid in using software.

a. fidelity
b. warranty
c. default
d. hard copy
e. media
f. menu
g. cassette
h. tuning
i. input
j. output

Transcription Guidelines

3

CHAPTER 3

Punctuation

OBJECTIVES

After reading this chapter and working the exercises, you should be able to

1. Demonstrate the ability to use reference materials to select the proper punctuation needed in unfamiliar copy.
2. List, in your own words, the reasons for the accurate use of punctuation marks.
3. State the grammatical terms for different parts of speech and for the various parts of a sentence and match these terms with a written example.
4. Use the vocabulary of punctuation by writing the rule, using your own words and the proper terms, while working with an illustration of the rule in use.
5. Demonstrate the ability to use proper punctuation marks accurately by inserting punctuation into unpunctuated copy.

INTRODUCTION

Transcriptionists have more trouble with punctuation than with any other aspect of document preparation. Many authorities disagree with one another and with common usage. The following rules and exercises adhere not only to traditional guidelines but also to use in popular contemporary lay magazines and medical journals; to style guides for medical writers, editors, and transcriptionists; and to the results of field studies regarding the material preferred by authors of medical dictation. The use of punctuation should be guided by well-established, accepted conventions of style. However, sometimes "well-established" uses change, sometimes dramatically, as time goes by. An attempt is made to show variations in practices and to alert you to possible future style changes. Often, current methods are shown, but information is given on a former style that may be preferred in your work environment. You need to learn to follow the basic principles and *be consistent.*

Because proper punctuation is vital to business writing and document preparation, this summary is included to help you establish the rules in your mind so that you will acquire good punctuation habits. Proper punctuation helps the reader understand which items belong together, when to pause, or what is being emphasized. Some of us never learned to punctuate correctly, and many keyboard operators simply add a comma when it seems time for the reader to take a breath!

Without proper punctuation, communication breaks down, meaning can be lost or distorted, or the flow of ideas is interrupted. For example, the comma is used to clarify or signal the writer's exact meaning for the reader; therefore, comma misuse may either mislead the reader or delay his or her comprehension. Undoubtedly, you have seen sentences in which the meaning changes when a comma is moved.

In reviewing, remember that punctuation is often simple, but also keep in mind that it is not always subject to precise and unchanging rules. Certain punctuation marks are simply common practice, so if you rely on *common sense* you may not always be right.

Finally, because this chapter is not, and cannot be, a guide to proper punctuation under all circumstances, a professional writer, typist, or transcriptionist should have a comprehensive guide book in his or her desk library.

This chapter is not easy. Some of the words described in the vocabulary may not have received your attention since grade school. Please take time to review any areas that may present a problem before going forward. Remember that the material here will not disappear, and you may want to refer back to it at some time.

Final notes for students: Typeset marks and symbols often appear different from those made with the typewriter, word processor, or computer. Follow the basic rule for size and placement of symbols and characters as given.

VOCABULARY

The following terms will be used freely and without further definition in the rules that follow, so you should be quite comfortable with them. Before you begin to punctuate a sentence, review some of the vocabulary pertaining to sentence formation. You need to develop knowledge of the parts of speech and how they are strung together to form simple, compound, or complex sentences.

Sentence: A group of words containing a subject and a verb that forms a complete statement and is able to stand alone. The subject need not always be expressed; it may be understood.

EXAMPLE

Get this to the lab STAT. (The subject *you* is understood.)

- The first step in acquiring sentence sense is learning to recognize verbs.

Verb: A word or a group of words that expresses action or otherwise helps to make a statement. It may be one or several words that are written together or separated by other words.

Notice the verbs written in italics in the following sentences.

EXAMPLES

The patient *needs* a complete blood count.

The patient *is scheduled* for a complete blood count.

The patient *had* a complete blood count.

Send the patient to the lab for a complete blood count and *ask* him to return.

Will you *advise* the patient to have a complete blood count?

Pick out the verb in this sentence: "Instructors may be critical of students' work."

If you selected *may be,* you are correct. It expresses action. This part of the sentence is called the predicate.

- The second step in acquiring sentence sense is learning to recognize the subject of verbs.

Subject: That part of a sentence about which something is being said. This part is properly called the *complete subject,* but within the complete subject there is always a word or group of words that is the principal word within the complete subject and is called the *simple subject.* The subject is usually a noun or pronoun.

Noun/pronoun: The name of a person, place, or thing.

Notice the subject written in italics in the following sentences.

EXAMPLES

The *patient* needs a complete blood count.

The *patient* is scheduled for a complete blood count.

The *patient* had a complete blood count.

He had a complete blood count.

The first three examples are nouns, and the fourth example is a pronoun.

A word used in place of a noun is called a pronoun.

Pick out the noun subject of the following sentence:

My goal is to become a certified medical transcriptionist.

If you picked the noun *goal*, you are correct. Now look at this sentence and identify the subject and then the verb.

Exactly one year ago, Janet was promoted.

If you selected *Janet* as the subject and *was promoted* as the verb, you are correct. Because the subject may appear at almost any point in a sentence, it is usually easiest to locate if you pick out the verb first.

We can also express a sentence as follows:

Exactly one year ago, *she* was promoted.

In this case, the pronoun *she* is used in place of the noun.

Select the subject of the following sentence:

Down the elevator on a broken wheelchair struggled my patient.

Good for you if you selected *patient* from this convoluted grouping! Did you remember to find the verb first and then ask yourself "who struggled"?

- Step three is recognizing the independent clause or main clause in a sentence and the dependent clause when there is one.

Clause: Any group of words containing a subject and a verb.

EXAMPLE

Everyone *who is learning to transcribe* should study punctuation.

Notice that in this sentence, there are two sets of clauses. The one in italics is dependent. It contains a subject and a verb like the remainder of the sentence, but it *depends* on the balance of the sentence to make sense. Pick out the subject and the verb in the following sentence:

Routine laboratory studies that we carried out on admission disclosed a white count of 19,200.

If you selected *studies* (or the complete subject, *routine laboratory studies*) as the subject, you are correct. The verb is *disclosed*. What about the clause *that we carried out on admission*? That is called a dependent clause. Continue with your vocabulary.

Independent clause: A group of words containing a subject and a verb, making a complete statement, and able to stand alone as a *complete sentence*.

EXAMPLE

There was a small area of fibrotic scarring involving the right uterosacral ligament.

NOTE: In this example *there* is the subject, and *was* is the verb.

Compound sentence: Two or more independent clauses together make up a compound sentence.

EXAMPLES

I understand that you will complete the history and physical for the admission, and *I will order the preoperative evaluation.*

Good English skills are essential to our secretary, and *she will study hard to ensure her success.*

Pick out the two independent clauses from this compound sentence:

The patient had a complete blood count and we asked him to wait for the results.

HINT: Remember to look for the verb first (*had* in the first clause and *asked* in the second).

You selected *The patient had a complete blood count* as the first independent clause and *we asked him to wait for the results* as the second. Notice that each of these clauses can stand alone and that neither depends on the other to express a complete thought.

Dependent clause: A group of words containing a subject and a verb that depends on some other word or words in the sentence for completeness of meaning.

EXAMPLES

He is a patient *who must have general anesthesia* because he does not respond normally to routine dental care.

Many students find transcribing easy *because they have prepared themselves well for it.*

3

NOTE: In this example, *Many students find transcribing easy* is the independent clause, and *because they have prepared themselves well for it* is the dependent clause. This is one of the common ways that sentences are formed. Notice how the dependent clause *depends* on other words for completeness of meaning.

Select the dependent clause in the following sentence:

She had a complete blood count because she was scheduled for surgery tomorrow.

The clause *because she was scheduled for surgery tomorrow* is the dependent or subordinate clause because it depends on the first part of the sentence to be complete. It cannot stand alone as the first part of the sentence (an independent clause) does.

Take a close look at the following sentence. Does it contain a dependent clause?

The patient had a complete blood count and was asked to wait for the results.

No. The phrase *was asked to wait for the results* does not contain a subject. This illustrates a compound predicate or two sets of verbs after the single subject. Because this is a very common structure, you need to be able to tell the difference between an independent clause, a dependent clause, and a compound verb. Do this by selecting the verb first and then find the noun that is the subject of the sentence; finally decide whether the subject-verb combination can stand alone (independent clause) or whether it depends on the independent clause to be complete (dependent clause). If there is no subject-verb combination, then you may have the third illustrated combination: a compound verb, which is two or more verbs with one subject. There are additional pieces of these sentences to explore.

Introductory phrase: A group of words that occurs at the beginning of a sentence. This phrase can be thought of as being out of order or transposed in the sentence.

EXAMPLE

By now, you should have decided what courses you will need for graduation.

NOTE: The simple order of the sentence would be *You should have decided what courses you will need for graduation by now.*

EXAMPLE

In view of the continuing excessive tone in the plantar flexor muscles, it will be necessary to continue with orthotic control.

Please select the introductory phrase from the following sentence:

One day after beginning treatment, the patient's sense of well-being markedly improved.

There are several clues here: *one:* the introductory phrase appears at the beginning of the sentence; and *two:* the sentence is correctly punctuated with a comma after the phrase (more about this later).

At this point, do not worry too much about the words themselves: *phrase* and *clause.* (Clauses have a subject and a verb; phrases do not.) The important point is to notice the action and position of these groups of words in the sentence and the impact that they have on the dynamics of the sentence itself.

Essential: A word, phrase, or clause that is vital to the meaning of the sentence. Sometimes these are called "restrictive."

EXAMPLES

Everyone *employed in the Medical Records Department* received a commendation from the administrator.

The patient *who was born with a meningomyelocele* underwent closure of his spinal dysraphia in the newborn period.

Nonessential: A word, phrase, or clause that is not vital to the meaning of the sentence and simply provides explanatory material. Sometimes these are called "nonrestrictive."

EXAMPLE

Marlene Bruno, *who took medical terminology with me last semester,* is on the Dean's List.

NOTE: It is interesting that Marlene Bruno took *medical terminology* with the writer, but it is not essential or vital to the meaning of the sentence.

EXAMPLE

The patient's weight was 83.5 kg, *up presumably as a result of inactivity,* and his height was 166 cm.

Determine in the following sentences whether the words in italics are essential or nonessential (restrictive or nonrestrictive):

Students *who wish to enroll in medical keyboarding* must be typing 45 words per minute.

Any health plan *where there is a broad selection of hospitals, clinics, and caregivers* stands a good chance for success.

Our health plan, *with a broad selection of hospitals, clinics, and caregivers,* is very successful in the community.

In the first two sentences, the italics illustrate essential elements. You must know *which* students and *what* kind of plan will be successful. In the third sentence, you are told that the plan is successful, and *additional* information is provided with the words in italics.

Parenthetical expression: An interrupting group of words that does not change or contribute to the meaning of a sentence. They may appear at the beginning, middle, or end of the sentence and are always nonessential.

EXAMPLES

It is important, *as you know,* for medical records to be typed accurately.

I do not question the diagnosis; *however,* the result of his urinalysis and culture is negative.

NOTE: Some very common words or groups of words used as parenthetical expressions are *therefore, however, furthermore, in my opinion, strictly speaking, for example, in the first place, on the other hand, indeed, I suppose, of course, after all, by the way, it seems,* and *to be sure.*

Select the parenthetical expression in the following sentences:

The patient will be seen, I suppose, as soon as the triage is complete.

The patient, I suppose, will be seen as soon as the triage is complete.

The patient will be seen as soon as the triage is complete, I suppose.

I suppose is the correct selection.

The expression, as you no doubt noticed, completes its purpose in a variety of places in the sentence.

Appositive: A noun or pronoun that closely follows another noun or pronoun to restate, rename, explain, or clarify it. It may be essential or nonessential. An appositive must always consist of a word or words that can be directly substituted for the noun or pronoun they follow.

EXAMPLES

Dr. Pappin, *my employer,* prefers to dictate all chart notes.

This 2-month-old male child, *a Hmong Laotian,* was admitted via the Emergency Room with a cough, fever, and congestion.

Please select the appositive in the following sentence:

The syringe was disposed of properly in the sharps container, the box for hazardous materials.

Your selection of *the box for hazardous materials* is correct.

Conjunction: These are words that are used to join other words, phrases, clauses, and independent clauses.

EXAMPLES

and, or, for, nor, so, but, yet

- Joining other words: The medical assistant **and** the medical transcriptionist . . .
- Joining phrases: The medical assistant and the medical transcriptionist *attended the lecture* **and** *participated in the discussion.*
- Joining independent clauses: The medical assistant and the medical transcriptionist attended the lecture, **and** they planned to participate in the discussion that followed.

Sometimes parenthetical expressions are used as conjunctions.

EXAMPLES

however, furthermore, therefore

The medical assistant and the medical transcriptionist attended the lecture; *therefore,* they planned to participate in the discussion that followed.

Select the conjunctions in the following sentence, and decide the nature of the word or words that they are joining.

I enjoyed Chapter 1 and Chapter 2 of my textbook, but it appears that Chapter 3 may be a bit more difficult.

You are correct if you selected *but,* which joins **two independent clauses,** and *and,* which joins **two sets of words.**

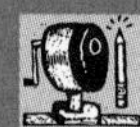 3–1: SELF-STUDY

3

Directions: Examine the sentences or parts of sentences that follow and write the part of the sentence or phrase that is requested on the line provided. The first exercise is completed for you.

1. Furthermore, I feel that a well-trained medical transcriptionist should be very well paid.

   Subject of the sentence I

   Parenthetical expression furthermore

   Independent clause I feel that a well-trained medical transcriptionist should be very well paid.

   Appositive none in this sentence

2. I appreciate my understanding of medical terminology.

   Subject of the sentence ____________________

   Independent clause ____________________

3. Please return this to Medical Records as soon as possible.

   Subject of the sentence ____________________

   Independent clause ____________________

4. After spending five hours in the operating room, the patient was sent to the recovery room.

   Introductory phrase ____________________

   Subject of the sentence ____________________

   Independent clause ____________________

5. The patient is a well-developed, well-nourished black female and reported that she has been well until this time.

   Subject of the sentence ____________________

   Independent clause ____________________

   Second verb clause ____________________

   Appositive ____________________

   Conjunction ____________________

6. Joan, the medical secretary, and Beth, the file clerk, are taking an evening college course in medical ethics.

   Subject ____________________

   Independent clause ____________________

   ____

   Appositive 1 ____________________

   Appositive 2 ____________________

   Parenthetical expression ____________________

7. The reception room is well lighted and stocked with current literature, so the patients do not mind their wait to see Dr. Jordan, who never seems to arrive on time.

   First subject ____________________

   Independent clause ____________________

   ____

Second subject ____________________

Independent clause ____________________

____

Conjunction joining independent clauses ____________________

Appositive ____________________

Nonessential clause ____________________

8. There is overwhelming evidence, however, to prove that the ability to spell is vital to success in this field.

Independent clause ____________________

Parenthetical expression ____________________

Appositive ____________________

9. The American Association for Medical Transcription, the national organization for medical transcriptionists, has a business and educational meeting every month.

Subject ____________________

Independent clause ____________________

____

Appositive ____________________

Parenthetical expression ____________________

Conjunction joining two independent clauses ____________________

10. Perfection, not speed, is the key word in medical transcription skills.

Subject ____________________

Verb ____________________

Independent clause ____________________

Appositive ____________________

Parenthetical expression ____________________

Nonessential phrase ____________________

11. Hospital transcriptionists often need to.

Subject ____________________

Independent clause ____________________

12. When you telephone the hospital, please have the patient's complete name, address, and telephone number and the admitting diagnosis.

Subject ____________________

Verb ____________________

Independent clause ____________________

____

Nonessential phrase ____________________

Introductory clause ____________________

Conjunction joining words in a series ____________________

3

13. Appointment scheduling, contrary to what you might think, requires skill; it should be, and can be, a real art.

    Independent clause ______________________________

    ____

    Nonessential clause or phrase ______________________________

    Parenthetical expression ______________________________

14. A perfectly typed resume, well-planned and prepared, should accompany your letter of application.

    Independent clause ______________________________

    ____

    Introductory phrase ______________________________

    Nonessential phrase ______________________________

15. He walks with his heel down with a varus tendency in the ankle but with no severe problem.

    Independent clause ______________________________

    Dependent group of words ______________________________

    Conjunction joining two independent clauses ______________________________

16. To minimize the chance of overlooking a recurrence of the infection, a CBC and sed rate were carried out today.

    Subject ______________________________

    Independent clause ______________________________

    Introductory phrase ______________________________

    Nonessential phrase ______________________________

Note: After you have completed the entire exercise, check your answers to the problems with those on page 89 of this chapter. Review the vocabulary if you have made any errors.

PUNCTUATION

The Comma

The comma is the most-used mark of punctuation and often causes the most problems for writers. At the same time, it is a very important aid in clarifying the meaning for the reader. Commas should be used appropriately and sparingly. Therefore, it is important to learn the rules for proper placement. Once the basic rules have been learned, the remainder of the punctuation marks should cause little problem.

■ Rule 3.1 Use a comma, or pair of commas, to set off nonessential words, phrases, or clauses from the remainder of the sentence.

These can also be called *parenthetical expressions* or *nonrestrictive phrases.* We need to take some time and examine them carefully.

EXAMPLE: *Nonessential clause*

Paul Otis, *who had a coronary last year,* came in for an examination today.

You may test yourself to be sure this is nonessential by asking the question: "Do I need to know which Paul Otis?" Unless we have several or even two patients with this name, we can say that the clause is nonessential to the meaning of the sentence. When you are in doubt, ask yourself if you need to know *which one.*

EXAMPLE: *Nonessential phrase*

Please notice, *if you will,* the depth of the incision.

EXAMPLE: *Nonessential word*

Yes, please type this before you leave this afternoon.

EXAMPLE: *Parenthetical expression*

She should have, *in my opinion,* immediate surgery.

NOTE: Nonessential or nonrestrictive descriptive phrases or clauses add information that is *not* essential to the meaning of the sentence. However, do not enclose *essential* material within commas. (Essential material will indicate the manner or condition or who, what, why, when, or where.)

EXAMPLES

I want to examine all of the children, *when they have been prepared.* (incorrect)

I want to examine all of the children when they have been prepared. (correct)

Medical staff members, *who fail to attend the meeting,* will lose their consulting privileges. (incorrect)

Medical staff members who fail to attend the meeting will lose their consulting privileges. (correct)

Do not create a comma fault by leaving out one of the commas when a pair is required.

Her temperature, *which has been high* fell suddenly. (incorrect)

Her temperature, which has been high, fell suddenly. (correct)

NOTE: Many people often have difficulty with correct usage of *who/whom/whose, that,* and *which* as function words in essential and nonessential clauses.

Who/Whom/Whose is used in both essential and nonessential clauses.

That is used in essential clauses.

Which is generally used in nonessential clauses.

EXAMPLES

This is a 26-year-old male *who* cut his left index finger on a pocket knife.

The patients *whose* Pap smears are Class II must be notified.

She twisted her left knee, *which* has an artificial prosthesis in it.

The recommendation *that* she undergo radiation therapy was rejected by the family.

■ Rule 3.1a Nonessential appositives are separated from the remainder of the sentence by commas.

Remember that appositives merely explain or add to the information about other nouns or pronouns in a sentence.

EXAMPLES: *Appositive*

John Munor, *your patient,* was admitted to Center City Hospital today.

Laralyn Abbott, *the head nurse,* summoned me to the phone.

As with phrases and clauses, appositives may be essential to the complete meaning of the sentence, and then they must not be separated from the remainder of the sentence by commas. Remember that there are appositives that help identify a word by limiting or restricting its meaning, so you must ask yourself if you need to know *which one.*

EXAMPLE: *Essential appositive*

Your patient Ralph Swansdown died at 3:45 a.m.

Notice that if *Ralph Swansdown* is separated from the rest of the sentence with a pair of commas, it appears that the person being addressed by this remark had only one patient, the lately deceased Mr. Swansdown. It is *essential* to know *which* patient. Likewise, one-word appositives do not require commas.

EXAMPLES

I *myself* will stay late and finish the report.

My cousin *Pat* just became a certified medical transcriptionist.

■ Rule 3.1b Use a comma, or pair of commas, to set off a short parenthetical expression from the remainder of the sentence.

These expressions may begin, interrupt, or end a sentence and are always nonessential.

EXAMPLES

However, I want this report typed.

I want this report typed, *however.*

These comma pairs can also be used to draw emphasis to a nonessential expression. The rule is not superseded in this case, of course.

EXAMPLE

He is an excellent surgeon, *whether or not you care for my opinion,* and I feel that you must trust his judgment.

Recall that some of the words used as parenthetical expressions are *indeed, for example, I suppose, of course, after all, by the way, it seems, to be sure, therefore, however, furthermore, in my opinion, strictly speaking,* and so on. However, no word or expression in itself is parenthetical. When closely con-

3

nected in meaning with other words in a sentence, they are not set off.

EXAMPLE

However upset she is, she will finish the report.

To restate these three similar rules: Set off nonessential words from the main body of thought. Commas must be placed before and after such words, phrases, or clauses. If they occur at the beginning of a sentence a single comma follows the expression. Your ability to recognize the difference between essential words, phrases, or clauses and those that are nonessential is important. Remember that an essential or a restrictive element identifies or further defines the meaning of the sentence and must *not* be separated from the sentence; a nonessential element is separated.

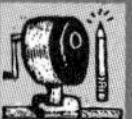 3–2: SELF-STUDY

Directions: Using Rule 3–1 and its subtopics a and b, add a comma or comma pair to the following sentences where required. Be careful not to enclose essential sentence parts. In the space provided, briefly state why you did or did not punctuate the sentence. A simple test for a nonessential element is to read the sentence without it. If the missing element does not change the basic meaning of the sentence, it should be set off by commas.

EXAMPLE

She said *if my memory serves me right* that she had graduated from medical school in 1975.

"if my memory serves me right" is nonessential. It is also a parenthetical expression.

1. John Munro your patient was admitted to Center City Hospital today.

___

2. He is an excellent surgeon whether or not you care for my opinion and I feel that you must trust his judgment.

___

3. She required trifocal not bifocal lenses at this time.

___

4. Dr. Mitchell having been in surgery since two this morning collapsed on the day bed.

___

5. The wound was closed with #3-0 silk sutures.

___

The answers to these self-study questions are at the end of this chapter on page 91. Check your answers before you continue.

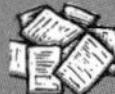 3–3: PRACTICE TEST

Directions: Using the directions found with Self-Study 3–2, complete the following problems.

1. Please telephone my nurse *if you are agreeable to postponing the surgery.*

___

3

2. He has done well following the transurethral resection of his prostate *with the exception of one episode of postsurgical hemorrhage.*

3. Our daughter Pat *who is a senior this year* is studying for a degree in rehabilitation therapy.

4. I want to examine all of the children *who have been exposed.*

5. Bill Birch's father *Ralph Birch* is Chief-of-Staff at Beech Hospital now.

6. His decision *not to operate* was a bit hasty if you ask me.

7. Only the second copy which is a carbon should be mailed to the referring physician.

8. I will contact the anesthesiologist *as soon as the operating room is free.*

9. *Essentials of Medical History* my textbook is excellent.

10. Nephritis *Bright's disease* will be the topic of his presentation at our meeting.

11. I had lunch with Alex St. Charles the new resident.

12. I would like to thank all of those patients *who donated blood.*

13. All patients wearing pacemakers should be told the good news.

14. Medical staff members *who fail to attend the meeting* will lose their consulting privileges however.

15. The secretary not the receptionist was promoted to office manager.

16. Furthermore she is to be prepped before Dr. Summers arrives.

17. Your patient Ethel Clifford saw me in consultation.

18. Ethel Clifford your patient saw me in consultation.

See Appendix A for the answers to Practice Test 3–3.

3–1: COMPUTER EXERCISE

3

Before proceeding, you may want to do more exercises based on the concepts you have learned. Additional practice material is on your computer diskette.

Directions: Insert the diskette into the computer and follow the instructions on the screen for Computer Exercise 3–1.

■ Rule 3.2a Use a comma to set off an introductory dependent phrase or clause.

EXAMPLES

After you have an x-ray, I will examine you.
(simple introductory clause)

Dr. Chriswell was having difficulty dictating; however, *after the equipment was adjusted,* she was able to finish her reports.
(part of the second independent clause)

Fully aware of his budget restrictions and with concern for the high cost of the equipment, Dr. Jellison approved the purchase of the word processor.
(compound introductory phrase)

NOTE: The comma follows the second phrase.

To transcribe this accurately the first time is the main goal.
(This introductory phrase serves as the subject of the sentence and must not be separated from the rest of the sentence by a comma.)

You will recall that this introductory element can be thought of as being "out of place" in the sentence. Many of these introductory dependent phrases or clauses begin with words such as *since, because, after, about, during, by, if, when, while, although, unless, between, so, until, whenever, as,* and *before* and with verb forms such as *hoping, believing, allowing, helping,* and *working.*

■ Rule 3.2b Do *not* use a comma when the essential or restrictive clause appears in natural order: at the end of the sentence or at the end of the independent clause.

Essential clauses limit the meaning of the main clause.

EXAMPLES

I will examine you *after* you have an x-ray.
(tells *when* the patient will be examined)

She was able to finish her report *after* the equipment was adjusted.

EXAMPLE: introductory

During the course of the procedure, a power failure occurred.

EXAMPLE: natural order

A power failure occurred *during* the course of the procedure.

OPTIONAL: The comma may be omitted after a very brief introductory element if clarity is not sacrificed.

EXAMPLE

If possible schedule the thoracotomy to follow the bronchoscopy.

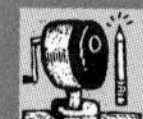

3–4: SELF-STUDY

Directions: Using the rules you have just learned, add a comma or comma pair where required. Be wary of separating the subject from the verb with a comma, which you might attempt to do when the subject is lengthy. Always check to be sure there is an intact independent clause. Please insert and circle optional commas.

EXAMPLE

After the surgery was completed, he dictated the operative report. (Note the comma after the introductory phrase.)

1. That you have lost your secretarial position is not my concern.
2. Although she had been in pain for some time she failed to seek medical attention.

3. If you are not feeling better by tomorrow take two aspirins and call Dr. Meadows.
4. When initially seen the patient was in restraints lying in bed.
5. To transcribe and complete the insurance billing is her responsibility.
6. Our receptionist whom I hired yesterday failed to come in today.

The answers to Self-Study 3–4 are at the end of this chapter on page 91. Check your answers before you continue.

3–5: PRACTICE TEST

Directions: Use the rules you have learned thus far and place commas, as needed, in the following problems. Then, briefly state the reason for the commas you have added.

1. She will go immediately into the operating room as soon as it is free.

   ______

2. Whatever he said to her was misunderstood.

   ______

3. Dr. Johnston the pathologist deserves the credit for that diagnosis.

   ______

4. The delivery of the baby a girl was uneventful.

   ______

5. Furthermore I will not be here to interview the new medical transcriptionist.

   ______

6. When you have the opportunity please dictate the operative note.

   ______

7. To be sure she was safe the nurse took her to the car in a wheelchair.

   ______

8. After lunch he must rest quietly.

   ______

9. Thinking he was at home the patient attempted to get out of bed.

   ______

10. Helping the blind transcriptionist research a word is Janet's responsibility.

    ______

The answers to Practice Text 3–5 are found in Appendix A at the end of the book.

■ Rule 3.3 Use a comma to set off a year date that is used to explain a preceding date of the month.

EXAMPLES

He was born on March 3, 1933, in Reading, Pennsylvania.

Make her an appointment for Wednesday, July 6, 199X.

Omit commas when the complete date is not given.

EXAMPLES

We will see the patient again on May 6.

He had surgery in April 1995 in Arizona.

3

Omit the comma with the military date sequence.

EXAMPLE

11 November 199X

■ Rule 3.4 Use a comma to set off the name of the state when the city precedes it.

EXAMPLE

The pacemaker was shipped to you from Syracuse, New York, by air express.

Use commas to separate all the elements of a complete address.

EXAMPLE

Please mail this to my home address: 132 Winston Street, Park Village, IL 60612.

NOTE: Do not place a comma between the state name and the ZIP code. The ZIP code is considered part of the state name.

■ Rule 3.5 Do not use a comma to set off "Inc." and "Ltd." following the name of a company unless the company prefers the usage.

EXAMPLES

I was employed by Thoracic Surgery Medical Group Inc., in Encino, California, for five years.

Headquarters for the American Association of Medical Assistants Inc. is Chicago, Illinois.

■ Rule 3.6 Use a comma or pair of commas to set off titles and degrees following a person's name.

EXAMPLES

John A. Meadows, MD, saw the patient in consultation.

Ms. Nancy Bishop, administrator, gave him ten days to bring his incomplete charts up to date.

If there are multiple degrees or professional credentials after a person's name, place them in the order in which they were awarded and separate them with commas.

EXAMPLES

Mary Watkins, BS, MS, JD

Nancy Casales, CMA, CMT, is the new president of AAMT, Mountain Meadows Chapter.

Frances Knight, LLB, MD, will be the speaker about risk management.

NOTE: There is a trend to eliminate commas, particularly when meaning is not sacrificed. Some writers are not using commas to separate degrees and titles following a person's name. As always, follow the wishes of the bearer of the name.

Do not place a comma before roman numbers indicating first, second, third, etc. or Jr. or Sr. following a name unless the bearer of the name prefers that usage.

EXAMPLES

Howard J. Matlock III

Carl A. Nichols Jr. was admitted to Ward B.

A Billroth I anastomosis was performed.

■ Rule 3.7 Use a comma after each element or each pair of elements in a series of coordinate nouns, adjectives, verbs, or adverbs.

OPTIONAL: You *may* omit the comma before the conjunction if clarity is not sacrificed. However, many writers avoid this option.

EXAMPLES

Please copy the patient's operative report, pathology report, and consultation report for Dr. Gifford.

The various hospital departments were decorated in green and yellow, blue and brown, and green and white.

There were papers to be filed, charts to be sorted, ledgers to be posted.

An adjective forming a noun phrase with the noun that it modifies is not separated from the immediately preceding adjective with a comma.

EXAMPLE

The patient is a well-developed, well-nourished, elderly, white female telephone operator.

The noun phrase is *female telephone operator,* and the adjective immediately preceding the noun phrase is *white.*

A test of whether commas are needed is to transpose the two modifiers. For example, one would not say *female white telephone operator.*

Furthermore, no comma is used before the ampersand (&).

EXAMPLE

The law firm is listed as Claborne, Franklin & Bowers.

NOTE: "Etc." in a series has a comma both before and after it unless it occurs at the end of a sentence; then its period ends the sentence.

■ Rule 3.8 Use a comma to separate two or more independent clauses when they are joined by the conjunction *and, or, nor, but, for, yet,* or *so.*

NOTE: The comma is placed in front of the conjunction.

EXAMPLE

Your appendix appears to be inflamed, but I do not believe that you need surgery at this time.

BUT: Your appendix appears to be inflamed but not acutely. *(not two independent clauses)*

EXAMPLE

The diagnosis of urinary tract infection was made, and he was treated with Septra.

BUT: The child weighed 7 pounds at birth and was the result of an uncomplicated pregnancy and delivery. *(not two independent clauses)*

Two of the preceding examples do not contain two independent clauses, and it would be incorrect and misleading if you placed commas in front of the conjunctions. Be careful not to make this error. Check the sentence to see if the clauses are independent by testing each clause to see if it expresses a complete thought and could stand alone as a sentence, omitting the conjunction. When the second (or third) clause is *dependent,* the subject is usually missing. There must be a subject in the second clause to make it independent. Do not make the mistake of using a comma just because there is a conjunction present. Know why you are punctuating; and when in doubt, leave it out!

OPTIONAL: You *may* omit a comma between two short, closely related independent clauses if there is no chance of the meaning being confused.

EXAMPLE

She came in just after noon so we invited her to lunch.

BUT: I kicked the ball, and John accidentally slipped reaching for it.

If you omit the comma after "ball" it appears, at first glance, as if you also kicked John accidentally.

3

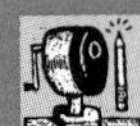

3–6: SELF-STUDY

Directions: Using Rules 3.3 through 3.8, add a comma or commas where required. Briefly state why you inserted the comma or commas.

1. The patient was first seen in my office on Wednesday July 14, 199X.

____

2. Please send this to Natalie Jayne RN Chief of Nurses Glorietta Bay Hospital.

____

3. Carl A. Nichols Jr. was admitted to Ward B.

____

4. The blood test included a white blood count red blood count hematocrit and differential.

____

5. There is a story of a mild head injury at age ten and she was in a moderately severe motorcycle accident about fifteen years ago.

____

6. The condition is now stationary and permanent and he should be able to resume his normal work load.

____

7. She was fully dilated at 2:30 a.m. but did not deliver the second twin until 2:55 a.m.

____

3

See page 92 at the end of the chapter for the answers to this Self-Study.

 3–7: PRACTICE TEST

Directions: In the following sentences, fill in the missing punctuation, and in the space after each sentence, fill in the letter or letters of the rule or rules you used from the list given after **Rule Review.** Each rule may be used more than once, and it is not necessary to refer back to the point in the chapter where the rule was introduced. Make a circle around any optional commas.

RULE REVIEW

Use a comma or pair of commas to

a. set off nonessential words from the remainder of the sentence
b. set off nonessential appositives
c. set off a parenthetical expression
d. set off an introductory phrase or clause
e. set off the parts of a date
f. set off "Inc." or "Ltd." in a company name only if the firm prefers
g. set off titles and degrees following a person's name
h. separate words in a series
i. separate two independent clauses
j. separate the name of the state from the name of the city

EXAMPLE

On auscultation, there are diffuse rhonchi and occasional rales heard.

Rule ___d___

1. He will be able to return to light work at any time but he should not be allowed to operate a jackhammer.

   Rule _______________

2. His wounds are all healing well and he has had no further pain.

   Rule _______________

3. In the preceding week he had had an automobile accident and was under the care of Dr. Finish.

   Rule _______________

4. The patient continued her labor and was closely monitored for fetal heart tones.

   Rule _______________

5. I have consulted with the Radiation Therapy Department at University Hospital and they have suggested that radiation therapy would be the best approach to this problem.

   Rule _______________

6. It is my understanding that you will do the history and physical for the hospital but not the consultation.

   Rule _______________

7. Please contact Charles Rick MD in Nogales Arizona as soon as possible.

   Rule ______________

8. He had surgery July 14 1994 for carcinoma of the prostate but is now free of disease.

   Rule ______________

9. Dr. Phillip is the newest member of St. Peter's Medical and Surgical Group Inc.

   Rule ______________

10. On physical examination I found a well-developed well-nourished white woman in no acute distress.

    Rule ______________

11. He noticed increasing dyspnea with effort extreme shortness of breath and night sweats.

    Rule ______________

12. She is to be admitted with your concurrence on Wednesday July 1 199X at 2 p.m.

    Rule ______________

13. Before you call surgery to schedule this and before you telephone Mrs. Jones will you report to me?

    Rule ______________

14. As you know John Briggs MD my partner is retiring on July 31 this year.

    Rule ______________

15. On March 26 199X she had a left lower lobectomy and postoperatively had bronchopneumonia which required intravenous antibiotics.

    Rule ______________

See Appendix A at the end of the book for a list of the rule or rules used in this exercise. After you have completed the assignment, you may consult this list to check yourself. If you chose the wrong rule, perhaps you have misplaced the comma!

3–2: COMPUTER EXERCISE

Before proceeding, you may want to do more exercises based on the concepts you have learned. Additional practice material is on your computer diskette.

Directions: Insert the diskette into the computer and follow the instructions on the screen for Computer Exercise 3–2.

■ Rule 3.9 Enclose names of persons used in direct address and the words *yes* and *no* in commas.

EXAMPLES

My thanks, Paul, for sending Mr. Byron in for a consultation.

No, it is not our policy to give out that information.

Now is the time, medical language specialists, to make your voices heard.

■ Rule 3.10 If two or more words independently modify the same noun, separate them with a comma if a mental "and" can be placed between them or if the order in which they are used can be reversed.

EXAMPLES

She is a tall, slender woman.

It was a wide, deep wound.

BUT: She is an efficient medical secretary.

3 Do not place a comma after the last modifier in front of the noun. In the following sentence, we would not place a comma in front of *memo.*

We received a poorly punctuated, rude memo from your department.

■ Rule 3.11 Use a comma or a pair of commas to avoid misleading or confusing the reader and to set off contrasts.

EXAMPLES

In 1984, 461 babies were delivered in our new obstetrics wing.

It is one thing to be assertive, another rigid.

We are here to work, not visit.

Soon after, he got up and discharged himself from the hospital.

He spells out difficult terms, for example, radioactive isotopes.

The day before, I had seen her in the emergency department.

Diagnosis: Fracture, third and fourth ribs on right.

Operation performed: Hemorrhoidectomy, radical.

Impression: Diverticulosis, moderate.

■ Rule 3.12 Use a comma after the complimentary close when using "mixed punctuation" in a letter.

EXAMPLE

Sincerely yours,

■ Rule 3.13 Use commas to group large numbers in units of three.

EXAMPLE

platelets 250,000; WBC 15,000

NOTE: Addresses, year dates, ZIP codes, four-digit numbers, and some ID and technical numbers are traditionally not separated by commas, nor are commas used with decimals or the metric system.

EXAMPLE

1000 ml (correct) 1,000 ml (incorrect)
My bill to Medicare was $1250.

CAUTION: Do not separate numbers that are parts of complete units.

EXAMPLE

She was in labor for *6 hours 40 minutes* before we decided to do a cesarean section.

NOT: 6 hours, 40 minutes

EXAMPLE

The infant weighed *4 lb 15 oz* on delivery.

NOT: 4 lb, 15 oz

EXAMPLE

The patient is a 24-year-old, unemployed, *gravida 2 para 1* white female in no acute distress.

NOT: gravida 2, para 1

■ Rule 3.14 Use a comma to separate the parts of a date in the date line of a letter.

EXAMPLE

November 11, 199X

BUT: 11 November 199X

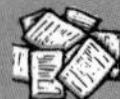 3–8: PRACTICE TEST

Directions: Using your text and any other reference materials, properly punctuate the letter on page 71. There are 18 commas missing. (Other punctuation marks, including two commas, are provided for you, so your completed letter will contain 20 commas including any optional commas.) In the margin, number each comma you insert, and on a separate sheet of paper, give your reason for using each comma.

This letter should be retyped on letterhead paper of your choice and punctuated, but it may be punctuated as is if there is a time problem or equipment is not available in the teaching lab. The correct version is given in Appendix A.

3

September 16 199x

Tellememer Insurance Company
25 Main Street, Suite R
Albuquerque NM 87122

Gentlemen:

RE: Ron Emerson

I understand from Mr. Emerson that the insurance company feels that the charges for my services on June 30 199X are excessive.

Mr. Emerson was seen on an early Sunday morning with a stab wound in his chest, which had penetrated his lung producing an air leak into his chest wall. In addition he had a laceration of his lung.

After consultation and review of his x-rays his laceration was repaired. He was observed in the hospital for two days to be sure that he did not have continuing hemorrhage or collapse of his lung.

I feel that the bill given to Mr. Emerson is a fair one. We received on July 31 199X a Tellememer Insurance Company check for $40 and I feel that your payment of $40 is unreasonable. It is doubtful that one could get a plumber to come out early Sunday morning to fix a leaky pipe for $40 and Mr. Emerson's situation in my opinion was much more serious than would be encountered by a plumber.

We will bill Mr. Emerson for the remainder of the $200 balance on his account but I want you to know that we feel that your payment is insufficient. If he feels that the bill is excessive we would be glad to submit to arbitration through the County Medical Society Fee Committee. If this fails I suggest we seek help through the New Mexico Insurance Commission.

Sincerely yours

William A. Berry MD

rl

Enclosed: X-ray report; history and physical report

Copy: Mr. Ron Emerson

3-9: REVIEW TEST

3 *Directions:* Place a comma or commas where needed in the sentences that follow. Please circle optional commas.

1. In the meantime he was discharged to his home.
2. She is scheduled to be seen again on February 3 at 10:30 a.m.
3. Laralyn Abbott the trauma team nurse issued a code blue.
4. Your patient Kay Hai Wong was readmitted to the Veterans Administration Hospital with a diagnosis of cholecystitis pancreatitis and mild gastritis.
5. As demonstrated earlier chemotherapy had little effect on the rate of tumor growth.
6. In 1995 461 cases were reviewed by the Tumor Board.
7. Soon after he got up and discharged himself from the hospital.
8. Dr. Powell not Dr. Franklyn delivered the infant.
9. After three surgeries are not scheduled.
10. I would like her to be and she probably will be a candidate for heart surgery.
11. She is a spastic retarded child.
12. He had crystal clear urine.
13. It has been a pleasure Winton to help you take care of Mr. Ibarra.
14. She required trifocal not bifocal lenses at this time.
15. Dr. Chriswell was having difficulty dictating; however, after the equipment was adjusted she was able to finish her reports.
16. He was indeed concerned about her progress.
17. Even though he was experiencing difficulty breathing we decided not to perform a tracheotomy.
18. Gastric lavage was carried out and the patient was placed in four-point restraints.
19. The surgery was completed in 2 hours 40 minutes.
20. The infant demonstrated normal reflexes of suck root and startle.

3-3: COMPUTER EXERCISE

Before proceeding, you may want to do more exercises based on the concepts you have learned. Additional practice material is on your computer diskette.

Directions: Insert the diskette into the computer and follow the instructions on the screen for Computer Exercise 3–3.

The voice of the speaker usually gives us clues to understanding the meaning of what is being said because of voice inflection, pauses, tone, and word emphasis. To convey this to the person to whom the dictator is communicating, the vocal clues must be translated into written clues.

You have just completed your study of the most used written clue: the comma. Now we will tackle the remainder of the basic aids to understanding the written word. Again, special emphasis has been placed on the punctuation rules you will use most often in medical transcribing.

The Period and Decimal

NOTE: Some dictators will indicate the end of a sentence by saying "period" or "full stop." Others drop their voice to indicate closure. You will need to learn the individual styles of your dictators.

■ Rule 3.15 Place a period at the end of a sentence and at the end of a request for action that is phrased as a question out of politeness.

EXAMPLES

His chest was clear to percussion and auscultation.

You must be seen by a surgeon at once.

Will you please send a copy of the operative report to Dr. Blanche.

NOTE: Use only one period at the end of a sentence, even if the sentence ends with a punctuated abbreviation.

EXAMPLE

The surgery is scheduled to begin at 7 a.m.

■ Rule 3.16 Place a period with the following:

1. Single capitalized words and single letter abbreviations

   Mr. Jr. Dr. Inc. Ltd. Joseph P. Myers

2. The name of the genus when it is abbreviated and used with the species

   E. coli M. tuberculosis E. histolytica

3. Lower case Latin abbreviations

   a.m. p.m. e.g. t.i.d. p.o.

4. After letters and numbers in alphanumeric outlines except those enclosed in parentheses

I. ....
  A. ....
  B. ....
    1. ....
    2. ....

Diagnoses:

1. Bilateral external canal exostoses.
2. Deafness, left ear, unknown etiology.

The following are **not** punctuated:

1. Metric and English units of measurement

   wpm mph ft oz sq in mg mL L cm km

2. Certification, registration, and licensure abbreviations

   CMA-A CMT RN RRA ART LPN

3. Acronyms

   CARE Project HOPE AIDS MAST

4. Most abbreviations typed in capital letters

   UCLA PKU BUN CBC COPD D&C T&A I&D PERRLA

5. Scientific abbreviations typed in a combination of capital and lower case letters

   Rx Dx ACh Hb IgG mEq mOsm Rh Na K pH

6. Abbreviations that are brief forms of words

   exam phenobarb sed rate flu Pap smear

7. Academic degrees and religious orders

   BVE DDS MD MS PhD RCSJ SJ

Some individuals prefer that these abbreviations be punctuated with a period. It is not incorrect to do this.

■ Rule 3.17 A period (decimal point) is used to separate a decimal fraction from whole numbers.

EXAMPLES

His temperature on admission was 99.8°F.
The new surgical instrument cost $64.85.
Epinephrine dose: 0.3 ml.
The wound measured 2.5 x 3.5 cm.

The Semicolon

The semicolon is always used as a mark of separation. It is frequently equivalent to a period; in this situation, both sides of the semicolon must be independent clauses. Sometimes the semicolon replaces a comma and tells the reader, "Keep reading; the second part is related."

■ Rule 3.18 Use a semicolon to separate two or more closely related independent clauses when there is no conjunction.

EXAMPLES

You have requested our cooperation; we have complied.

The nose is remarkable for loud congestive breathing; there is no discharge visible.

■ Rule 3.19 Use a semicolon to separate independent clauses if either one or both have already been punctuated with two or more commas.

3

EXAMPLE

Around the first of July, he developed pain in his chest, which he ignored for several days; and, finally, he saw me, at the request of his family doctor, on July 16.

■ Rule 3.20 Use a semicolon before a parenthetical expression when it is used as a conjunction between two independent clauses. (A comma is placed after the expression.)

EXAMPLE

I attempted a labor induction with Pitocin, and contractions occurred; however, the patient failed to develop an effective labor pattern, and I discharged her after eight hours.

NOTE: Some of the most common parenthetical (transitional) expressions used as conjunctions are *however, furthermore, therefore, consequently, nevertheless,* and *accordingly.*

■ Rule 3.21 Use a semicolon between a series of phrases or clauses if any item in the series has internal commas. (This gives a clear indication of where one word group ends and another begins.)

EXAMPLES

Among those present at the Utilization Committee Meeting were Dr. Frank Byron, chief-of-staff; Mrs. Joan Armath, administrator; Ms. Nancy Speeth, medical records technician; and Mr. Ralph Johnson, director of nurses.

Medications: He will continue his 1800-calorie ADA diet and usual medicines, which include estradiol, 2 mg/d for 25 of 30 days; flurazepam HCl, 30 mg h.s.; hydrocodone bitartrate, 5 mg; and ibuprofen, 600 mg q.i.d.

The Colon

Think of the colon as a pointer, drawing your attention to an important and concluding part. It is a mark of *anticipation.* It helps to couple separate elements that must be tied together but emphasized individually. Often, the material to the right of the colon means the same as the material to the left of the colon.

■ Rule 3.22 Use a colon followed by a double space to introduce a *list* preceded by a *complete sentence.* These lists are often introduced by the following expressed or implied words: *as follows, such as, namely, the following.*

EXAMPLE

Please bring the following items with you to the hospital: robe, slippers, toilet articles, and two pairs of pajamas.

INCORRECT: The patient had: a history of chronic obstructive lung disease and congestive heart failure.

CORRECT: The patient had a history of chronic obstructive lung disease and congestive heart failure.

■ Rule 3.23 Place a colon after the salutation in a business letter when "mixed" punctuation is used.

OPTIONAL: When the salutation is informal and the person is addressed by his first name, you *may* use a comma.

EXAMPLES

Gentlemen:
Dear Dr. Berry:
Dear Bill: (or) Dear Bill,
To Whom It May Concern:
Dear Sir or Madam:

■ Rule 3.24 Use a colon with numbers in expressing ratios, dilute solutions, and between the hours and minutes indicating the time in figures.

EXAMPLE

Her appointment is for 10:30 a.m.

NOTE: The colon is not used in expressions of military time.

EXAMPLE

The patient was seen at 1430.

NOTE: The colon and double zeros are not used with the even time of day.

EXAMPLE

10 a.m.

EXAMPLE

The solution was diluted 1:100.

EXAMPLE

The odds are 10:1.

■ Rule 3.25 Place a colon after the introductory word or words in preparing a written history and physical, in introducing a reference line, in listing the patient's vital signs, or with the introductory words in an outline.

EXAMPLES

Chief complaint: Hyperemesis.

Past history: Usual childhood diseases; no sequelae.

Allergy: Patient denies any drug or food sensitivity.

EXAMPLE

Re: Mrs. Blanche Mitchell.
Reference: #306-A.
Subject: Stress test.

EXAMPLE

Vital Signs:
  Temperature: 101°.
  Pulse: 58.
  BP: 130/90.
  Respirations: 18.

EXAMPLE

Diagnoses: 1. Gastritis.
  2. Pancreatitis.
  3. Rule out cholecystitis.

NOTE: Close your listed items with a period.

■ Rule 3.26 Use a colon to introduce an example or a clarification of an idea.

EXAMPLES

I see only one alternative: chemotherapy.
You have only one goal here: accuracy.

NOTE: These examples are often introduced by the expressions "thus" or "that is," or the expression could be supplied mentally.

Colons are generally used in sentences in which the second set of words amplifies or clarifies the first. A *capital letter* is used to begin the set of words after the colon if it is a formal statement.

EXAMPLE

This is how the transcribers are stored: Insert the headset loosely in the plastic bag provided and place it next to the transcriber itself.

3–10: SELF-STUDY

Directions: Using Rules 3.15 through 3.26, add a semicolon, colon, or period where required.

1. Mr Clark E Rosamunde is scheduled to arrive at 4 30 pm
2. Josephine Tu, MD, will present six cases to the Oncology Review Board Dr Richland will be unable to attend.
3. Would you please send this on to Ralph Desmond Jr
4. Please place the following warning on the door to Room 16 "Caution Radioactive materials in use."
5. The ambulance arrived at precisely 2110
6. The patient was treated for the following problems insomnia, malaise, depression.
7. The consultation fee of $85 was not covered by insurance

Turn to the end of the chapter, page 92, for the answers to these problems.

3–11: PRACTICE TEST

Directions: In the following exercises, fill in the missing punctuation, and in the space after each exercise, fill in the letter of the rule you used from the list given after **Rule Review.** Each rule may be used more than once, and it is not necessary to refer back to the point in the chapter where the rule was introduced.

RULE REVIEW

Use a period:
a. with single capitalized word abbreviations.
b. to separate decimal fractions.

3

Use a semicolon:
c. between two independent clauses that have internal punctuation.
d. between two independent clauses with a parenthetical expression acting as a conjunction.
e. between two independent clauses with no conjunction.
f. to simplify reading the sentence because of other punctuation marks.

Use a colon:
g. to introduce a series of items.
h. to clarify an idea.
i. with introductory words in an outline.
j. with a reference notation.

EXAMPLE

The child had a full-term gestation; his birth weight was 9 lb 4 oz.

Rule e

1. She hasn't quite returned to full physical activity yet therefore, I will want to see her again in a month to re-evaluate her status.

   Rule __________

2. As you recall, Mr Scout is a 41-year-old man with severe angina, myocardial ischemia, and triple artery disease but he does have a well-functioning ventricle.

   Rule __________

3. The procedures performed were as follows bronchoscopy, bronchography, scalene node biopsy, right pneumonectomy. The insurance reimbursement (welcome as it was) amounted to only $65075. *(Six hundred fifty dollars and seventy-five cents.)*

   Rule __________

4. The panel members included the following staff Dr Mary A Jamison, chief resident Dr Peter R Douglas Jr, surgical director Mrs Nancy Culpepper, operating room supervisor and Jane Morris, RN, ICU supervisor.

   Rule __________

5. One fact stands out in all this discussion about this young man he has a great element of fear about being anesthetized.

   Rule __________

6. The patient was admitted with a temperature of 1012° *(one hundred and one and two tenths degrees),* chills, and nausea she also complained of low back pain and cervical pain.

   Rule __________

7. The operative site was injected with 05% *(point five per cent)* Xylocaine and epinephrine.

   Rule __________

8. Her neurologic examination now, as in the past, has been completely normal and there has never been any evidence of cerebral injury as a result of the gunshot wound.

   Rule __________

9. Her neurologic examination is normal she has full rotation of her neck, with flexion and extension unlimited.

   Rule __________

10. Final clinical diagnosis Acute cervical sprain, resolved. Condition on discharge Improved.

    Rule __________

Answers are given in Appendix A at the end of the book.

3

The Hyphen

■ Rule 3.27 Use a hyphen when two or more words have the force of a single modifier before a noun.

EXAMPLES

figure-of-eight sutures
self-addressed envelope
seizure-inducing drug
end-to-end anastomosis
self-inflicted knife wound
well-known speaker
ill-defined tumor mass
large-for-dates fetus
non-English-speaking patient

He was seen today in follow-up examination.

The resident consulted the alcoholism counselors on his two MAST-positive patients.

That was an ill-advised remark written in the medical record. (See also Rule 3-28.)

NOTE: Omit the hyphen when the compound follows the noun.

EXAMPLES

The patient is a well-developed, well-nourished black male.

HOWEVER: The patient is well developed.

This is a very up-to-date reference for drug names.

HOWEVER: This reference needs to be brought up to date.

This 19-year-old Mayview College student was injured in the accident.

HOWEVER: This Mayview College student is 19 years old.

During her pregnancy she experienced a 45-pound weight gain.

HOWEVER: She gained 45 pounds during her pregnancy.

NOTE: An adverb ending in "ly" is not hyphenated before the adjective and noun.

EXAMPLES

She is a moderately obese waitress.
That was a poorly dictated report.
He is an exceptionally gifted diagnostician.

NOTE: *Common* compound expressions as well as essential parts of disease descriptions are not hyphenated.

EXAMPLES

low cervical incision
normal sinus rhythm
pelvic inflammatory disease
congestive heart failure
right upper quadrant
chronic obstructive pulmonary disease
central nervous system
intensive care unit
Social Security check
civil rights issue
special delivery letter
deep tendon reflexes
ad hoc committee
in vitro testing
amino acid residue
rapid frozen section
atrial septal defect
low back pain

■ Rule 3.28 Use a hyphen between coordinate expressions after the verb.

EXAMPLES

The waiting room was painted a sort of yellow-orange.

That remark was well-taken.

The patient's expression was happy-sad.

The receptionist appeared ill-humored.

There was blood pooling in the cul-de-sac.

That remark was ill-advised.

This drug is not a cure-all.

■ Rule 3.29 Use a suspending hyphen in a series of compound modifiers.

EXAMPLES

There were small- and large-sized cysts scattered throughout the parenchyma.

He has a two- or three-month convalescence ahead of him.

A 1- to 2-cm longitudinal incision will be made just above the umbilicus.

■ Rule 3.30 Use a hyphen when numbers are compounded with words and they have the force of a single modifier.

EXAMPLES

He is a 56-year-old janitor in no acute distress.

We work a 35-hour week.

3

Four-vessel angiography showed a narrowing of the left carotid artery.

A 2-mm drill bit was selected for the craniotomy.

■ Rule 3.31 Hyphenate compound numbers 21 to 99 when they are written out.

EXAMPLES

Fifty-five medical transcriptionists attended the meeting last night.

Ninety-nine percent of the time I am confident of the diagnosis.

■ Rule 3.32 Use a hyphen when there is a prefix before a proper noun.

EXAMPLES

anti-American pseudo-Christian

The estimated date of confinement is mid-May.

■ Rule 3.33 Use a hyphen after the prefixes *ex, self,* and *vice* and after other prefixes to avoid an awkward combination of letters, such as two or three identical vowels in a sequence.

EXAMPLES

salpingo-oophorectomy
self-inflicted
ex-patient
anti-immune
vice-president
co-op

BUT:
coordinate
intraarterial
preeclampsia
preelection
preemergent
preempt
preenzyme
preepiglottic
preeruptive
reemploy
reenact
reenlist
reenter
reexamine

■ Rule 3.34 Use a hyphen after a prefix when the unhyphenated word would have a different meaning.

EXAMPLES

re-collect (collect again)
re-cover (cover again)
re-create (create again)
re-present (present again)
re-sign (sign again)
re-sort (sort again)
re-treat (treat again)

One should also hyphenate a word for ease of reading, comprehension, and pronunciation.

EXAMPLES

re-do
co-op
re-type

■ Rule 3.35 Do not use a hyphen with the prefixes *bi, tri, uni, co, extra, infra, inter, intra, mid, mini, multi, pseudo, sub, super, supra, ultra, out, over, ante, anti, semi, un, non, pre, post, pro, trans,* and *re* unless there are identical letters in a sequence.

EXAMPLES

preoperative
pre-evaluation
antenatal
semiprone
postoperative
post-traumatic
antidepressant
nondrinker

BUT: non-Hodgkin's (see Rule 3.32)
transsacral
preeclampsia
reexamine
reemploy

NOTE: Because hyphens are not generally used with prefixes, it is easiest to remember the few that **are** hyphenated: *ex, self,* and *vice,* along with the suffixes that take the hyphen: *odd, elect, type,* and *designate.*

EXAMPLES

ex-husband
twenty-odd
self-made
president-elect
vice-chair
papal-designate

■ Rule 3.36 Use a hyphen with the letters or words describing chemical elements except with subscripts or superscripts.

EXAMPLES

I-131 or 131-I
Uranium-235

BUT: ^{131}I
^{235}U

■ Rule 3.37 Use a hyphen to take the place of the words "to" and "through" to identify numeric and alphabetical ranges.

EXAMPLES

Rounds were made in Wards 1-4.

Check V2-V6 again.

Take 100 mg Tylenol, 1-2 h.s.

■ Rule 3.38 Use a hyphen following a single letter joined to a word forming a coined word.

EXAMPLES

x-ray Z-plasty S-shaped T-shirt
U-bag X-Acto K-wires

BUT: 3M T square

■ Rule 3.39 Place a hyphen between compound nouns and compound surnames.

EXAMPLES

Nonne-Milroy disease

Arnold-Chiari type II malformation

Legg-Calvé-Perthes disease

A Davis-Crowe mouth gag was used.

Mary Smyth-Reynolds was in today for her yearly Pap smear.

Antonia is the secretary-treasurer for our local chapter of the American Association for Medical Transcription.

Refer to Chapter 8, Rules 8–1 through 8–22, for further discussion on use of the hyphen.

The Dash

A dash is made on the keyboard with two hyphens. There is no space before, between, or after the two hyphens. The dash indicates a sudden shift in thought and should be used very sparingly.

■ Rule 3.40 Use a dash as a forceful break for emphasis or to call attention to explanations not closely connected with the remainder of the sentence.

EXAMPLES

I want you to--no, I insist that you--consult a surgeon about the lump in your breast.

We may be so busy analyzing physical signs that we miss--or dismiss--clues to frame of mind.

For this patient, a polyp meant a fatal malignancy--and all the awful experiences that attend it.

■ Rule 3.41 Use a dash for summary.

NOTE: A dash is sometimes used instead of a colon. It works well if the list is in the middle of a sentence because the second dash shows clearly where the list ends. Dashes are also helpful with appositives that are already punctuated with commas.

EXAMPLES

Red, white, and blue--these are my favorite colors.

She soon became bored with the nontranscription details of her job--editing, printing, collating--but finally realized it was part of the fabric of the position.

NOTE: Never begin a new line with a dash. You must carry the last word before the dash to the following line along with the dash.

The Apostrophe

■ Rule 3.42 Use an apostrophe to show singular or plural possession of nouns, relative pronouns, and abbreviations.

EXAMPLES (singular possessive)

the typist's responsibility (one typist)
Bob's doctor
Dr. Farnsworth's office

EXAMPLES (singular nouns that end in an *s* or in a strong *s* sound are made singular possessive by adding an apostrophe)

the waitress' table (multiple syllable noun)
for appearance's sake (multiple syllable noun)
Mr. Moses' surgery (multiple syllable noun)
James Rose's appointment (single syllable noun)
Mr. Jones's medical record (single syllable noun)

NOTE: Concerning Mr. Walters:
Mr. Walter's point of view (incorrect)
Mr. Walters' point of view (correct)

EXAMPLES (plural forms of nouns)

Singular	*Plural*
woman's watch	women's watches
child's toy	children's toys
man's shoe	men's shoes

EXAMPLES (plural nouns ending in *s* are formed by adding an apostrophe)

typists' responsibility (more than one typist)

the Joneses' medical records (more than one Jones)

the employees' records

EXAMPLES (hyphenated noun)

my brother-in-law's book
my brothers-in-law's book (one book, two owners)

EXAMPLES (pronouns)

nobody's fault
anyone's guess
somebody else's responsibility

EXAMPLES (understood noun)

The stethoscope is Dr. Green's. (stethoscope)

I consulted *Dorland's.* (dictionary)

EXAMPLES (possession involving two persons)

Dr. Pate and Dr. Frank's office (one office)
Dr. Pate's and Dr. Frank's offices (two offices)
Dr. Thomas's associate's diagnosis

EXAMPLE (abbreviation)

Proofreading is the CMT's responsibility.

Personal pronouns such as *its,** *hers, yours, his, theirs, ours, whose,*† or *yours* do not require an apostrophe.

EXAMPLES

The next appointment is hers.

The dog injured its foot.

You're coat is soiled. (incorrect)

Your coat is soiled. (correct)

NOTE: Probably one of the most common errors made concerns the misuse of the apostrophe with *it.* Because *its* and *it's* are both correct when used in the proper context, writers often make an improper choice. Remember that *it's* means *it is.*

There are many eponyms (adjective derived from a proper noun) used in medical typing. When they are used to describe parts of the anatomy, diseases, signs, or syndromes they may show possession. However, for names of places, patients, or surgical instruments, the possessive is not used, nor is it used in a compound eponym. Because this is often confusing—how does one recognize the name of a place or patient in contrast to that of a researcher or physician?—some authorities suggest its eventual elimination. In addition, if the eponym is preceded by the article *an, a,* or *the,* one can eliminate the possessive as well. In the meantime, follow the guidelines as best you can and consult your dictionary; if you hear the possessive dictated, use it. If not, you may feel free to eliminate it. Refer to Chapter 10 for further discussion on eponyms.

EXAMPLES (eponyms with possessive)

Signs and tests
Romberg's sign
Hoffmann's reflex
Babinski's sign
Ayer's test

Anatomy
Bartholin's glands
Beale's ganglion
Mauthner's membrane

Diseases and syndromes
Fallot's tetralogy
Tietze's syndrome
Hirschsprung's disease

EXAMPLES (where you can eliminate the possessive)

Use of the article
A Pfannenstiel incision . . .
The Babinski sign . . .

EXAMPLES (eponyms without the possessive)

Surgical instruments
Mayo scissors
Richard retractors
Foley catheter
Liston-Stille forceps

Names of places or patients
Christmas factor
Lyme disease
Chicago disease

Compounds
Stein-Leventhal syndrome
Adams-Stokes disease
Leser-Trélat sign
Bass-Watkins test
Gruber-Widal reaction

But this is not a compound
Blackberg and Wanger's test

NOTE: Be careful to check the correct spelling of the name. Is it Homan's sign or Homans' sign? Is it Water's view or Waters' view? (The second choice is correct in both cases.)

* Notice these contractions, however: It's time for your next appointment. (*It's* is a contraction for *it is.*)

† Notice these contractions, however: Who's going to clean the operatory? (*Who's* is a contraction for *who is.*)

■ Rule 3.43 Use an apostrophe in contractions of words or figures.

EXAMPLES

'84, won't, can't, she'll, o'clock, doesn't, couldn't

NOTE: *Avoid* the use of contractions of words or figures except for "o'clock" in all medical reports and formal business letters.

EXAMPLES

You hear	*You type*
'84	1984
won't	will not
she'll	she will
doesn't	does not
couldn't	could not
nine o'clock	nine o'clock

■ Rule 3.44 Use an apostrophe in possessive expressions of time, distance, and value.

EXAMPLES

He should be able to return to work in a month's time.

You should have full range of motion in your elbow in two months' time.

The bullet came within a hair's breadth of the thoracic aorta.

I want the patient to feel that she got her money's worth.

■ Rule 3.45 Use an apostrophe to form the plural of the capital letters *A, I, O, M,* and *U;* of all lower case letters; and after a lower case letter in an abbreviation.

NOTE: The reason for this rule is to avoid making what might appear to be a word with the combination of some letters and "s," such as *Is, Ms, Us, is,* and *as.* It is not necessary to use the apostrophe to form the plural of numbers or capital letter abbreviations.

EXAMPLES

When you make an entry in a chart, be careful that your 2s don't look like z's.

You used four I's in that first paragraph.

He has a note for three Rx's on his desk.

The TMs were intact.

Quotation Marks

■ Rule 3.46 Use quotation marks to enclose the exact words of a speaker.

EXAMPLE

The patient said, "There has been hurting in the pelvic bones."

BUT: The patient said there has been some pain in the pelvic bones.

■ Rule 3.47 The titles of minor literary works are placed within quotation marks.

EXAMPLE

His photographic entry "The Country Doctor" won first place in the contest.

NOTE: Underline the titles of published books, magazines, and articles. Place in quotation marks the titles of chapters, papers, sections, and subdivisions of published work.

EXAMPLE

Your homework assignment is to read "Causes of Disease" in <u>Diseases of the Human Body.</u>

■ Rule 3.48 Use quotation marks to single out words or phrases for special attention.

EXAMPLES

I can see no need for "temper tantrums" in the operating suite.

"Accommodate" is at the top of the list of "most frequently misspelled words."

The technical term for Lou Gehrig disease is "amyotrophic lateral sclerosis."

■ Rule 3.49 Use quotation marks to set off slang, coined, awkward, whimsical, or humorous words that might show ignorance on the part of the author if it is not known that the writer is aware of them.

EXAMPLE

See if you can schedule a few "well" patients for a change.

NOTE: Punctuation with quotation marks is as follows: periods and commas go *inside* the quotation mark; semicolons and colons go *outside* the quotation mark. Question marks and exclamation marks belong inside the quotation marks when they are part of the quoted material; they are placed outside the final quotation marks when they are part of the entire sentence.

EXAMPLES

The third chapter, "Punctuation," is the most difficult for me.

The patient related that she spoke with her hands "like an Italian."

The medical report answers my original question, "What is the secondary diagnosis?"

3

Parentheses

Introduction. Parentheses, commas, and dashes are used to set off incidental or nonessential elements in text. Which you choose will be determined either by the dictator/writer of the material or by the closeness of the relationship between the material enclosed and the remainder of the sentence. In general, commas are used to set slightly apart closely related material, and parentheses are used when commas have already been used within the nonessential element or the material itself is neither grammatically nor logically essential to the main thought. The dash is a more forceful and abrupt division and draws attention to a statement; parentheses de-emphasize. Material enclosed within parentheses can range from a single punctuation mark (!) to several sentences.

■ Rule 3.50 Use parentheses to set off words or phrases that are clearly nonessential to the sentence. These are often definitions, comments, or explanations.

EXAMPLES

She felt that she had inhaled some sort of ornamental dust (gold, silver, bronze, etc.) while working in her flower shop.

The administrative medical assistant (receptionist, secretary, bookkeeper, insurance clerk, transcriptionist, file clerk) requires the same length of training as the clinical medical assistant.

■ Rule 3.51 Use parentheses around figures or letters indicating divisions.

NOTE: You may elect to use a period after figures or letters indicating divisions as long as they do not occur within a sentence.

EXAMPLES

(1) Sterile field	*or*	1. Sterile field
(2) Suture materials		2. Suture materials
(3) 4 x 4 sponges		3. 4 x 4 sponges

However, only the parentheses are acceptable in the following illustration:

EXAMPLE

It is my impression that she has (1) progressive dysmenorrhea, (2) uterine leiomyoma, and (3) weakness of the right inguinal ring.

The Slash (also called the bar or diagonal)

■ Rule 3.52 Use the slash in writing certain technical terms. The slash sometimes substitutes for the words "per," "to," or "over."

EXAMPLES

She has 20/20 vision. *(indication of visual acuity)*

His blood pressure is 120/80. (120 *over* 80)

The dosage is 50 mg/day. (milligrams *per* day)

■ Rule 3.53 Use the slash to offer word choice.

EXAMPLES

and/or
Mr./Mrs./Miss/Ms.

■ Rule 3.54 Use the slash to write fractions or to create a symbol.

EXAMPLES

2/3 c/o 1 1/2

Spacing with Punctuation

■ Rule 3.55 NO SPACE

following a period within an abbreviation
following a period used as a decimal point
between quotation marks and the quoted material
before or after a hyphen
before or after a slash
before or after a dash (two hyphens)
between parentheses and the enclosed material
between any word and the punctuation following it
between the number and the colon in a dilute solution
before an apostrophe
before or after a comma used within numbers
before or after an ampersand in abbreviations, e.g., L&W
on either side of the colon when expressing ratios
on either side of the colon when expressing the time of day
after the closing parenthesis if another mark of punctuation follows

EXAMPLE

If Mrs. Ross is promoted (to lead transcriptionist), she will leave this department.

■ Rule 3.56 ONE SPACE

after a comma
after a semicolon
after a period following an initial

after the closing parenthesis
on each side of the "x" symbol in an expression of dimension

EXAMPLE

a 2 x 2 sponge

■ Rule 3.57 TWO SPACES

after a period, question mark, or exclamation point at the end of a sentence
after a quotation mark at the end of a sentence
after a colon (except when used with the time of day, ratio, or when expressing a dilute solution)

NOTE: When keyboarding, it is becoming common practice to leave only one space after the closing period at the end of a sentence.

Do not be intimidated by the large number of rules. You must already be comfortable with a great many of them, so some of this instruction is just a review for you. Take a little time to re-examine those rules that cause you problems.

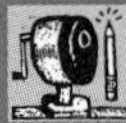 3–12: SELF-STUDY

Directions: Using Rules 3–27 through 3–54, add a hyphen, dash, apostrophe, quotes, parentheses, or slash where required.

1. Her favorite response is that weve always done it this way.
2. It was an ill defined tumor mass.
3. The diagnosis is grim I feel helpless.
4. Her temperature peaked at 106.5 degrees we were relieved when this occurred, and the seizures subsided.
5. There were no 4 x 4s left in the box.
6. Because of his condition emphysema and age 88, he is a poor risk for anesthesia at this time.
7. Eighty five of the patients were seen first in the outpatient department.
8. The patient with the self inflicted gun shot wound had a poorly applied bandage.
9. The blood pressure ranged from 120 to 140 over 80.
10. This is a very up to date drug reference.

Please turn to the end of the chapter, page 92, for the answers to these problems.

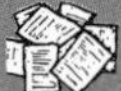 3–13: PRACTICE TEST

Directions: In the following exercises, fill in the missing punctuation and indicate which of the rules you used. (Refer to the brief rule review.) In the space following the sentence, write the letter of the rule or rules used. Each rule is used more than once.

RULE REVIEW

Use a hyphen:	a. when two or more words have the force of a single modifier.
	b. when figures or letters are mixed with a word.
	c. between compound names or words.
	d. between coordinate expressions.
Use an apostrophe:	e. to show possession.
	f. to show letters are missing.
	g. to form the plurals of lower case letters.
Use quotes:	h. to show slang or awkward wording.
Use parentheses:	i. to set off a strongly nonessential phrase.
Use a slash:	j. to divide certain technical terms.

3

EXAMPLE

"Accommodation" is spelled with two c's, two m's, and three o's.

Rule g

1. Mrs. Gail R. Smith Edwards was hospitalized this morning. She is the 47 year old woman Dr. Blank admitted with a self inflicted knife wound. Her blood pressure was 60 40. *(sixty over forty)*

   Rule ______________

2. Barbara Ness happy go lucky personality was missed when she was transferred from Medical Records.

   Rule ______________

3. Glen Mathews, the well known trial lawyer, and the hospitals Chief of Staff, Dr. Carlton Edwards, will appear together if you can believe that on TVs latest talk show tonight. Its the only subject on the hospitals gabfest.

   Rule ______________

4. I want a stamped, self addressed envelope enclosed with this letter and sent out with todays mail.

   Rule ______________

5. Dr. Davis said his promotion was a good example of being kicked upstairs. He obviously didnt want to leave his job in the X ray Department.

   Rule ______________

6. Havent you ever seen a Z fixation? Bobbi Jo will be happy to explain it to you.

   Rule ______________

7. Were all going to the CCU at 4 oclock for instructions on mouth to mouth resuscitation.

   Rule ______________

8. Right eye vision: 20 20
   Left eye vision: 10 400
   Right retinal examination: Normal
   Left retinal examination: Inferior retinal detachment

   Rule ______________

9. You were seen on September 24 at which time you were having some stiffness at the shoulders which I felt was due to a periarthritis a stiffness of the shoulder capsule; however, xray of the shoulder was negative.

   Rule ______________

10. After he completed the end to end anastomosis, he closed with #1 silk through and through, figure of eight sutures.

    Rule ______________

11. Dr. Chriswells diagnosis bears out the assumption that the red green blindness is the result of an X chromosome defect.

    Rule ______________

12. After his myocardial infarction MI, his blood test showed high level C reactive protein.

    Rule ______________

Refer to Appendix A at the back of the book for the answers to this exercise.

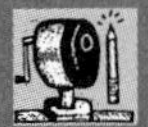 3–14: SELF-STUDY

3

Directions: In the following exercises, the marks of punctuation are missing, but the number of marks that are needed has been provided. This number includes any optional marks and the periods needed at the end of a sentence. Some periods are indicated for you with an asterisk (*). Parentheses and quotes will count as 2. You may use your text or reference materials as your instructor directs. The exercise is to be retyped and double spaced for proper placement.

1. Dr Younger couldnt find the curved on flat scissors therefore all heck broke loose* (Needs 9 marks)
2. The patients admission time is 330 *(three thirty)* pm* When he comes in please call me for a face to face confrontation with him about his visitors* (Needs 8 marks)
3. This 68 year old right handed Caucasian retired female telephone operator was well until mid February* While sitting in a chair after dinner she had the following symptoms paralysis of her left arm and left leg paresthesia in the same distribution bilateral visual blurring and some facial numbness* (Needs 14 marks)
4. The patient was admitted to the Ward at one oclock in the morning screaming Alls fair in love and lust the attending physician sedated him with Thorazine 600 mg day* *(600 mg per day)* (Needs 7 marks)
5. The following describes a well prepared business letter neat accurate well placed correctly punctuated and mechanically perfect* The dictator expects to see an attractive letter with no obvious corrections smudges or unevenly inked letters* It is an insult in my opinion to place a letter that appears other than described on your employers desk for signature* (Needs 15 marks)

See page 93 for the answers to this Self-Study.

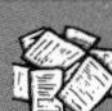 3–15: PRACTICE TEST

Directions: Follow the directions given in Self-Study 3–14 and type the following exercises.

1. She inadvertently sterilized the Smith Petersen nail instead of the V medullary* (Needs 3 marks)
2. She has had no further spells but she did have two episodes prior to this one several years ago* (Needs 4 marks)
3. The patient presents as a well developed asthenic elderly extremely bright and oriented Caucasian female* She is fully alert and able to give an entirely reliable history however she is somewhat anxious and concerned over her present condition* (Needs 9 marks)
4. The patient has just moved to this community from Anchorage Alaska where he was engaged in the lumber industry* He had an emergency appendectomy performed at some remote outpost in January 1986* According to the patient he has always felt like somethings hung up in there* Roentgenograms taken July 17 199X failed to reveal anything unusual* (Needs 12 marks)
5. He is a 35 year old well developed well nourished black truck driver oriented to time place and person* (Needs 10 marks)
6. The X chromosome defect resulted in her ovarian aplasia undeveloped mandible webbed neck and small stature Morgagni Turner syndrome* (Needs 7 marks)
7. Vital signs Blood pressure 194 97 pulse 127 respirations 32 regular and gasping* General Healthy appearing male looking his stated age in moderately severe respiratory distress with slightly dusky colored lips* (Needs 17 marks)

Turn to Appendix A at the end of the book for the answers to this Practice Test.

3–16: REVIEW TEST

3

Directions: Follow the directions given in Self-Study 3–14 and complete the following exercises.

1. His heart is in regular sinus rhythm without murmurs or thrills the distal pulses are all palpable and Phalens maneuver is negative* (Needs 5 marks)
2. I want to raise the charge for office calls to $15 this is long overdue and hospital calls to $25* Please explain this to all the patients including the new ones when they call for an appointment* (Needs 6 marks)
3. I took the samples of the powder to Dr Peterson White pathologist and he has not as yet made any report* As you can see from the initial report there is no evidence of powder in the biopsy specimen* (Needs 9 marks)
4. Really the prognosis is not too good but well hope that maybe shell defy the usual course of events* (Needs 5 marks)
5. I will restate the situation Mr Goodman has a right superior mediastinal widening which has proven to be secondary to some dilatation and lateral displacement of the superior vena cava* (Needs 3 marks)
6. It is anticipated that following completion of this radiation therapy and your recovery from it in a period of 4 to 6 weeks you should be able to return to your former employment without difficulty* (Needs 3 marks)
7. Dr Lopez advice was to transfer the patient* Please see that his x rays are sent with him to the Veterans Administration Hospital* (Needs 5 marks)
8. She is a spastic retarded child with bilateral hip bowing greater on the right than on the left whose mother is very very anxious for noninvasive correction* (5 marks)
9. Notice please There will be no further parking allowed in the staff lot without an up to date sticker violators will be towed away at the owners expense* (6 marks)
10. According to the pathology report see enclosed there is no evidence of Mr Neibauer my patient having active pulmonary tuberculosis at this time* The debate concerning the approval of his attending the Contagious Disease Conference became heated we had to recess several times once for 40 minutes and we finally adjourned with no definite policy established* Ann Reynolds my administrative assistant will get in touch with Mr Neibauer to let him know* (16 marks)

Let's Have a Bit of Fun

1. In which sentence is Miss Hamlyn in trouble?
   a. Miss Hamlyn, the medical assistant failed to report for work.
   b. Miss Hamlyn, the medical assistant, failed to report for work.
2. Which shows a breach of ethics?
   a. Five nurses knew the diagnosis, all told.
   b. Five nurses knew the diagnosis; all told.
3. Which shows compassion?
   a. I left him, feeling he'd rather be alone.
   b. I left him feeling he'd rather be alone.
4. Which is harder for the interns?
   a. Down the hall came four interns carrying equipment and several doctors with their patients.
   b. Down the hall came four interns, carrying equipment, and several doctors with their patients.
5. Which is unflattering to the hostess?
   a. The party ended, happily.
   b. The party ended happily.
6. In which does the writer know about the private lives of her fellow workers?
   a. Every secretary, I know, has a secret ambition.
   b. Every secretary I know has a secret ambition.
7. Where would you prefer to work?
   a. The hospital employs a hundred odd men and women.
   b. The hospital employs a hundred-odd men and women.

8. Who's late?
   a. The receptionist said the nurse is late.
   b. The receptionist, said the nurse, is late.

9. Which is the worse problem?
   a. All my money, which was in my billfold, was stolen.
   b. All my money which was in my billfold was stolen.

10. Who filled up the emergency ward?
   a. All of the students who ate in the snack bar got food poisoning.
   b. All of the students, who ate in the snack bar, got food poisoning.

11. Who is the best leader?
   a. I intend to serve you fairly energetically and enthusiastically.
   b. I intend to serve you fairly, energetically, and enthusiastically.

The answers are given in Appendix A.

3

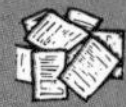 3–17: PRACTICE TEST

Directions: Using your text and reference materials, punctuate the letter on page 88. Use mixed punctuation for the salutation and complimentary close. The letter is to be retyped, but you may proofread it by marking your text before you copy the letter.

Turn to Appendix A at the end of the text to see this letter punctuated correctly. Optional commas have been circled.

PUNCTUATION RULE SYNOPSIS

Use a Comma or Pair of Commas	*Rule*	*Page*
To set off a nonessential word or words from the rest of the sentence	3.1	60
To set off nonessential appositives	3.1a	61
To set off a parenthetical expression	3.1b	61
To set off an introductory phrase or clause	3.2a (See also Rule 3.2b)	64
To set off the year in a complete date	3.3	65
To set off the name of the state when the city precedes it	3.4	66
To set off "Inc." or "Ltd." in a company name	3.5	66
To set off titles and degrees following a person's name	3.6	66
To separate words in a series	3.7	66
To separate two independent clauses	3.8	67
To set off the name of a person in a direct address	3.9	69
To separate certain modifiers	3.10	69
To avoid confusion	3.11	70
After the complimentary close	3.12	70
In certain long numbers	3.13	70
To separate the parts of a date in the date line of a letter	3.14	70

Use a Period	*Rule*	*Page*
At the end of a sentence	3.15	73
With single capitalized word abbreviations	3.16	73
When the genus is abbreviated	3.16	73
In certain lower case abbreviations	3.16	73
To separate a decimal fraction from whole numbers	3.17	73

Use a Semicolon		
Between two independent clauses when there is no conjunction	3.18	73
Between independent clauses if either or both are already punctuated	3.19	73
Before a parenthetical expression when it is used as a conjunction	3.20	74
Between a series of phrases or clauses when any item in the series has internal commas	3.21	74

Use a Colon		
To introduce a list or series of items	3.22	74
After the salutation in a business letter when using "mixed" punctuation	3.23	74
Between the hours and minutes indicating the time in figures	3.24	74

3

William A. Berry, MD
3933 Navajo Road
San Diego California 92119
463-0000

August 13 199X

John D. Mench MD
455 Main Street
Bethesda MD 20034

Dear Dr Mench

Re Debra Walters

This letter is to bring you up to date on Mrs Walters who was first seen in my office on March 2 199X at which time she stated that her last menstrual period had started August 29 199X. Examination revealed the uterus to be enlarged to a size consistent with an estimated date of confinement of June 5 199X.

The pregnancy continued uneventfully until May 19 at which time the patient's blood pressure was 130 90. Hygroton was prescribed and the patient was seen in one week. Her blood pressure at the next visit was 150 100 and additional therapy in the form of Ser-Ap-Es was prescribed in addition to other antitoxemic routines. Her blood pressure stabilized between 130 and 140 90.

The patient was admitted to the hospital on June 11 199X with ruptured membranes mild preeclampsia and a few contractions of poor quality. Intravenous oxytocics were started and after two hours of stimulation there was no change in the cervix with that structure continuing to be long closed and posterior. The presenting part was at a -2 to a -3 station and the amniotic fluid had become brownish-green in color suggesting some degree of fetal distress.

Consultation was obtained and it was recommended that a low cervical cesarean section be performed. A female infant was delivered by cesarean section. It was noted at the time of delivery that the cord was snugly wrapped around the neck of the baby three times and this might have contributed to the evidence of fetal distress as evidenced by the color of the amniotic fluid.

The patients postoperative course was uneventful and she and the baby were discharged home on the fifth postpartum day.

Sincerely yours

William A Berry MD

mlo

Use a Colon (Continued)	Rule	Page
In ratios and dilutions	3.24	74
After the introductory word or words in a history and physical report	3.25	74
With the introductory words in an outline	3.25	74
To introduce an example or clarify an idea	3.26	75

Use a Hyphen	Rule	Page
When two or more words have the force of a single modifier	3.27	77
Between coordinate expressions	3.28	77
In a series of modifiers	3.29	77
When numbers are compounded with words	3.30	77
In certain chemical expressions	3.36	78
Within compound numbers 21 to 99 when they are written out	3.31	78
Between a prefix and a proper noun	3.32	78
After prefixes *ex, self,* and *vice;* to avoid awkward combinations of letters	3.33	78
After a prefix when the unhyphenated word would have a different meaning (Exceptions, see Rule 3.35)	3.34	78
To take the place of the words "to" and "through"	3.37	78
Following a single letter joined to a word, forming a coined word	3.38	79
Between compound nouns and compound surnames	3.39	79

Use a Dash	Rule	Page
For a forceful break	3.40	79
For summary	3.41	79

Use an Apostrophe	Rule	Page
To show singular or plural possession	3.42	79
In contractions	3.43	81
In possessive expressions of time, distance, and value	3.44	81
To form the plural of some letters	3.45	81

Use Quotation Marks to	Rule	Page
Enclose the exact words of a speaker	3.46	81
Enclose the titles of minor literary works	3.47	81
Single out words or phrases	3.48	81
Set off slang, coined, awkward, whimsical words	3.49	81

Use Parentheses	Rule	Page
To set off clearly nonessential words or phrases	3.50	82
Around figures or letters indicating divisions	3.51	82

Use a Slash	Rule	Page
In certain technical terms	3.52	82
To offer a word choice	3.53	82
To write fractions	3.54	82

Spacing with Punctuation Marks	Rule	Page
No space	3.55	82
One space	3.56	82
Two spaces	3.57	83

3-4: COMPUTER EXERCISES

Before proceeding, you may want to do more exercises based on the concepts you have learned. Additional practice material is on your computer diskette.

Directions: Insert the diskette into the computer and follow the instructions on the screen for Computer Exercise 3–4.

A *Answers to* 3-1: SELF-STUDY

Note: Material in parentheses may be included in your answers.

2. ***Subject*** I

Independent clause I appreciate my understanding of medical terminology

3

3. ***Subject*** You (this is "understood")

Independent clause Please return this to Medical Records (as soon as possible)

4. ***Introductory phrase*** After spending five hours in the operating room

Subject (the) patient

Independent clause the patient was sent to the recovery room

5. ***Subject*** (the) patient

Independent clause The patient is a well-developed, well-nourished black female

Second verb clause reported that she has been well until this time

Appositive (none)

Conjunction and

6. ***Subject*** Joan (and) Beth

Independent clause Joan and Beth are taking an evening college course in medical ethics

Appositive 1 the medical secretary

Appositive 2 the file clerk

Parenthetical expression (none)

7. ***First subject*** (the) reception room

Independent clause the reception room is well lighted and stocked with current literature

Second subject (the) patients

Independent clause the patients do not mind their wait to see Dr. Jordan

Conjunction joining independent clauses so

Appositive (none)

Nonessential clause who never seems to arrive on time

8. ***Independent clause*** There is overwhelming evidence to prove that the ability to spell is vital to success in this field

Parenthetical expression however

Appositive (none)

9. ***Subject*** (the) American Association for Medical Transcription

Independent clause The American Association for Medical Transcription has a business and educational meeting every month.

Appositive the national organization for medical transcriptionists

Parenthetical expression (none)

Conjunction joining two independent clauses (none)

10. ***Subject*** Perfection

Verb is

Independent clause Perfection is the key word in medical transcription skills

Appositive (none)

Parenthetical expression (none)

Nonessential phrase not speed

11. *Subject* (hospital) transcriptionists

    Independent clause (none) This is not a complete sentence

12. *Subject* the second "you," which is understood as occurring just before "please"

    Verb have

    Independent clause please have the patient's complete name, address, and telephone number and the admitting diagnosis

    Nonessential phrase (none)

    Introductory clause When you telephone the hospital

    Conjunction joining words in a series and

13. *Independent clause* Appointment scheduling requires skill/it should be a real art

    Nonessential clause or phrase and can be/contrary to what you might think

    Parenthetical expression contrary to what you might think

14. *Independent clause* A perfectly typed resume should accompany your letter of application

    Introductory phrase (none)

    Nonessential phrase well-planned and prepared

15. *Independent clause* he walks with his heel down (with a varus tendency in the ankle)

    Dependent phrase with no severe problem *also* with a varus tendency in the ankle

    Conjunction joining two independent clauses (none)

16. *Subject* a CBC and sed rate

    Independent clause a CBC and sed rate were carried out today

    Introductory phrase To minimize the chance of overlooking a recurrence of infection

    Nonessential phrase (none)

A *Answers to* **3–2: SELF-STUDY**

1. Commas around *your patient.* It is a nonessential appositive.
2. Comma after surgeon and after opinion. *Whether or not you care for my opinion* is a parenthetical expression.
3. Comma after *trifocal* and after *bifocal* to enclose a nonessential expression.
4. Comma after *Mitchell* and *morning* to enclose a nonessential expression.
5. No commas in this sentence.

A *Answers to* **3–4: SELF-STUDY**

1. No comma. Be careful not to separate the subject from the verb by placing a comma after *position.* Be alert when you consider placing a comma in front of a verb.
2. Place a comma after *time.* This is an introductory phrase.

3. Place a comma after *tomorrow.* This is an introductory phrase. (The subject, "you," is understood.)
4. Place a comma after *seen.* This is an introductory phrase.
5. No comma. Be careful not to separate the subject from the verb by placing a comma after *billing.*
6. Enclose *whom I hired yesterday* in commas. This is nonessential.

A Answers to 3–6: SELF-STUDY

1. The patient was first seen in my office on Wednesday, July 14, 199X. *Separate all parts of a complete date.*
2. Please send this to Natalie Jayne, RN, Chief of Nurses, Glorietta Bay Hospital. *Separate degrees and titles following a person's name.*
3. Carl A. Nichols Jr. was admitted to Ward B. *No comma is used before Jr. or Sr. unless the user prefers it.*
4. The blood test included a white blood count, red blood count, hematocrit, and differential. *Separate words in a series. The comma after "hematocrit" is optional.*
5. There is a story of a mild head injury at age ten, and she was in a moderately severe motorcycle accident about fifteen years ago. *Separate two independent clauses with a comma before the conjunction.*
6. The condition is now stationary and permanent, and he should be able to resume his normal work load. *Separate two independent clauses with a comma before the conjunction.*
7. She was fully dilated at 2:30 a.m. but did not deliver the second twin until 2:55 a.m. *No comma because the second clause is dependent.*

A Answers to 3–10: SELF-STUDY

1. Insert period after *Mr.*, the *E.*, the *p.*, and the *m.* at the end of the sentence. Place a colon between the 4 and the 30.
2. Insert an optional period after the *M* and *D* and insert a period after *Dr.*, and a semicolon after *Board.* (Periods are not required with MD.) Do not place a period after *Board* making two sentences.
3. A period serves both to close the sentence and to punctuate the abbreviation. This is a polite question so no question mark is required.
4. A colon is placed after 16 and after *caution.*
5. A period closes the sentence. No punctuation mark used with military time of day.
6. A colon is placed after *problems.*
7. A period closes the sentence. No decimal point needed with the $85.

A Answers to 3–12: SELF-STUDY

1. Insert an apostrophe in the contraction "we've." Enclose *we've always done it this way* in quotes.
2. Place a hyphen between *ill* and *defined.*
3. Insert a dash between *grim* and *I.*
4. Place parentheses around *we were relieved when this occurred.*
5. No marks placed in this one.
6. Place parentheses around *emphysema* and *88.*
7. Place a hyphen after *eighty.*
8. Place a hyphen after *self.* There is no hyphen after poorly.

9. Place a slash between 140 and 80, e.g., 140/80. (It is also correct to write 120-140/80.)
10. Place a hyphen after *up* and after *to.*

A *Answers to* **3–14: SELF-STUDY**

1. Dr. Younger couldn't find the curved-on-flat scissors; therefore, "all heck broke loose." *(It would also be correct to just place "heck" in quotes.)*
2. The patient's admission time is 3:30 p.m. When he comes in, please call me for a face-to-face confrontation with him about his visitors.
3. This 68-year-old, right-handed, Caucasian, retired female telephone operator was well until mid-February. While sitting in a chair after dinner, she had the following symptoms: paralysis of her left arm and left leg, paresthesia in the same distribution, bilateral visual blurring, and some facial numbness.
4. The patient was admitted to the Ward at one o'clock in the morning screaming "All's fair in love and lust"; the attending physician sedated him with Thorazine 600 mg/day.
5. The following describes a well-prepared business letter: neat, accurate, well-placed, correctly punctuated, and mechanically perfect. The dictator expects to see an attractive letter with no obvious corrections, smudges, or unevenly inked letters. It is an insult, in my opinion, to place a letter that appears other than described on your employer's desk for signature.

4

CHAPTER

4

Capitalization

OBJECTIVES

After reading this chapter and working the exercises, you should be able to

1. Demonstrate the ability to capitalize words accurately from copy prepared in lower case letters.
2. Explain the special uses of capital letters in the preparation of medical reports and correspondence.
3. Use the reference materials to check unfamiliar medical and business terms.

INTRODUCTION

This review of capitalization rules should be a pleasant interlude after your study of punctuation. Only a few capitalization rules cause problems for transcriptionists, so we will review those and emphasize where they most commonly occur in medical and business transcription.

The purpose of capitalizing a word is to give it emphasis, distinction, authority, or importance. Avoid unnecessary capitalization, and do not use capital letters to highlight something unnecessarily, e.g., a person's name on a document. Words completely composed of capital letters often are more difficult to read because there is not as much "white space" around them.

EXAMPLES

Hazel Tank, CMT (correct)
HAZEL TANK, CMT (incorrect)

Like rules regarding punctuation, rules regarding capitalization can differ. The current trend is toward less, rather than more, capitalization. Consequently, as with a punctuation mark, be sure you have a reason for using a capital letter, and when in doubt, check your references.

VOCABULARY

4

Capital Letter: Upper case letter, also called "Caps."

Small Letter: Lower case letter, noncapital letter.

Eponym: An adjective derived from a proper noun.

EXAMPLES

Bright's disease
Skene's glands

Acronym: A word formed from the initial letters of other words.

EXAMPLES

NOW (National Organization for Women)
HOPE (Health Opportunities for People Everywhere)
WHO (World Health Organization)
CARE (Cooperative for American Remittances to Everywhere)

Lower case letters are used when the acronym is commonly used in the language.

EXAMPLES

laser, radar, scuba

Proper Noun: The name of a specific person, place, or thing.

Some *common nouns* may be used to name a specific person, place, or thing but are often modified by *my, your, his, our, their, these, the, this, that,* or *those.*

EXAMPLES OF COMMON NOUNS:

my mother, the doctor, your patient, our president.

NOTE: They refer to specific persons, yet they are not proper nouns.

EXAMPLES OF PROPER NOUNS:

Secretary Lewis, Dr. Smith, Mary Tunnell, President Lincoln, the Brooklyn Bridge.

RULES

The following five rules pertain to typing business letters:

■ Rule 4.1 Capitalize the first word of the salutation and the complimentary close.

EXAMPLES

Dear Dr. Reynolds:
Sincerely yours,
Yours very truly,

■ Rule 4.2 Capitalize boulevard, street, avenue, drive, way, and so on, when used with a proper noun.

EXAMPLES

321 Westvillage *Drive*

One of the most attractive *streets* in La Mesa is Palm *Avenue.*

■ Rule 4.3 Capitalize a person's title in business correspondence when it appears in the inside address, typed signature line, or envelope address.

EXAMPLES

Sincerely yours,
Ms. Marilyn Alan, *President*

W. Peter Deal, MD, *Director*
ATTENTION Ralph Cavanaugh, *Buyer*
Gene Ham, *Instructor*

■ Rule 4.4 Capitalize the first letter or all of the letters in the word *Attention* when it is part of an address; capitalize the first letter of each word or all the letters in the title *To Whom It May Concern.*

EXAMPLES

ATTENTION Reservation Clerk
(or)
Attention Paul Glenn, MD, Dean

TO WHOM IT MAY CONCERN:
(or)
To Whom It May Concern:

■ Rule 4.5 Capitalize both letters of the state abbreviation in the inside address and the envelope address.

EXAMPLES

District Heights, *MD* 20028
San Diego, *CA* 92119

Appendix B contains a complete list of U.S. Postal Service abbreviations for state names. You should remove this from your book and place it in your reference notebook or photocopy it for your reference book.

The next eight rules are often used in transcribing medical letters and reports.

■ Rule 4.6 Capitalize professional titles, political titles, family titles, and military ranks when they immediately *precede* the name.

EXAMPLES

Military and professional titles
Capt. Max Draper, USN Medical Corps, will be the guest speaker at the annual meeting of the AMA. *Dr.* Smith, the *president,* plans to meet his plane. The *doctor* will leave for the airport at four o'clock. We will meet with *President* Austin at the university this evening. *Dean* Caldwell may not be able to join us, however.

EXAMPLES

Professional and political titles
Dr. Randolph, the *president* of the medical society, was invited to speak at the joint meeting with the local bar association. *Rev.* John Hughes will give the invocation.

The *attorney* will be here at 9:30 a.m. to meet with the *doctor* about his testimony.

DO NOT capitalize the names of medical or surgical specialties or the type of specialist.

NOTE: Only titles of high distinction are capitalized *following* a person's name except in the address and typed signature line. "High distinction" can be very subjective, depending on who is doing the writing. "High distinction" often refers to the persons of rank in one's own firm and to high government officials.

EXAMPLES

The internist referred him to a thoracic surgeon.

He is studying to be an emergency room specialist.

We asked for a second opinion from the cardiologist.

EXAMPLE

Parkland Community College
3261 Parkview Drive
Boise, ID 83702

ATTENTION Ms. P. Lombardo, *Administrator*

EXAMPLES

Family titles
My *father* is bringing *Aunt* Mary here this afternoon for her flu shot.

The patient's *mother* died of carcinoma of the breast at age 56, and his *father* is living and well.

EXCEPTION: A title is not capitalized when followed by an appositive.

EXAMPLE

My *uncle,* William Peters, moved here recently from Cleveland.

■ Rule 4.7 Capitalize proper nouns, well-known nicknames for proper nouns, and eponyms.

4

EXAMPLES

Proper nouns
Dr. Watson was a fictional hero in *Sherlock Holmes's* classics.

I couldn't remember if he joined the *Air Force* or the *Navy.*

Do you realize that *Mother* will have to be placed in a nursing facility if she is unable to care for herself?

COMPARE WITH: Our *mother* will have to be placed in a nursing home.

Proper nouns and well-known nicknames for proper nouns
Josephine Holman just moved here from the *Rockies* and is looking for a job as a medical assistant.

We learned that valley fever is endemic to *Imperial Valley, San Joaquin Valley,* and the *Sonoran* deserts.

She moved to the *Bay Area* after winning the *Nobel Prize.*

Ellen wanted to return to the *Deep South* after working in *California* for just a few years.

Eponyms
We need a #15 *Foley* catheter.

The diagnosis proved to be *Hodgkin's* disease.

It is interesting that *Christmas* disease was named for a family with a particular type of hereditary condition.

The procedure was performed through a *McBurney* incision.

Some interesting names from mythology are used to describe parts of the anatomy, such as "*Achilles* tendon," or conditions, such as "*Oedipus* complex."

Newcomers to medicine often misspell *Burow's* solution and think that the *Sippy* diet is one you sip!

NOTE: Words *derived* from eponyms are not capitalized, nor are those that have acquired independent common meaning. (When in doubt, check the dictionary.)

4

EXAMPLES (nouns derived from eponyms)

Parkinson's disease but *parkinsonism*
Cushing's syndrome but *cushingoid* facies
Gram stain but *gram-positive* results
Addison's disease but *addisonian* crisis

EXAMPLES (common nouns and adjectives formed from proper nouns)

arabic number
atlas
braille symbol
brussels sprouts
cesarean section
chinese blue
curie unit
epsom salt
eustachian tube
french fries
freudian slip
graafian follicle
haversian system
hippocratic clubbing
india ink
joule
klieg light
kocherize
koebnerization
manila folder
mendelian genetics
mullerian duct
paris green
pasteurized milk
petri dish
plaster of paris
politzerize
portland cement
roentgen unit
roman numeral
siamese twins
watt

EXCEPTION: Americanization

■ Rule 4.8 Capitalize the names of races, people, religions, and languages.

EXAMPLE

He is a well-developed, well-nourished *Asian* businessman in no acute distress.

EXAMPLE

She is a *Catholic,* but they decided to be married in the *Jewish* temple.

EXAMPLE

We are taking an evening course in medical *Spanish* because we have many *Hispanic* patients who do not speak *English.*

NOTE: Designations based on skin color are not capitalized.

EXAMPLES

She is a well-developed, well-nourished *black* female student.

This 43-year-old *white* farm worker fell from the back of a truck at 3:55 a.m.

■ Rule 4.9 Capitalize the name of the genus when used in the singular form (with or without the species name) but do not capitalize the name of the species that follows it.

EXAMPLE

The patient was admitted by the ophthalmologist with *Onchocerca* volvulus.

EXAMPLE

Ralph saw the doctor because he had a bad reaction to *Cannabis* sativa.

NOTE: The genus may be referred to by its first initial only; this is capitalized with a period and followed by the species name.

EXAMPLES

E. coli (Escherichia coli)
M. tuberculosis (Mycobacterium tuberculosis)
H. influenzae (Hemophilus influenzae)

Remember not to capitalize the plural or adjectival form of a genus name.

EXAMPLES

Giardia lamblia but *giardiasis*
Diplococcus but *diplococci* and *diplococcal*
Streptococcus but *streptococci* and *streptococcal*

Refer to Appendix B for a list of the most frequently used genus and species names.

■ Rule 4.10 Capitalize trade names and brand names of drugs and other trademarked materials.

NOTE: It is often difficult for the beginning medical transcriptionist to recognize a brand name (capitalized) in contrast to a generic name (lower case). Until you become familiar with these and various suture materials and instruments, it will be necessary to use reference books.

After completing Chapter 8, you will have more competence in determining which terms for drugs are capitalized.

EXAMPLES

Generic names of drugs and suture materials
nitroglycerin, analgesic, hydrocortisone, potassium iodide, alcohol, ether, silk, catgut, cotton

EXAMPLES

Trade names of drugs and suture materials
Nitora, Darvon, Cortisporin, Theokin, pHisoHex, Gelfoam, Surgicel, Dermalon, Ser-Ap-Es, HydroDiuril

NOTE: See Rule 4.22.

■ Rule 4.11 Capitalize the names of *specific* departments or sections in the hospital.

EXAMPLES

Please see that the records are sent to St. Joseph's Hospital *Admitting Department.*

The *admitting department* was overwhelmed with 45 new admissions yesterday.

Albertson City Hospital *Pathology Department* received an award from the Greater Albertson County Industrial Council.

The specimen was sent to *pathology.*

All *pathology departments* should have this notice posted.

The *Emergency Department* at Westside General Hospital has just received a new hyperbaric unit.

Some *emergency departments* are sending patients to *acute care centers* after triage.

The baby was born in the hallway somewhere between the pharmacy and *The Women's Center.*

■ Rule 4.12 Capitalize specific designations used with numbers.

EXAMPLES

You have a reservation on *Flight* 707.

Please examine *Figure 3* on page 14.

We ordered a *Model* 14 Medtronic pacemaker.

NOTE: Some of the following common nouns are not capitalized when used with numbers. Those with an asterisk *may be* capitalized when used with a roman number because the roman numeral is a capital letter.

case, chapter, chromosome, column, experiment, factor,* fraction, grade,* gravida,* grant, group, lead, line, method, note, page, para,* paragraph, part, patient, phase, section, sentence, series, size, stage,* type, volume, wave

There is an error in your copy on *page* 27, *paragraph* 2, *line* 3.

Sometimes we let appearance make the choice when we have one.

EXAMPLES

Kennedy *Class II.*

The patient was a *Gravida II Para I* white female.

The patient was a *gravida 2 para 1* white female.

The patient had a *Stage III* burn with full-thickness loss of skin.

The *stage III* tumor had invaded the chest wall and the nodes in the supraclavicular area.

We found a deficiency in *Complex I.*

4

■ Rule 4.13 Capitalize the first word of each line in an outline or subheading of a report and the entire main heading of a formal report.

NOTE: Often the fully capitalized *main heading* is also underlined; the *topic* is fully capitalized and not underlined; and the *subtopic* begins with a single capital letter.

EXAMPLE

Diagnoses:
(1) *Stress* incontinence of urine.
(2) *Monilial* vaginitis.

EXAMPLE

HEENT:

HEAD: Normal.
EYES: Pupils round and equal, react to L&A.
EARS: Hearing normal, TMs intact, canals patent.

EXAMPLE

PHYSICAL EXAMINIATION:

HEENT:

Head: Normal.
Eyes: Pupils round and equal, react to L&A.
Ears: Hearing normal, TMs intact, canals patent.
Nose: Canals patent.
Throat: Trachea in the midline.

EXAMPLE

OPERATIVE REPORT

PREOPERATIVE DIAGNOSIS: Glaucoma, chronic, simple, bilateral.

POSTOPERATIVE DIAGNOSIS: Glaucoma, chronic, simple, bilateral.

OPERATION PERFORMED: Iridencleisis, right eye.

The next eight rules are used in all kinds of writing.

■ Rule 4.14 Capitalize the first word of the sentence, the first word of a complete direct quotation, and the first word after a colon if that word begins a complete thought.

EXAMPLES

The instructor said, "*Strive* for mailable copy even when you are practice-typing."

These are your directions: *Begin* typing as soon as you hear the signal and stop when the timer rings.

4

■ Rule 4.15 Capitalize the first and last words and all other words in the titles of articles, books, and periodicals with the exception of conjunctions, prepositions, or articles.

NOTE: Remember, book titles are also underlined.

EXAMPLE

Do you use the reference The Medical Word Book by Sheila Sloane?

■ Rule 4.16 Capitalize the names of the days of the week, months of the year, holidays, historic events, and religious festivals.

EXAMPLE

There will be no class on *Friday, November* 11, because it is *Veterans'* Day.

EXAMPLE

Do we get an *Easter* holiday or *Passover* vacation? Neither. It's called *"Spring Vacation."*

BUT: I am taking an advanced transcription class in the *spring* semester; I wish I had taken it this *fall.*

■ Rule 4.17 Capitalize both the noun and the adjective when they make reference to a specific geographic location.

EXAMPLE

The patient was born and raised in the *Southwest;* he has lived in the *Deep South* only a short while.

EXAMPLE

We plan to stay at a resort by the *Atlantic Ocean* when we go *east* for the medical meeting this fall.

EXAMPLES

the Great Lakes
Cape of Good Hope
Apache Reservation
Statue of Liberty

EXCEPTION: The names of places are not capitalized when they appear before the names of a specific place or are general directions.

EXAMPLE

New York State
(but)
the state of New York

■ Rule 4.18 Capitalize abbreviations when the words they represent are capitalized. Capitalize most abbreviations of English words; capitalize each letter in an acronym.

EXAMPLES

ECG is the preferred abbreviation for "electrocardiogram."

Ronda A. Drake, MD, graduated from UCSD.

Dr. Bowman is working with Project HOPE and UNICEF.

Our patient JB has converted from being HIV positive and now has AIDS.

Dr. Ashamed is scheduled to assist with the T&A.

The DTRs are intact.

NOTE: Metric and English forms of measurement or Latin abbreviations are not capitalized.

EXAMPLES

e.g. t.i.d. ft cm oz mph mg
p.o. q.4h.

■ Rule 4.19 Capitalize the abbreviation of academic degrees and religious orders.

EXAMPLES

MD PhD DDS MS SJ BVE
DPM LLB AS

Please refer to Chapter 5 for a complete review of the use of abbreviations and Chapter 3 for the use of punctuation with abbreviations.

■ Rule 4.20 Capitalize the names of all organizations, institutions, business firms, government agencies, and conferences as well as the names of their departments and divisions and the title of officers in the organizations' minutes, bylaws, and rules.

NOTE: The word "the" is not capitalized when it immediately precedes the name of the organization unless it is an official part of the name.

EXAMPLES

The *Secretary* read the minutes, and they were approved as read.
Dr. Sanderson has recently retired from *the Navy.*

International Clinical Congress
American College of Internal Medicine
American Cancer Society
Knights of Columbus
Toastmasters, Inc.
Eastridge *Clinic*

BUT: She went to the *clinic* for her annual physical.

■ Rule 4.21 Capitalize the names of specific academic courses.

BUT: Academic subject areas are not capitalized unless they contain a proper noun.

EXAMPLE

I am enrolled in *Medical Assisting* 103; I am also taking *typing* and *business English.*

These last three rules are frequently used in medical writing.

■ Rule 4.22 Capitalize each letter in the name of a drug, use bold print, or both when reporting drug allergies in a *chart note* or in a patient's *history.*

EXAMPLES

Allergies: Patient is allergic to PHENOBARBITAL and CODEINE.

Allergies: The patient reports a sensitivity to **SULFA.**

■ Rule 4.23 Capitalize the names of diseases that contain proper nouns, eponyms, or genus names. The common names of diseases and viruses are not capitalized.

EXAMPLES

The patient tested positive for *Rocky Mountain* spotted fever. (proper noun)

She was given the final series of *diphtheria, pertussis,* and *tetanus.* (common diseases)

She is now suffering from *postpoliomyelitis syndrome* and is unable to breathe without the use of her respirator. (virus name)

There has been an increase in *Chlamydia* infections in this age group. (genus)

We have had the usual problems with *rubella, rubeola,* and *chickenpox* in the kindergarten population. (common diseases)

We do not know if he should be designated as showing signs of early senility or *Alzheimer's* disease. (eponym)

■ Rule 4.24 Capitalize cardiologic symbols and abbreviations that are used to express electrocardiographic results.

EXAMPLES

The P waves are slightly prominent in V_1 to V_3. (or V_1-V_3)(or V1-V3)

It is not clear whether it contains a U wave.

The QRS complexes are normal, as are the ST segments.

There are T-wave inversions in LI, aVL, and V1-4.

4–1: SELF-STUDY

Directions: Draw a single line under each letter that should be capitalized. You may refer to your reference materials.

1. after i finish medical transcription 214, i will take a class in medical insurance billing. i want to get a job with goodwin-macy medical group.
2. all the patients were reminded that the office will be closed on labor day, monday, september 7.
3. dr. albert k. shaw's address is one west seventh avenue, detroit, michigan.
4. two of the commonly sexually transmitted pathogens are chlamydia trachomatis and neisseria gonorrhoeae.
5. it was mr. geoffry r. leslie, vice president of medical products, inc., who returned your call.
6. dr. johnson exclaimed, "it is necessary for me to leave for the coronary care unit at once!"
7. patsy, who works in the valley view medical center, is studying to become a certified medical transcriptionist.
8. the dorcus travel bureau arranged dr. berry's itinerary through new england last fall.
9. keep this in mind: accuracy is more important than speed.
10. the following are my recommendations:
    (1) continuing treatment through the spinal defects clinic.
    (2) evaluations at 2-month intervals during the first year of life.
    (3) physical therapy reevaluation at six months of age.
11. the patient has four siblings, all living and well; his mother died of heart disease at age 45 and his father of an automobile accident when he was 24; there is no history of familial disease.
12. we expect judge willard frick to arrive from his home on the pacific coast for the memorial day weekend.
13. i find current medical terminology by vera pyle, cmt, to be an excellent reference book for the x-ray department transcribing station.
14. my uncle, sam, is a thoracic surgeon in houston.
15. mr. billingsgate wrote to say that he had moved to 138 old highway eight, space 14.

Turn to page 108 for the answers to this assignment.

4–2: PRACTICE TEST

Directions: Draw a single line under the letters that should be capitalized in the sentences below.

1. the right rev. michael t. squires led the invocation at the graduation ceremony for greenlee county's first paramedic class.
2. nanci holloway, a 38-year-old caucasian female, is scheduled for a cesarean section tomorrow.
3. the internist wanted him to have meprobamate, so he wrote a prescription for miltown.
4. johnny temple had chickenpox, red measles, and german measles his first year in school.
5. unfortunately, the patient in icu whom dr. berry saw this morning has hodgkin's disease.
6. the pathology report showed a class IV malignancy on the pap smear.
7. some patients have been very sick with kaposi's sarcoma, the rare and usually mild skin cancer that seems to turn fierce with aids victims.
8. the mustard procedure is often used to reroute venous return in the atria.
9. the young man was an alert, asthenic, indochinese male who was well-oriented to time and place.
10. the gynecologist wrote a prescription for flagyl for the patient with trichomonas vaginalis.
11. please note on mrs. stefandatter's chart that she is allergic to phenobarbital.
12. dr. collier recommended a combination of gentamicin and a penicillin, such as bicillin, for our patient with endocarditis.
13. barbara, our lpn, is the new membership chairman for the local now chapter; she asked me to join.
14. the od victim was brought to the er by his roommate.
15. rhonda keller, mr. zimmer's executive secretary, spoke to the aama about good telephone manners.

The answers to these problems are in Appendix A. Do not be concerned with your progress if you had trouble with some of the abbreviations; the next chapter provides an in-depth study.

4–3: SELF-STUDY

Directions: Retype the following letter, inserting capital letters where necessary. You may use your reference materials. Use the U.S. Postal Service abbreviations for the state name in the address. After you have retyped the letter, turn to page 109 at the end of the chapter.

4

William A. Berry, MD

3933 Navajo Road
San Diego, California 92119

463 - 0000

may 17, 199x

barbara h. baker, md
624 south polk drive
boothbay harbor, maine 04538

dear dr. baker:

at the request of dr. thomas brothwell, i saw mrs. brenda woodman in the office today. he, apparently, felt that her thyroid was enlarged.

mrs. woodman stated that she is on tedral, 1/2 tablet q.i.d.; sski drops, 10 t.i.d.; choledyl b.i.d.; and prednisone. she has had asthma for twelve years and, other than a t & a in childhood, has never been hospitalized.

on physical examination her thyroid was 2+ enlarged, especially in the lower lobes, and smooth. the heart was in regular sinus rhythm of 110, and she had findings of moderate bronchial asthma at this time. on pelvic examination, she had a virginal introitus and a moderate senile vaginitis. she had heberden's nodes on the fingers and vibration sense was decreased by about 25 seconds.

the laboratory tests, a copy of which is enclosed, showed a normal thyroid function. the urinalysis was negative; and the electrocardiogram, a copy of which is enclosed also, showed some nonspecific st and t-wave changes and some positional change suggestive of pulmonary disease.

in summary, i do not feel that the lady has hyperthyroidism but simply an enlarged thyroid due to the prolonged iodide intake.

it was my pleasure to see your sister in the office and i hope that the above findings will reassure her family in the northeast.

sincerely,

william a. berry, md

jr

enclosures

cc: thomas b. brothwell, md

4-4: PRACTICE TEST

Directions: Retype the following two letters, inserting capital letters where necessary. Use the correct U.S. Postal Service abbreviations for the state name in the address.

See Appendix A for the correct version of these letters.

4

William A. Berry, MD
3933 Navajo Road
San Diego California 92119

463-0000

may 6, 199X

mrs. adrianne l. shannon
316 rowan road
clearwater, florida 33516

dear mrs. shannon:

dr. berry asked me to write to you and cancel your appointment for friday, may 15. we hope this will not inconvenience you, but dr. berry has made plans to attend the american college of chest physicians meeting in kansas city at that time. i have tentatively rescheduled your appointment for monday, may 18, at 10:15 a.m.

by the way, you might be interested to know that dr. berry has been asked to read the paper that he wrote, entitled "the ins and outs of emphysema." i believe that you asked him for a copy of this article the last time you were in the office.

sincerely yours,

(ms.) laverne shay
secretary

4

William A. Berry, MD
3933 Navajo Road
San Diego California 92119

619-463-0000

Fax 619-463-0000

march 3, 199X

state compensation insurance fund
p. o. box 2970
winnetka, illinois 60140

attention ralph byron, inspector

gentlemen:

re: james r. gorman

the above-referenced patient was seen today for presurgical examination in the office. he has an acute upper respiratory infection with a red left ear and inflamed tonsils. therefore, his surgery was cancelled, and he was placed on keflex, 250 mg every six hours.

mr. gorman's surgery was rescheduled for march 15 at mercy hospital. he will be rechecked in the office on march 14.

very truly yours

william a. berry, m d

ref

4–1 COMPUTER EXERCISE

Before proceeding, you may want to do more exercises based on the concepts you have learned. Additional practice material is on your computer diskette.

Directions: Insert the diskette into the computer and follow the instructions on the screen for Computer Exercise 4–1.

4

CAPITALIZATION RULE SYNOPSIS

Capitalize	*Rule*	*Page*
Abbreviations	4.18	100
Abbreviations for state names	4.5	96
Academic courses	4.21	101
Academic degrees	4.19	100
Acronyms	4.18	100
Allergies	4.22	101
Article titles	4.15	100
"Attention" lines	4.4	96
Avenue in addresses	4.2	96
Book titles	4.15	100
Boulevard in addresses	4.2	96
Brand names for drugs	4.10	98
Brand names for products	4.10	98
Capitals with colons	4.14	99
Cardiologic abbreviations	4.24	101
Cardiologic symbols	4.24	101
Colons with capital letters	4.14	99
Complimentary closes	4.1	96
Days of the week	4.16	100
Degrees	4.19	100
Departments in hospital	4.11	98
Direct quotes	4.14	99
Diseases	4.23	101
Drugs	4.10 and 4.22	98 and 101
Eponyms	4.7 and 4.23	97 and 101
Family titles	4.6	97
Genuses	4.9 and 4.23	98
Geographic locations	4.17	100
Headings	4.13	99
Historic events	4.16	100
Holidays	4.16	100
Languages	4.8	98
Military ranks	4.6	97
Months of the year	4.16	100
Names	4.7 and 4.23	97 and 101
Names for courses	4.21	101
Nicknames	4.7	97

Capitalize	*Rule*	*Page*
Nouns	4.7	97
Nouns used as adjectives	4.9	98
Nouns with letters	4.12	99
Nouns with numbers	4.12	99
Numbers with words	4.12	99
Officers' titles	4.20	100
Organizations' names	4.20	100
Outlines	4.13	99
People's titles	4.3	96
People	4.8	98
Periodical titles	4.15	100
Place names	4.17	100
Political titles	4.6	97
Professional titles	4.6	97
Proper nouns	4.7 and 4.23	97 and 101
Quotes	4.14	99
Races	4.8	98
Religions	4.8	98
Religious festivals	4.16	100
Religious orders	4.19	100
Salutations	4.1	96
Sentences	4.14	99
Signature lines	4.3	96
Species	4.9	98
Specific departments	4.11	98
State abbreviations	4.5	96
Street name in addresses	4.2	96
Title of articles	4.15	100
Title of periodicals	4.15	100
Titles	4.6	97
Titles for people	4.3	96
Title in addresses	4.3	96
Title of books	4.15	100
Title of officers	4.20	100
Title on envelopes	4.3	96
Title with signatures	4.3	96
"To Whom It May Concern" lines	4.4	96
Trade names	4.10	99
Viruses	4.23	101

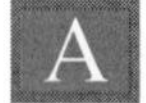

Answers for 4–1 Self-Study

1. after i finish medical transcription 214, i will take a class in medical insurance billing. i want to get a job with goodwin-macy medical group.
2. all the patients were reminded that the office will be closed on labor day, monday, september 7.
3. dr. albert k. shaw's address is one west seventh avenue, detroit, michigan.
4. two of the commonly sexually transmitted pathogens are chlamydia trachomatis and neisseria gonorrhoeae.
5. it was mr. geoffry r. leslie, vice president of medical products, inc., who returned your call.
6. dr. johnson exclaimed, "it is necessary for me to leave for the coronary care unit at once!"
7. patsy, who works in the valley view medical center, is studying to become a certified medical transcriptionist.
8. the dorcus travel bureau arranged dr. berry's itinerary through new england last fall.
9. keep this in mind: accuracy is more important than speed.
10. the following are my recommendations:
    (1) continuing treatment through the spinal defects clinic.
    (2) evaluations at 2-month intervals during the first year of life.
    (3) physical therapy reevaluation at six months of age.
11. the patient has four siblings, all living and well; his mother died of heart disease at age 45 and his father of an automobile accident when he was 24; there is no history of familial disease.
12. we expect judge willard frick to arrive from his home on the pacific coast for the memorial day weekend.
13. i find current medical terminology by vera pyle, cmt, to be an excellent reference book for the x-ray department transcribing station.
14. my uncle, sam, is a thoracic surgeon in houston.
15. mr. billingsgate wrote to say that he had moved to 138 old highway eight, space 14.

William A. Berry, MD
3933 Navajo Road
San Diego, California 92119

463-0000

may 17, 199x

barbara h. baker, md
624 south polk drive
boothbay harbor, ~~maine~~ 04538 — ME substituted

dear dr. baker:

at the request of dr. thomas brothwell, i saw mrs. brenda woodman in the office today. he, apparently, felt that her thyroid was enlarged.

mrs. woodman stated that she is on tedral, 1/2 tablet q.i.d.; sski drops, 10 t.i.d.; choledyl b.i.d.; and prednisone. she has had asthma for twelve years and, other than a t & a in childhood, has never been hospitalized.

on physical examination her thyroid was 2+ enlarged, especially in the lower lobes, and smooth. the heart was in regular sinus rhythm of 110, and she had findings of moderate bronchial asthma at this time. on pelvic examination, she had a virginal introitus and a moderate senile vaginitis. she had heberden's nodes on the fingers and vibration sense was decreased by about 25 seconds.

the laboratory tests, a copy of which is enclosed, showed a normal thyroid function. the urinalysis was negative; and the electrocardiogram, a copy of which is enclosed also, showed some nonspecific st and t-wave changes and some positional change suggestive of pulmonary disease.

in summary, i do not feel that the lady has hyperthyroidism but simply an enlarged thyroid due to the prolonged iodide intake.

it was my pleasure to see your sister in the office, and i hope that the above findings will reassure her family in the northeast.

sincerely,

william a. berry, md

jr

enclosures

cc: thomas b. brothwell, md

Note: The letters that you see underlined should be capitalized.

CHAPTER 5

Transcribing Numbers, Figures, and Abbreviations

OBJECTIVES

After reading this chapter and working the exercises, you should be able to

1. Explain when a number should be typed as a figure, typed in spelled-out form, or typed as a roman numeral.
2. Type medical and business symbols and abbreviations when appropriate.
3. Demonstrate your ability to prepare accurately typed material containing numbers, symbols, and abbreviations commonly found in medical writing.

INTRODUCTION

This chapter continues the discussion of the various typing techniques peculiar to medical and scientific reports, also known as style. We are going to be working with rules, and they, like those we have been studying previously, are not sacred; however, they are sound and practical. When you master the techniques presented in this chapter, you will have the mechanical skill necessary to type medical and scientific papers with confidence.

One of the most difficult tasks in studying machine transcription is learning the technical and mechanical manner of writing used by those already working in the field. Therefore, even a mastery of medical terminology may not give you the confidence that what you are typing is being done exactly the way it should be.

Furthermore, absence of basic mechanical skill results in copy that lacks refinement or accuracy. Unfortunately, errors can occur because the transcriptionist "thought" he or she heard a certain word and then typed a senseless remark or a fragment of material. A more thorough understanding of the topic helps to prevent such an error. It is important for the transcriptionist to be both grammatically and technically proficient.

If you want to be able to avoid mistakes in your work, you must learn correct terms and practices, and, at the same time, keep "current" by reading medical reports, papers, and journals. You do not have to understand the complete technical content of an article, but you must read to become familiar with how the copy is prepared. Some formats that are used in journal writing (for example, the use of italics for foreign words) are not generally used in medical transcription unless something is being transcribed for publication. When this is so, then one must be sure to follow all the stylistic rules used by that journal or publication.

You will find that there may be several ways of doing something—not several ways of doing something "right," just several ways of doing something. Some of the ways are preferred, although other methods might be acceptable. The extra trouble that you take to learn the "best" way will make the extra difference in your work—that touch of polish. You may hear a veteran transcriptionist say "I have always done it this way" with a tone of voice indicating that it therefore makes it correct. This may not always be so. Many people learn by copying other people's work whom they trust and admire. However, those persons may just have "invented" a format, setup, or method of transcription. Years of doing something incorrectly does not make it correct. Learn now which references and role models are trustworthy. Learn to question practices that do not look or sound exactly right.

There are some ways of writing numbers for which no set rule exists. There is an increased tendency to write as many numbers as possible with symbols (1, 2, 3, and so on). In general, figures may be easier to understand than numbers in written-out form. Because medical typing is technical, numbers in the form of figures are often preferred because they stand out clearly, are emphatic, and are easier to read in that they are quickly and easily understood. Only vague or approximate numbers are consistently written out, e.g., "There were hundreds present." One needs to stay alert to the changing styles and always use what is preferred by the dictator or author of the material.

TYPING NUMBERS

The first set of rules has to do with typing numbers. We have already discussed punctuating numbers and even capitalizing words that appear with them. Now the spotlight is on the numbers themselves. Numbers can be expressed in a variety of ways: We have the terms *numeral, arabic numeral, figure, numeric term, roman numeral, cardinal number,* and *ordinal number.* Each one describes a different way that numbers themselves are expressed or written. Numbers can be spelled out, written as figures, or written in a combination of a figure and a part of a word (e.g., 3rd).

Numeral and *arabic numeral* mean the *figures* and combinations of the figures 0, 1, 2, 3, 4, 5, 6, 7, 8, and 9.

Numeric term refers to written-out numbers.

Roman numerals refer to the use of certain letters of the alphabet, most frequently certain capital letters and combinations of the letters I, V, and X.

Cardinal numbers refer to the quantity of objects in the same class. It may be a whole number, a fraction, or a combination, e.g., 3 days, $15, and so forth.

Ordinal numbers express position, sequence, or order of items in the same class. They can be spelled out or written as a figure plus a word part, e.g., first, 1st, third, eleventh, 14th, and so forth. The following rules will be separated into these different groups, with some numbers being expressed in more than one way.

Ordinal Numbers (first, second, third, and so on)

■ Rule 5.1 *Spell out* ordinal numbers (first through ninth) when used to indicate a time sequence and numbered streets under ten. Use *figures* for ordinals when they are part of a series that includes a higher ordinal (10 and above), street numbers 10 and above, and when the number indicates any other technical term.

EXAMPLES

spelled out numbers

This is her *second* visit to the clinic.

The patient was discharged to his home on the *fifth* postoperative day.

The *first* stage of the disease went by relatively unobserved.

Most spontaneous abortions occur during the *first* or *second* week of pregnancy, just after the *first* menstrual cycle is missed.

Her new office is located at 924 *Fifth* Avenue, Suite 10.

figures

The clinic was for children in the *1st* through *12th* grades.

The *4th, 5th,* and *6th* ribs were fractured.

The injury was between the *1st* and *2nd* cervical vertebrae.

It occurred sometime between the *14th* and *30th* week of pregnancy.

Change the mailing address from PO Box 254 to 1335 *11th* Street.

Give the patient an appointment for the *6th* of August.

HOWEVER: Give the patient an appointment for August 6.

NOTE: As with all numbers, use a spelled-out ordinal number to begin a sentence or recast the sentence to avoid beginning with a number. See Rule 5.2.

EXAMPLE

Twelfth-grade students in the honor programs are simultaneously enrolled in community college classes.

Numbers Spelled Out (Written as Words) (one, two, three, and so on)

■ Rule 5.2 Spell out numbers at the beginning of a sentence.

EXAMPLE

Fourteen patients were studied at the request of the staff, *four* were studied at the request of their physicians, and *eleven* were studied as interesting problems for discussion.

NOTE: When several related numbers are used in a sentence, be consistent; type all numbers in figures or write them all out. Normally, it is easier to type all of them in figures. If the number beginning the sentence is large (more than two words), it may be necessary to rewrite the sentence so that the number may be used as a figure within the sentence. *However, if you must begin a sentence with a numeric term, you are not bound to write out the other large numbers in the sentence.*

EXAMPLE

Seventy-one percent responded to the questionnaire; *33%* were positive, *21%* were negative, and *17%* gave a "no opinion" response.

NOTE: Be sure to spell out an abbreviation or symbol used with a number if the number has to be spelled out for some reason, e.g., the word "percent" in the previous example.

■ Rule 5.3 Spell out all whole numbers *one* through and including *ten* when they do not refer to technical terms.

EXAMPLES

She had pulmonary tuberculosis *three* years ago and spent *seven* months in a sanitorium.

The EEG was run for *three* minutes with no activity.

BUT: The EEG was run for *20* minutes with no activity.

ALSO: The EEG was run for *5 1/2* minutes with no activity.

The address for our risk management team is *One* East Wacker Drive, Chicago, IL 60601.

He will have to convalesce for *five* to *six* weeks before returning to work.

■ Rule 5.4 Spell out numbers that are used for indefinite expressions.

EXAMPLES

I received *thirty-odd* applications.

He had diphtheria in his *mid-forties.*

Hundreds thronged to see my "celebrity" patient.

■ Rule 5.5 Spell out fractions when they appear without a whole number or are not used as a compound modifier.

EXAMPLES

He smoked a *half*-pack of cigarettes a day.

He smoked *one-half* pack of cigarettes a day.

BUT: He smoked *1 1/2* packs of cigarettes a day.

A 1/2-inch incision was made in the thenar eminence. (use of modifier)

There was damage to one-fourth of the distal phalanx. (no use of modifier)

NOTE: Make all fractions on the keyboard using the whole number, the slash, and the second whole number, with no spacing. Mixed fractions are made with a space between the whole number and the first number of the fraction.

EXAMPLES

1/2 inch

1 1/2 inch (not 1 and 1/2 inch, which the dictator might say)

1/2-inch incision (compound modifier)

■ Rule 5.6 Spell out the first number and use a figure for the second number when two numbers are used together to modify the same noun.

EXAMPLES

two 1-liter solutions
six 3-bed wards
fifty 3-gallon tanks

5

NOTE: Remember Rule 3.30, page 77, and use the hyphen when words are compounded with figures.

■ Rule 5.7 Spell out the *even time of day* when written without o'clock or without a.m. or p.m.

EXAMPLES

The staff meeting is scheduled to begin at *three.*

He is due at *nine* this evening.

ALSO: Give her an appointment for half-past two.

NOTE: Figures are used for all other expressions of time. See Rule 5.9. The phrases *in the morning, in the afternoon,* and *at night* are written with "o'clock" and not with a.m. or p.m. Do not use *o'clock* with *a.m.* or *p.m.* or when both hour and minutes are expressed.

EXAMPLES

I met her in the emergency room at *3* o'clock in the morning.

She is expected at *3* o'clock p.m. (incorrect)

She is expected at *3* o'clock. (correct)

She is expected at *3:30* o'clock. (incorrect)

She is expected at *3:30* p.m. (correct)

NOTE: It is also acceptable to write out an even time of day with the expression *o'clock.*

EXAMPLES

Please ask her to come at *three* o'clock. (correct)

Please ask her to come at *3* o'clock. (correct)

■ Rule 5.8 Spell out large round numbers that do not refer to technical quantities.

EXAMPLE

There were *eighteen hundred* physicians present at the symposium.

NOT: There were one thousand, eight hundred present.

HOWEVER: He was given *600,000* units of penicillin. (technical)

Numbers as Figures (Also Called Cardinal Figures or Arabic Figures—1, 2, 3, and so on)

■ Rule 5.9 Use figures to express the time of day with a.m. or p.m. and the time of day when *both* hours and minutes are expressed alone.

NOTE: Even times of day are written without the colon and zeroes.

EXAMPLES

He arrived promptly at *2:30.*

Office hours are from *10:00 a.m.* to noon. (incorrect)

Office hours are from *10 a.m.* to noon. (correct)

NOTE: Do not use *a.m.* or *p.m.* with 12. You may use the figure 12 with the word *noon* or *midnight* or use the words alone without the figure 12.

EXAMPLES

We close the office at *12 noon.* (or simply *noon*)

My shift is over at *midnight.*

■ Rule 5.10 Use figures to write numbers larger than ten.

Use a comma to punctuate large numbers when there are five or more digits represented. Addresses, year dates, ZIP codes, fax numbers, four-digit numbers, and some ID and technical numbers are traditionally not separated by commas, nor are commas used with decimals or the metric system.

EXAMPLES

The piece of equipment is valued at *$12,300.*

Piedmont Hospital Association serves a population of *150,500.*

Please send this to Union Annex Box *87543.*

All of the ZIP codes changed in our area; please note that the new one is *06431.*

Some very large numbers are written using scientific notation. (See page 117 and the use of superscript.)

EXAMPLE

2.5×10^8 (not 25,000,000)

■ Rule 5.11 Use figures to write numbers under ten when they occur with a larger number on the same subject.

EXAMPLE

There are *3* beds available on the maternity wing, *14* on the surgery wing, and *12* on the medical floor.

■ Rule 5.12 Use figures to write numbers with the expression "o'clock" when used to designate areas on a circular surface.

NOTE: Only whole numbers are used.

EXAMPLES

The sclera was incised at about the *3 o'clock* area.

The cyst was in the left breast, just below the nipple at the *5 o'clock* position.

■ Rule 5.13 Use figures to write dollar amounts. (Even amounts are written without the period and zeroes.)

EXAMPLE

The initial consultation is *$85.*

NOTE: Not *$85.00*

■ Rule 5.14 Use figures in writing vital statistics such as age, weight, height, blood pressure, pulse, respiration, dosage, size, temperature, and so on.

You Hear: he is a sixteen year old well developed well nourished white male height is seventy two inches weight is one hundred forty five pounds blood pressure is one hundred twenty over eighty pulse is seventy two and respirations are eighteen.

You Type: He is a 16-year-old, well-developed, well-nourished white male. Height: 72″. Weight: 145 lb. Blood pressure: 120/80. Pulse: 72. Respirations: 18.

NOTE: In the above example, the transcriptionist eliminated the verbs "is/are" and substituted the colon when the vital statistics were given. Each set of "vitals" is closed off with a period (a semicolon would also be correct).

EXAMPLE

Height: 72″. (correct)
Height: is 72″. (incorrect)

You Hear: this is a three day old black female infant with a rectal temperature of one hundred two degrees weighing seven pounds and nine ounces and measuring twenty one inches in length.

You Type: This is a 3-day-old black female infant with a rectal temperature of 102°, weighing 7 lb 9 oz, and measuring 21 inches in length.

You Hear: he is to take tofranil seventy five milligrams per day for three days to be increased to one hundred to one hundred fifty milligrams per day if there is no response.

You Type: He is to take Tofranil, 75 mg/day for three days to be increased to 100-150 mg/day if there is no response.

You Hear: the patient has twenty forty vision in the right eye and twenty one hundred in the left eye.

You Type: The patient has 20/40 vision in the right eye and 20/100 in the left eye.

■ Rule 5.15 Use figures when numbers are used *directly* with symbols, words, or abbreviations.

There is a space between the number and the words or the abbreviation; there is *no space* between the symbol and the number.

5

EXAMPLES

Number and abbreviation

15 mmHg (mm Hg also correct)
1 q.i.d.
400 mOsm of solute
6 inches (but 6″)
6 mL
8 lb 3 oz
5 ft 6 inches
3 a.m.
1.5 cm

EXCEPTION: q.4h. (Abbreviations concerning *"every* so many *hours"* are written closed up.)

Number and symbol

1+ protein
at a –2 station
36°C (notice that there also is no space between the symbol and the abbreviation)
+2.50
120/80
Rh–
2%
$10 (not $10.00)
#14 Foley
6″
#3-0
1:100
20/40

EXCEPTION: 3 × 5 (Spaces are used because the symbol crowds the figures.)

NOTE: Do not use symbols and hyphens together.

EXAMPLE

a *3″-incision* (incorrect)
a *3-inch* incision (correct)

You Hear:	*You Type:*
one plus protein	1+ protein
fifteen millimeters of mercury	15 mmHg (also 15 mm Hg)
two percent	2%
seventy five milliliters per kilogram per twenty four hours	75 mL/kg/24 hours

5

You Hear:	*You Type:*
one "cue eye dee"	1 q.i.d.
ten milligrams "tee eye dee"	10 mg t.i.d.
the "bee you en" is forty five milligrams percent	the BUN is 45 mg%
ninety nine degrees fahrenheit	99°F *or* 99 degrees Fahrenheit
a ten day history	a 10-day history
ten dollars	$10 *not* $10.00
sixty three cents	63 cents *not* 63¢ *or* $.63
number fourteen foley	#14 Foley *or* No. 14 Foley
thirty to thirty five milliequivalents	30-35 mEq (also 30 to 35 mEq)
four hundred milliosmol of solute	400 mOsm of solute
oh-ess equals plus two point five oh plus oh point seven five	O.S. = +2.50 + 0.75

■ Rule 5.16 Use figures for the day of the month and the year; write out the month when used in narrative text and the date line of a letter. Use figures separated by hyphens in other formats.

NOTE: Hyphens are generally preferred to slashes with numbers because the slash could be confused with the number one and cause crowding of figures.

EXAMPLES

Date line for letter or report
November 3, 199X

3 November 199X *(military and foreign style; not used in text format)*

Text use
The patient was first seen in the emergency department on *March 3, 199X.* (correct)

The patient was first seen in the emergency department on *3-3-9X.* (incorrect)

The patient was first seen in the emergency department on *3/3/9X.* (incorrect)

The patient was first seen in the emergency department on *3 March 199X.* (not correct in nonmilitary documents)

The patient was first seen in the emergency department on *March 3* last year. (not correct. Find out the correct year and insert it.)

In reports
Office visit: *3-3-9X.* (preferred)

Office visit: *03-03-9X.* (double-digit method also acceptable)

DOB: *3-3-93.* (date of birth)

Office visit: *3/3/9X.* (not preferred)

D: *11-3-9X.* (date of dictation)
T: *11-4-9X.* (date of transcription)

The double-digit dating system
D: *11-03-9X.*
T: *11-04-9X.*

■ Rule 5.17 Use figures when writing the military time of day.

You Hear:	*You Type:*
oh three fifteen *(3:15 a.m.)*	0315
twelve hundred hours *(noon)*	1200
fourteen hundred hours *(2 p.m.)*	1400
sixteen thirty *(4:30 p.m.)*	1630

EXAMPLES

Your appointment is set for 16:30. (incorrect)

Your appointment is set for 1630 p.m. (incorrect)

Your appointment is set for 1630. (correct)

NOTE: Military time is not used with a.m., p.m., or o'clock.

■ Rule 5.18 Use figures in writing suture materials.

NOTE: When the dictator says "three oh" or "triple oh" in referring to suture materials, you may type 000 or 3-0. For reading ease, use only the number, hyphen, and the zero when the number is larger than three, that is, from 4-0 through 11-0.

EXAMPLES

The incision was closed with #6-0 fine silk sutures. (correct)

The incision was closed with #000000 fine silk sutures. (incorrect)

The incision was closed with #60 fine silk sutures. (incorrect)

She used 000 chromic catgut for suture material. (correct)

She used 3-0 chromic catgut for suture material. (correct)

She used #3-0 chromic catgut for suture material. (correct)

NOTE: It is optional to insert the # symbol or "No." unless dictated.

■ Rule 5.19 Use figures and symbols when writing dimensions.

You Hear:
eight point five by five by four

NOTE: Add a zero after the decimal point and whole numbers for consistency in the *set* of numbers. Leave a space on each side of the "x."

You Type:
8.5 x 5.0 x 4.0 (correct)
8.5 x 5 x 4 (incorrect)

Subscript and Superscript

At one time, many numbers were typed in subscript or superscript (slightly below or above the line). With the advent of word processing equipment, this technique has become somewhat easier, but it can still be time consuming to locate the proper formatting. For example, using Microsoft Word on a Macintosh computer, one can either select the icon for superscript or subscript on the mini-menu bar or select FORMAT, then CHARACTER, and then POSITION (subscript or superscript). Using WordPerfect 5.1 on an IBM-compatible computer, one must place the cursor where the superscript or subscript is to be inserted. Press Control + F8, S (font size). Select 1 (superscript) or 2 (subscript) and then type in the number you need. Press the right arrow. This will not appear on the screen, but it will print out correctly. This helps you understand why it is usually acceptable to execute *most* subscript and superscript symbols on-line. Numbers are more easily read when typed on-line because most reports are single spaced. Again, some dictators or authors may insist on proper formatting, so be alert to this.

EXAMPLES

H_2O *(the symbol for water)*

A_2 is greater than P_2 *(the aortic second sound is greater than the pulmonic second sound)*

The L_4 area was bruised *(reference to the fourth lumbar vertebra)*

^{131}I was given *(reference to radioactive iodine)*

You might want to learn this technique. It is shown in the examples, along with numbers typed on the line. An exception to the general rule of avoiding subscripts and superscripts is in the case of numbers given to the power of 10, e.g., *"urine culture grew out 10^5* colonies of E. coli." It is obvious that in this case, to write the superscript on the same line would change the value of the number.

■ Rule 5.20 Use figures with capital letters to refer to the vertebral (spinal) column.

NOTE: C is used for the cervical vertebrae 1-7
T (or D) is used for the thoracic (or dorsal) vertebrae 1-12
L is used for the lumbar vertebrae 1-5
S is used for the sacral vertebrae 1-5

Normally the physician would not say "thoracic six" but "tee six."
You Type: T6 or T_6

You Hear: he has a herniated disk at el four five.
You Type: He has a herniated disk at L4-5 (*or* $L_{4\text{-}5}$).

You Hear: there was an injury to the spine between see seven and tee one.
You Type: There was an injury to the spine between C7 and T1 (or C_7 and T_1).

NOTE: Reference to the spinal nerves is made in the same manner.

5

■ Rule 5.21 Use figures when writing electrocardiographic *chest* leads. These leads are V_1 through V_6 and aV_L, aV_R, and aV_F.

Leads for recording electrocardiographic tracings are designated by numbers and letters. The standard leads are indicated by roman numerals; the central terminal lead is designated by "V" for the central terminal and a letter for right or left arm or foot.

EXAMPLES

lead I
lead III
VR
aVR
aVF

Chest leads are indicated with a "V" for the central terminal and an arabic number for the chest electrode and a roman numeral for intercostal space positions.

EXAMPLES

lead V1
lead VR1
lead V3III

You Hear: lead vee-r-two
You Type: lead VR2

You Hear: lead vee-three-three
You Type: lead V3III

You Hear: there is es tee elevation in leads vee two and vee six.
You Type: There is ST elevation in leads V2 and V6 (*or* V_2 and V_6)

You Hear: the leads one, two, "a vee el," and "a vee ef" are missing in this sequence.
You Type: The leads I, II, aV_L (aVL also correct), and aV_F (aVF also correct) are missing in this sequence.

5

NOTE: Roman numerals are used with *limb* leads. See page 120.

■ Rule 5.22 Use figures in writing technical ratios and ranges.

You Hear: the solution was diluted one to one hundred.
You Type: The solution was diluted 1:100.

You Hear: there is a fifty-fifty chance of recovery.
You Type: There is a 50-50 chance of recovery.

NOTE: A *ratio* expresses the elements of a proportion and expresses the number of times the first contains the second.* A *range* is the linking of a sequence of values or numbered items by expressing only the first and last items in the sequence or the difference between the smallest and the largest varieties in a statistical distribution.

Ratios made up of words are expressed with a slash, a hyphen, or the word "to."

EXAMPLES

The odds are ten to one.
the female/male ratio or female-male ratio

Numerical ratios are expressed using a colon.

EXAMPLES

The odds are 10:1.

The solution was diluted 1:100,000.

Symbolic ratios are written with a slash.

EXAMPLE

The a/b ratio

The word "to" or a hyphen may be used in expressions of range.

EXAMPLES

The projected salary increases are $2.75 to $3.00 per hour.

The projected salary increases are $2.75-$3.00 per hour.

We released all the medical records from 1980-1985 to microfilm storage.

There is a waiting period of 3-6 months.

NOTE: Do not use the hyphen when the range includes a plus and/or minus sign.

EXAMPLES

There was a weight change expected of anywhere from –6.5 kg to +10.5 kg.

The presenting part was at a –2 to a –3 station.

The symbol or abbreviation is used with each of the figures in the range.

EXAMPLES

The survival rate was consistent at 20% to 25%.

The fever fluctuated daily between 100° and 103°.

■ Rule 5.23 Use figures and symbols when writing plus or minus with a number.

You Hear: one to two plus
You Type: 1 to 2+

You Hear: pulses were two plus
You Type: pulses were 2+

You Hear: the presenting part was at a minus two station
You Type: The presenting part was at a -2 station.

You Hear: visual acuity with correction was increased to twenty two hundred by plus eight point fifty lens
You Type: Visual acuity with correction was increased to 20/200 by +8.50 lens.

Mixed Numbers

■ Rule 5.24 Use figures to write both technical and nontechnical mixed numbers (whole numbers with a fraction).

NOTE: Fractions are not used with the metric system nor with the percent (%) sign. Decimals are used with the metric system to describe portions of whole numbers.

EXAMPLE

You Hear: three-fourths percent
You Type: 0.75% (not 3/4%)

EXAMPLE

The patient moved to this community 2 1/2 years ago. (mixed number)

BUT: The patient moved to this community two years ago. (whole number less than ten)

You Hear: one and one half years ago
You Type: 1 1/2 years ago

* An example in making lemonade might be the following: Water:lemon juice:sugar ratio: 10:1:2 tablespoons.

You Hear: one and a half centimeters
You Type: 1.5 cm (not 1 1/2 cm)

NOTE: To type fractions, type the numerator, the slash, and the denominator. Leave a space between the whole number and the numerator of the fraction: 2 1/4.

■ Rule 5.25 Use figures in writing numbers containing decimal fractions.

EXAMPLE

The incision site was injected with *0.5%* Xylocaine. (not 1/2%)

NOTE: A zero is placed before a decimal that does not contain a whole number so it will not be read as a whole number. Be very careful with the placement of the zero and decimal. Incorrect placement could result in a 10- or 100-fold error.

EXCEPTION: By tradition and custom, no zero is used when expressing the caliber sizes of weapons.

EXAMPLE

He used a .22-caliber rifle.

Unrelated Numbers and Other Combinations

■ Rule 5.26 Unrelated numbers in the same sentence follow the rules governing the use of each one.

EXAMPLE

He has *three* offices and employs *21* medical assistants, including *2* transcriptionists. (Rule 5.3 and Rule 5.11)

5

■ Rule 5.27 Round numbers in millions and billions are expressed in a combination of figures and words.

EXAMPLE

Do you know that Keane Insurance sold over *$3 1/2 billion* of medical insurance last year? ($3.5 billion is also correct.)

Spacing

The symbols +, –, %, #, $, °, ', ", and / are typed directly in front of or directly after the number to which they refer, with no spaces.

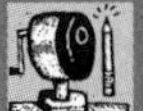 5–1: SELF-STUDY

Directions: Imagine that you hear the following "phonetic" phrases or sentences. On a separate sheet of paper, retype the phrases properly. Do not copy the quote marks that are placed around the "phonetic" phrase. Watch for the proper use of capitalization and punctuation. There is a synopsis of rules on page 131 to help you locate the rules quickly.

EXAMPLE

the patient was seen in the emergency room at twenty hundred hours on eleven august nineteen ninety

The patient was seen in the emergency room at 2000 hours on August 11, 1990.

1. the wound was closed in layers with "two oh" and "three oh" black silk sutures
2. the three month premature infant was delivered by cesarean section
3. he is a twenty four year old black male with an admitting blood pressure of one hundred eighty over one hundred
4. paresis is noted in four fifths of the left leg
5. it was then suture ligated with chromic number one catgut sutures
6. there were multiple subserous fibroids ranging in size from point five to two point five centimeters in diameter
7. there are a thousand reasons why i wanted to be a doctor but at three "ay em" after i have been awakened from a deep sleep it is hard to think of any
8. my charge for the procedure is seven hundred and fifty dollars and the median fee in the community is eight hundred dollars
9. the patient received four units of blood
10. the bullet traveled through the pelvic plexus into the spinal cord shattering "es" two "es" three and "es" four

After you have typed this exercise, check the end of the chapter on page 131 to see if you completed it properly. *Retype* any problems that you missed so that you get the "feel" of producing them correctly and another chance to see them written accurately.

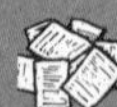 5–2: PRACTICE TEST

Directions: Follow the directions given in Self-Study 5–1.

1. on september twenty six nineteen ninety she had a left lower lobectomy
2. two sutures of triple oh cotton were placed so as to obliterate the posterior cul de sac
3. he smoked one and one half packs of cigarettes a day
4. there was a tear in the iris at about six oh clock
5. the resting blood pressure is seventy six over forty
6. please mail this to doctor ralph lavton at ten dublin street bowling green ohio four three four oh two
7. we had seven admissions saturday twenty four sunday and three this ay-em
8. In the accident the spine was severed between see four and five
9. the child was first seen by me in the x ray department on the evening of eleven may nineteen ninety
10. i recommend a course of cobalt sixty radiation therapy

The answers to these problems are in Appendix A at the back of the book. Retype any that you missed so that you have the opportunity of producing them correctly.

Roman Numerals

Roman numerals are generally used as noncounting numbers. There are many medical phrases *traditionally* expressed with capital roman numerals. These are made on the keyboard with the capital letters I, V, and X. Lower case roman numerals are used in the preparation of prescriptions and are made with the lower case i, v, and x; however, they are seldom required in typing. Capitalize a proper noun occurring with a roman numeral, a noun occurring with a roman numeral at the beginning of a sentence, and other nouns occurring with roman numerals if the dictator or author chooses this style. Because the use of roman numerals is based only on tradition, some professionals prefer the use of arabic numbers. Always follow the desires or customs of your employer; however, the examples that follow show only the use of the roman numerals.

■ Rule 5.28 Type numbers with the following expressions using roman numerals.

Expressions	*Examples*
Type	type I hyperlipoproteinemia
Factor (blood clotting)	missing factor VII (I to XIII)
Stage	stage II carcinoma
	stage I coma
	lues II (secondary syphilis) (I to III)
	Billroth I (first stage of an operative procedure)
Phase	phase II clinical trials
Class	class II malignancy
	cardiac status: Class IV
Grade	grade II systolic murmur
cranial nerves	cranial nerves II-XII are intact (I to XII)
cranial leads (EEG)	lead I reading
limb lead (ECG)	lead II reading (I to III)
technique	Coffey technique III
with Greek alphabet	alpha II*

*The symbols for the Greek alphabet cannot be made on the standard keyboard, so the names are written out. The most commonly used letters are lower case alpha, beta, gamma, delta, lambda, and theta.

Pregnancy and delivery are expressed using the words *gravida* for the number of pregnancies and *para* to indicate the number of deliveries. Occasionally, the dictator will also dictate the number of abortions. Again, follow the preference of the author of the material in using these traditional expressions. These may be written in the following manner:

Gravida II Para II

gravida II para II

gravida 2 para 2

gravida 2 para 2 abortus 0

At no time are numerals mixed or is the set punctuated. Some dictators will abbreviate the three main topics with GPA after the topic "obstetrics."

EXAMPLE

OB: G3 P3 A0

Another method for representing a patient's obstetric history is the use of a set of four arabic numbers to indicate the number of pregnancies resulting in term deliveries, of deliveries of premature infants, of abortions, and of living children. These numbers are separated with a hyphen.

EXAMPLE

OB: Gravida 5 para 4-1-0-5

This expression indicates that the patient delivered four infants at term, one prematurely; had no abortions; and has five living children.

5

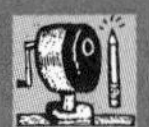

5–3: SELF-STUDY

Directions: Imagine that you hear the following phonetic words, phrases, or sentences. On a separate sheet of paper, retype the sentences properly. Watch for the proper use of capitalization and punctuation.

1. there is a loud grade three musical bruit over the bifurcation of the left carotid artery. there is a soft grade one to two over the right internal carotid artery
2. bleeding was controlled with two oh ties
3. she is a gravida four para zero
4. the doctor's callback time is every day at four oh clock
5. i was called to the "ee" "are" at three in the morning where i performed an emergency tracheotomy on a four day old male infant. i remained in attendance for two hours to be sure he was out of danger
6. he came in for a class three flight physical
7. he has passed the five year mark without any evidence of a recurrence
8. he has a grade two beta strep infection
9. send my mail to post office box six not my home address
10. this is her fourth admittance this year

After you have typed this exercise, check the end of the chapter on page 132 to see if you completed the sentences properly. Retype any that you missed so that you will get a chance to produce them correctly.

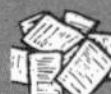

5–4: PRACTICE TEST

Directions: Follow the directions given in Self-Study 5–3.

1. he has a grade one arteriosclerotic retinopathy and a grade four hypertensive retinopathy
2. she was gravida five para one abortus four and denied venereal disease but gave a history of vaginal discharge
3. i can see only fifteen to twenty patients a day

4. please order twelve two gauge needles
5. use only one eighth teaspoonful
6. the dorsalis pedis pulses were two plus and equal bilaterally
7. the ear was injected with two percent xylocaine and one to six thousand adrenalin
8. please check the reading in "vee four" again
9. this is her third "see" section
10. she quickly advanced from a stage two to a stage four lymphosarcoma

After you have checked your answers in Appendix A, retype any that you missed so that you will have the opportunity of producing them correctly.

USE OF SYMBOLS

You will notice many symbols printed in medical journals and texts, but the only symbols we consider here are those generally used in medical transcription. However, there are many symbols on the "hidden keyboard" of computers. One needs to be able to find these and use them when appropriate. For example, some typists will avoid using the degree symbol because it is not represented on the standard keyboard. This may be unacceptable to some dictators, so learn how to access this symbol on your computer. For example, the degree symbol (°) is found under shift-option-8 on the Macintosh and is found under Alt + 248 using WordPerfect 5.1 (hold down Alt and the number on the number pad, not the keyboard).

Symbols are substitutes for words and may be useful and desirable to speed up reading and comprehension.

Symbol	*Means*	*Explanation*
&	and	symbol is called an "ampersand"
°C	degree Celsius	degree symbol
°F	degree Fahrenheit	
=	equals	on the keyboard
′	feet	made with the apostrophe
″	inches	made with quotation marks
–	minus *or* to	made with the hyphen
#	number	on the keyboard
/	per *or* over	made with the slash
:	ratio	made with the colon
%	percent	on the keyboard
+	plus	on the keyboard
x	times *or* by	the lower case x

■ Rule 5.29 Use symbols *only* when they occur in immediate association with a number.

EXAMPLES

You Hear:	*You Type:*
eight by three	8 x 3
four to five	4-5 *or* 4 to 5
number three oh	#3-0
pulses are two plus	pulses are 2+
vision is twenty twenty	vision is 20/20

You Hear:	*You Type:*
six per day	6 per day
diluted one to ten	diluted 1:10
at a minus two	at a -2
sixty over forty	60/40
grade four over five	Grade IV/V
patient had nocturia times two	patient had nocturia x 2
performed a tee and a	performed a T&A
25 millimeters per hour	25 mm/h *or* 25 mm per hour
extension limited by 45 percent	extension limited by 45%
thirty degrees celsius	30°C *or* 30 degrees Celsius
lost a few see sees	lost a few cubic centimeters

NOTE: You may spell out *degrees Celsius* or *degrees Fahrenheit,* but do not use the word *degree* with the abbreviation *C* or *F.* It is also correct to simply type the temperature with or without the symbol.

EXAMPLES

The patient's admitting temperature was 99 (or 99° or 99 degrees or 99°F)

The patient's admitting temperature was 99 degrees F. (incorrect)

The patient's admitting temperature was 99° Fahrenheit. (incorrect)

Be consistent when you have a choice. Further illustration of symbol usage will be combined with the discussion of abbreviations.

USE OF ABBREVIATIONS

There are some abbreviations and symbols that we use so often that we no longer think of them as abbreviations but rather as complete words. We hear "percent," and we see %. "Mister" and "Doctor" look a bit out of place because Mr. and Dr. are such familiar titles. Medicine, like other technical fields, involves the use of many abbreviations and symbols that are particularly familiar to the medical writer and reader; this section is a guide to their proper use.

It is difficult for the beginning transcriptionist to know exactly how abbreviations should be typed. In addition, some abbreviations are typed in full capital letters, some in lower case, and some in a combination. They are written with or without periods. Chapter 3 contains a punctuation rule for the use of periods with abbreviations; that rule is repeated in this chapter so you need not turn back for review.

Symbols and abbreviations can save time, space, and energy and can prevent the needless duplication of repetitious words. The overuse of abbreviations is to be avoided, however, with only standard abbreviations appearing in the patient's record where permitted. Office and hospital "shortcuts" and hieroglyphics should be confined to memos and telephone messages. Furthermore, abbreviations of any type should never be used when there is a chance of misinterpretation. To add further to the problem, many reference books disagree on both the capitalization and the punctuation of abbreviations. When in doubt (and you know the meaning of the abbreviation), spell it out.

The medical transcriptionist in the medical office is permitted far greater latitude in using abbreviations than either the hospital transcriptionist or those employed by transcription services.

■ Rule 5.30 Do not use abbreviations in the following parts of the patient's medical record: admission and discharge diagnoses, preoperative and postoperative diagnoses, and names of surgical procedures.

EXAMPLES

Incorrect
Discharge diagnosis: PID

Correct
Discharge diagnosis: Pelvic inflammatory disease

Incorrect
Postoperative diagnosis: OMChS

Correct
Postoperative diagnosis: Otitis media, chronic, suppurating

Incorrect
Operation performed: T&A

Correct
Operation performed: Tonsillectomy and adenoidectomy

5

■ Rule 5.31 Use symbols and abbreviations in the medical record only when they have been approved by the medical staff and there is an explanatory legend available to those authorized to make entries in the medical record and to those who must interpret them.

NOTE: These lists will vary, of course, among institutions. Obtain lists from the institutions for which you work and refer to them carefully.

■ Rule 5.32 Spell out an abbreviation when you realize there could be a misunderstanding in the interpretation of the definition. You must be positive, of course, that *your* interpretation is correct; otherwise leave it alone or flag the transcript for the dictator to interpret.

EXAMPLE: The patient had a history of CVRD. (cardiovascular renal disease?, cardiovascular respiratory disease?)

■ Rule 5.33 Use an abbreviation to refer to a test, committee, drug, diagnosis, and so on in a report or paper *after* it has been used once in its completely spelled-out form.

EXAMPLE: "All newborns are routinely tested for phenylketonuria (PKU). As a result, the incidence of PKU as a cause of infant . . ."

■ Rule 5.34 Check any unfamiliar abbreviations or those that seem inappropriate with your reference lists. Individual letters in spoken form can sound alike.

EXAMPLE: "I performed an IND . . ." (or I&D or IMD or IMB or IMP or IME) (This could go on and on.)

■ Rule 5.35 Type as abbreviations familiar, common abbreviations and words that are usually seen as abbreviations.

EXAMPLES

Mr. Dr. Mrs. oz a.m. p.m. CBC
C-section DNA ER pH Rh

5

Appendix B contains a brief list of some abbreviations that are commonly used in office chart notes and hospital records. You may wish to remove it from the book or photocopy it and place it in your standard-size, three-ring binder for a quick reference. Later, you may wish to add new abbreviations that you discover as well as an institution-approved lists. Some abbreviations are said as a word (*cabbage* for *CABG* and *hope* for *HOPE*); others are said as an entire word but are typed as an abbreviation (*milligram* for *mg* and *see section* for *C-section*); and for others, each letter of the abbreviation is spoken (*b.i.d.* or *L&W*). *Bedtime* can mean *h.s.* if the dictator says either *one h s* or *one at bedtime.* A few pronunciation hints are added to your Appendix B list from time to time.

■ Rule 5.36 Use abbreviations for all metric measurements used *with* numbers.

EXAMPLES

You Hear:	*You Type:*
one millimeter	1 mm
five millimeters	5 mm
ten centimeters	10 cm
point five millimeters	0.5 mm
six cubic centimeters	6 cc
seven milliliters	7 mL *or* ml
twenty kilograms	20 kg (not kilos)
thirty seven degrees celsius	37°C

NOTE: Notice the zero (0) in front of the decimal point. Refer to Rule 5.25. Also notice that metric abbreviations are always written in lower case letters, are typed with one space after the number, and are not made plural. An exception is the capital C for *Celsius* and capital L for *liter.* In addition, some physicians use the word *centigrade* rather than *Celsius.* Use the capital C as the abbreviation for both.

BUT: There was only *a centimeter* difference between the two. (no abbreviation)

NOTE: Do not separate the figure from the abbreviation that follows it. If the figure occurs at the end of a line, insert a space in front of the figure so that it will carry to the next line and appear with the abbreviation.

EXAMPLES

.... was 1400 mL
of serosanguineous fluid (correct)

.... was
1400 mL of serosanguineous fluid (correct)

.... was 1400
mL of serosanguineous fluid (incorrect)

For example, you can keep this set together when using WordPerfect 5.1 by typing the *1400* + home key + space + *mL.* The entire expression will carry to the next line. This is likewise true for the hyphen. When you have *x-ray* at the end of the line and do not want it to separate, type the *x* + the home key + hyphen + home key + *ray.* The expression will be intact on the next line. Some people prefer to do a carriage return (or "hard return") in front of the set to be carried to the next line. This works fine if there is no additional internal editing that could throw off the character count.

■ Rule 5.37 Periods are used with single capitalized words and single letter abbreviations:

EXAMPLES

Mr. Jr. Dr. Inc. Ltd. Joseph P. Myers E. coli

- lower case abbreviations made up of single letters:

a.m. p.m. e.g. t.i.d.

NOTE:

- Units of measurement are *not* punctuated.

wpm mph ft oz sq in

- Certification, registration, and licensure abbreviations are *not* punctuated.

CMA-A CMT RN RRA ART LVN

- Acronyms and metric abbreviations are *not* punctuated.

CARE Project HOPE AIDS mg mL L cm km

- Most abbreviations typed in full capital letters are *not* punctuated.

UCLA PKU BUN CBC WBC COPD D&C T&A I&D P&A NBC FICA KEZL TV FM

EXCEPTION: Some transcriptionists prefer to punctuate I.V. (intravenous) so it is not confused with the roman numeral IV.

- Scientific abbreviations written in a combination of capital and lower case letters are *not* punctuated.

Rx Dx ACh Ba Hb IgG mEq mOsm Rh

- Academic degrees and religious orders are now *generally* not punctuated.

MD PhD DDS BVE MS SJ

(This is also Rule 3.16.)

■ Rule 5.38 Chemical and mathematical abbreviations are written in a combination of both upper and lower case letters without periods.

EXAMPLES

CO_2 (CO2)	*(carbon dioxide)*
Hb	*(hemoglobin)*
Hg	*(mercury)*
Na	*(sodium)*
T_4 (T4)	*(thyroxine)*
O_2 (O2)	*(oxygen)*
Ca^{++}	*(calcium ion)*
NaCl	*(sodium chloride)*
pH	*(hydrogen ion concentration)*
DNA	*(deoxyribonucleic acid)*
HCl	*(hydrochloric acid)*
10^4	*(ten to the fourth)*
K	*(potassium)*

NOTE: The pH of a substance is a measure of its acidity or alkalinity (ranging from 0 to 14). It is indicated with a whole number or a whole number and a decimal fraction. If there is no following fraction, this is indicated with a zero (0).

Dictated: pee h was seven.
Transcribed: The pH was 7.0. (not hydrogen ion concentration)

Dictated: the patient had a pee h of five point two.
Transcribed: The patient had a pH of 5.2.

Dictated: The dee en a is unavailable for further study.
Transcribed: The DNA is unavailable for further study.

Dictated: stat report shows sodium one hundred thirty eight milliequivalents per liter potassium three point three milliequivalents per liter chloride ninety seven milliequivalents per liter and a total see oh two of five milliequivalents per liter blood glucose is seven hundred milligrams percent.
Transcribed: STAT report shows sodium (or Na) 138 mEq/L, potassium (or K) 3.3 mEq/L, chloride (or Cl) 97 mEq/L, and a total carbon dioxide (CO_2 or CO2 also correct) of 5 mEq/L. Blood glucose is 700 mg% (not mg percent or milligrams percent).

■ Rule 5.39 Latin abbreviations are typed in lower case letters, with periods.

EXAMPLES

i.e. (that is)	etc. (and so forth)
et al. (and other people)	e.g. (for example)
op. cit. (in the work cited)	a.m. (ante meridian)
b.i.d. (twice a day)	p.m. (post meridian)
t.i.d. (three times a day)	p.c. (after meals)
q.i.d. (four times a day)	a.c. (before meals)

EXCEPTION: A.D. (in the year of Our Lord)

NOTE: It has become acceptable to write "a.m." and "p.m." in capital letters. This form is not punctuated: AM and PM.

5

■ Rule 5.40 Do not abbreviate names unless the name is abbreviated in the correspondent's letterhead. Shortened forms of a person's name, such as a nickname, are allowed in the salutation.

EXAMPLE

Steven J. Clayborn *and* Dear Steve:

NOTE: Do not use "Geo." or "Chas." with a last name unless thus abbreviated in the letterhead.

NOTE: Some "nicknames" might not be a shortened form but rather the entire name.

EXAMPLES

Ray, Gene, Will, Al, Alex, Ben, Ed, Fred, Sam, Pat, Beth, Hugh, Betty

Do not abbreviate in some other cases:

1. Titles other than Dr., Mr., Mrs., and Ms., unless a first name or initial accompanies the last name.

   EXAMPLES

   Maj. Ralph Emery *but* Major Emery

   Hon. John Wilson *but* Honorable Wilson

   Rt. Rev. Donald Turnbridge *but* Right Reverend Turnbridge

2. The words *street, road, avenue, boulevard, north, south, east,* and *west* in an inside address. However, *Southwest (SW), Northwest (NW),* and so on are abbreviated *after* the street name.

   EXAMPLES

   936 North Branch Street

   1876 Washington Boulevard, NW

3. Days of the week and months of the year. To avoid confusion, numbers should not be substituted for the names of the months in correspondence; however, they are acceptable in some records and reports.

   EXAMPLE

   January 11, 199X (narrative copy)

   NOT: Jan 11, 199X, *or* 1-11-9X *or* 1/11/9X *or* 01-11-9X

5

Typing Drugs

As a review of some of the rules, these are some hints for typing drugs into documents using numbers and symbols.

- Metric units of measure are used in abbreviated form with numerals.

  25 mg 0.50 mg

- Dosage instructions are preferably written in lower case letters with periods separating the initials.

  p.o. t.i.d. q.i.d. b.i.d. p.r.n. q.4h.

- Do not separate the number at the end of the line from the symbols that may follow

  25 mg (correct) 25
  mg (incorrect)

  NOTE: On your computer, either use the hard return in front of the 25 in the above example or press Home + space bar to keep the set together.

- Do not use either the lower case or capital "o" on the keyboard for zero; use the zero symbol.

  50 mg (correct) 5O mg, 5o mg (incorrect)

- Brand or trade name drugs and methods of administration are capitalized; generic and chemical names are not.

  Dalmane *(brand name)*
  Fero-Gradumet Filmtab *(brand name and method of administration)*
  captopril *(generic name)*

- It is not necessary to follow an unusual capital letter–small letter combination or all capital letter spelling given by the drug company unless you or your employer wish it. However, one might like to keep a name like *pHisoHex* intact. Use a capital letter after a hyphen in a brand-name drug.

  Di-Delamine (correct)
  HydroDIURIL (Hydrodiuril is also correct)

- Drugs in a simple narration, especially without dosages given, are separated by commas.

  The patient was discharged home on Lanoxin, Calan, and Solu-Medrol.

- In a more complex combination, when commas are needed within a string of information concerning a single drug, the units are separated by semicolons.

  MEDICATIONS: He will continue his 1800-calorie ADA diet and usual medicines, which include the following: estradiol, micronized, 2 mg/d for 25 of 30 days; propoxyphene HCl, 65 mg q.i.d., which is an increase from his current t.i.d. regimen; flurazepam HCl, 30 mg h.s.; hydrocodone bitartrate, 5 mg; ibuprofen, 600 mg q.i.d.

- A complex string can be typed in list format:

  MEDICATIONS:

  1. Continue his 1800-calorie ADA diet.
  2. Estradiol (micronized) 2 mg/d for 25 of 30 days.
  3. Flurazepam HCl, 30 mg h.s.
  4. Hydrocodone bitartrate, 5 mg b.i.d.
  5. Acetaminophen, 500 mg b.i.d.
  6. Ibuprofen, 600 mg q.i.d.
  7. Levothyroxine sodium, 0.15 mg/d.
  8. Metoprolol tartrate, 25 mg/d.
  9. Prednisone, 5 mg/d.
  10. Propoxyphene HCl, 65 mg q.i.d. (which is an increase from his current t.i.d. regimen).

ABBREVIATION REFERENCE

See Appendix B for a list of some abbreviations commonly used in the completion of office letters and chart notes and in transcribing hospital reports of all types. This is not a comprehensive list of abbreviations but will be helpful to you when completing the exercises. This will serve as a reference for your exercises and to illustrate the variety of ways that many common abbreviations are typed: full capital letters, combination of capital letters and lower case letters, and lower case letters. The italics will indicate how the abbreviation is generally said, when it is not said as the individual letters of the abbreviation itself. Furthermore, you should know that abbreviations, symbols, and contractions are used far more freely in chart notes (progress notes) and history and physical reports than they are in a discharge summary, operative report, legal report, or formal correspondence. For example, you would type "The GU tract was clear" in the patient's medical office record but would type "The genitourinary tract was clear" in a report to an insurance examiner. The medical office record might note that "the *pt* had an *appy* on *7-1-9X*" and "*she's* waiting for the results of a *cysto*." The letter to another physician reports that "the *patient* had an *appendectomy* on *July 1, 199X*"; likewise, "*she is* waiting for the results of a *cystoscopy*."

5

5–5: SELF-STUDY

Directions: Study the Abbreviation Reference and type the answers to the questions on a separate sheet of paper.

1. You hear: eye gee gee

   You type: ____________________

2. You hear: fifteen millimeters of mercury

   You type: ____________________

3. You hear: ten to the fourth

   You type: ____________________

4. You hear: are-h negative

   You type: ____________________

5. You hear: clear to pee-en a

   You type: ____________________

6. You hear: h double e en tee

   You type: ____________________

7. You hear: take one bee eye dee pee are en for pain

   You type: ____________________

8. You hear: hen pee

   You type: ____________________

9. You hear: pee oh two

   You type: ____________________

10. You hear: acetylcholine

    You type: ____________________

After you have typed this exercise, refer to the end of this chapter, page 132, to check your answers.

5–6: SELF-STUDY:

Directions: Imagine that you hear the following phonetic phrases or sentences. On a separate sheet of paper, retype the sentences and phrases properly. Watch for proper use of symbols, numbers, abbreviations, punctuation, and capitalization.

EXAMPLE

the "pee-h" was seven: neutrality; just between alkalinity and acidity

The pH was 7.0: neutrality; just between alkalinity and acidity.

1. flexion was limited to fifteen degrees extension to ten degrees adduction to ten degrees and abduction to twenty degrees
2. by use of a half inch osteotome one centimeter of the proximal end of the proximal phalanx was removed
3. "dee tee ares" are one to two plus

4. range of motion of the neck is limited to approximately seventy percent of normal
5. the date on the cholecystogram was nine one ninety one
6. estimated blood loss was one hundred "see-sees" none was replaced
7. at two "ay-em" the patients temperature was thirty eight point nine degrees celsius
8. the "pee-ay" and right lateral roentgenograms show a fracture of the right third and fourth ribs
9. lenses were prescribed resulting in improvement of his visual acuity to twenty thirty in the right eye and twenty forty five in the left eye. the visual field examination was normal and the tension is seventeen millimeters of mercury of schiotz with a five point five gram weight
10. the number twenty two foley with a thirty "see-see" bag was then inserted
11. i removed six hundred milliliters of serosanguineous fluid from the abdomen

After you have typed this exercise, check the end of the chapter, page 132, to see if you completed it properly. Retype any portions that you missed so that you get the "feel" of producing them correctly and another chance to see them written accurately.

5–7: PRACTICE TEST

Directions: Follow the instructions given in Self-Study 5–6.

1. hemoglobin on seven twenty seven was eleven point two grams hematocrit was thirty seven
2. did you know that the postal rates were twenty five cents for the first ounce and twenty cents for each additional ounce to mail something first class in nineteen eighty nine
3. the protein was sixty five milligrams percent
4. electromyography shows a three plus sparsity in the orbicularis oris
5. an estimated point two cubic centimeters of viscid fluid was removed from the middle ear cavity
6. he entered the "e-are" at four "ay-em" with a temperature of ninety nine degrees fahrenheit
7. there was a reduction of the angle to within a two degree difference
8. take fifty milligrams per day
9. i then placed two four by four sponges over the wound
10. the "tee-bee" skin test was diluted one to one hundred
11. drainage amounts to several "see-sees" a day

After you have checked your answers with Appendix A, retype any that you missed so that you will have the opportunity of producing them correctly.

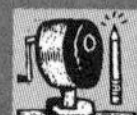

5–8: SELF-STUDY

Directions: Follow the instructions given in Self-Study 5–6.

1. the urine was negative for sugar, "pee-h" was seven and specific gravity was one point zero one two
2. the "bee-you-en" is forty five milligrams percent, one plus protein
3. i excised a small well circumscribed tumor two millimeters in diameter
4. use a three "em" vi-drape to cover the operative site
5. she received her second dose of "five-ef-you"

6. the culture grew one hundred thousand colonies of e coli per cubic centimeter
7. the surgeon asked for a number seven jackson bronchoscope
8. there were high serum titers of "gee" immunoglobulin antibodies
9. the phenotype "a-two-b" was found consistently in the family blood history
10. respirations sixteen per minute

After you have typed this exercise, check the end of the chapter on page 133 to see if you completed it properly. Retype any portions that you missed before you go on to your final exercise.

5

5-9: REVIEW TEST

Directions: Follow the instructions given in Self-Study 5–6.

1. the patient has a "pee-h" of six point ninety six "pee oh two" of twelve and "pee see oh two" of fifty four
2. there is a one by point five centimeter area of avulsed tissue and a three centimeter gaping deep laceration of the chin
3. lungs: clear to "pee and a." heart: not enlarged, "ay-to" is greater than "pee-to" there was a grade one to two over six decrescendo early diastolic high frequency murmur
4. cycloplegic refraction: "oh-dee" equal plus three point two five plus oh point seven five times one hundred twenty five equals twenty thirty minus one
5. the patient received a six thousand gamma roentgen dose
6. iodipamide sodium i one hundred thirty one was used
7. we used a concentration of five times ten to the fifth per milliliter
8. a dilute solution of one to one was used
9. he was scheduled for a "tee three" uptake
10. aqueous procaine penicillin "gee," four point eight million units intramuscularly with one gram of probenecid orally, is still recommended for uncomplicated gonorrhea
11. she returned today for her vitamin "bee-twelve"
12. my plan was to give her six hundred thousand units of penicillin on the first day and give her half that on the second
13. he denied symptoms of dysuria hematuria and urgency but did report nocturia times two
14. she is to take her medication "cue-four-h" with an additional one half dose "a-see"
15. i have an appointment for the eleventh of june and i need to change it to the first of july
16. six case histories were presented at the tumor board meeting today for a total of ninety seven this year
17. we expect that thousands of students will be able to participate in this surgery through the use of closed circuit "tee vee"
18. he has been a two pack a day cigarette smoker for the last forty years
19. please order six twenty gauge catheters
20. plan the surgery to begin at seven "ay em" sharp
21. i feel that my fee of twelve hundred dollars is fair
22. the jury awarded one point two million dollars in damages to the parents of the child
23. i removed a forty five slug from the left lower liver margin

24. how many centimeters long was that tear in her thumb
25. the hemoglobin was eight point eight, hematocrit twenty six point five white blood cells eight thousand one hundred with eighty segs and eighteen lymphs
26. you will notice that the standard leads one, two, "a vee el" and "a vee ef" are missing in the "ee-see-gee" lead-sequencing formats
27. then five to ten milliliters of one percent lidocaine was injected into the right breast at the four oclock and eight oclock areas
28. call back all "are-h" negative women with no demonstrable antibody titer for an injection of "row-gam"

5–1 COMPUTER EXERCISE

Before proceeding, you may want to do more exercises based on the concepts you have learned. Additional practice material is on your computer diskette.

Directions: Insert the diskette into the computer and follow the instructions on the screen for Computer Exercise 5–1.

POSTSCRIPT

Some of the phrases and expressions discussed in this chapter occur frequently in dictation and are worthy of mention one more time. Be sure that you are able to use them correctly.

You Hear:	*Properly Transcribed:*
it was her fifth admission	It was her fifth admission.
will be admitted at four pee em	will be admitted at 4 p.m. (PM)
came to see me at four o clock	came to see me at 4 o'clock (or four o'clock)
ay two is greater than pee two	A2 is greater than P2 (or A_2, P_2)
vision is twenty twenty	vision is 20/20
a twenty nine year old	a 29-year-old
weight is six pounds five ounces	weight is 6 lb 5 oz
taken tee i dee for three days	taken t.i.d. for three days
ninety nine degrees	99° (99 degrees)
diluted one to ten	diluted 1:10
sixty-five milligrams percent	65 mg%
bee pee is one hundred over eighty	BP is 100/80
sutured with three oh chromic	sutured with 3-0 (or 000) chromic

You Hear:	*Properly Transcribed:*
injected with point five percent	injected with 0.5%
used three four by fours	used three 4 x 4s
nocturia times two	nocturia x 2
one plus protein	1+ protein
drink seven hundred fifty milliliters per twelve hour period	drink 750 mL/12-hour period
herniated disk at tee three four	herniated disk at T3-4 or T_{3-4}
dorsalis pedis pulses were two plus	dorsalis pedis pulses were 2+
class two infection	class II infection
cranial nerves two through twelve	cranial nerves II-XII
cut was ten centimeters long	cut was 10 cm long
fifteen millimeters of mercury	15 mmHg (or mm Hg)
the pee h was seven	the pH was 7.0
he takes two pee see	he takes 2 p.c.
seen on four twenty-one	seen on April 21

SYMBOL AND NUMBER RULE SYNOPSIS

	Rule	Page
General		
Abbreviations and numbers	5.15	115
Date	5.1, 5.16	112, 116
Decimals	5.24, 5.25	118, 119
Dimensions	5.19	116
Fractions	5.5, 5.24	113, 118
Indefinite expressions	5.4	113
Large numbers	5.8, 5.10, 5.27	114, 114, 119
Money	5.13	115
Multiple use of numbers	5.2, 5.6, 5.11, 5.24, 5.26	113, 113, 114, 118, 119
Numbers in the address	5.1	112
Ordinal numbers (first, second)	5.1	112
Spelling out numbers	5.2 to 5.8	113 to 114
Time of day	5.7, 5.9, 5.17	114, 114, 116
Unrelated numbers	5.26	119
Written-out numbers	5.2 to 5.8	113 to 114
Technical		
Abbreviations	5.30 to 5.40	123 to 125
Capitalization of abbreviations	5.37	124
Chemical abbreviations	5.38	125
Dilute solutions	5.22	118
Electrocardiograph leads	5.21, 5.28	117, 120
Figures with plus or minus	5.23	118
Foreign abbreviations	5.39	125
Greek letters	5.28	120
Metric abbreviations	5.36	124
Military time	5.17	116
Miscellaneous abbreviations		123
O'clock area	5.12	114
Punctuation with abbreviations	5.37	124
Ranges	5.22	118
Ratios	5.22	118
Roman numerals	5.28	120
Spacing with symbols	5.15	115, 119
Spinal column and nerves	5.20	117
Subscript and superscript		117
Suture materials	5.18	116
Symbols	5.15, 5.29	115, 122
Units of measurement	5.14, 5.19, 5.22	115, 116, 118
Vital statistics	5.14	115
When not to abbreviate	5.30 to 5.32, 5.40	123, 125

A *Answers to* 5–1: SELF-STUDY

1. The wound was closed in layers with *2-0* and *3-0* black silk sutures. (*00* and *000* also correct)
2. The *3*-month-premature infant was delivered by cesarean section. (note hyphens)
3. He is a *24-year-old* black male with an admitting blood pressure of *180/100.* (note hyphens and slash)
4. Paresis is noted in *four-fifths* of the left leg. (note hyphen)
5. It was then suture ligated with chromic *#1* catgut sutures. (*No. 1* also correct)
6. There were multiple subserous fibroids ranging in size from *0.5* to *2.5 cm* in diameter.
7. There are a *thousand* reasons why I wanted to be a doctor; but at *3 a.m.*, after I have been awakened from a deep sleep, it is hard to think of any. (check your commas and semicolon too; capital *AM* also correct)
8. My charge for the procedure is *$750*, and the median fee in the community is *$800.* (not $750.00 and $800.00; nor is 750 dollars correct)
9. The patient received *4* units of blood.
10. The bullet traveled through the pelvic plexus into the spinal cord, shattering S_2, S_3, and S_4. (*S2, S3,* and *S4* also correct)

5

A *Answers to* **5–3: SELF-STUDY**

1. There is a loud *grade III* musical bruit over the bifurcation of the left carotid artery. There is a soft *grade I-II* over the right internal carotid artery. (*grade I to II* also correct) (Some prefer to use a capital letter for "Grade.")
2. Bleeding was controlled with *2-0* ties. (*00* also correct)
3. She is a Gravida *IV* Para *0.* (gravida and para also correct) (gravida 4 para 0 also correct)

5

4. The doctor's callback time is every day at *4* o'clock. (four o'clock also correct)
5. I was called to the *ER* at *three* in the morning where I performed an emergency tracheotomy on a *4-day-old* male infant. I remained in attendance for *two* hours to be sure he was out of danger.
6. He came in for a *class III* flight physical. (A dictator may prefer a capital letter for "Class.")
7. He has passed the *five-year* mark without any evidence of a recurrence.
8. He has a *grade II* beta strep infection. (A dictator may prefer a capital letter for "Grade.")
9. Send my mail to Post Office Box *Six*, not my home address. (*PO Box 6* also correct)
10. This is her *fourth* admittance this year.

A *Answers to* **5–5: SELF-STUDY**

1. IgG
2. 15 mmHg or 15 mm Hg
3. 10^4
4. Rh-
5. clear to P&A
6. HEENT
7. take 1 b.i.d., p.r.n. for pain
8. H&P
9. pO2 or pO_2
10. acetylcholine (chemical words used alone are written out)

A *Answers to* **5–6: SELF-STUDY**

1. Flexion was limited to *15°*, extension to *10°*, adduction to *10°*, and abduction to *20°*. (degrees can also be written out, e.g., *15 degrees*)
2. By use of a *half-inch* osteotome, *1 cm* of the proximal end of the proximal phalanx was removed.
3. *DTRs* are *1-2+*. (also *1 to 2+*)
4. Range of motion of the neck is limited to approximately *70%* of normal. (70 percent also correct)
5. The date on the cholecystogram was *September 1, 1991.*
6. Estimated blood loss was *100 cc;* none was replaced. (note semicolon)
7. At *2 a.m.*, the patient*'s* temperature was *38.9°C*. (also *38.9 degrees Celsius;* also capital *AM*)
8. The *PA* and right lateral roentgenograms show a fracture of the right *third* and *fourth* ribs.

9. Lenses were prescribed resulting in improvement of his visual acuity to *20/30* in the right eye and *20/45* in the left eye. The visual field examination was normal and the tension is *17 mmHg* of Schiotz with a *5.5-gm* weight. (also *17 mm Hg*) (Note: The medical office record could use the right eye and left eye abbreviations in that sentence so the phrase would appear as follows: 20/30 OD and 20/45 OS.)
10. The *#22* Foley with a *30-cc* bag was then inserted. (*No. 22* also correct)
11. I removed *600 mL* of serosanguineous fluid from the abdomen. (*ml* also correct)

5

A *Answers to* **5–8: SELF-STUDY**

1. The urine was negative for sugar, *pH* was *7.0*, and specific gravity was *1.012*.
2. The *BUN* is *45 mg%*, *1+* protein.
3. I excised a small, well-circumscribed tumor, *2 mm* in diameter.
4. Use a *3M Vi-Drape* to cover the operative site. (3-M might be how you typed it, but this company does not print it that way. *Vi-Drape* is a brand name that you now know. Always expect that words of this sort that are not in the dictionary are brand names. The letter after the hyphen in a brand name is generally capitalized.)
5. She received her *second* dose of *5-FU*.
6. The culture grew *100,000* colonies of *E. coli/cc.* (*E. coli per cubic centimeter* is also correct. In the first example, the abbreviation is used correctly with a symbol (/), and in the second example, the word is written out following the word "per." Consistency is important.)
7. The surgeon asked for a *#7 Jackson* bronchoscope. (also *No. 7*)
8. There were high serum titers of *IgG* antibodies.
9. The phenotype A_2B was found consistently in the family blood history. (A2B also correct)
10. Respirations: *16/min.* (*16 per minute* also correct) (Don't forget to check your punctuation.)

6

Letter Transcription

OBJECTIVES

After reading this chapter and working the exercises, you should be able to

1. Appraise the value of an attractive letter to a business.
2. Assess how the business letter reflects the public image of a medical practice.
3. Describe the specific qualities that make a letter mailable.
4. Demonstrate the three basic mechanical formats of letter preparation.
5. Demonstrate the ability to paragraph properly and to place a letter attractively on a page.
6. Use a specific letter format in preparation of a letter from copy typed as a single paragraph.
7. Prepare envelopes using the recommended U.S. Postal Service procedure.
8. Prepare a two-page letter following the rules for multiple-page letters.
9. Identify the unique format for "To Whom It May Concern" documents.

INTRODUCTION

Letter preparation is unique in many ways and has several special attributes that may make it difficult to plan. These include the following:

1. The overall appearance, which is challenging; unlike documents that are meant only for the medical record, the letter must be attractive. It is the personal representative of the writer and expresses his or her professional standing

through its contents as well as its appearance. You control its appearance, and you may in part control how it reads; thus, it also represents you. The placement of the letter on the page must be considered, with top and bottom white areas taken into account and even and equal margins maintained.

2. Formats are important; traditionally, they are followed exactly.
3. Paragraphing is also important, but it is not easy for the beginner to recognize when shifts to new subject matter occur.
4. Correct punctuation, although important in all documents, can be a particular challenge in letters.
5. Shifts of emphasis and format often are confusing. For example, the dictator may decide to place an abbreviated version of the patient's physical examination within the body of the letter. In this situation, the transcriptionist cannot expect to provide a strictly traditional document and must know how to handle variations in paragraphing.
6. Lengthy lists of enclosures and/or courtesy copies can make it difficult to maintain an attractive overall appearance.
7. Confusing opening and closing remarks often bewilder the novice. For example, the dictator may give both street address and post office box address, dictate a lengthy reference line that is not in the proper sequence, address the recipient of the document by a name other than the one previously dictated (this may be a mistake or a nickname), close the letter with unusual or non-traditional greetings or salutations (e.g., Shalom! Happy New Year! Kindest personal regards) that were not covered in the "placement rules," or sign off with just a first name instead of the usual full name.

In this chapter, all of the standard letter transcription practices are discussed, and some variations are introduced, so you can be confident that you are setting up the document in the best possible order. It should be obvious to you by now that you are the key factor in turning out a product: the letter.

It is important that the letter be perfect in every way, beginning with "eye appeal" and with great attention paid to details. Your success depends on your ability to produce a mailable letter. Therefore, in learning to identify the specific qualities that make a letter mailable, you should also be able to recognize errors in form, grammar, punctuation, typing, and spelling.

VOCABULARY

Open Punctuation: Style of letter punctuation in which no punctuation mark is used after the salutation or complimentary close. (See Fig. 6–1*B*, page •••.)

Mixed Punctuation: Style of letter punctuation in which a colon or a comma is used after the salutation and a comma is used after the complimentary close. (See Fig. 6–1*A*, page 138.)

Letter Format: The mechanical set-up of a letter, which dictates placement of the various letter parts. (See Fig. 6–2, page 141.)

Continuation Sheets: The sheets of paper used to type a second and subsequent pages of a letter. These are often called second sheets.

Full Block: The name of a particular letter format. (See Fig. 6–1*A*, page 137.)

Modified Block: The name of a particular letter format. (See Fig. 6–1*B*, page 138.)

QUALITIES OF A MAILABLE LETTER

1. *Placement.* The letter should:
   a. be attractively placed on the page with the right margin fairly even. Because the right margin is not justified on medical documents, ragged right margins often occur. No more than five characters in variation is ideal, but sometimes this is not possible.
   b. have "eye appeal," with the letterhead taken into consideration when format is chosen.
   c. have picture-frame symmetry as an achievable ideal.
2. *Form.* The following should be taken into consideration:
   a. correct format (such as full block or modified block).
   b. double spacing between paragraphs.
   c. consistent punctuation (open or mixed).
   d. correct use of enclosure and copy notations.
3. *Typing techniques.* There should be no typing, keyboarding, formatting, or printout errors, such as improper word wrapping to the next line; incorrect spacing; transposition of words; typographic errors; material omitted; or words divided incorrectly at the end of a line.
4. *Proper mechanics.* You should show proper knowledge of technical writing techniques (e.g., abbreviations, numbers, and symbols). (See Chapter 5.)
5. *Grammar use.* The words in the letter should be

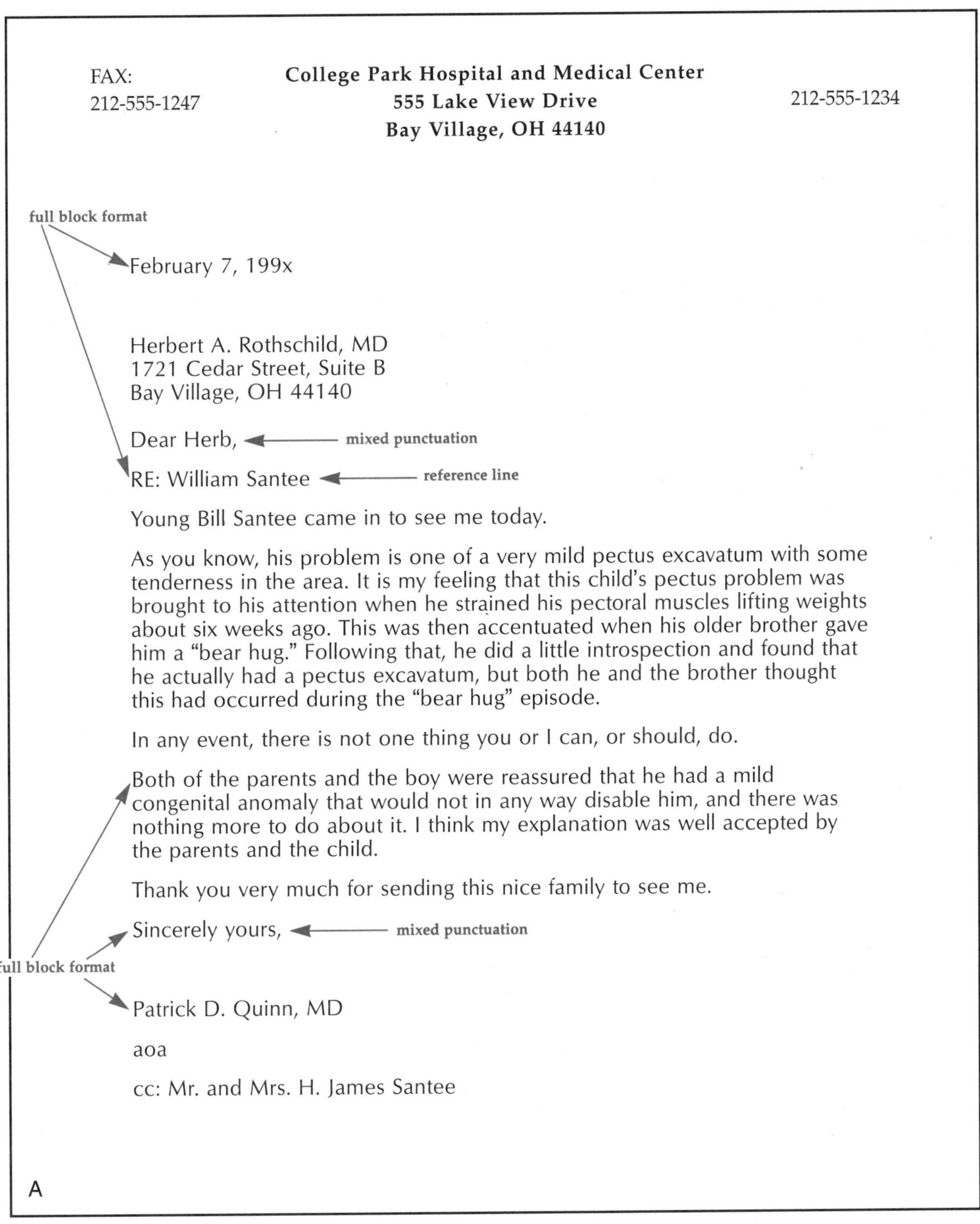

FAX:
212-555-1247

College Park Hospital and Medical Center
555 Lake View Drive
Bay Village, OH 44140

212-555-1234

February 7, 199x

Herbert A. Rothschild, MD
1721 Cedar Street, Suite B
Bay Village, OH 44140

Dear Herb,

RE: William Santee

Young Bill Santee came in to see me today.

As you know, his problem is one of a very mild pectus excavatum with some tenderness in the area. It is my feeling that this child's pectus problem was brought to his attention when he strained his pectoral muscles lifting weights about six weeks ago. This was then accentuated when his older brother gave him a "bear hug." Following that, he did a little introspection and found that he actually had a pectus excavatum, but both he and the brother thought this had occurred during the "bear hug" episode.

In any event, there is not one thing you or I can, or should, do.

Both of the parents and the boy were reassured that he had a mild congenital anomaly that would not in any way disable him, and there was nothing more to do about it. I think my explanation was well accepted by the parents and the child.

Thank you very much for sending this nice family to see me.

Sincerely yours,

Patrick D. Quinn, MD

aoa

cc: Mr. and Mrs. H. James Santee

Figure 6–1. Letters illustrating various styles and punctuation. *A*, Full-block style and mixed punctuation.

Illustration continued on following page

used correctly in accordance with their meaning (e.g., all ready/already).

Homonyms should be used correctly (e.g., their/there, site/sight/cite).

Contractions should be avoided whenever possible.

6. *Spelling.* There must be no doubt about the correct spelling of a word, and a dictionary must be consulted without hesitation. (See Chapter 8.)
7. *Overall appearance.* Be sure to check the following:
   a. printout is easily readable.

6

FAX: 212-555-1247

College Park Hospital and Medical Center
555 Lake View Drive
Bay Village, OH 44140

212-555-1234

February 7, 199x

modified block

Herbert A. Rothschild, MD
1721 Cedar Street, Suite B
Bay Village, OH 44140

RE: William Santee

Dear Herb ← open punctuation

reference line (breaking the placement rule)

Young Bill Santee came in to see me today.

As you know, his problem is one of a very mild pectus excavatum with some tenderness in the area. It is my feeling that this child's pectus problem was brought to his attention when he strained his pectoral muscles lifting weights about six weeks ago. This was then accentuated when his older brother gave him a "bear hug." Following that, he did a little introspection and found that he actually had a pectus excavatum, but both he and the brother thought this had occurred during the "bear hug" episode.

In any event, there is not one thing you or I can, or should, do.

Both of the parents and the boy were reassured that he had a mild congenital anomaly that would not in any way disable him, and there was nothing more to do about it. I think my explanation was well accepted by the parents and the child.

Thank you very much for sending this nice family to see me.

open punctuation

Sincerely yours

modified block

Patrick D. Quinn, MD

aoa

cc: Mr. and Mrs. H. James Santee

B

Figure 6–1 *Continued.* *B,* Modified-block style and open punctuation. Illustrates reference line that breaks the placement rule.

b. page start up and page breaks are correct.
c. letterhead is not in conflict with printout.

8. *Content.* Be sure of the following:
   a. accurate as dictated.
   b. no material is omitted.
   c. no material is changed to alter the meaning of the letter.

LETTER FORMATS

Secretarial manuals illustrate and name many different formats in which letters may be prepared. There are variations in the names given to these arrangements, but the formats are standard.

The following formats have been named to match closely those names you might already have

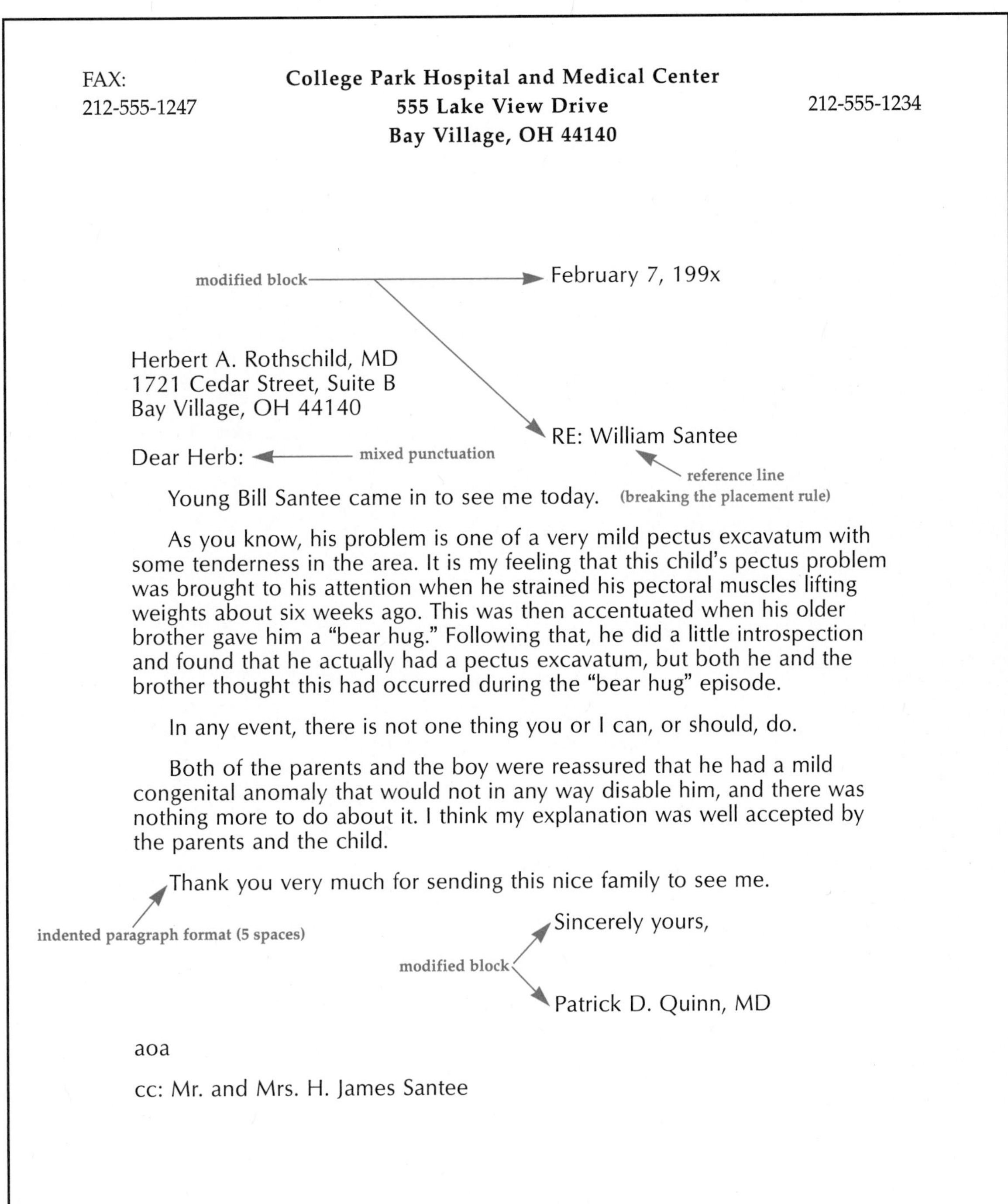

FAX:
212-555-1247

College Park Hospital and Medical Center
555 Lake View Drive
Bay Village, OH 44140

212-555-1234

February 7, 199x

Herbert A. Rothschild, MD
1721 Cedar Street, Suite B
Bay Village, OH 44140

RE: William Santee

Dear Herb:

Young Bill Santee came in to see me today.

As you know, his problem is one of a very mild pectus excavatum with some tenderness in the area. It is my feeling that this child's pectus problem was brought to his attention when he strained his pectoral muscles lifting weights about six weeks ago. This was then accentuated when his older brother gave him a "bear hug." Following that, he did a little introspection and found that he actually had a pectus excavatum, but both he and the brother thought this had occurred during the "bear hug" episode.

In any event, there is not one thing you or I can, or should, do.

Both of the parents and the boy were reassured that he had a mild congenital anomaly that would not in any way disable him, and there was nothing more to do about it. I think my explanation was well accepted by the parents and the child.

Thank you very much for sending this nice family to see me.

Sincerely yours,

Patrick D. Quinn, MD

aoa

cc: Mr. and Mrs. H. James Santee

Figure 6–1 *Continued.* *C*, Modified-block style with indented paragraphs and mixed punctuation.

learned and, at the same time, to describe as nearly as possible the appearance of the letter:

Full Block (Fig. 6–1*A*). This is the most frequently used format. Notice that the date line, address, salutation, reference line, all lines of the body of the letter, complimentary close, and typed signature line are flush with the left margin. This is a popular format because no tab stops are needed. As long as it is compatible with the letterhead and the wishes of the dictator, you may use it.

Modified Block (Fig. 6–1*B*). The date line, reference line, complimentary close, and typed signa-

PERFECT PUNCTUATION COMPANY
2526 LA MAL AVENUE
SAN VALLEY, CA 92014
(714) 555-7185

July 16, 199x

Ms. Amy L. WIng
1234 College Avenue
Columbus, OH 43201

Dear Ms. Wing:

1

Sincerely yours,

Robert T. Bowhay, President

mlo

cc: Eric T. Myhre

PERFECT PUNCTUATION COMPANY
2526 LA MAL AVENUE
SAN VALLEY, CA 92014
(714) 555-7185

May 29, 199x

Ms. Amy L. WIng
1234 College Avenue
Columbus, OH 43201

Dear Ms. Wing

2

Sincerely

(Mrs.) Nora George
Secretary

Enclosure

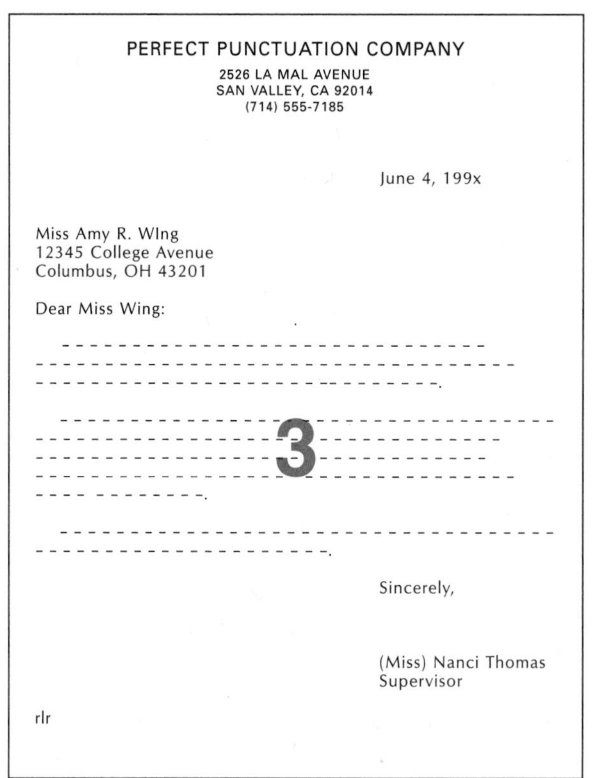

PERFECT PUNCTUATION COMPANY
2526 LA MAL AVENUE
SAN VALLEY, CA 92014
(714) 555-7185

June 4, 199x

Miss Amy R. WIng
12345 College Avenue
Columbus, OH 43201

Dear Miss Wing:

3

Sincerely,

(Miss) Nanci Thomas
Supervisor

rlr

D

Figure 6–1 *Continued.* *D-1,* Full-block style and mixed punctuation. *D-2,* Modified block style and open punctuation. *D-3,* Modified-block style with indented paragraphs and mixed punctuation.

ture line are typed to begin just to the right of the middle of the page. This format has a little more "personality" and is compatible with most letterheads. Most dictators are comfortable with the signature area.

Notice that placement of the date line sets your format. If you place the date at the left margin, you must continue with full-block format. If you place your date at the center point, you must follow through with this format, making sure that the complimentary close and typed signature line are lined up with it.

Modified Block with Indented Paragraphs (Fig. 6–1*C*). The third and final format is not as popular as the first two because of the tab stop necessary at each paragraph. It is a traditional format and might be preferred by the dictator. Additional formats you may have learned in business typing classes are not used for medical letters because they are too informal.

Many general business offices have one letter format that is used by all the secretaries in the company. However, you may find that there are few formal rules about letter styles in a hospital or medical office. Figure 6–1*D* illustrates all three variations.

Each of the following items refers to the corresponding number in Figure 6–2; refer to this figure as we examine a business letter and discuss its components.

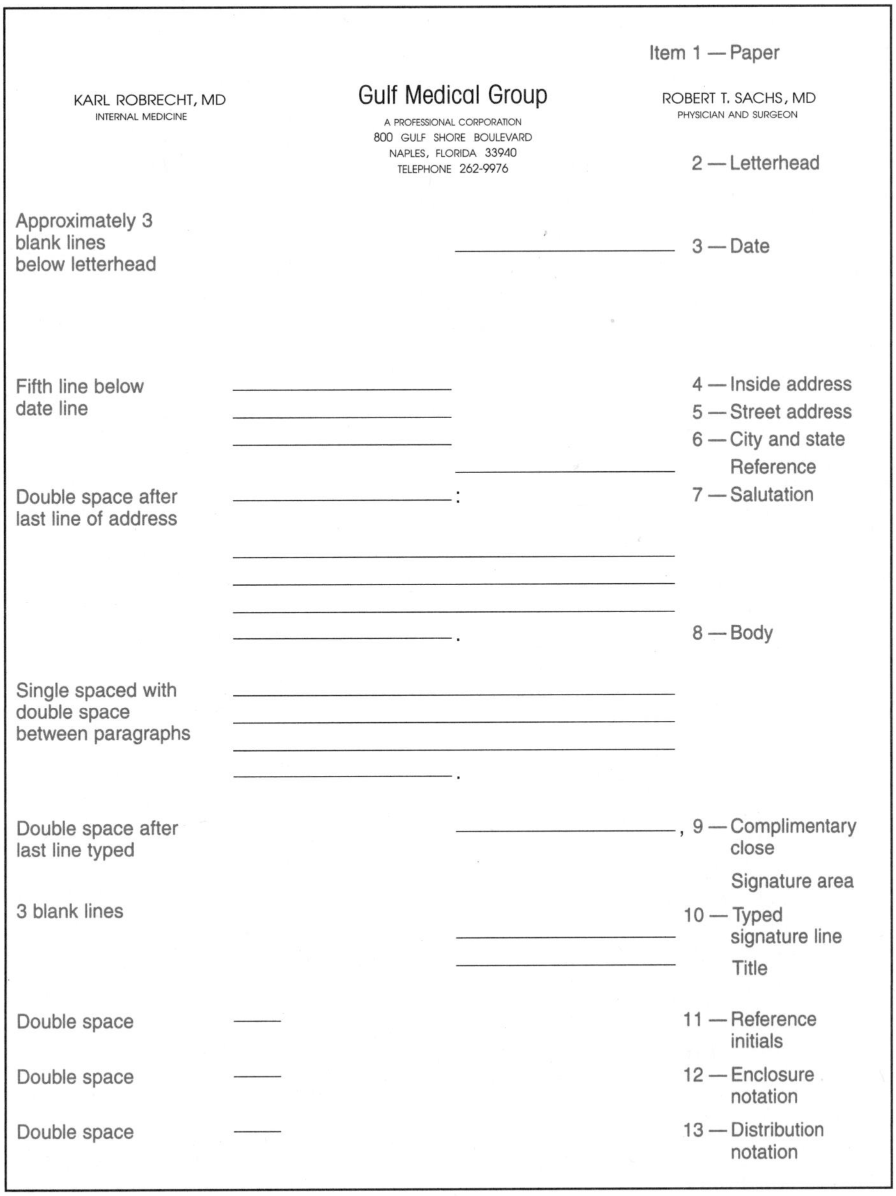

6

Item 1 — Paper

KARL ROBRECHT, MD
INTERNAL MEDICINE

Gulf Medical Group
A PROFESSIONAL CORPORATION
800 GULF SHORE BOULEVARD
NAPLES, FLORIDA 33940
TELEPHONE 262-9976

ROBERT T. SACHS, MD
PHYSICIAN AND SURGEON

2 — Letterhead

Approximately 3 blank lines below letterhead ________ 3 — Date

Fifth line below date line ________ 4 — Inside address
________ 5 — Street address
________ 6 — City and state
________ Reference

Double space after last line of address ________: 7 — Salutation

____
____
____
________. 8 — Body

Single spaced with double space between paragraphs
____
____
____
________.

Double space after last line typed ________, 9 — Complimentary close

Signature area

3 blank lines ________ 10 — Typed signature line
________ Title

Double space ___ 11 — Reference initials

Double space ___ 12 — Enclosure notation

Double space ___ 13 — Distribution notation

Figure 6–2. Business letter set-up mechanics showing modified-block format and mixed punctuation. (See text for a description of each item illustrated.)

Item 1—Paper

Standard 8 1/2 × 11 inch, 25 percent cotton content bond paper is most often used. The paper is usually white, although off-white or eggshell may be preferred. Be sure that the paper is compatible with the printer and inserted properly.

Item 2—Letterhead

6

The letterhead must be appropriate and current. The physician will use stationery with his or her name (or the corporate name) and address printed on it. Other information, such as the telephone number, fax number, medical specialty, or board membership, is often included. The letterhead should be confined to the top 2 inches of the page. Avoid a letterhead that is continued to the bottom of the page because it makes placement difficult, and the style is unnecessary. Printed borders on the paper are equally distracting.

Many physicians choose to have steel die engraved letterheads. Engraving makes the finest quality letterhead; it looks very professional and will further enhance the appearance of the correspondence. Thermographing (raised printing) is also popular.

Embossing and color art, which are very popular on business letters, were seldom seen on physicians' letterheads until recently. However, these are gaining in popularity. Be sure to obtain the approval of your employer before you change the letterhead, the type of printing, or the quality of the paper you have been using.

Continuation sheets do not have a letterhead but are of the same color and quality as the first sheet. When using continuation sheets, be careful to print out on the face of the paper. You can tell the face from the back by holding the paper to the light. The watermark (a faint symbol that is part of the paper) will be visible and can be read from the front. If you print out on the back, the paper may appear to be of a different color and texture and will not match your letterhead paper.

Number 10 (4 1/8 × 9 1/2) envelopes should match the paper in color and quality. The return address is engraved or printed to match the letterhead. Because the envelope is the first impression one makes on a correspondent, deliberate care must be taken in its preparation.

A variety of typefaces and set-up styles are available (Fig. 6–3). The secretary may be asked to set up an appropriate letterhead when a change is made in what is currently being used. A reputable printer will provide you with a list of available typefaces and will help you design an attractive letterhead.

Item 3—Date

The date is in keeping with the format of the letter and is placed in line with the complimentary close and typed signature line. It is typed approximately three lines below the letterhead (no closer but you may drop it farther down for a brief letter). The date used is the day on which the material was dictated and *not* the day on which it was transcribed. This is very important because comments made in the document could reflect on this date. Spell out the date in full in either the traditional or the military style. Note the use of the comma in the example of the traditional style below.

EXAMPLES

December 22, 199X (traditional style)
22 December 199X (British and military style)

Item 4—Inside Address

The inside address is typed flush with the left margin and is begun on approximately the fifth line below the date (it may be moved up or down a line or two depending on the length of the letter). The name of the person or firm is copied exactly as printed on their letterhead or as printed in the medical society directory or the telephone book. A courtesy title is added to a name. If you do not know whether the person is a man or woman, use the title "Mr." The title "Ms." is used when you do not have a title for a woman; it is also used as a substitute for "Miss" or "Mrs." because many women prefer this use. The degree is preferred over a title in the case of a physician, and in no case should a title and a degree be used together. Use the middle initial when it is known.

EXAMPLES

Ms. Mary T. Jordan
Professor Otis R. Laban
Drs. Reilly, Lombardo, and Hamstead
Dora F. Hodge, MD
Captain Denis K. Night
Glenn M. Stempien, DDS
Neal J. Kaufman, MD, FACCP
Rabbi Bernice Gold
Paul Kip Barton, MD, MAJ, USN

Or when title and/or name is lengthy:

William Peter Sloan-Wilson, MD
Captain, USN, USCG

KARL ROBRECHT, MD
INTERNAL MEDICINE

ROBERT T. SACHS, MD
PHYSICIAN AND SURGEON

Gulf Medical Group
A PROFESSIONAL CORPORATION
800 GULF SHORE BOULEVARD
NAPLES, FLORIDA 33940
TELEPHONE 262-9976

College Park Hospital and Medical Center
555 Lake View Drive
Bay Village, OH 44140

Patrick D. Quinn, Administrator
(216) 871-9486
Fax (216) 555-9486

THORACIC SURGERY MEDICAL GROUP, INC.
ROBERT T. STIENWAY, MD
STEPHEN R. CLAWSON, MD
CHRISTIAN M. LOW, MD
MARY SUE LOW, MD

504 WARFORD DRIVE
SYRACUSE, NEW YORK 13224
TELEPHONE 466-4307

19098 CHATAM ROAD
SYRACUSE, NEW YORK 13203
TELEPHONE 279-2345

Kwei-Hoy Wong, MD
1654 PIIKEA STREET
HONOLULU, HAWAII 96818
TELEPHONE 534-0922

DIPLOMATE, AMERICAN BOARD
OF OTOLARYNGOLOGY

EAR, NOSE THROAT,
HEAD AND NECK SURGERY

Figure 6–3. Letterhead styles and type faces.

NOT: Dr. Clifford F. Adolph, MD
Dr. Bertrum L. Storey, PhD

If a business title accompanies the name, it may follow the name on the same line, or, if lengthy, it may appear on the next line. (Note the punctuation in the examples.)

EXAMPLES

F. E. Stru, MD, Medical Director

Ms. Sheila O. Wendall
Purchasing Agent

Adrian N. Abott, MD
Chief-of-Staff
Sinai-Lebanon Hospital

Item 5—Street Address

Following the name of the person or firm is the street or post office box address. (If both are given, use the post office box address. The street address has been provided for those visiting the firm; they may not even have the facilities for receiving mail there. If the post office box is given, they have indicated that they prefer post office box delivery.) Abbreviations are permitted *after* the street name only; they include NW, NE, SW, and so on. Do not abbreviate North, South, East, West, Road, Street, Avenue, or Boulevard. "Apartment" is abbreviated only if the line is unusually long. The apartment, suite, or space number is typed on the same line with the street address, separated by a comma.

6

EXAMPLES

321 Madison Avenue
1731 North Branch Road, Suite B
845 Medford Circle, Apartment 54
8895 Business Park NW
P.O. Box 966
P.O. Box 17433, Foy Station

If all of the delivery address line information cannot be typed in a single line above the city, state, and ZIP code, then place the secondary address information (e.g., suite, apartment, building, room, space numbers) on the line immediately *above* the delivery address line. This may seem awkward, but this is the correct placement. The envelope address is generally a copy of the inside address, and post office personnel read only the last two lines of the address, so these lines must contain the street address, city, state, and ZIP codes. The mail carrier is the only one interested in the suite, apartment, or space number. When you do not know whether a suite or apartment is indicated, use the pound sign (#), space, and the number you have been given.

EXAMPLES OF ENTIRE ADDRESS

Mrs. Lila Hadley
Apartment 21
1951 52nd Street
Tucson, AZ 85718

Mrs. Marijane Simmons
8840 Marshall Place #5
Jamestown, NY 14701

Item 6—City and State

The name of the city is spelled out and separated from the state name with a comma. The state name may be spelled out or abbreviated and is separated from the ZIP code by one to three spaces and no punctuation. The U.S. Postal Service abbreviations are not used without the ZIP code. (See Appendix B.)

EXAMPLE

Honolulu, Hawaii 96918 or Honolulu, HI 96918

NOT: Honolulu, HI

Item 7—Salutation

The salutation is typed a double space below the last line of the address, as follows:

1. Open punctuation format: no mark of punctuation used.
2. Mixed punctuation format (formal): followed by a colon.
3. Mixed punctuation format (informal—first name used): followed by a comma or a colon.

EXAMPLES

Open: Dear Mr. Walsh
Mixed (formal): Dear Mr. Walsh:
Mixed (informal): Dear Don: or Dear Don,

See Figure 6–1*A* and *C* for examples of mixed punctuation and Figure 6–1*B* for an example of open punctuation.

EXAMPLES OF SALUTATIONS USED FOR MEN, SHOWING MIXED PUNCTUATION

Gentlemen:
Dear Mr. Sutherland:
Dear Dr. Hon:
Dear Drs. Blake and Fortuna:
Dear Dr. Blake and Dr. Fortuna:
Dear Rabbi Ruderman: (likewise Father, Bishop, Reverend, Monsignor, Cardinal, Brother, Deacon, Chaplain, Dean, and so on)
Dear Mr. Tony Lamb and Mr. Peter Lamb:

EXAMPLES OF SALUTATIONS USED FOR WOMEN, SHOWING MIXED PUNCTUATION

Ladies:
Mesdames:
Dear Dr. Martin:
Dear Mrs. Clayborne:
Dear Ms. Robinson:
Dear Judge Peterson: (likewise Reverend, Rabbi, Chaplain, Dean, Deacon, Bishop, Captain, Professor, and so on)
Dear Sister Rose Anthony:
Dear Miss Thomas and Mrs. Farintino:

EXAMPLES OF SALUTATIONS USED FOR ADDRESSING MEN AND WOMEN TOGETHER

Dear Sir or Madam:
Ladies and Gentlemen:
Dear Doctors:
Dear Mr. and Mrs. Knight:
Dear Dr. and Mrs. Wong:
Dear Professor Holloway and Mr. Blake:
Dear Drs. Candelaria or Dear Dr. Lois Candelaria and Dr. Fred Candelaria:
Dear Mr. Clayborne and Mrs. Steen-Clayborne:
Dear Dr. Petroski and Mr. Petroski:
Dear Captain and Mrs. Philips:
Dear Dr. Mitchelson et al.: (used for addressing large groups of men and/or women)

Item 8—Body

The body of the letter is begun a double space from the salutation or the reference line (when used here) and is single spaced. (Even very brief letters are single spaced.) The first and subsequent lines are flush with the left margin unless indented paragraphs are used, in which case the first line of each paragraph is indented five spaces. There is always a double space between paragraphs.

Make use of tabulated copy when it is appropriate. This will add emphasis to the material, make the letter easier to read, and add visual interest. This part of the letter is indented at least five spaces from *each* margin. Figure 6–4 illustrates two examples of appropriate use of tabulated copy.

6

William A. Berry, MD
3933 Navajo Road
San Diego California 92119

619-463-0000 Fax 619-463-0000

March 27, 199x

Mrs. Lila Hadley
1951 52nd Street, Apartment 21
Tucson, AZ 85718

Dear Mrs. Hadley:

This is in reply to your letter concerning the results of your tests that were done here and by Dr. Galloway.

1) Intestinal symptoms, secondary to a lactase deficiency.

2) Generalized arteriosclerosis.

3) Mitral stenosis and insufficiency.

4) History of venous aneurysm.

You were seen on February 2, at which time you were having some stiffness at the shoulders which I felt was likely to be due to a periarthritis. This is a stiffness of the shoulder capsule.

Figure 6–4. Letters illustrating use of tabulated copy.

Illustration continued on following page

Kwei-Hoy Wong, MD

1654 PIIKEA STREET
HONOLULU HAWAII 96818
TELEPHONE 534-0922

DIPLOMATE, AMERICAN BOARD
OF OTOLARYNGOLOGY

EAR, NOSE THROAT,
HEAD AND NECK SURGERY

6

March 27, 199x

Roy V. Zimmer, MD
6280 Jackson Drive
San Antonio, TX 78288

Re: Mrs. Florida Sanchez

Dear Roy:

Thank you for referring Mrs. Florida Sanchez to my office. She was first seen on February 17, 199x.

Her past history is of no great significance and will not be reiterated at this time.

Physical examination revealed the following:

Thyroid: Normal to palpation, with no cervical adenopathy.

Breasts: No masses, tenderness or axillary adenopathy.

Abdomen: Flat. Liver, kidneys, and spleen not felt. There is a well-healed McBurney scar present. No masses, tenderness, or

Figure 6–4 *Continued*

When the dictator decides to include an outline for the proposed plan for the care of the patient, an abbreviated version of the patient's past or present history, or a brief physical examination, prepare it in the form as illustrated. Be sure you carry the block indentation to continuing pages when necessary, and remember to return to the established margin when this material is complete.

Item 9—Complimentary Close

The complimentary close is lined up with the date and is typed a double space below the last typed line. Only the first word is capitalized. A comma is used after the close if a colon appears with the salutation (mixed punctuation). No punctuation mark is used with the "open" format. If the author of the document dictates some other greeting at the end of the letter, such as "Kindest personal regards," "Merry Christmas to Janet and the children," "Happy New Year!" "Regards in the holiday season," and so on, type it as a final paragraph, and use the complimentary close as usual.

EXAMPLES OF MIXED PUNCTUATION

Sincerely,
Yours very truly,

EXAMPLES OF OPEN PUNCTUATION

Sincerely
Yours very truly

See Figure 6–1 for mixed and open punctuation examples.

Item 10—Typed Signature Line

The dictator's or writer's name is typed exactly as it appears in the letterhead, with three blank lines inserted after the complimentary close. Press the return/enter key four times after you type the complimentary close. Then type the name lined up with the complimentary close. If an official title accompanies the name, it may appear on the same line, preceded by a comma, or be typed on the line directly below the signature without a comma. If the dictator signs off with just a first name, type his or her complete name (and title, if there is one).

EXAMPLE

Sincerely,

Samuel R. Wong, MD
Chief-of-Staff

EXAMPLE

Yours very truly,

Kathryn B. Black, MD, Medical Director

Note the punctuation.

NOTE: An office employee using the letterhead stationery will always identify his or her position in the firm and provide a courtesy title. The title enables the correspondent to have a title to use in writing or telephoning. The title is enclosed in parentheses.

EXAMPLES

(Ms.) Lynmarie Myhre, CMT, Secretary

(Mrs.) Elvira E. Gonsalves
Receptionist

(Miss) Paula de la Vera, CMA-A
Office Manager

Item 11—Reference Initials

The transcriptionist's initials are typed a double space below the typed signature, flush with the left margin. Only two or three of the transcriptionist's initials are used, and humorous or confusing combinations are avoided. Do not type your initials when you type a letter for your own signature.

EXAMPLES

crc (rather than cc)
db (rather than dmb)
dg (rather than dog)

NOTE: If the dictator wants his or her initials used, they will precede the initials of the typist, or if the dictator differs from the person who signs the document, the dictator's, the signer's, and the typist's initials are used.

EXAMPLES

lrc/wpd or lrc:wpd
RF:BJT:wpd

6

Item 12—Enclosure Notation

If the dictator is enclosing one or more items with the letter, attention is called to the item or items with a notation. The notation is typed flush with the left margin, and the number of enclosures should be noted if there are more than one. A wide variety of styles is acceptable. We have underlined the example most commonly used.

EXAMPLES

Enc.   <u>Enclosure</u>   Check enclosed
Enc. 2   2 Enc.   2 enclosures
Enclosures
Enclosures: 2
Enclosed: (1) Operative report
(2) Pathology report
(3) History and physical

NOTE: This last notation can help you ensure that all items are enclosed before the letter is sealed. The recipient's secretary should also check the enclosure line when the letter is opened to ensure that he or she has all of the mentioned items before the envelope is discarded.

Item 13—Distribution Notation

It is understood that a file copy is made of every item prepared by the secretary/transcriptionist. If a copy of the correspondence is sent *to someone else,* this is noted on the original copy. The notation is typed flush with the left margin a double space below the reference initials or last notation made. A variety of styles is used, and all are followed by the complete name of the recipient. A colon may be used with the notation. Even though most copies mailed out today are photocopies rather than carbon copies of the original, the abbreviation "cc" remains correct and popular. It used to mean "carbon copy" and now means "courtesy copy."

6

EXAMPLES

cc: Frank L. Naruse, MD
c: Ruth Chriswell, Business Manager
CC Hodge W. Lloyd
Copy: Carla P. Ralph, Buyer
Copies: Kristen A. Temple
Anthony R. McClintock

Because most copies mailed out today are photocopies, some people prefer to use the abbreviation "pc."

EXAMPLE

pc: John Smith

NOTE: You *never* type a copy notation without a name following it.

If you have a very lengthy list of copy notations, consider making a two- or three-column list rather than a long string that could affect another page.

EXAMPLE

CC:	Claire Duennes, MD	Norman Szold, MD
	Sharon Kirkwood, MD	James Tanaka, MD
	Amrum Lambert, MD	Robert Wozniak, MD
	Clifford Storey, MD	Vell Yaldua, MD

OTHER LETTER MECHANICS

Blind Carbon Copy

If the sender wishes a copy of the correspondence to be sent to a third party and does not wish the recipient of the original copy to know that this was done, he will direct that a "blind copy" be mailed. Do *not* make a copy notation on the original but do make a notation on the file copy with the name of the recipient following the notation. Use of a removable adhesive note on the original letter will show the "bcc" notation on your filed photocopy.

EXAMPLE
(typed on file copy only)

bcc: Ms. Penelope R. Taylor

Postscript

The postscript is typed one double space below the last reference notation and is flush with the left margin. The abbreviation "P.S." usually introduces the item. You may use P.S.: or PS:

NOTE: The P.S. can be an afterthought or a statement deliberately withheld from the body of the letter for emphasis or a restatement of an important thought (e.g., a telephone number in a letter of application). A handwritten afterthought, added by the dictator, does not need to be introduced with "P.S."

EXAMPLE
(afterthought)

P.S. By the way, I saw Flo Douglas in the elevator in St. Michael's Hospital the other day. She has certainly recovered nicely from her surgery.

EXAMPLE
(emphasis)

P.S. Please do not hesitate to call on me if I can help you in any way.

If the postscript is longer than one line, indent any subsequent lines to align with the first word of the message.

If the transcriptionist has made a rough copy of the letter, he or she may insert an "afterthought P.S." in the appropriate place in the final copy. If the original P.S. reads "By the way, I will return the x-rays to your office after I see Mrs. Theobald next week," you insert the same statement in the body of the letter where the x-rays were last mentioned and then eliminate the P.S. This is very easy to accomplish with the "cut and paste" feature of the word processing software.

Attention Line

The attention line is typed two spaces below the last line of the address. "Attention" may be spelled out in full caps or with only the first letter capitalized. It is not abbreviated, nor is any punctuation used with it. The attention line is used so that the letter will receive attention by a specific person if he or she is available; if not, another member of the firm will take care of the matter. The appropriate salutation with an attention line is "Gentlemen" or "Dear Sir or Madam," because the letter is addressed to the firm. The salutation should agree with the first line of the address. See example on page 149.

Avoid the use of the attention line unless it is necessary. A letter should be addressed to the person you wish to receive it; in the following example, that would be Josephine Simmons, and it would be awkward to begin your letter "Dear Dr. Parsons:".

John R. Parsons, MD
321 Fifth Avenue, Suite B
Altamont Springs, FL 32716

Attention Josephine Simmons, Administrator

PERFECT PUNCTUATION COMPANY
2526 LA MAL AVENUE
SAN VALLEY, CA 92014
(714) 555-7185

August 18, 199x

Engraved Letterhead Company
2171 Lincoln Boulevard
Philadelphia, PA 19105

ATTENTION Mr. Charles P. Trask, Buyer

Gentlemen:

However, "Dear Dr. Parsons:" is the correct greeting for the above example. Therefore, place Josephine Simmons' name above Dr. Parsons' name in the address and place the "in care of symbol" (c/o) in front of Dr. Parsons' name, as shown.

Ms. Josephine Simmons, Administrator
c/o John R. Parsons, MD
321 Fifth Avenue, Suite B
Altamont Springs, FL 32716

Now, "Dear Josephine" *or* "Dear Ms. Simmons" would be the correct greeting.

To Whom It May Concern

This line is used when you have no person or place to send a document. It is typed in full capitals or the first letter of each word is capitalized. It may be typed flush with the left margin or centered on the page. Open or mixed punctuation is used with it. Generally, the complimentary close is not used with this format.

When a reference line is used with this document, it is double spaced below the "To Whom It May Concern."

EXAMPLE

TO WHOM IT MAY CONCERN:

RE: Rudy Carpenter, SS # 576-39-9654

Reference Line

This is very commonly used in medical correspondence and medicolegal reports. However, it is misplaced so often in documents that transcriptionists who place it correctly not only are in the minority but also begin to think that they are in error. There is no arbitrary rule about this line. Remember that it is considered a part of the body of the letter. The problem with misplacement began when custom dictated that the "rule could be broken" when using modified-block format and the reference line was very brief. The second part of the problem occurred when dictators, unconcerned with style or format, gave information for the reference line before pronouncing the salutation. Finally, instead of taking a single space and then inserting the reference followed by another single space, a double space was made both before and after the reference in the "break the rule" format. Take care to place this line correctly, and begin by looking closely at and studying the examples below, which show both incorrect and correct placements.

EXAMPLES OF REFERENCE LINES INCORRECTLY PLACED

Matthew R. Bates, MD
7832 Johnson Avenue
Denver, CO 80241

RE: Leah Hamlyn

Dear Dr. Bates:

ALSO INCORRECT

Matthew R. Bates, MD
7832 Johnson Avenue
Denver, CO 80241

RE: Leah Hamlyn

Dear Dr. Bates:

6

CORRECT PLACEMENT

Matthew R. Bates, MD
7832 Johnson Avenue
Denver, CO 80241

Dear Dr. Bates:

RE: Leah Hamlyn

ALSO CORRECT (NOTE THE SPACING BETWEEN THE ADDRESS AND SALUTATION)

Matthew R. Bates, MD
7832 Johnson Avenue
Denver, CO 80241

RE: Leah Hamlyn

Dear Dr. Bates:

LENGTHY REFERENCE LINES SHOULD ALWAYS FOLLOW THIS FORMAT

Matthew R. Bates, MD
7832 Johnson Avenue
Denver, CO 80241

Dear Dr. Bates:

RE: Leah Hamlyn, Accident report E 14-78-9865

LINE UP A LONG SET OF REFERENCES

Matthew R. Bates, MD
7832 Johnson Avenue
Denver, CO 80241

Dear Dr. Bates:

RE: Leah Hamlyn
Horizons Insurance Company
Accident report E 14-78-9865

A reference line is used to save time and delay by giving the addressee a specific named reference. It also assists when filing the document. Placement is determined by the letter format chosen. In full-block format it is *always* placed at the left margin. It is typed a double space *below* the salutation because it is considered part of the body of the letter. In modified-block format, one has two choices: (1) flush with the left margin a double space *below* the salutation (this is best used when the line is lengthy) and (2) lined up with the date line of the letter on *the next line* after the city, state, and ZIP code of the address. This final style is called "breaking the format rule" and is popular because it saves two lines of space. It is technically out of place because it appears above the salutation. (See Fig. 6–1*B* and *C*.)

A colon is typed after the RE (or Re), which is used to introduce the reference. After typing the reference line, *single space down one line* and type the salutation.

See Figure 6–1*A*, *B*, and *C* for more examples of reference line placement.

TWO PAGE LETTERS

If a letter is too long for one page, it must be appropriately continued on a second page. The following rules apply:

1. Continue to the second page at the end of a paragraph whenever possible.
2. Carry at least two lines of the paragraph to the second page.
3. Leave at least two lines of a paragraph on the first page.
4. Type no closer than 1 inch from the bottom of the page.
5. Do not divide the last word on the page.
6. Place headings 1 inch from the top of the page.
7. Leave two blank lines between the last line of the heading and the first line of the continuation of the letter. To do this, press the return or enter key three times at the end of the typed data in the heading.

The second sheet or continuation sheet is plain paper that is identical to the letterhead paper. Headings are placed on the second sheet to identify it as belonging to the first sheet. There are two styles for page headings.

EXAMPLE (FOR HORIZONTAL FORM)

RE: Leah Hamlyn	2	October 3, 199X
(patient's name)	*(page number)*	*(date)*

EXAMPLE (FOR VERTICAL FORM)

RE: Leah Hamlyn
Page 2
October 3, 199X

NOTE: The page number is centered in the horizontal form. In a nonmedical letter, the name of the correspondent is listed in place of the patient's name.

Always check your printout to be sure that the page 2 markings appear where they were intended. It is an insult to ask the document author to sign a letter in which new page markings are on the bottom of the page or a few lines into a paragraph on page 2. If documents are printed off-site and you do not have the opportunity to review the final printed document, be sure that someone on-site checks them and the printer set-up for you.

COPIES

The transcriptionist makes a copy of every item he or she types. One needs to ensure with great care that a copy is made of every corrected original before it is mailed. A document may need to be rushed to the mail after signature, so make it a habit to photocopy the letter *before* it is signed. If there are corrections or additions, make another copy and discard the first photocopy. Be sure that good quality paper is used for copies that are mailed out of the office. The office copy becomes part of the patient's permanent record and is filed in his or her chart.

PLACEMENT

Placement should have picture-frame symmetry and balance of the three blank margins and the letterhead. A good rule to follow for margins is to use 2-inch margins with short letters (fewer than 100 words), 1 1/2-inch margins with medium-length letters (100 to 200 words), and 1-inch margins with long (200+ words) letters.

To achieve symmetry and to squeeze a letter onto one page, you may adjust the spacing at the end of the letter (beginning with the typed signature line). Leave two, rather than three, spaces for the signature and single space between the typed signature line, the reference initials, and other notations. If you are using the modified-block format, you may type the reference initials on the same line as the typed signature line to save more space. If you still find that you cannot fit the letter on one page, reformat the letter, widen the margins, and type the final paragraph on a second page.

The visual appeal of the letter is very important. Try to keep the right margin as even as possible, and try not to vary the line length by more than five characters.

Figure 6–5 is a complete letter typed in modified-block format with mixed punctuation; it illustrates proper spacing and margin width. Note the placement of the reference line in particular because it was typed using the "break the rule" placement. (Note: the bottom of the page was cut off to fit the figure size, so it does not properly reflect bottom spacing.)

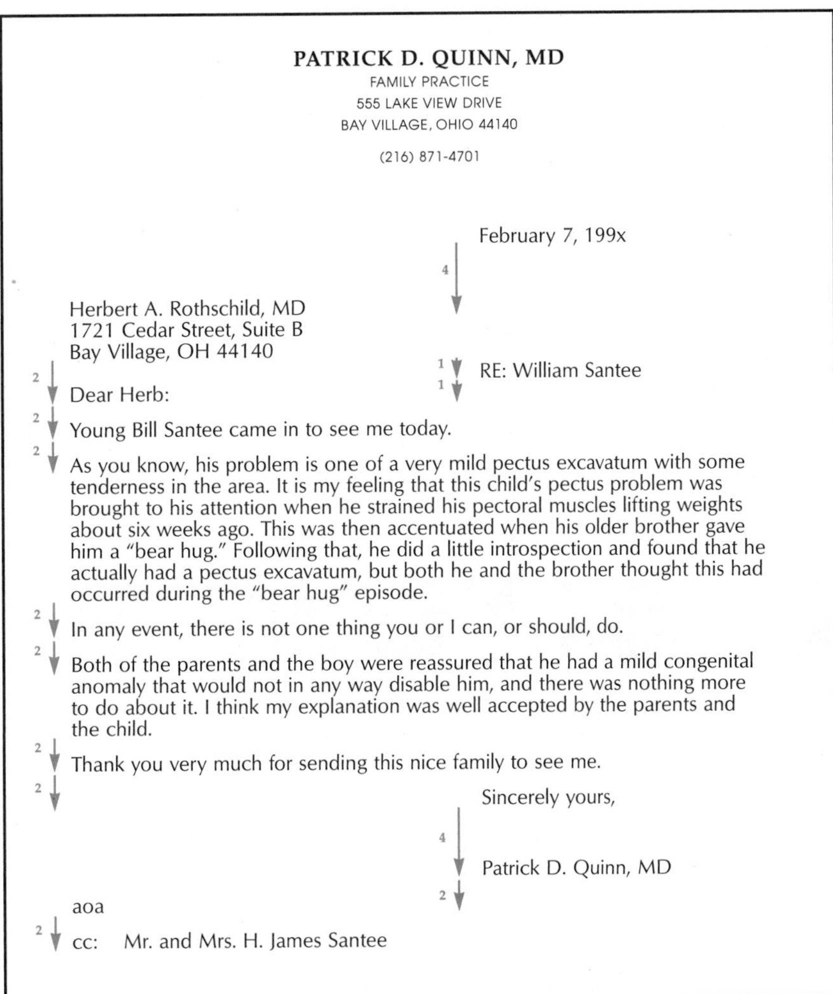

PATRICK D. QUINN, MD
FAMILY PRACTICE
555 LAKE VIEW DRIVE
BAY VILLAGE, OHIO 44140
(216) 871-4701

February 7, 199x

Herbert A. Rothschild, MD
1721 Cedar Street, Suite B
Bay Village, OH 44140

RE: William Santee

Dear Herb:

Young Bill Santee came in to see me today.

As you know, his problem is one of a very mild pectus excavatum with some tenderness in the area. It is my feeling that this child's pectus problem was brought to his attention when he strained his pectoral muscles lifting weights about six weeks ago. This was then accentuated when his older brother gave him a "bear hug." Following that, he did a little introspection and found that he actually had a pectus excavatum, but both he and the brother thought this had occurred during the "bear hug" episode.

In any event, there is not one thing you or I can, or should, do.

Both of the parents and the boy were reassured that he had a mild congenital anomaly that would not in any way disable him, and there was nothing more to do about it. I think my explanation was well accepted by the parents and the child.

Thank you very much for sending this nice family to see me.

Sincerely yours,

Patrick D. Quinn, MD

aoa

cc: Mr. and Mrs. H. James Santee

Figure 6–5. Letter typed in modified-block format and mixed punctuation to illustrate proper spacing and margin width. The illustration is smaller than the standard 8 1/2 × 11 inch paper.

6–1: TYPING ASSIGNMENT

Directions: Retype the following material into letter form. Make a letterhead using a computer macro to match the name of the dictator, inventing an appropriate address, or use any prepared letterhead paper as your instructor directs. Use full-block format, open punctuation, a reference line, and the current date. Refer to the vocabulary list at the beginning of the chapter if necessary. Pay close attention to placement and mechanics. Remember to use the proper state abbreviations you learned in Chapter 4. (See Appendix B.)

6

To help you with placement, notice the length of the material (164 words equals medium length) and place your margins accordingly. Paragraph beginnings are indicated by the symbol ¶. Save this letter after your instructor has checked it because you will need it for Self-Study 6–3.

The letter is from Laurel R. Denison, MD, and is to Gregory O. Theopolis, MD, 4509 Roessler Road, Detroit, Michigan 48224, and is in reference to Bobby West.

Dear Dr. Theopolis ¶ This one-month-old baby was seen in my office yesterday for evaluation of difficulty with the right foot. ¶ The mother reports that this is the third sibling in the family. The older two siblings have no difficulty with the feet. When this baby was born, there was obvious deformity of the right foot which has not corrected itself. ¶ Physical examination reveals that the hips are normal. There is internal tibial torsion. There is pes equinus; there is hindfoot supination and forefoot adduction. It is obvious that this baby has a congenital talipes equinovarus in the right foot. ¶ He was casted in the office yesterday. ¶ We do not know the prognosis yet since this is the first experience with the child. Prognosis depends on the congenital factors that caused the deformity, in the first place, and the elasticity of the tissues, in the second place. We will follow the child at weekly intervals. ¶ Thank you for the opportunity of seeing this baby. Sincerely

6–2: TYPING ASSIGNMENT

Directions: Retype the following material into letter form. Use letterhead paper as your instructor directs. Use modified-block format, mixed punctuation, and a reference line that "breaks the placement rule" placement. (See pages 149 and 150.) Use the current date and the state abbreviation. Pay close attention to placement and mechanics. Notice that the letter contains ________ words, which equals a ________ size letter requiring ________ inch margins. Paragraph beginnings are indicated by the symbol ¶. Remember, we are not making office copies of our documents, but one would *always* do this in the workplace.

This letter is from Emery R. Stuart, MD, to Walter W. von der Meyer, MD, 6754 Sunrise Circle, Ft. Lauderdale, Florida 33312. Copies should be sent to Dr. Barney P. Haber and Dr. Herbert W. Delft. (It is not necessary to make these copies, just the notation.) The patient is Mrs. Nora George.

Dear Walter. ¶ This is a final follow-up letter on Nora George who you will recall was admitted to Sunrise View Hospital in February 199X for aortic valve replacement with a diagnosis of aortic stenosis. ¶ Nora has done well; she is in normal sinus rhythm, and she is well controlled on her Coumadin. She, at times, has some swelling of her hands and feet and has gained considerable weight since surgery. She needs continued close medical observation of her prothrombin level, which should be maintained at about 20% of normal, indefinitely. She should also be maintained on Lanoxin and may possibly require diuretics intermittently. ¶ We will not follow Nora any further for her heart disease. She has had an uneventful postoperative course and can continue her medical follow-up through your office or that of Dr. Herbert Delft, whichever you decide. ¶ Thank you very much for letting us see this patient with you and perform her surgery. We will be glad to see her at any time if there are any questions regarding her valve function or clinical course. Sincerely yours.

Save this letter after your instructor has checked it.

PARAGRAPHING

Paragraphs give the letter shape. The subject is divided into topics, and these topics are paragraphs, which aid the reader by signaling a *new* idea with each division.

The paragraphing will contribute to the visual appeal of the letter and should be well balanced. Therefore, the first and last paragraphs are usually brief, and the middle paragraphs are longer. Nevertheless, a paragraph may be of any length, and you should not hesitate to make one sentence a paragraph when it is appropriate. A series of brief paragraphs in a row, however, can be distracting to the reader. On the other hand, with a brief letter a long paragraph may appear uninviting, and you may have to break it up to provide visual appeal.

Many dictators will not directly indicate the beginning (or end) of a paragraph, but they may give indirect clues with voice inflections or other subtle voice changes. Each new paragraph is begun with a sentence that suggests the topic or further explains it in a different way.

Correct paragraphing is not difficult with most medical letters because the letters generally follow a well-established pattern. The knowledge of this pattern will help you determine the paragraph breaks with or without vocal hints.

Physicians' letters dealing with patient care are usually narrative reports to workers' compensation carriers, consultation reports, follow-up notes, or discharge summaries.

The first paragraph is normally a brief introduction or explanation for the letter. In patient-related letters, the patient and his or her chief complaint are introduced in the initial brief paragraph. The next paragraph may contain the history of the complaint, along with a general description of any contributing problems in the patient's past history. This is followed in the third or fourth paragraph with the findings on examination of the patient. (At times, these remarks may be so brief that they constitute only one sentence.)

The next-to-last paragraph is confined to a medical opinion, prognosis, diagnosis, recommendation, report of tests, results of surgical procedures, detailed outlines for proposed care or treatment, evaluation of return-to-normal status, or summary. Then, the subject is closed in the final paragraph. At this time, the dictator may thank a referring physician, indicate what will take place next with the patient, or request some action on the patient's behalf.

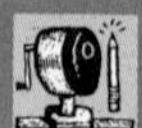 6–3: SELF-STUDY

6

Directions: Obtain your copy of Typing Assignment 6–1. Notice the paragraph breaks. Answer the following questions here or on a separate sheet of paper as your instructor directs.

1. Notice that paragraph 1 is only one sentence long. What does the dictator do with this sentence?

 ______
2. Notice that paragraph 2 is three sentences long. Could the first of these sentences have been placed in the first paragraph? ______ Why or why not? ______
3. What is the dictator *doing* in paragraph 2? ______
4. Could any part of paragraph 3 logically be part of the second or fourth paragraph? ______ Why or why not? ______

 ______
5. What is the dictator *doing* in paragraph 3? ______

 ______
6. Again, we have one sentence in paragraph 4. Could the typist have joined this sentence to paragraph 3? ______ What did the dictator *do* in this paragraph? ______
7. What is the subject of paragraph 5? ______

 Could this paragraph be joined to paragraph 4? ______ Why or why not? ______

 ______
8. Notice the last line of paragraph 5. Could this have been a paragraph on its own? ______ Why or why not? ______ Could you make it a part of the last paragraph? ______ Why or why not? ______

 ______
9. What is the dictator doing in the final paragraph, number 6? ______ Do you think it is appropriate to have this single sentence standing as an entire paragraph? ______ Why or why not? ______

Turn to the end of the chapter for answers to these questions.

6–4: SELF-STUDY

Directions: Obtain your copy of Typing Assignment 6–2. Notice the paragraph breaks. Answer the following questions here or on a separate sheet of paper as your instructor directs.

1. Paragraph 1 tells us the type of document this is. What is it? ______
2. Paragraph 1: What is the subject(s) of this paragraph? ______
3. Paragraph 2. What is the dictator *doing* in this paragraph? ______

 ______

 Could the last two sentences of this paragraph be used to form a new paragraph? ______

 ______

 Why or why not? ______

 ______

4. Paragraph 3. What is the dictator saying in this paragraph?

____

Could this one have been combined with the last two sentences of paragraph two? ________

Why or why not? ____

____

5. Paragraph 4. Subject of this paragraph? ______________________________

Should this be arranged as two short paragraphs? __________________________

See the end of the chapter for the answers.

6

6–5: TYPING ASSIGNMENT

Directions: Retype the following material into letter form using full-block format, mixed punctuation, and the current date. Watch for proper paragraphing, placement and mechanics. Use letterhead paper. Carefully mark your book where you think the paragraph breaks should be. Ask yourself if they follow the pattern you have just learned. If not, consider some different breaks. Remember that there is sometimes more than one choice for a new paragraph break. On your final draft, print a number by each paragraph break. On a separate sheet of paper, type an explanation for that paragraph break, and turn it in with your letter.

The letter is from Steven A. Flores, MD, and is to another physician, Willard R. Beets at 7895 West Sherman Street, San Diego, California 92111. Dear Dr. Beets. I saw Mr. Tim Molton, your patient, in my office yesterday afternoon. As you will recall, Mr. Molton is a 49-year-old professional gardener who came to see you with a chronic cough and a history of expectoration of a whitish material. He brought the x-rays from your office with him, and I noted a fossa on the superficial surface of his lung. He was afebrile today and stated that he had been so since the onset of his symptoms. He did not complain of pain but did experience some dyspnea on exertion and some shortness of breath. I did not carry out a physical examination, but I did skin test him for both tuberculosis and coccidioidomycosis. I did not give him a prescription for any medication and will wait until we get the results of his skin tests. It seems to me that your diagnosis of his problem is correct, so we will proceed with that in mind. As you probably know, valley fever is endemic to San Diego; and since Mr. Molton was born and raised in New York State, he could be very susceptible. You may tell his employer that if he does have valley fever, he will have to convalesce for a month to six weeks, after which time he should be fully able to return to his normal duties. I will keep you posted on the results of his tests. Thank you very much for letting me help you with Mr. Molton's problem. Sincerely.

6–6: TYPING PRACTICE TEST

Directions: Retype this material in letter form. Use modified-block format with indented paragraphs, mixed punctuation, and a reference line. Use letterhead paper. You will have to supply proper punctuation, capitalization, paragraphing, and mechanics. Good luck!

6

may 1 199X ian r wing m d 2261 arizona avenue suite b milwaukee wisconsin 53207 dear dr wing i saw your patient mrs elvira martinez in consultation in my office today. she brought the x-rays from your office with her. she was afebrile today but on questioning admitted a low grade fever over the past few days i removed the fluid as seen on your film of april 30 from the right lower lung field and she felt considerably more comfortable, on thoracentesis there was 50 cc of straw colored fluid her history is well known to you so i will not repeat it. on physical examination i found a well developed well nourished white female with minimal dyspnea there was no lymphadenopathy breath sounds were diminished somewhat on the right there was dullness at the right base the left lung was clear to percussion and auscultation. the remainder of the examination was negative. because of her history of chronic asthma i suggested she might consider bronchoscopy if this fluid reaccumulates. because she is a heavy smoker i insisted she stop smoking completely. if she does not she will not enjoy continuing good health although i have no idea of the actual prognosis. mrs martinez has been returned to you for her continuing care i will be glad to see her again at any time you think it necessary thank you for letting me see this pleasant lady with you sincerely yours jon l mikosan m d ps i am enclosing a copy of the pathology report on the fluid as you can see it is negative

This letter, prepared properly, is in Appendix A. Do not refer to it until your document is complete and printed.

ENVELOPE PREPARATION

A No. 10 (4 1/2 × 9 1/2 inch) envelope, printed to match your letterhead stationery, is always used with your 8 1/2 × 11 inch paper.

The U.S. Postal Service can process mail using an optical character reader (OCR) to read, code, and sort the mail mechanically. However, mail must be prepared properly in a format that the OCR can "read." Nothing other than the address must appear in the "read zone," or it will confuse the scanner. Furthermore, proportional spacing and script type styles should not be used because they do not "read" well.

Here are the guidelines for typing the envelope properly:

1. Type all envelopes in the *block format,* single spaced, 2 inches from the top (12 lines down) and aligned 4 inches from the left edge (Fig. 6–6).

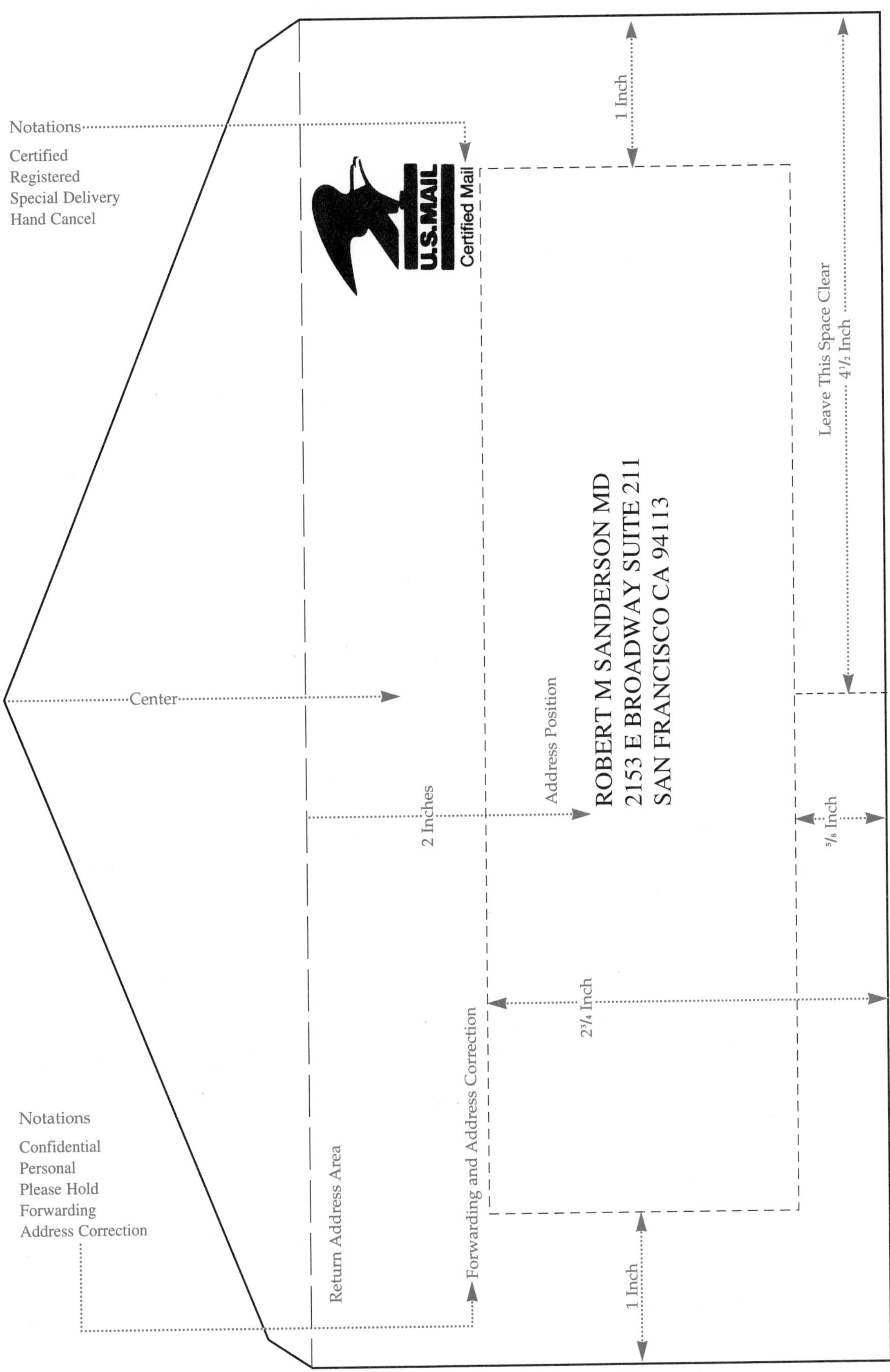

Figure 6–6. Address placement on a No. 10 envelope, showing location for notations. The illustration is smaller than a No. 10 envelope, which is 9 1/2 × 4 1/8 inches.

2. Capitalize *everything*.
3. Eliminate *all* punctuation (periods, commas).
4. Use the standard two-letter state code and the ZIP code.
5. The last line of the address must contain the name of the city, state code, and ZIP code.
6. The address should end at least 5/8 inch from the bottom, parallel with the bottom edge of the envelope (not slanted), and it must end within at least 1 inch from the right edge of the envelope; a near-center location is best. No printing can appear to the left, right, or below the address.

Practice with a No. 10 envelope: Fold it in half and then in half once again. Unfold it and place it in the typewriter. Type your name and address beginning your first line five spaces to the left of your midline crease and directly under your horizontal crease. Type each line beneath the one before. Remove it from the typewriter and examine your placement.

The OCR "reads" only the last two lines of the address and can read only the city, state, and ZIP code as the last line. Therefore, the last line of the address must contain only these items spelled accurately, and nothing must be typed below the last line. The next-to-the-last line must contain the address and street name only. An "Attention" line, when necessary, must be placed as the first or second line of the address, out of the "read zone." Special notations, such as "Special Delivery" or "Certified Mail," should be typed two lines below the postage area. "Personal" or "Confidential" may be typed two lines below the return address.

The only abbreviations permitted are those found in the Abbreviations section of the National ZIP Code Directory. It is unacceptable to abbreviate any city name containing 13 or fewer letters because the OCR will not be able to read a nonstandard abbreviation. The directory gives standard abbreviations for the city names containing more than 13 digits.

Mail addressed to occupants of multiunit buildings should include the number of the apartment, room suite, or other unit. The unit number should appear immediately after the street address on the same line or the line directly above the street address and never below or in front of the street address.

Many computer printers have the capability of copying the address from the letter and printing it directly onto the envelope. Generally, you highlight or block the address to be transferred, access the envelope preparation format, insert an envelope in the printer, and direct the address to print. If you want to use the U.S. Postal Service format, first direct the computer to change your inside address to comply with the guidelines. Usually, this is used for bulk mailings. This format requires you to highlight the address, remove punctuation, change to full capital letters, and make abbreviations where appropriate. There are some font styles that the OCR can read in upper and lower case formats, but the elimination of punctuation and the insertion of abbreviations would be time consuming and probably not worth the effort.

Notice these envelope addresses. Which ones appear neater and will speed their way through the postal service routing machines?

DEMOREST, SEDWICH, AND TRALL
224 East Van Buren Street
Room 22B
FT. WAYNE, INDIANA 46818
ATTN: JOHN DEMOREST, ATTORNEY-AT-LAW

or

JOHN DEMOREST
DEMOREST SEDWICH AND TRALL
224 E VAN BUREN ST ROOM 22 B
FT WAYNE IN 46818

or

DEMOREST SEDWICH AND TRALL
ATTN JOHN DEMOREST
224 E VAN BUREN ST ROOM 22 B
FT WAYNE IN 46818

The "attorney-at-law" title does not have to be placed on the envelope; however, ESQ may be placed after Mr. Demorest's name.

EXAMPLES

Traditional Style	*Recommended Style*
Mrs. Anne Potts Post Office Box 7893 Littleton, Colorado 80120	MRS ANNE POTTS PO BOX 7893 LITTLETON CO 80120
Frank W. Paulson, MD 1335 11th Street Tucson, Arizona 85715	FRANK W. PAULSON MD 1135 11 ST TUCSON AZ 85715

Mrs. Sheila Meadows 8765 Broadway, Suite 16 Los Angeles, CA 90057	MRS SHEILA MEADOWS 8765 BROADWAY SUITE 16 LOS ANGELES CA 90057
National Paper Company 1492 Columbus Avenue, North Syracuse, NY 13224 Attention: Frank Honeywell	ATTN FRANK HONEYWELL NATIONAL PAPER CO 1492 COLUMBUS AVE N SYRACUSE NY 13224 or NATIONAL PAPER CO ATTN FRANK HONEYWELL 1492 COLUMBUS AVE N SYRACUSE NY 13224

6

Mail addressed to a foreign country should have the name of that country as the last line of the address block, placing it a double space below the city, state, and ZIP code line. Coding will vary from country to country.

EXAMPLE

PROF WOLFGANG HINZ
ART DIRECTOR RHINELAND INST
SCHULSTRASSE 21
SIEGELBACH
PFALZ 6751

GERMANY

Mail addressed to members of the military using APO or FPO addresses are set up as follows:

EXAMPLE

JONATHAN R PEZINOSKI WO
COMPANY R
5th INFANTRY REGT
APO NEW YORK NY 09801

6–7: PRACTICE TYPING TEST

Directions: Using the following names and addresses, prepare four No. 10 envelopes using the method recommended by the U.S. Postal Service for OCR processing. Pay close attention to placement, and consult the list of common address abbreviations above. Do not forget to practice with the folded envelope and your own name and address first. Answers are in Appendix A.

1. Noam L. Flickenger, MD
   435 North Michigan Avenue
   Chicago, Illinois 60611

   Special Delivery

2. Mr. Steven R. Madruga
   Post Office Box 9982
   Philadelphia, Pennsylvania 19101

3. Occidental Life Insurance Company
   1150 South Olive, Suite 16
   Los Angeles, California 90015

   ATTENTION Mrs. Sylvia Farquar

4. Ms. Marijane N. Woods
   Manager, Desert Realty
   2036 East Camelback Road
   Phoenix, Arizona 85018

   Confidential

SIGNING AND MAILING

When the letter is ready for signature, use a paper clip to attach the envelope (and any enclosures) to the top of the letter, with the flap over the letterhead. Until you present the letter for signature, keep it in a folder to keep it clean and out of the view of any passerby. After the letter is signed and

No. 10 Envelope (9-1/2 x 4-1/8 Inches)

DO bring up the bottom third of the sheet, and crease. Fold down the upper third of the sheet so the top edge is a one-inch from the first fold, and crease. Insert the last creased edge into the envelope first.

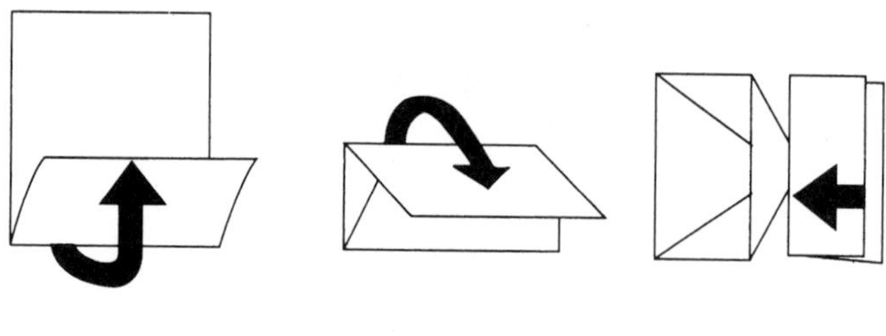

Window Envelope

DO bring up the bottom third of the sheet and fold. Fold the top of the sheet *back* to the first fold so that the inside address is on the outside, and crease. Insert the sheet so the address appears in the window.

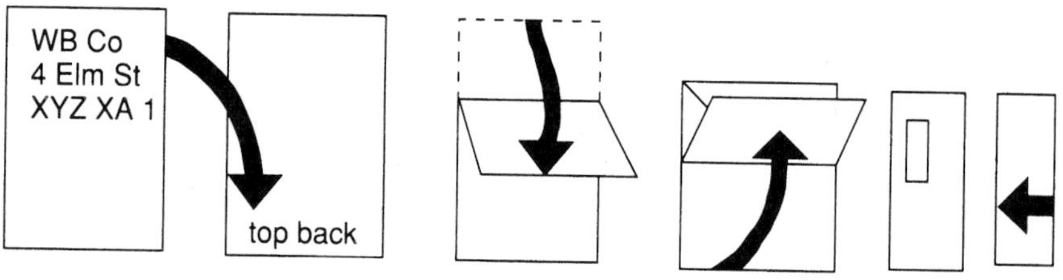

Figure 6–7. Proper ways to fold letters for different types of envelopes. (From Fordney MT, Diehl MO.: *Medical Transcription Guide: Do's and Don'ts*, Philadelphia, WB Saunders, 1990.)

before you place it in its envelope, make sure that there are no smudges and that all enclosures are attached.

Fold the letter by bringing the bottom of the page one third up the page and then creasing. Next, fold the upper third down to within 1/2 inch of the first crease and make the second crease. Insert the letter into the envelope so that when it is removed it will open right side up. Bundle your OCR mail separately and label it "OCR." Figure 6–7 illustrates folding letters.

On occasion, the dictator will be unavailable to sign the mail after dictation but will request that it be sent out rather than delayed for his or her signature. You should handle this as directed, by signing his or her name followed by your initials, by typing below the signature area "Dictated but not signed" followed by your initials, or by simply signing his or her name. Be particularly careful that the letter is completely error free in every way. Keep the copy available for the dictator's return rather than filing it immediately.

A FINAL NOTE

Letterhead stationery in addition to the standard 8 1/2 × 11 inch type is often kept in the office for brief letters or secretarial correspondence. There are two standard sizes: Monarch (7 1/2 × 10 1/2 inches) and Baronial (5 1/2 × 8 1/2 inches). Envelopes are printed to match these two sizes, and papers and envelopes should *not* be mixed. Follow the same general guidelines in preparing the envelopes, except that you should begin the address 2 1/2 inches from the left edge of the envelope rather than 4 inches.

6–8: TYPING REVIEW TEST

Instruction sheet for retyping the following material into letter form.

1. Paper: use letterhead, size 8 1/2 × 11
2. Envelope: use No. 10
3. Copies: single

4. Equipment: typewriter, word processor, computer
5. Format: Modified block, open punctuation
6. Date: May 16 plus current year
7. Mechanical needs: proper paragraphing, placement on page, *some* internal punctuation, other mechanics as may be required
8. Placement on page: proper alignment for attractiveness and "eye appeal"
9. Patient's name: LeeAnn Jensen
10. Dictator: Dr. Randolph R. Bever
11. Addressed to: Dr. Norman C. Kisbey Jr, at Post Office Box 1734, Washington, DC 20034

Dear Dr. Kisbey. Today I have seen your patient Mrs. LeeAnn Jensen in neurosurgical consultation at your request. As you know, she is a very pleasant 40-year-old, right-handed lady who comes in with a history of seizure-like episodes beginning in January of 199X. These seizures consist of a sense of unreality and a feeling as though she were observing herself as an actress on a stage. Prior to the onset of, or associated with, these seizure-like episodes, she has noted a smell of heavy fragrant flowers. She describes the smell of the flowers as slightly unpleasant, almost funereal. Each of these so-called seizure states lasts only a few seconds and is followed by a tremendous feeling of unreality. This is also associated with a great fear that she won't be able to move and she always gets up and walks around afterward to make sure she is not paralyzed. During the episode there is no loss of cognitive ability and she is able to converse with her husband and she has virtually total recall for the entire episode. She had episodes, as described, in January and February of 199X, four in March and five in April. There is no family history of seizures. There is a story of a mild head injury at age ten and apparently she was in a moderately severe motorcycle accident about fifteen years ago which resulted in a broken mandible. The neurological examination at this time is essentially normal. The extraocular movements and fundi show no abnormalities. The visual fields and confrontation testing are intact. There is no Babinski sign. The only abnormality that I could detect in the entire examination was a stiffened right shoulder which she tells me came on after a lengthy game of tennis. I could palpate no masses over the head and there were no audible bruits over the head or over either carotid bifurcation. She had been on a dose of phenobarbital, gr 1, b.i.d. and did not care to add any Dilantin. The phenobarbital keeps her in a drowsy state consequently she is not able to think creatively or participate in sports activities. She brought with her the skull x-rays and brain scan taken at University Hospital and I have reviewed them. In my opinion, they are within normal limits. In addition, she brought with her several EEG records which I have gone over. The neurologist's summary is enclosed. I thought there was a slight abnormality present in the right temporal area. At this time, I do not believe there is evidence of intracranial mass lesion or of focal neurologic deficit. A number of features argue against interpreting her spells as true psychomotor seizures: Firstly, the fact that the aura is unusual, and secondly the fact that she has total recall for the entire episodes. Thirdly, there is the fact that she has no postictal abnormality. My tendency at this time would be to gradually switch her over to Dilantin gr 1 1/2 t.i.d. and, in addition, place her on Diamox, 25 mg each morning. I suggest the Diamox because she tells me that the "seizure" episodes tend to come on within a few days of her menstrual periods. We have agreed that if she is not markedly improved within a period of one month on this regimen she would come into the hospital for 4-vessel angiography. Thank you for the privilege of seeing this interesting patient and for thinking of me in connection with her problems. Yours sincerely. Randolph R. Bever, MD Professor of Neurosurgery, Weeks Medical School.

TRANSCRIPTION EXERCISE

To begin transcribing simple letters, documents 1 through 12 may be found on *Sound Tapes to Accompany Medical Keyboarding, Typing, and Transcribing: Techniques and Procedures, Cassette 1, Side A.*

FOOD FOR THOUGHT

Directions: Imagine for a few minutes that you have just received the letter on page 163 in the mail. Try to read it with the assumption that it is to you personally. What is your reaction to the letter? How many errors can you find?

If nothing else, you have formed a definite opinion about this company based entirely on the written representation of themselves. It is doubtful that you would consider asking them for any information about their tours. Nor would you give them further thought other than to wonder how they stay in business. Certainly, you would not feel they could be trusted to handle a tour because they are unable to handle their correspondence.

The recipients of your office correspondence will be equally affected by the preparation and thought that go into the letters they receive from your office. It is inconsistent to ignore the fact that careless preparation could affect their opinion of *your* employer.

B L O T C H E T T   T O U R S

8888 Malarky Drive

Fun Valley, UT 99999

4/1/9x

Ms.. Glendora Kirsch
211 Elm Ave. Apt a
Losangeles, Cal. 99999

Dear Miss Kirsch,

It seems that each year about this time we send~~ed~~ you a letter inquiring about your plans for this sumer. Each year for the passed three years now we have had no answer.

According to our records, you wrote Blotchett Tours inquiring about some information concerning different tours. We sent you our price lists, departure date list, special off season excursions, etc. Wouldn't it be nice if you could plan to travel this summer. Why not reserve a place for yourself in one of our package deals.

Enclosed herewith please find an application blank for you to fill out. Just return it in the business reply envelope with your small check for only $35 and your place will be assured. Naturally your deposit will aply toward the fu-ll purchase of your tour. We are guaranteed and bonded.

We will be looking for your response soon.

Very Truly Yours,

Hank Behn, Sales rep.

6–1: COMPUTER EXERCISE

Before proceeding, you may want to do more exercises based on the concept you have learned. Additional practice material is on your computer diskette.

Directions: Insert the diskette into the computer and follow the instructions on the screen for Computer Exercise 6–1.

A *Answers to* 6–3: SELF-STUDY

1. Notice that paragraph 1 is only one sentence long. What does the dictator do with this sentence? *She introduces the patient with his age, problem, and date first seen.* (Notice that the reference line is the only place that the patient's name is mentioned.)

2. Notice that paragraph 2 is three sentences long. Could the first of these sentences have been placed in the first paragraph? *Yes.* Why or why not? *The other sentences would need to go along with it, however, since they are part of the past history of the patient. It is better as it stands.* (By this final statement, one sees that "no" is the better answer.)
3. What is the dictator doing in paragraph 2? *Giving a brief past history.*
4. Could any part of paragraph 3 logically be part of the second or fourth paragraph? *No.* Why or why not? *This is a definite change from past to present.*
5. What is the dictator doing in paragraph 3? *Giving the physical evidence of the patient's problem.*
6. Again, we have a one-sentence paragraph in paragraph 4. Could the typist have joined this sentence to paragraph 3? *Yes, but why? Is the typist afraid of one-line paragraphs?* What did the dictator do in this paragraph? *She told how she handled the patient's problem.*
7. What is the subject of paragraph 5? *The prognosis.* (What the expected outcome will be.) Could this paragraph be joined to paragraph 4? *No.* Why or why not? *Because there is a definite shift from "treatment" to "prognosis." It would weaken the impact of each paragraph.*
8. Notice the last line of paragraph 5. Could this have been a paragraph on its own? *Yes.* Why or why not? *It could have stood alone since it is the "plan" to be followed in the treatment program; however, because there are so many brief paragraphs it is fine where it is.* Could you make it a part of the last paragraph? *Yes.* Why or why not? *It could be done, but there is no reason for it. Actually, it would serve to weaken the final paragraph. No.* Why or why not? *It will weaken the final paragraph. Leave it alone.*
9. What is the dictator doing in the final paragraph? *Saying "Thank you," which is standard protocol and acknowledges that the recipient of the letter is the patient's primary physician.* Do you think it is appropriate to have this single sentence standing as an entire paragraph? *Yes.* Why or why not? *It gives impact.* *Note:* Your words do not have to match the answers exactly, but the ideas expressed should be the same or similar.

A *Answers to* **6–4: SELF-STUDY**

1. Paragraph 1 tells us the type of document this is. What is it? *A final follow-up letter.*
2. Paragraph 1: What is the subject(s) of this paragraph? *An introduction of the patient about whom the letter is written and a reminder about what has transpired with her. We could call this her "immediate past history."*
3. Paragraph 2: What is the dictator *doing* in this paragraph? *Stating the patient's present status and proposed plan of treatment.* Could the last two sentences of this paragraph be used to form a new paragraph? *Yes.* Why or why not? *Because it indicates a new subject: the proposed plan. However, that would make three very short paragraphs in a row, which is somewhat unattractive. One must think of appearance as well as content when it is possible to do so. (Therefore, "no" would be the better answer.)*
4. Paragraph 3. What is the dictator saying in this paragraph? *What his involvement with the patient is now.* Could this one have been combined with the last two sentences of paragraph two? *Yes.* Why or why not? *This would be appropriate because it all pertains to plans for the patient's future care. (Note that the typist's choice here is probably best as a result of the strong opening of paragraph 3: "we will NOT follow Nora. . . . "*
5. Paragraph 4. What is the subject of this paragraph? *A brief thank you and close.* Should this be arranged as two short paragraphs? *No. That would not be appropriate.*

CHAPTER

7

7

Proofreading and Making Corrections

OBJECTIVES

After reading this chapter and working the exercises, you should be able to

1. Explain where errors may occur in your work.
2. Illustrate how important it is to check your copy very carefully for possible errors.
3. Demonstrate the ability to use and recognize formal proofreader's symbols.
4. Demonstrate the ability to proofread and mark your own work for revision.
5. Redo a document that has been corrected and marked.
6. Prepare a document for corrections by using the revision marks.
7. Explain the variety of methods for correcting different types of errors.
8. Identify and correct errors after editing phrases, sentences, and documents.

INTRODUCTION

Now that you are beginning to learn to produce good medical typing, it is important that you also learn sound proofreading skills. The largest medical vocabulary, the fastest fingers, and the latest equipment all mean nothing if the final document does not reflect the professional quality for which you are striving. Proper proofreading skills can give you this quality, and the lack of it can cause embarrassment and poor self-image. You need these skills now because you will have to check your work carefully to earn high marks on the copy you submit for grading. Later, you will want to have excellent skills when you begin your career as a transcriptionist. Because accurate written communication is so important, the abilities to proofread your own work and to work without supervision will give you an advantage: on these bases you may well be promoted to supervisory capacity.

A great deal of self-discipline is required of the transcriptionist who wants to turn out perfect copy. No matter how accurate a speller you are and no matter how well honed are your punctuation, capitalization, and mechanical skills, errors can and do occur, and it is necessary to approach every document you prepare with the attitude that errors may be present. A systematic search for errors is then begun. More than half of the mistakes made are due not to ignorance or to carelessness but rather to the inability to "see" the mistake or recognize it or because we become too familiar with the material or, in contrast, are dealing with unfamiliar material.

Because you have progressed this far, you know where many mistakes can be found. It is unlikely that you will make errors in format; if you learned your punctuation, capitalization, and mechanical rules well, these areas should not bother you. If you are careful to stop and check spelling each time you have a doubt about accuracy, where will you look for errors?

Let's find out.

WHERE ERRORS OCCUR

There are differences of opinion among teachers, students, and your prospective employers as to what an error is and how important different errors are. For example, transposed letters in the name of a drug could be very serious, whereas the incorrect use of a capital letter, although upsetting to a fastidious instructor, would hardly be grounds for dismay on the part of an employer, and there are many other kinds of errors that are value judgments on the part of the student, teacher, or employer checking the paper.

There are, in fact, some kinds of errors that are "permissible" and with which the copy is still useable; other errors are easily corrected; and, finally, some errors can be eliminated only by redoing the material.

On the other hand, you do not want to work so slowly to avoid making errors that your production drops or you become nervous about the errors you "might" be making. Instead, try to keep your errors to a minimum, learn to find those you do make, and learn to correct them quickly and easily.

When transcribing from equipment (in contrast to copy typing or transcribing from notes), you can look at your work while typing; therefore, you can see mistakes and correct them as they occur.

On-screen proofing itself is not as easy as proofreading hard copy (the printed page) because you may overlook some errors (e.g., punctuation marks, letters that tend to blend together). You must train your eyes to spot the smallest of errors. In the classroom, always proof your work on screen until you feel it is perfect; then, print it out and proofread it, and notice what, if anything, has slipped past your notice. Your skills will improve in time, and it is easier and less time consuming than redoing your work. Listen ahead to avoid grammar problems.

A beginning student is often concerned with whether he or she should stop and research unfamiliar material as it occurs or should continue with the work and thoroughly proofread it later, making corrections and insertions. One point in favor of continuing to work is that some "mystery words" are no longer mysteries when seen in the overall context; also, the dictator may use the word again, and the second time it is understandable. Becoming accustomed to a dictator's voice as one progresses into a document clears up misunderstood words. If you decide to try this approach, highlight the area to which you must return and carefully leave clues for yourself concerning the missing material. Certainly it is wise to completely punctuate a sentence when you have the sentence in front of you. Clues such as drops and inflections of the voice help with the punctuation as you progress, but it is usually necessary to review the material later for final punctuation. Never rely on a spell checker to correct the overall document, but stop as you go along and check any words about which you are in doubt. It is not a good idea to research these later because you could overlook them and they may not be picked up in spell checking.

ACCURACY

Medical records must be as accurate as you can possibly type them. This requires accuracy on the part of *both* dictator and transcriptionist. The problem with accuracy sometimes is the meaning of the word "accuracy." Who determines what is accurate? For example, you have just learned some basic letter formats, yet the dictator asks that the reference line be placed at the top right edge of the page, canceling the professional appearance of the letter. You know this is incorrect, and you know that those who receive the document will also question your skills, yet you must do as the dictator directs. To him or her, that is accuracy.

Likewise, you have just completed a thorough study of punctuation, capitalization, and abbreviations. An employer may insist that all drug names be typed in full capitals, all abbreviations be punctuated, or inappropriate dashes be used in every other sentence. When you comply with these directions, you are being accurate. In certain circumstances, you might consider discussing these and any similar problems with the dictator, always remembering that the employer's version of accuracy must be followed.

Finally, rules may have been set up by a governing body, either the hospital or its governing body. The physician may dictate an abbreviation in the final diagnosis that you know is incorrect. However, both you and the dictator must comply with these rules; therefore, accuracy demands that you spell out these abbreviations and that you check with the dictator to be sure you have the correct words if you have any doubts.

The transcriptionist needs to develop a trust relationship with the dictator, and when he or she becomes aware of inappropriate, incomplete, or inconsistent use of grammar, abbreviations, and so on, the transcriptionist needs to inform the dictator or supervisor and discuss this with him or her. If possible, discuss these possible problem areas when you are hired so that you will know exactly how they are to be transcribed.

TYPES OF ERRORS

■ Rule Always consult a dictionary when you have the slightest doubt about the spelling of any word.

Misspelling. Whether a word is misspelled or just mistyped, it results in the same thing: a spelling error that can mislead or distract the reader. A misspelling can be the result of a dropped letter, an added letter, transposed letters, wrong letters, substituted letters, or a homonym used in place of the word dictated. For simplicity's sake, we will just call the word "misspelled," and you might want to analyze on a personal basis the "why" and "how" of your spelling errors.

Most computer software has built-in English spell-checking abilities. Medical dictionaries and medical spell-check systems are also available for installation into your computer. As previously mentioned, do not depend on running a spell check at the end of your document. As you progress, stop and check the spelling and the definition when you do not understand what the word means. It is foolish to have a correctly spelled word that sounds like the word you want but makes no sense. Spell-check systems give a false sense of security by indicating that the word is correct when actually it signifies that "this is a word and this word is spelled correctly." It does not say that "this is the correct word." This can create a particular hazard for drug names that sound alike. Because most drug manuals do not provide the phonetic pronunciation of a drug, it is possible for a variety of drug names to be substituted for the one dictated. Do not depend on the drug name that the spell checker provides, but check your drug reference for additional information concerning the drug to be sure that you have made the proper selection. Some dictators will carefully spell drug names (or medical words they feel you may have trouble locating). It is important to double check orally spelled words if you have any doubts about their accuracy.

Homonyms, of course, are not recognized as misspelled words, and the spelling checker will not recognize a wrong word substitute or other grammatical errors.

■ Rule If you must divide a word, divide it only at the proper point.

Word Division. Words may be divided only between syllables or word parts. There are preferred places to divide a word, and every effort must be made to divide at these points (consult a dictionary). Some words may not be divided (see Chapter 8, pages 200–202). Professionals avoid dividing words because it slows down production and usually requires checking with reference materials.

■ Rule Always check printouts to be sure they conform to proper placement protocol.

Spacing. Rules concerning the spacing after certain punctuation marks, abbreviations, and symbols should be carefully followed; however, the spacing error that is frequently overlooked may be made by hitting the space bar at the wrong time. Notice what can occur with this spacing error.

EXAMPLE: The patient was prepped andd raped in the usual manner.

Spacing problems often occur with word processing and computer printouts that automatically take material to another line (or page) when we did not intend to do so. Always check your printout to be sure that the headers appear where they were intended. If documents are printed off-site so you do not have an opportunity to review the print, be sure that someone on-site checks them and the printer set-up for you.

7

When you type or make changes to something you have entered into the word processor, it is possible to create a new error in the process. Double check your correction! One common "newly created" error is to repeat a word on the line following the word, such as "and and." Some spell checkers will alert you to the "double-word" entry.

■ Rule Always know why you are placing a punctuation mark.

Punctuation. Placing punctuation marks where they do not belong and omitting others that should be included are obvious problems. A comma fault (e.g., one comma missing from a comma pair, a comma separating a dependent clause, or commas enclosing essential elements) is a common error to check for. The improper use and substitution of marks (e.g., a colon for a semicolon or a comma for a semicolon) are examples of other errors. Punctuation errors are often made because the transcriptionist has not listened far enough ahead in the material to grasp the sense of the sentence, or forgot to look at the entire sentence and return to insert or delete marks.

■ Rule Always know why you are using a capital letter.

Capitalization. Most capitalization errors are caused by a failure to capitalize; however, you should be careful not to capitalize unless there is a reason for the capital letter. In medical typing, the two areas where capitalization problems most often occur are with drug names (see Chapter 8, page 211) and abbreviations (see Chapter 5, page 123).

■ Rule Know the technical symbols for your specialty area and use them correctly.

Figures and Symbols. Errors with figures and symbols are usually caused by writing out numbers rather than using figures. Remember to express age, drug dosage, time of day, and other technical terms in figures (see Chapter 5). Omission of a symbol is certainly a minor error and usually occurs because the typist is unaware of the symbol or abbreviation.

Occasionally, symbols and abbreviations may be used incorrectly. For example, sometimes a symbol is avoided and the word is spelled out because it is difficult to stop and make that symbol. However, this is not an error if the dictator approves of this substitution. The improper use of symbols and abbreviations, rather than the failure to use them, is usually where errors occur.

EXAMPLES

Postoperative diagnosis: PID (incorrect)

Postoperative diagnosis: Pelvic inflammatory disease (correct)

a 3-cm. incision was carried along the . . . (incorrect, no period)

a 3-cm incision was carried along the . . . (correct)

Cultures grew out 10 to the fifth per mL (incorrect)

Cultures grew out 10^5/mL (correct)

■ Rule Recheck any vital materials you transcribe.

Accuracy. Errors occur when figures, dates, times, names, positions, and types and kinds of procedures and treatments are changed slightly or transposed with other similar material. As stated, drug names can be particularly confusing because of the wide variation in pronunciation.

Accurately obtain all social data, including the correct spelling of the patient's name, the record number, hospital number, x-ray number, pathology specimen number, Social Security number, and so on. Verify that the name dictated is the full and correct legal name of the patient, and confirm unusual names (e.g., nicknames that may be actual given names, foreign names, names that could be easily transposed, and so on). Be sure to verify the correct and complete names of the attending physicians and all others involved in patient care. Confirm the accuracy of all dates, including dates of admission, discharge, and procedures. Be alert to problems and conditions, admissions and discharges, procedures, and so on that were described as having taken place *last year, two days ago, last month,* and so on. Research records to find out when exactly *yesterday* was when it is dictated and insert the correct date. You may use inexact dates such as *the day after surgery* or *the day before he came into the emergency department* if those dates appear in the report (e.g., the day of the surgery or the day he came into the emergency department).

■ Rule Proofread carefully and correct all typographical errors.

Typographical. As you correct your work, watch to see whether your typographical errors form a pattern. When you can recognize the types of errors you make (e.g., transposing the last two letters of a four-letter word), pay particular attention to overcoming the problem.

Electronic. Many pieces of equipment today have the ability to convert certain codes or symbols that are typed within the text to complete words, phrases, sentences, or paragraphs. Codes or "boiler plates" are also used by some programs to indicate a certain style, set-up, or format. The inadvertent use or mistyping of these symbols will result in a printout containing an incorrect format (e.g., set-up, underlining, spacing, centering, indenting, and so on) or an inappropriate word, phrase, or even an entire paragraph or two.

■ Rule Use all electronic shortcuts slowly and with caution. Carefully check the final printout.

EXAMPLE

Conclusion:

Relatively

severe

L4-5

spinal

stenosis.

(Somehow a code was given to the computer to print this format.)

Alphabet expanders are wonderful time savers because they permit you to type in an abbreviation that, with a cue, becomes a complete word or series of words. One needs to complete the process carefully, or bizarre printouts result. Seasoned transcriptionists have collections of these slip-ups. They may be funny unless YOU are the responsible party.

EXAMPLES

Memphis, Tenderness (TN, the abbreviation for *Tennessee,* is also the cue for *tenderness.*)

San Ramon, Carcinoma (or condyloma acuminatum) (*CA,* the abbreviation for *California,* is also the cue for these expressions.)

Patients' names have carelessly been printed as follows:

Iron deficiency anemia Robinson (Her first name was *Ida.*)

Rectal examination Morris (His first name was *Rex.*)

Diagnoses have been printed as follows:

Diagnosis: Struck with a pancreas (a *pan*)

Diagnosis: Sterile saline solution (instead of *sick sinus syndrome*)

The dictator may also provide you with a list of predictated paragraphs, which may be stored in your computer. You insert these where appropriate in the dictation. However, you must check to be sure that they are accurate. A simple change of a number by the dictator or transcriptionist may place a paragraph pertaining to the closure of an abdominal incision in a transcription about the closure of an eye incision. Do not assume that the dictator is incapable of making a mistake about the accuracy of these directions.

Computers provide wonderful editing features: you can change and rearrange words, insert and remove punctuation, manipulate and rearrange entire sentences or paragraphs, increase or decrease the size of the margins, add or delete tab stops, and so on. However, while you are busy with these tasks, you could change a sentence so that there is no longer a subject, the verb is missing or now is a singular instead of a plural form, a paragraph appears in the wrong place, instead of electronic "cut and paste" a duplicate paragraph is added, subscripts become superscripts, headers appear other than where they were intended, and so on. A nightmare can be created. Particular care must be taken whenever you perform these procedures.

7

EDITING

The area we have been examining in your transcript has been material you have produced. Now we must look at the words themselves and see what, if any, control you have over the "sound" of the transcript. To a certain extent, the medical transcriptionist must edit the transcription. The term "edit" means making minor corrections in certain areas of the transcript *while preserving the exact meaning, style, and personality* of the author or dictator. We will now examine where these problems lie.

Grammar

Skilled transcriptionists change, delete, and clean up work, often unaware that they are doing so. They would not consider this to be an integral part of their job, but it is. Dictators for whom they work consider them invaluable or are often unaware that they have carried out this function. There is no argument about correcting improper grammar; never leave in a grammar error with the misguided notion that you are transcribing "exactly what was said." Here are a few grammar rules:

■ Rule Make sure that the verb and noun match in number.

EXAMPLES

There *was* fifteen members present. *(were)*

The Language of Medicine, stacked with three other terminology texts, *are* sitting on my desk. *(is)*

Sections of the cervical tissue *shows* mild dysplasia. *(show)*

Bronchoscopy of the right upper lobe bronchus, right lower lobe bronchus, and left lower lobe bronchus *reveal* bronchiectasis. *(reveals)*

7

Collective nouns often cause problems:

EXAMPLES

This group of diagnoses *are* proposed. *(is)*

Then, 2 cc *was* injected . . . *(were)*

Review of systems *were* negative . . . *(was)*

■ Rule Use proper parts of speech.

EXAMPLE:

The patient was found *laying* on the floor. *(lying)*

Give this to *whomever* sees the patient. *(whoever)*

The Tumor Board agreed that *they* would meet on the first Friday. *(it)*

She neither smokes *or* drinks. *(nor)*

■ Rule Use proper words.

EXAMPLE:

There was no *reoccurrence* of his tumor. (*recurrence*)

It's the *worse* possible diagnosis. *(worst)*

He should *of* been admitted immediately. *(have)*

It looked *like* he would begin the procedure unassisted. *(as if)*

The patient was seen yesterday and *is* doing well. *(was)*

■ Rule Use nouns and adjectives correctly.

EXAMPLE:

He was scheduled for replacement of his *aorta* valve. (*aortic*)

She had a *vesicle* fistula to her vagina. (*vesical*)

■ Rule Use proper singular or plural nouns.

EXAMPLE:

The *conjunctiva* were bilaterally inflamed. (*conjunctivae*)

■ Rule Position the modifiers correctly.

EXAMPLE

The patient had a hysterectomy leaving one tube and ovary in Jacksonville. (incorrect)

The patient had a hysterectomy in Jacksonville, leaving one tube and ovary. (correct)

■ Rule Use the proper tense:

Past tense is used:
in the *past history* portion of a report
in discharge summaries to discuss an expired patient.

Present tense is used:
in the current illness or disease
in the history and physical.

EXAMPLE:

The patient *has had* left sciatica for the past two years; this *is* now exacerbated.

■ Rule Check unfamiliar words to be sure that you are using them correctly.

Homonyms and sound-alike words may be dictated incorrectly, but often the transcriptionist perceives the word incorrectly or is unaware that another word exists that sounds like or similar to what was said. (Refer to Appendix B and become familiar with some of the more common homonyms.)

EXAMPLES

mucous membranes were intact (correct use of the adjective form)

mucus membranes were intact (incorrect use of the noun form)

After delivery of the placenta, the *perineal* tear was suture ligated . . . (correct)

After delivery of the placenta, the *peroneal* tear was suture ligated . . . (incorrect because *peroneal* pertains to the fibula, a bone in the lower leg.)

A *culdocentesis* was performed, which revealed pooling of blood . . . (correct)

A *colpocentesis* was performed, which revealed pooling of blood . . . (incorrect as *colpocentesis* is not a word but sounds logical because "colpo" has to do with the vagina and the dictation concerns a gynecologic problem)

BE ALERT: When you cannot locate a common word in your dictionary, further research is necessary.

Inconsistencies, Redundancies, and Technical Errors

Physicians do not dictate in the same manner that they would write out material, often editing as they go along. John Dirckx, MD, expressed it well in the Summer 1990 issue of *Perspectives on the Medical Transcription Profession:* "By choosing to dictate a document rather than write it out, the dictator not only sidesteps many of the mechanical tasks associated with composition but implicitly delegates these tasks to the transcriptionist. No dictators have such perfect powers of concentration that they never accidentally repeat themselves, never inadvertently substitute one word for another, never leave a sentence unfinished. Sooner or later, the most alert and cautious dictator makes each of these mistakes, and others besides. Clearly, these normal human lapses ought not to be reproduced in the transcript; and just as clearly, the duty of identifying and correcting them devolves on the transcriptionist."

Careful editing is necessary to good risk management, and the dictator appreciates the time and trouble taken to retain accuracy and grammar.

Editing for medical accuracy often requires skill that even some experienced transcriptionists have not acquired. The physician may be discussing a tendon in the hand and use the term for a tendon found in the foot. The transcriptionist who is alert to this either has an excellent knowledge of terms or in researching the proper spelling for the tendon sees that the incorrect term was used. Either way, the desired result is achieved. The researching transcriptionist uses the *lack* of knowledge to obtain more knowledge, and this is what the beginner must focus on. Another example is when, through a slip of the tongue, the dictator says "hypotension" when "hypertension" has been the subject of the report and the meaning for hypertension is implied, the transcriptionist notes and corrects this immediately. Attendance at medical lectures helps the transcriptionist not only to acquire knowledge about new medical materials, techniques, and procedures but also to reinforce anatomy and physiology skills. An educated transcriptionist is prepared to recognize potential errors because of an increased understanding of medicine.

■ Rule Adjust or rephrase inconsistencies.

EXAMPLE

The patient drinks several beers per day, occasional cigars and cigarettes. (incorrect)

The patient drinks several beers per day and occasionally smokes cigars and cigarettes. (correct)

■ Rule Delete redundancies.

EXAMPLE

The patient has no sisters and no siblings. (incorrect)

The patient has no siblings. (correct)

When you become more proficient at transcription, you will be able to recognize that there are other medical inconsistencies that you have the ability to correct. At this point, you will recognize them, but you might not know what to do. You do have the obligation to ask when in doubt.

■ Rule Spell out slang or short-form expressions.

Unlike abbreviations in which letters take the place of whole words, slang or short-form expressions are abbreviated forms of complete words. Slang expressions are used to avoid the real word (substitutes for death are very common) or because the dictator is comfortable with a colloquial expression and does not notice its use.

EXAMPLES

After repeated attempts at resuscitation, the patient *was flat line* and was *pronounced.*

Substitute *expired* and finish the sentence with *dead* and the time of day.

After three hours of labor, this *primip's* contractions *fizzled out* and she was sent home.

Change to *primipara's* and consider the use of *stopped* or *diminished.*

She was sent to the mental health unit for a *psych eval.*

Insert *psychiatric evaluation.*

Check the list of short forms or slang expressions in Appendix B and see which of these are acceptable in transcription. Expressions that may be fine in an office chart note or emergency department note are not acceptable in a letter or consultation report.

NOTE: There are some unusual words used in medicine that may appear strange the first time you hear them. The physician may use "peanuts," "fat" towels, "Dandy" scissors, and "cigarette" drains during surgery. Neurologists may make note of "gull-wing" signs and "dolls' eye" movements. See Appendix B for a list of more of these unusual medical terms.

■ Rule Correct technical errors.

EXAMPLES

A *2-mm* incision was closed above the left eyebrow. (too small)

A *2-cm* incision was closed.

The baby weighed 3 1/2 kg. (incorrect use of metric)

The baby weighed 3.5 kg.

There was a 2 × 3 × 3 ovarian tumor.

There was a 2 × 3 × 3 cm ovarian tumor. (This information is confirmed by the pathology report, operative report, or dictating physician.)

We removed 1800 mg of serosanguinous fluid. (wrong unit of measurement)

We removed 1800 mL of serosanguinous fluid.

EXAMPLE

The *suture* was closed with #6-0 silk sutures. (incorrect)

7

The *wound* was closed with #6-0 silk sutures. (correct)

NOTE: When you are working and errors such as this one occur, you will have to ask your supervisor or the dictator for the correct word unless you are *positive* you know what word was intended but not dictated.

EXAMPLE

The tonsils were removed by blunt and sharp *diagnosis.* (dissection)

Most physicians depend on the medical transcriptionist to discover dictation errors, and they appreciate being alerted to possible errors or inconsistencies so they can make appropriate corrections if necessary. Consider these sentences:

"This 33-year-old woman had her gallbladder removed in 1950."

"The patient presented with diffuse infiltrate in the left lower lung fields and bronchography confirmed her lower lobe bronchiectasis; therefore, a right thoracotomy and right lower lobectomy were performed the following day."

You may have access to the patient's medical record and be able to determine the correct age of the woman or the date of her cholecystectomy. Examination of the actual x-ray films or the medical record should help you clarify the right/left problem in the second sentence. If not, you must check these with the dictator. Other mistakes dictators make are "he/she" substitutions or substitution of the referring physician's name for the patient's name.

Abbreviations

Take particular care with abbreviations and use them only when appropriate. Remember that the letters *d, p, g, t,* and *e* sound very much alike, and *n* sounds like *and* or *in,* and vice versa.

Misunderstandings

One problem that even the most experienced medical transcriptionist confronts is that of not quite hearing, or not being able to understand, a word or phrase that is dictated. Because you can back up the tape over and over again, the word or words may eventually "come to you." Sometimes it helps to listen ahead; the word may be used again and said more clearly, or the meaning of the word may become obvious because of other words or other parts of the document. Many transcribing units have controls that permit the operator to increase and decrease the speed of play back. The use of this may facilitate the understanding of a word. Here are some simple examples of such words or phrases:

EXAMPLES

The lab withdrawn on June 1, 199X . . .
The lab work drawn . . .

Lot sa snow how can I help you in the future
Let us know . . .

The middlehear was hair containin'
The middle ear was air containing

Such problems become increasingly difficult as the words or phrases become more complex.

Foreign dictators, speaking according to the grammatical rules governing their own language, know what they want to say but may make odd English word choices. These expressions indicate a language barrier, not poor patient care. It is your responsibility to determine what the dictator intended to say and type it that way, again taking care to preserve the integrity of the meaning of the sentence.

EXAMPLES

The incision was *prolonged.* (change to *extended.*)

The patient's *painful feets had disappeared.* (change to *foot pain had disappeared.*)

This is easier to accomplish if you are working in a setting in which you have regular conversation with a dictator whose first language is not English. Then, you become used to the nuances of his or her English translation problems. Each language is structured in a particular way; when we know or understand that structure, it is easier for us to work with such problems as omitting the past tense particle, making all words plural by adding an "s" to the singular, transposition, or choosing the incorrect synonym. Many foreign-born physicians have extensive English vocabularies and speak perfect English; however, a heavy accent or the

Dear Doctor ______________________:

RE: Patient name ______________________

Report name ______________________

Date dictated ______________________

- ☐ Please see blank on page ___, paragraph _____ of this report. It sounded like ______________
- ☐ Dictate more slowly and distinctly.
- ☐ Spell proper names.
- ☐ Spell unusual words in address.
- ☐ Spell patient names.
- ☐ Spell new and unusual surgical instruments.
- ☐ Spell new drug names.
- ☐ Spell new laboratory tests.
- ☐ Indicate unusual punctuation.
- ☐ Indicate closing salutation.
- ☐ Indicate your title.
- ☐ Indicate end of letter.
- ☐ Give dates of reports.
- ☐ Speak louder.
- ☐ Give patient's hospital number.
- ☐ Please read the area of this report indicated by the penciled checkmark for accuracy.
- ☐ Your dictation was cut off. Please fill in the rest of the report or redictate.

Thank you. Please return this note with corrections via hospital mail to:
Transcriptionist ______________________

Telephone No. ______________ Date __________

Figure 7–1. Example of a flagging or tagging note to be appended to a medical manuscript for solving problem dictation. This form can be printed on colored paper. (From Fordney, M. T., and Diehl, M. O.: Medical Transcription Guide: Do's and Don'ts. W. B. Saunders Company, Philadelphia, 1990.)

inability to pronounce certain letters in our language makes it difficult to understand them until we have "tuned in our ears." You have the obligation to assist the dictator and make him or her sound good. Actually, the dictator trusts that you will make his or her dictation appear as correct and professional as possible.

Flagging

We can "get away with" many bad habits in our spoken language that are not correct in written form. Avoid using contractions. Do not type material that does not make sense to you. If you cannot understand a word and the dictator is unavailable, ask your supervisor or another transcriptionist for help. If they cannot help, leave a blank space in your material that is long enough to allow you to insert the correct word later and attach a flag sheet to the material. This flagging (also called carding, tagging, or marking) can best be done by using the repositionable adhesive notes. They have just enough adhesive on the back to hold them firmly in place until removed. You can also staple or paperclip your card or flag. The flag should include the patient's name, the page number, the paragraph, and the line of the missing word. If you are in a large organization, add your name. It will help the dictator if you put the missing word in context, that is, include a few words that come before and after it.

EXAMPLE

Williams, Maribeth #18-74-78. Under PX, Respiratory (page 2, line 8) "   respirations present." Sounds like "chain smokes." Judy, 5-17-9X

The reply to this will read "*Cheyne-Stokes* respirations present." Students, remember to also follow this format on your practice transcripts. See Fig. 7–1 for an example of a preprinted note that can be attached to your transcript.

Do not type in an underlined blank or a series of periods, asterisks, or question marks; do leave an obvious blank space. Do not type in something about the missing word; this must be done on the attached or electronic flag. If your material is printed off-site and you are not able to properly flag or tag it, then you must leave an electronic flag with the transcript to alert the editor in charge of the print-out process. For example, you may have a built-in flagging mechanism in the computer that you can use, and it will print out at the beginning or end of the document. Some transcriptionists have a phobia about leaving blanks. Vera Pyle, CMT, a founding member of AAMT and author of *Current Medical Terminology* has this to say about blanks: "To me a blank is an honorable thing; it means you don't know. If you have tried everything you can try to fill in that blank and can't, leaving a blank is preferable to guessing. Guessing is bluffing and to me it is more honest to admit, 'I don't know; I couldn't hear.' It is filled in in a doctor's handwriting in ink and is entirely legal and entirely acceptable."

Some transcriptionists use a full sheet of paper for a flag, forcing the signer of the document to lift it from the signature area to sign, in the hope that it will be noticed. Do whatever works.

Slang and Vulgar and Inflammatory Remarks

When you are employed in the word processing department of a large clinic or hospital, your supervisor will be able to assist you in the handling of questionable material. Those transcribing for a service whose policy demands verbatim transcription can likewise ask a supervisor or director for help. In a private medical office, you may, of course, approach the dictator directly. Very few physicians make derogatory or inflammatory remarks, but they may speak in this manner because of frustrations with the care of the patient. A surgeon may have just lost his or her patient to cancer and tears through the hospital, leaving a path of destruction behind. The "stupid physician" referred to in the dictation he or she leaves behind in your department reflects the frustration in not having a cure. That remark, obviously, is not meant to appear in print.

Questionable remarks can reflect on you and your judgment, the physician, the hospital, and the patient. The dictator may refer to patients, patients' families, or other members of the health care team as *stupid, crocks, dumb, lousy surgeons, quacks, "too dumb to know any better,"* and so on. The dictator will usually have forgotten the irritation that precipitated the problem in the first place by the time you transcribe it. Some institutions provide written policies to deal with inappropriate or inflammatory remarks written or dictated into the record. Transcriptionists must discover whether there are any written directions or rules for handling these kinds of remarks and follow these directives. Because most physicians are not legal experts, they may put themselves and the institution at risk if they are unaware of unprofessional language in the dictation. In addition to inappropriate comments about the patient, statements referring to hospital personnel or physicians, comments made regarding injury to the patient during a procedure, or comments made regarding complications or aborted procedures need to come to the attention of risk management personnel, who must be involved in any decision concerning what is written into the records. Do you transcribe it? Consider these alternatives:

1. Check with your supervisor before transcribing it.
2. Contact the dictator and diplomatically and tactfully ask about it.
3. Make two transcripts, flag the problem, and ask the dictator to make a choice, destroying the original and copies of the rejected transcript (very costly and time-consuming).
4. Leave a blank with a flag that says "I'm sorry, but I couldn't quite make out the first three words in paragraph 2."

It is better to leave a blank than to type a questionable remark. How you handle the problem will depend on your work situation and your personal contact with the dictator.

Consider this example:

"This patient's condition would never have deteriorated to this extent if the nitwit charge nurse on four had brought it to my attention instead of taking it upon herself to practice medicine without a license."

Inflammatory remarks have no place in a medical record and could place innocent people in jeopardy. You were not there when the incident occurred, and you have no idea what precipitated this remark, so it would not be your responsibility to edit or delete it. Your responsibility *is* to bring it to the attention of the dictator, supervisor, or risk manager *before* it becomes a permanent part of the patient's medical record. The risk manager is responsible for reporting, analyzing, and tracking any atypical occurrence in a hospital or other facility.

Your ability to analyze and polish and to proofread effectively and accurately will reflect your professional development. Remember: Follow the protocol available, master the intricacies of English, and become familiar with reference materials and how to use them.

One must remember that medical records are legal documents, and although they are vital in the care of the patient, they are also vital historically and could be the major protection for the physician in the case of a misunderstanding or a professional liability lawsuit. It is imperative that they be current, accurate, legible, unaltered, and clear.

A conclusion to the art of making corrections may be Dr. Dirckx's comment in the Summer 1990 issue of *Perspectives on the Medical Transcription Profession:* "A permanent medical document dictated by one professional and transcribed by another is expected to conform to certain norms of precision, clarity, coherence, and taste. Most transcriptionists perform this operation so deftly and unobtrusively that the majority of dictators never even suspect that their dictation has undergone revision (or that it needed it)."

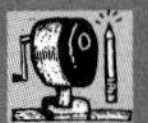

7–1: SELF-STUDY

Directions: In the following sentences, locate and underline any error, and then write the correct word or words in the blank provided. If the sentence is correct, write "C" after it. It may be necessary to rewrite an entire sentence to correct some errors.

EXAMPLE

The nurse said the count of the instruments *were* correct. *(was)*

1. The patient was all ready anesthetized when the resident arrived.

____

2. Congradulations. You have just been promoted. _______________
3. Dr. Thomas, a Thoracic Surgeon, has been setting in the reception room for over 1 hour waiting.

____

4. He was transported by the Paramedics to Brookview hospital.

____

5. Three students passed the transcriptionist's test with no mistakes.

____

6. The patient was first seen in November of last year.

____

7. The patients hobbies are knitting, painting, and to read in her spare time.

____

8. Closing the wound, the bladder was nicked.

____

9. *Dorland's Dictionary,* along with three other medical references, are sitting on my desk.

____

10. The number of surgeries we can accomodate because of the new surgery wing are increased.

____

11. The patient was mad as hell because of the delay in being seen.

____

12. She has the option, does she not, of still going ahead with the surgery?

____

13. Send copies of the operative report to Dr. Stuart Jamison, Dr. Claude Weiss and myself.

____

14. Neither the patient nor his wife have discussed the prognosis with me.

15. Neither the surgeon or the referring doctor have been notified.

16. The diagnosis of three of our staff members are listed on the report.

17. Each of the instruments have been tested.

18. The raise policy has certainly boosted the morale of all who work here.

19. She experienced numb and swollen in her left leg.

7

20. The sputum grew out H. flu.

21. The adnexa was negative.

22. Patient has chest pain if she lies on her left side for over a year.

23. The patient is edentulous and the teeth are in poor repair.

24. He was seen by whomever was on duty in the Emergency Department.

25. A intravenous pyelogram demonstrated functioning lower tracts.

26. He was seen on November 7 and is doing quite well.

27. 4-0 plain chromic catgut was used to secure and reapproximate the skin edges of both incisions.

28. He had two episodes of basilar pneumonia in 1994.

29. The specimen was removed and sent to pathology in total.

30. When three weeks old, his mother first noticed he was not responding to loud noises.

Turn to the end of this chapter for the answers to some of these problems and suggestions for some of the others.

HOW TO PROOFREAD

Establish good proofreading habits now and follow these general rules:

1. Always proofread as you go along. This is easy to do, unlike copy typing, because you are able to look at your work as you transcribe. Production typists do not have time for complex editing. Some sophisticated equipment, however, makes error correction very easy, and little thought is given to errors until final hard copy is ready to be printed out.

2. Do not proofread too fast. Read aloud, if you can, because this will keep you from skimming over material.
3. Read everything on the screen before you print it. Print out a fast, low-quality copy on machines with this feature. Check for typographical errors, mechanical errors, style, spelling, grammar, and meaning. If possible, do not look for everything at once. In one reading, look for the typographical errors and mechanical errors. Then, in a second reading, check for style, grammar, and meaning.
4. On long, complicated material, have someone read your work back to you, spelling out difficult words as you check the copy, or replay the tape and check your work as you listen again.
5. To check for spelling alone, try reading each line backward, a word at a time.
6. After a "cooling off" period, when you are not as familiar with the material, read it again. "Cold" errors are easier to spot.
7. Read everything before the final printout or sending it off-site for printing. Check carefully for placement, appearance, and format.

When you proofread your material, you will not mark it unless it is a rough draft. Rough draft material is double spaced, leaving room for corrections and comments.

Most professionals have their own set of marks indicating their revisions. When your employer asks you to prepare a rough draft so that he or she can revise it and mark it before it is typed in final form, informal marks and symbols are generally used. If, however, your employer is writing for publication, it will be necessary for you to recognize and use the more formal symbols. We consider this particular problem in Chapter 16.

Proofreader's Marks

When copy is prepared for printing, it is corrected and marked, with correction symbols placed either in the margin or between the lines to indicate the changes to be made. If more than one marginal note is necessary, a slash mark (/) divides the notes. Either or both margins are used.

In proofreading your own copy, you may be more informal, using marginal notes only when there is no room on the single-spaced copy to indicate the change.

While you are a student, your instructor will proofread your work and may mark the copy and use marginal notes in a variety of ways. Therefore, let us examine the proofreader's marks as they are used formally and see how we may modify them for our own use. Your instructor may wish to add his or her marking symbols as well.

The following examples will introduce you to the formal proofreader's marks (Fig. 7–2) and will show you how the copy is marked, as well as illustrating how the correction is highlighted with

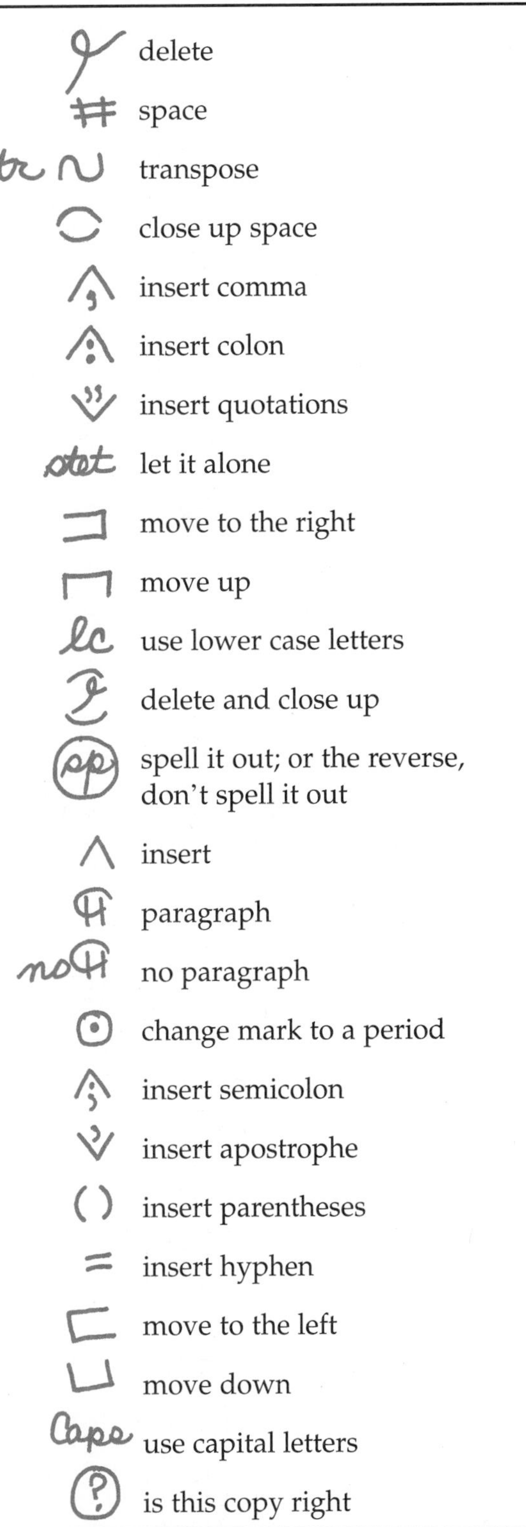

Figure 7–2. Formal proofreader's marks.

margin symbols. In addition, we will show you how you might use some of the symbols in a less formal way to mark your own copy.

The following abbreviations are used to indicate each example:

1. E = Error or incorrect copy
2. FM = Formal markings with the correction indicated
3. IM = Informal markings that you, your employer, or instructor might use. These should probably be done with a contrasting color (teachers love red!)
4. C = Copy as it appears when corrected

Spacing. The proofreader's margin symbol # indicates that spacing is to be increased. A slash (/) is made on the copy to indicate where the correction is to be made. The mark ⁐ indicates that there is too much space and that the copy should be closed up.

7

E		John Jonesis scheduled.
FM	#	John Jones/is scheduled.
IM		John Jones/is scheduled.
C		John Jones is scheduled.
E		Look at this.See how it is typed.
FM	#	Look at this./See how it is typed.
IM		Look at this./See how it is typed.
C		Look at this. See how it is typed.
E		Too much spa ce here.
FM	⁐	Too much spa ce here.
IM		Too much spa ce here.
C		Too much space here.

Delete. The margin symbol to take out a word, a line, or a punctuation mark looks something like this ℓ. A line is drawn through the copy to be deleted and a "tail" is added to the top of the line.

E		There are too many patients waiting.
FM	ℓ	There are ~~too~~ many patients waiting.
IM		There are ~~too~~ many patients waiting.
C		There are many patients waiting.
E		I will dictate the summary, but not the formal report.
FM	ℓ	I will dictate the summary/ but not the formal report.
IM		I will dictate the summary/ but not the formal report.
C		I will dictate the summary but not the formal report.

Insert Bottom Punctuation. The symbol ^ is drawn in the margin with the correct punctuation mark to be inserted within it.

Comma: ^ Colon: ^ Semicolon: ^

NOTE: Often one punctuation mark is deleted and another is added. When two or more margin notes are used they are separated by a slash (/).

E		Jean Bradley your patient, came in
FM	^	Jean Bradley^your patient, came in
IM		Jean Bradley, your patient, came in
C		Jean Bradley, your patient, came in
E		He agreed to the surgery I scheduled it.
FM	^	He agreed to the surgery^I scheduled it.
IM		He agreed to the surgery; I scheduled it.
C		He agreed to the surgery; I scheduled it.
E		I wanted to remove the tumor, however, he refused.
FM	/ ^	I wanted to remove the tumor/^however, he refused.
IM		I wanted to remove the tumor; however, he refused.
C		I wanted to remove the tumor; however, he refused.
E		Gentlemen;
FM	/ ^	Gentlemen/^
IM		Gentlemen:
C		Gentlemen:
E		Diagnosis Bronchogenic carcinoma.
FM	^/#	Diagnosis^Bronchogenic carcinoma.
IM		Diagnosis:Bronchogenic carcinoma.
E		Diagnosis: Bronchogenic carcinoma.

7

Insert Top Punctuation. The symbol ∨ is drawn in the margin with the correct punctuation mark to be inserted within it. Notice how this symbol for the margin differs from the three we just examined.

Apostrophe: ’∨ Quotation Marks: ”∨

E		The patients incision has healed quickly.
FM	’∨	The patients incision has healed quickly.
IM		The patient’s incision has healed quickly.
C		The patient’s incision has healed quickly.
E		She had these seizures frequently.
FM	”∨	She had these seizures frequently.
IM		She had these “seizures” frequently.
C		She had these “seizures” frequently.

7

Insert a Period. A circle is drawn around a period in the margin and is drawn around the punctuation mark in the copy that is to be changed to a period.

E		Joaquin R, Navarro, MD
FM	⊙	Joaquin R, Navarro, MD
IM		Joaquin R• Navarro, MD
C		Joaquin R. Navarro, MD

Insert a Hyphen. The symbol = in the margin indicates a hyphen is to be inserted in the copy.

E		She is a well developed, well nourished
FM	=/=	She is a well developed, well nourished
IM		She is a well-developed, well-nourished
C		She is a well-developed, well-nourished

Insert a Word. When you wish to indicate that a word is missing from a single-spaced copy, the missing word is written in the margin and a line is drawn to the place where it is to be inserted. When the copy is double spaced, it is fairly easy to insert the word above the copy with the ∧ symbol showing where it belongs.

E		The blood pressure was 160/90.
FM		The blood pressure ∧ was 160/90. (on admission)
IM		The blood pressure was 160/90. on admission
C		The blood pressure on admission was 160/90.

7

Transpose. This symbol ∩∪ is placed around the letters, words, or other marks to be transposed and *tr* is written in the margin.

E		He was credited with savign
FM	tr	He was credited with savign
IM		He was credited with savign
C		He was credited with saving
E		A new medication was prescribed and, she seemed
FM	tr	A new medication was prescribed and, she seemed
IM		A new medication was prescribed and, she seemed
C		A new medication was prescribed, and she seemed
E		She was, however, seen as an outpatient.
FM	tr/	She was, however, seen as an outpatient.
IM		She was/ ~~however~~/ seen as an outpatient, however.
C		She was seen as an outpatient, however.

Let It Alone. Occasionally, after a correction is made the proofreader will change his or her mind. The formal marking is to place dots under the material that was originally marked and to write the word *stet* (let it stand) in the margin.

E		He should have cobalt-65 radiation therapy.
FM	stet	He should have cobalt-65 radiation therapy.
IM		He should have cobalt-65 radiation therapy.
C		He should have cobalt-65 radiation therapy.

Use Capital Letters. Three lines are drawn under the lower case letters that should be capitalized and the word *Caps* is written in the margin.

E		I called the Admitting department
FM	Caps	I called the Admitting department
IM		I called the Admitting department
C		I called the Admitting Department

7

Use Small (Lower Case) Letters. A slash (/) is drawn through the capital letter and the letters *lc* are written in the margin.

E		The patient's Mother died of heart disease.
FM	lc	The patient's Mother died of heart disease.
IM		The patient's Mother died of heart disease.
C		The patient's mother died of heart disease.

Spelling. Misspelled words, symbols that should be expressed as words, words that should be expressed as symbols, numbers that should be spelled out, and spelled-out numbers that should have been written as figures are circled. The margin notation is *sp*. If the editor is not sure what the writer meant with the circled word in question, a question mark appears in the margin.

E		The patient's temperature was ninety-nine degrees.
FM	sp	The patient's temperature was ninety-nine degrees.
IM		The patient's temperature was ninety-nine degrees.
C		The patient's temperature was 99°.
E		3 of the most serious problems
FM	sp	3 of the most serious problems
IM		3 of the most serious problems
C		Three of the most serious problems
E		Move her to the ICU immediately.
FM	sp	Move her to the ICU immediately.
IM		Move her to the ICU immediately.
C		Move her to the Intensive Care Unit immediately.

Paragraphing. The symbol ¶ is used in the margin and the copy is also marked to indicate where a new paragraph should begin. If the paragraph beginning is incorrect, the symbol no¶ is used at the beginning of the paragraph to indicate it should be a continuation of the preceding paragraph.

E		Her history is well known to you, so I will not repeat it. On physical examination, I found
FM	¶	Her history is well known to you, so I will not repeat it.^On physical examination, I found
IM		Her history is well known to you, so I will not repeat it.¶On physical examination, I found
C		Her history is well known to you, so I will not repeat it. On physical examination, I found

Move the Copy. The following symbols indicate that copy is to be moved to the right ⊐, to the left ⊏, up ⊓, or down ⊔

E	On physical examination, I found
FM	5] On physical examination, I found
IM	5] On physical examination, I found
C	On physical examination, I found

FINAL EXAMPLE

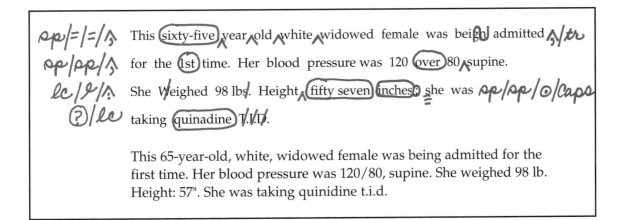

sp/=/=/^ This (sixty-five) year^old^white^widowed female was beign admitted^ ^/tr
sp/sp/^ for the (1st) time. Her blood pressure was 120 (over) 80^supine.
lc/ℓ/^ She Weighed 98 lbs. Height^(fifty seven)(inches) she was sp/sp/⊙/Caps
?/lc taking (quinadine) T.I.D.

This 65-year-old, white, widowed female was being admitted for the first time. Her blood pressure was 120/80, supine. She weighed 98 lb. Height: 57". She was taking quinidine t.i.d.

7

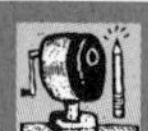 7–2: SELF-STUDY

Directions: Now try to interpret these symbols yourself. All formal marks are used with marks in the margin. Retype this paragraph on a separate piece of paper and use single spacing. After you have retyped your paper, compare it with the corrected copy at the end of the chapter.

> At cystoscopy their were multiple urethral polyps small
> in calibre and an irritated bladder neck; the urethral
> orifices were normal & the remainder of the bladder wall
> was no remarkable. I will have to presume that the bleeding
> is coming from the urethral polyps. I don't think this
> accounts for all this womans symptoms however. I am returni-
> ng her to your care and will follow her along for awhile
> to see what we can do about the hematuria.

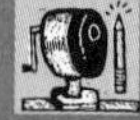 7–3: SELF-STUDY

Directions: Retype the letter on page 185 correctly following the proofreader's symbols. You will notice that the symbols used are a combination of formal and informal markings, just as your instructor or employer might use. Use letterhead paper and your own initials but please be careful not to create any new mistakes! Check the end of the chapter to see the corrected copy and compare it with your work.

7

PATRICK D. QUINN, MD
FAMILY PRACTICE
555 LAKE VIEW DRIVE
BAY VILLAGE, OHIO 44140

(216) 871-4701

July 17, 199x

Northern Ohio Gas & Electric Co.
Post Office Box 1831
Bay Village, Oh 44140

Attention/ T. J. Thompson Insurance Analyst

RE: Richard Wright

Gentlemen

Mr. Richard Right was seen in my office on July 9 199x. He was still having considerable pain in the right shoulder area but there was full range of passive motion and he felt likehe was gradually improving, although he was not hearly as pain free as before the recent surgery. The surgical wound was well healed on inspection. Their continued to be considerable tenderness to palpation in the depths of the surgical incision sight. There was no swelling or increased heat or readness and as noted above, there was a full range of passive motion of the right shoulder.

Because of the continuing rather excessive pain symptons, xrays were reexposed and felt to be completely within normal limits.

I continue to have no real good explanation for the patients continuing right shoulder symptosm, particularly in there present degree of severity. It would seem to me that the would be much improved what he was prior too his recent surgery.

I have asked him to use the part as much as possible and to retrun in 2 weeks. Hopefully at that time some consideration can be given to a return to work date. Further reports will be forwarded as indicated. Thank you for the plresure of careing for this patient.

Very Truly Yours,

Patrick D. Quinn, m.d.

ref

right margin too uneven and narrow

Kwei-Hay Wong, MD
1654 PIIKEA STREET
HONOLULU, HAWAII 96818
TELEPHONE 534-0922

DIPLOMATE, AMERICAN BOARD
OF OTOLARYNGOLOGY

EAR, NOSE, THROAT,
HEAD AND NECK SURGERY

1 Sept. 15 199x

2 Dr. Carroll W. Noyes M.D.
3 2113 4th Ave.
4 Suite 171
5 Houston, Tex. 77408

6 Dear Dr. Noyes;

7 I first saw Erma Hanlyn your patient on July 18 199x with a
8 history of a thyorid nodule since March of this year. This
9 thirty five year old woman had it diagnosed at Alvarado
10 Hospital where they urged her to have surgery I guess.

11 She gave a history that the nodule was quite tender when she
12 was seen there and that she was on thyroid when they took her
13 scan. However when I saw her the tenderness was gone. I
14 couldnt feel any nodule.

15 We have had her stay off of the thyroid so that we could
16 get an accurate reading and on Sept 8 199x we had another
17 scintigram done at Piikea General hospital which revealed a
18 symmetrical thyroid it was free of any demonstrable nodules.

19 All of the tenderness is gone and she feels well. She is
20 elated over the fact that she has avoided surgery

21 In my opinion Mrs. Hannlynn probably had a thyroiditis when
22 she was seen at Alvarado and the radioactive iodine that she
23 was given for the test is responsible for the cure.

24 Thank you very much for letting me see her with you and I will
25 will be happy to see her again at any time you or she feel
26 its necessary.

27 Sincerely

28 Kwei-Hay Wong, MD

29 lmp

30 cc

31

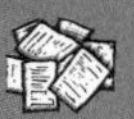 7-4: PRACTICE TEST

Directions: Identify all errors in the letter on page 186 by marking them in red, using the informal proofreader's marks. (You do not have to make margin markings.) The letter should have been typed in modified block format, using a reference line and using mixed punctuation. After you have proofread it, retype it properly. See the corrected version in Appendix A. *Clue:* There are 45 corrections to make, including errors of style, spelling, and punctuation.

Certainly, your letters will not look like those in the previous exercises, and you will be able to correct any errors while your copy is still on the screen or being processed by the computer. You will mark your copy only when it has to be redone.

In the beginning, you will want to transcribe letters and other documents in rough form. However, even in the beginning, try to make your rough copy look as much as possible like the finished product as far as placement and spacing go. It is much easier to work with double-spaced material, but you lose your placement advantage when you type a document this way. Also, if you are trying to save paper and begin to type on the first inch of paper, another opportunity to achieve proper placement is lost. As you prepare your copy, use letterhead paper, or a letterhead macro, place the date, space properly, and work from there.

However, when the dictator or writer asks for a rough draft, double space so that there will be plenty of room for editing.

An accomplished medical transcriptionist learns to make rough drafts "in his or her head" by learning how far ahead to listen. One day you will find that what started out as a rough copy was actually polished as you typed. However, do not be dismayed if you never accomplish this. There are some dictators whose dictation is so disjointed that it is always necessary to type it first in rough and then revise and edit. The use of a word processor makes the job of revision an easy task.

Every medical transcriptionist or proofreader sees and hears a variety of interesting remarks that never (we hope) find their way into print exactly as spoken or written. Hazel Tank, CMT, in San Diego, California, collected the following:

The child had a fever tugging at his right ear.
Return to the ED if worse or better.
I was beginning to lose patients with the patient.
The patient had her front end bent.
DX: Multiparous female who desires fertility.
She stepped wrong on her right hip.
The patient has Multi orgasm disease.
The baby was in the bass net all day.
The patient has trouble lying flat, particularly on his left side.
The patient was sleeping on my initial evaluation.
The end is almost in site.
The staff residence were called.

7-5: PRACTICE TEST PROOFREADING AND EDITING

Correct the word or words in the phrases below so they properly reflect what the physician dictated or how it should have been transcribed.

EXAMPLE

normal post-operative coarse — postoperative course

1. he had one slight dyspnea ____________
2. she uses oxygen binasal prongs ____________
3. the neck is subtle ____________

4. he had a mild cardial infarction ____________________
5. sutured along the buckle sulcus ____________________
6. Dx: Hypertension: ideology unknown ____________________
7. palette and tongue are normal ____________________
8. by manual examination of the uterus ____________________
9. no change in gate or stance ____________________
10. unable to breath ____________________
11. pressure at the sight of the bleeding ____________________
12. one sinkable episode ____________________
13. bleeding of the amniotic fluid ____________________
14. the right plural space ____________________
15. receptive aphagia for verbal commands ____________________
16. planter reflex is negative ____________________
17. deep tendon refluxes are in tact ____________________
18. no rales or bronchi ____________________
19. retinal exam revealed papal edema ____________________
20. a grey whirling tumor ____________________

See Appendix A for the answers.

7–1: COMPUTER EXERCISE

Before proceeding, you may want to do more exercises based on the concepts you have learned. Additional practice material is on your computer diskette.

Directions: Insert the diskette into the computer and follow the instructions on the screen for Computer Exercise 7–1.

A *Answers to* 7–1: SELF-STUDY

1. already
2. Congratulations!
3. thoracic surgeon/sitting/one
4. paramedics/Hospital
5. No errors (C)
6. 199X (in other words, the year date for last year)
7. patient's/reading

8. The bladder was nicked when closing the wound. (The verbal phrase must logically and clearly refer to the subject of the sentence. The bladder did not close the wound.)
9. is sitting
10. accommodate/is increased
11. very angry or "mad as heck" or very upset or "mad as hell" (insert the quotes)
12. No errors (C)
13. and me
14. has discussed
15. *nor* the referring doctor *has*
16. *is listed* or change *diagnosis* to *diagnoses* and keep the *are listed*
17. has been tested
18. no errors (C)
19. numbness and swelling
20. H. influenzae or Haemophilus influenzae
21. were negative
22. For over a year, the patient has had chest pain if she lies on her left side.
23. Check the medical record to see if the patient is edentulous or the teeth are in poor repair; they cannot be both.
24. whoever
25. An intravenous
26. was doing quite well
27. Number 4-0 (Don't begin a sentence with a figure.) You can recast the entire sentence to read as follows: The skin edges of both incisions were secured and reapproximated with 4-0 plain chromic catgut.
28. no errors (C)
29. in toto
30. His mother first noticed that he was not responding to loud noises when he was three weeks old. OR: When he was three weeks old, his mother noticed that he was not responding to loud noises.

A *Answers to* 7–2: SELF-STUDY

At cystoscopy, there were multiple urethral polyps, small in caliber, and an irritated bladder neck. The ureteral orifices were normal, and the remainder of the bladder wall was not remarkable. I will have to presume that the bleeding is coming from the urethral polyps. I do not think this accounts for all this woman's symptoms, however.

I am returning her to your care and will follow her along for a while to see what we can do about the hematuria.

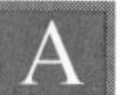

Answers to 7–3: SELF STUDY

PERFECT PUNCTUATION COMPANY
2526 LA MAL AVENUE
SAN VALLEY, CA 92014
(714) 555-7185

July 17, 199x

Northern Ohio Gas and Electric Company
Post Office Box 1831
Bay Village, OH 44140

Attention T. J. Thompson, Insurance Analyst

Gentlemen:

RE: Richard Wright

Mr. Richard Wright was seen in my office on July 9, 199x .

He was still having considerable pain in the right shoulder area but there was full range of passive motion and he felt like he was gradually improving, although he was not nearly as pain free as before the recent surgery.

The surgical wound was well healed on inspection. There continued to be considerable tenderness to palpation in the depths of the surgical incision site. There was no swelling or increased heat or redness and, as noted above, there was a full range of passive motion of the right shoulder.

Because of the continuing rather excessive pain symptoms, x-rays were reexposed and felt to be completely within normal limits.

I continue to have no good explanation for the patient's continuing right shoulder symptoms, particularly in their present degree of severity. It would seem to me that he would be much improved over what he was prior to his recent surgery. I have asked him to use the part as much as possible and to return in two weeks. Hopefully, at that time, some consideration can be given to a return-to-work date. Further reports will be forwarded as indicated.

Thank you for the pleasure of caring for this patient.

Very truly yours,

Patrick D. Quinn, MD

ref

CHAPTER

8

Spelling, Word Division, and Using References

OBJECTIVES

After reading this chapter and working the exercises, you should be able to

1. Locate the spelling of medical terms by using a medical dictionary.
2. Find medical terms by the use of cross references.
3. State the type of book(s) used to locate medical words to enhance research skills.
4. List the limitations of computer software spell checkers.
5. Name resources for locating newly coined medical terms.
6. Identify where English words and medical words are divided.
7. Select correct English and medical words to increase spelling skills.
8. Identify appropriate compound English and medical words in a sentence.
9. Identify French and other unusual medical terms.
10. Use the *Physicians' Desk Reference* as a drug speller and to identify generic and brand-named drugs.
11. State whether a laboratory result is high, low, or within the normal range.

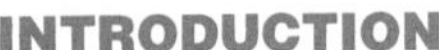

INTRODUCTION

In general, word processing computer programs include an ability to spell check individual words and entire documents as well as allow the user to add words to an electronic dictionary. Many medical word books or spellers are available in computer software format that allow the user to search for a word on screen while working in a document. However, these devices are of little use if you do not have any idea how to "try to spell a word." Electronic spell check systems cannot find an unknown word for you; they can only make certain that the word you select is spelled correctly. Sometimes, a spell check will provide a noun when an adjective is needed, so you must learn good research and word selection skills. Remember that a medical spell checker only alerts you to misspelled words; users must refer to dictionaries or drug books to ensure that the proper word is selected and that the word makes sense. If you do not have a medical spell check system, then your word spelling skills for both medical terms and drug words must be excellent.

8

This chapter is designed to increase your spelling, hyphenation, and capitalization skills. It will introduce you to the most common and helpful references for the medical transcriptionist, especially the medical dictionary, medical word books, and drug reference books.

Remember how hard it is to find the correct spelling of a word in the dictionary if you cannot spell it to begin with? Appendix B contains a Sound and Word Finder Table. This will provide you with some phonetic clues so that you can locate words more easily both in the medical dictionary and in the regular dictionary. When you cannot find a word, look up the sound in the Sound and Word Finder Table and it will guide you to some possible letters or letter combinations with the same sound.

EXAMPLE

The physician has dictated "kon-DRO-ma." Refer to the Sound and Word Finder Table and look under the K. Notice the clues given are *cho,*

PRONUNCIATION PLURAL FORM

THE WORD → **ar·thri·tis** (ahr-thri'tis) pl. *arthrit'ides* [Gr. *arthron* joint + *-itis*] — ORIGIN (Greek, Latin, French, Old English)

inflammation of joints; see also *rheumatism.*

Descriptive words with definitions of different types of diseases or illnesses related to the key medical term.

acute a., arthritis marked by pain, heat, redness, and swelling, due to inflammation, infection, or trauma.
acute gouty a., acute arthritis associated with gout.
acute rheumatic a., rheumatic fever.
acute suppurative a., inflammation of a joint by pus-forming organisms.
bacterial a., infectious arthritis, usually acute, characterized by inflammation of synovial membranes with purulent effusion into a joint(s), most often due to *Staphylococcus aureus, Streptococcus pyogenes, Streptococcus pneumoniae,* and *Neisseria gonorrhoeae,* but other bacteria may be involved, and usually caused by hematogenous spread from a primary site of infection although joints may also become infected by direct inoculation or local extension. Called also *pyoarthritis, septic a.,* and *suppurative a.*
Bekhterev's a., ankylosing spondylitis.
chronic inflammatory a., inflammation of joints in chronic disorders such as rheumatoid arthritis.
chronic villous a., a form of rheumatoid arthritis due to villous outgrowths from the synovial membranes, which cause impairment of function and crepitation; called also *dry joint.*
climactic a., menopausal a.
cricoarytenoid a., inflammation of the cricoarytenoid joint in rheumatoid arthritis; it may cause laryngeal dysfunction and rarely stridor.
crystal-induced a., that due to the deposition of inorganic crystalline material within the joints; see *gout* and *calcium pyrophosphate deposition disease.*
a. defor'mans, severe destruction of joints, seen in disorders such as rheumatoid arthritis.
degenerative a., osteoarthritis.
exudative a., arthritis with exudate into or about the joint.
fungal a., a. fungo'sa, mycotic a.
gonococcal a., gonorrheal a., bacterial arthritis occurring secondary to gonorrhea, often characterized by migratory polyarthritis that usually involves one and sometimes two joints, and commonly associated with erythematous skin lesions and tenosynovitis.
gouty a., arthritis due to gout; called also *uratic a.*
hemophilic a., bleeding into the joint cavities.
hypertrophic a., osteoarthritis.
infectious a., arthritis caused by bacteria, rickettsiae, mycoplasmas, viruses, fungi, or parasites.
Jaccoud's a., see under *syndrome.*
juvenile a., juvenile chronic a., juvenile rheumatoid a.
Lyme a., see under *disease.*

Figure 8–1. A typical word entry from *Dorland's Illustrated Medical Dictionary,* 28th edition. (W. B. Saunders Company, Philadelphia, 1994, p. 140.)

co, and *con.* Using your medical dictionary, locate the correct spelling of the term.

THE MEDICAL DICTIONARY

The medical transcriptionist's primary reference is, of course, the medical dictionary in book format and then, if possible, as computer software. No matter how expert you become, you will always need a dictionary. Because of this, it is important to obtain the most comprehensive and recent edition (no more than 10 years old) or, if working with software, to be sure to periodically upgrade it. A good dictionary may contain 100,000 words, but medical vocabulary contains 215,000 words. Many words not included in dictionaries relate to drugs, eponyms, instruments, acronyms, and so on; additional reference books are a must. Thousands of new terms are coined each year by researchers, scientists, geneticists, and others; therefore, the usefulness of a medical dictionary as a reference will diminish in time. A beginning transcriptionist must spend time becoming familiar with the arrangement of the dictionary because it will be an important asset in ensuring accuracy.

The best dictionaries usually include word origins, phonetics, abbreviations, and anatomic illustrations for each medical term (Fig. 8–1). Numerous words are not spelled exactly as they sound, so learn to check the phonetic spelling to determine the correct word to use. Because there are some variations in reference books, we base our exploration of the medical dictionary on *Dorland's Illustrated Medical Dictionary,* published by W. B. Saunders Company. All answers to Self-Study exercises, Practice Tests, and Reviews are based on the 28th edition. If you have another medical dictionary, follow along with this explanation as closely as you can.

Check the index for the tables and plates (illustrations) so that you will have a better idea of what anatomic pictures and lists are present. Look through and review the pertinent information in the tables themselves. If you have not had a formal course in medical terminology, check your dictionary for a listing of prefixes, suffixes, combining forms, and roots (e.g., "Fundamentals of Medical Etymology" at the beginning of the Dorland's dictionary) and become familiar with them.

In some dictionaries, there may also be a listing of the muscles, nerves, and arteries grouped together in one place. In Dorland's, a table is found in the appendices that lists the common name and three or more descriptive features of arteries, bones, muscles, nerves, and veins. These tables are helpful for quick reference of anatomic parts.

CROSS REFERENCE

Many times, the physician will dictate a word or combination of words that you cannot find when you consult your dictionary. An example is *"biferious pulse."* Because *biferious* is difficult to spell, it may be hard for you to find under the "Bs"; therefore, the first step is to look under *"pulse,"* which is easy to spell. You will find that *"biferious"* is listed alphabetically under this heading. In other words, this term is located under the NOUN rather than the adjective. Many other medical terms can be found in similar fashion. This knowledge is very helpful for you because the noun is often much easier to spell than the adjective, and the adjective spelling may be what brought you to the dictionary in the first place. It should be mentioned, however, that in some medical phrases the adjective is not necessarily the first word, as in *biferious pulse.* In Latin terms it is usually the second (e.g., *pulsus biferiens*) (Fig. 8–2).

Some physicians use complete Latin terms to designate muscles and nerves. In these instances, consult the Table of Muscles or the Table of Nerves to obtain the correct spelling.

pulse (puls) [L. *pulsus* stroke] 1. the rhythmic expansion of an artery which may be felt with the finger. The *pulse rate* or number of pulsations of an artery per minute normally varies from 50 to 100. See also *beat.* 2. a brief surge, as of current or voltage.
abdominal p., the pulse over the abdominal aorta.
abrupt p., a pulse which strikes the finger rapidly; a quick or rapidly rising pulse.
allorhythmic p., a pulse marked by irregularities in rhythm.
alternating p., pulsus alternans.
anacrotic p., one in which the ascending limb of the tracing shows a transient drop in amplitude, or a notch.
anadicrotic p., one in which the ascending limb of the tracing shows two small additional waves or notches.
anatricrotic p., one in which the ascending limb of the tracing shows three small additional waves or notches.
atrial liver p., a presystolic pulse corresponding to the atrial venous pulse, sometimes occurring in tricuspid stenosis.
atrial venous p., atriovenous p., a cervical venous pulse having an accentuated "a" wave during atrial systole, owing to increased force of contraction of the right atrium; a characteristic of tricuspid stenosis.
biferious p., bisferious p., pulsus bisferiens.
bigeminal p., a pulse in which two beats follow each other in rapid succession, each group of two being separated from the following by a longer interval, usually related to regularly occurring ventricular premature beats.
cannon ball p., Corrigan's p.
capillary p., Quincke's p.
carotid p., the pulse in the carotid artery, tracings of which are used in timing the phases of the cardiac cycle.
catadicrotic p., one in which the descending limb of the tracing shows two small additional waves or notches.

Figure 8–2. An example of a noun, "pulse," showing some adjective entries associated with this noun. (From *Dorland's Illustrated Medical Dictionary,* 28th edition. W. B. Saunders Company, Philadelphia, 1994, p. 1387.)

The following is a list of some frequently used nouns that have descriptive adjectives listed alphabetically under them in the dictionary.

Using your dictionary, look up *syndrome.* How many adjectives did you find as subheadings of this word?

NOTE: The same entity may be referred to as a disease or a syndrome (as Fabry's disease—Fabry's syndrome) or as a sign or a phenomenon (as Gowers' sign—Gowers' phenomenon). In some instances, the physician may have dictated a noun that does not list the adjective modifier you need. In this case, you will need to know the synonym for another choice. Here are some synonyms.

test (sign)
phenomenon (sign)
test (reaction)
syndrome (disease)
procedure (operation)
method (operation)

8

aberration
abortion
abscess
acid
acne
agglutination
alcohol
alopecia
anastomosis
anemia
anesthesia
aneurysm
artery
atrophy
bacillus
bacterium
bandage
block
body
bone
bougie
bursa
canal
capsule
carcinoma
cartilage
cataract
cavity
cell
center
circulation
cirrhosis
clamp
condyle
conjunctivitis
corpus
crisis
culture
cycle
cyst
deafness
degeneration
dermatitis
diabetes
diarrhea
diet
disease
duct
ductus
dysplasia
dystrophy
edema
embolism
erythema
facies
factor
fascia
fever
fiber
fissure
fistula
fold
formula
fossa
fracture
ganglion
gland
graft
gout
granule
groove
heart
hemorrhage
hernia
hormone
immunity
incision
index
inflammation
jaundice
joint
keratitis
lamina
law
layer
ligament
line
maneuver
margin
membrane
method
microscope
muscle
nerve
node
nucleus
oil
operation
os
paralysis
pars
pericarditis
phenomenon
plane
plate
plexus
pneumonia
point
position
pressure
process
pulse
ramus
rate
ratio
reaction
reflex
region
respiration
rule
serum
shelf
shock
sign
sinus
sodium
solution
space
speculum
spine
splint
sprain
stimulant
stomatitis
strain
substance
sulcus
surgery
suture
symptom
syndrome
system
tendon
test
theory
therapy
tic
tissue
tongue
tooth
tourniquet
tract
treatment
tremor
triangle
tube
tubercle
tuberculosis
tuberculum
tumor
tunica
tunnel
typhus
ulcer
unit
urine
vaccine
valve
vas
vein
vena
vertebra
virus
wave
wax
zone

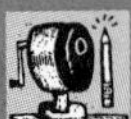 8–1: SELF-STUDY

Directions: Try the following exercises to get some experience with cross references.

First Word Dictated	*Second Word Dictated*	*Look Under*	*Spelling*
EXAMPLE			
KROOR-al	ligament	ligament	crural
1. bi-PEN-ate	muscle	____________	____________
2. pi″lo-MO-tor	nerve	____________	____________
3. mi-en-TER-ik	reflex	____________	____________
4. os	per″o-NE-um	____________	____________
5. SHIL-erz	test	____________	____________
6. lab″i-RIN-thīn	symptom	____________	____________
7. HOR-nerz	syndrome	____________	____________
8. de-KU-bi-tus	paralysis	____________	____________
9. tik	do-loo-ROO	____________	____________

Turn to the end of the chapter for the answers.

 8–2: PRACTICE TEST

Directions: Use your medical dictionary and locate the noun to see how to spell the adjective that has been dictated. If there is no listing, see whether the adjective is listed to obtain the correct spelling.

First Word Dictated	*Second Word Dictated*	*Look Under*	*Spelling*
1. pe-NAHRZ	maneuver	____________	____________
2. sal″i-SIL-ik	acid	____________	____________
3. WOS-er-man	test	____________	____________
4. BAR-to-linz	duct	____________	____________
5. vas	spi-RA-le	____________	____________
6. dif″the-RIT-ik	membrane	____________	____________
7. id″e-o-PATH-ik	disease	____________	____________
8. SKIR-us	carcinoma	____________	____________
9. TU-ni-kah	ad″ven-TISH-e-ah	____________	____________
10. ALTZ-high-mers	disease	____________	____________

The answers to these are in Appendix A.

MEDICAL WORD BOOKS

Medical word books that are used as spellers are available in two formats: (1) a single, comprehensive book divided according to all medical specialties with additional lists and (2) a dictionary-style word or phrase book. Many of the books are available in computer software. The books are inexpensive and compact and provide a simple method of locating a term quickly because the words are alphabetically arranged. Computer software may differ in price depending on whether the word book is on CD-ROM or 3.5-in diskettes.

Word books list commonly used and uncommon medical terms without definitions to ease the burden of searching through many books (e.g., *The Medical Word Book* (Sheila B. Sloane, W.B. Saunders Co., Philadelphia; updated periodically). It is divided into three major parts. The first covers anatomy, general medical and surgical terms, radionuclides, chemotherapeutic agents, experimental drugs for immune diseases, and laboratory terms; the second part is divided into 15 specialties or organ systems. Words are listed so that the familiar term will lead to the unfamiliar term given as a subentry; the third section gives abbreviations and symbols, combining forms, and rules for forming plurals. It is quicker and easier to use a book arranged by specialty because it limits the number of available words. For example, if the troublesome unknown word concerns the eye, you would locate it faster and easier by searching through the ophthalmology section in this type of book.

A regular medical speller has the same general format of a dictionary but has no definitions, and often the dictionary must be used after you find the word to check the meaning or to determine whether the term is part of the anatomy, a disease, an operation, a pathology term, and so on. These books are invaluable if you are transcribing in a specialty or doing many surgical reports. Because the terms are well organized in these books, the time needed to find a specific word is greatly reduced. Almost every medical specialty has its own speller reference. Specialty reference books can be found for the following: cardiology, dental, dermatology, gastroenterology, immunology/AIDS, internal medicine, laboratory medicine, neonatology, neurology and neurosurgery, obstetrics and gynecology, oncology/hematology, ophthalmology, oral and maxillofacial surgery, orthopedics, otorhinolaryngology, pathology, pediatrics, pharmaceutical, plastic surgery, podiatry, psychiatry, radiology and nuclear medicine, rehabilitation/physical therapy, speech/language/hearing, surgery, and urology.

Some of the publishers of the most popular word books are

F.A. Davis Co.
1915 Arch Street
Philadelphia, PA 19103
800-523-4049
fax 215-568-5065

Health Professions Institute
P.O. Box 801
Modesto, CA 95353
209-551-2112
fax 209-551-0404

W.B. Saunders Co.
6277 Sea Harbor Drive
Orlando, FL 32887
800-545-2522
800-433-0001 (Florida)

Williams & Wilkins
351 W. Camden Street
Baltimore, MD 21202-3393
800-882-0483
fax 800-447-8438

Medical word books or general medical speller books are by no means a complete listing of medical terms, and you may still encounter a problem when a new term or slang expression is dictated. When you first pick up a general medical word book, read the preface first so you will learn how to find the terms; each has a unique format. There also are format and style guides to show you how reports are set up, how to properly transcribe numbers, and so on.

8–3: PRACTICE TEST

Directions: This exercise will help you further develop research skills for finding the correct spelling of a technical word. You will be given a list of reference books. Each question gives a target word, sometimes within a phrase, that is underlined and spelled correctly. Report which reference book you would select if you needed to find the word or phrase to verify spelling, capitalization, punctuation, or meaning. Write in your choices on the lines using the letters that identify the book from the list of references given. Then write in the section of that book to which you will turn. There may be several methods to your research, so you may make more than one selection and write down any comments you feel are necessary.

Reference Book List

A Comprehensive drug book
B Drug speller

C Abbreviation book
D Medical speller with words listed by body systems
E Full-size medical dictionary
F Standard English dictionary
G English word speller
H Comprehensive medical speller
I Book of eponyms
J Medical phrase book
K Surgical word book
L Style guide
M Your textbook: *Medical Keyboarding, Typing, and Transcribing: Techniques and Procedures*
N Your own reference notebook
O Other (please name)

If you have any of the above types of books, you may want to write in the name of the book after the type of reference listed. This will reinforce your understanding of how and when to use these books.

8

EXAMPLE

After the diagnosis of benign prostatic hypertrophy was made, a TURP was scheduled.

First Choice: Book C Section T

Second Choice: Book D Section male

Comment: I actually have that abbreviation in my own reference note book (N).

1. The patient sustained a Colles' fracture.

First Choice: Book _______ Section __________

Second Choice: Book _______ Section __________

Third Choice: Book _______ Section __________

Comment: ______________________________

2. She recently relocated here from Albuquerque, New Mexico.

First Choice: Book _______ Section __________

Second Choice: Book _______ Section __________

Comment: ______________________________

3. with the employment of the Castroviejo scissors

First Choice: Book _______ Section __________

Second Choice: Book _______ Section __________

Third Choice: Book _______ Section __________

Comment: ______________________________

4. I do not think that extirpative surgery will be needed.

First Choice: Book _______ Section __________

Second Choice: Book _______ Section __________

Third Choice: Book _______ Section __________

Comment: ______________________________

5. You cannot understand if the dictator said 15 mg or 50 mg of a medication.

First Choice: Book _______ Section __________

Second Choice: Book _______ Section __________

Comment: ______________________________

6. There was a great deal of mucous discharge.

   First Choice: Book _______ Section ___________

   Second Choice: Book _______ Section ___________

   Comment: ____

7. There was considerable narrowing at the pylorus, with some reflux into the stomach.

   First Choice: Book _______ Section ___________

   Second Choice: Book _______ Section ___________

   Comment: ____

8. A D&C was performed after the spontaneous abortion.

   First Choice: Book _______ Section ___________

   Second Choice: Book _______ Section ___________

   Comment: ____

9. The patient experienced receptive aphasia after her last stroke.

   First Choice: Book _______ Section ___________

   Second Choice: Book _______ Section ___________

   Comment: ____

10. Darvocet-N was prescribed for the pain.

    First Choice: Book _______ Section ___________

    Second Choice: Book _______ Section ___________

    Comment: ____

11. Blood pressure was 120 over 80.

    First Choice: Book _______ Section ___________

    Second Choice: Book _______ Section ___________

    Comment: ____

12. The pH was 7.0.

    First Choice: Book _______ Section ___________

    Second Choice: Book _______ Section ___________

    Comment: ____

13. Diagnosis: Mycobacterium tuberculosis.

    First Choice: Book _______ Section ___________

    Second Choice: Book _______ Section ___________

    Comment: ____

14. Examination of the ears: TMs intact

    First Choice: Book _______ Section ___________

    Second Choice: Book _______ Section ___________

    Comment: ____

15. Eyes: PERRLA

    First Choice: Book _______ Section ___________

Second Choice: Book _______ Section ___________

Comment: ____

Answers are found in Appendix A.

SOFTWARE SPELL CHECKER

As mentioned, spell checkers have their limitations. A spell check can only tell you whether the word you select is spelled correctly. For example, the following sentences *Its knot all ways rite any whey. Its only a machine.* would appear to be without error when checked for accuracy. Therefore, it is up to you to decide what is correct and what makes sense as far as selection of noun, adjectives, or homonyms. Some software programs can help you find the spelling of drug names when you are not able to hear all of the word. For example, WordPerfect has this feature, and it can be accessed at any point while typing. Press *CTRL-F2* to spell. Type *5* or *L* for *Lookup.* Then, enter a pattern of letters that the spell check can look up for you. Type an asterisk for multiple missing letters and a question mark for single missing letters. For example, to spell a drug with the suffix *caine,* type in **caine,* and all of the words in the dictionary that end in *caine* will appear on the screen. Then, type the beginning of the word that you need, and it will be inserted into the document. Type in *V*cillin,* and drug names beginning with *V* and ending in *cillin* will be shown. You may also put the asterisk at the end of a prefix; for example, type in *peri*,* and words beginning with *peri* will be shown. Type in *rece?ve,* and *receive* will appear. This tool is excellent when you think that you would recognize the word if you could only hear all of it or see it. Remember to never rely totally on a spell check but to develop good research and word selection skills.

JOURNALS AND NEWSLETTERS

New words or words coined as they are born are available by membership or subscription before they appear in standard reference books or software. As a working transcriptionist, it is wise to have access to such publications to obtain information on new terminology and pharmaceuticals as well as articles of interest to a practicing transcriptionist. Examples of such publications include the following:

Journal of the American Association for Medical Transcription (JAAMT), a journal published bimonthly by the American Association for Medical Transcription, P.O. Box 576187, Modesto, CA 95357-6187.

Stedman's WordWatch, a newsletter published biannually by Williams & Wilkins, P.O. Box 1496, Baltimore, MD 21298-9724.

MT Monthly, a newsletter published by Computer Systems Management, 1633 NE Rosewood Drive, Gladstone, MO 64118.

The Latest Word, a newsletter published bimonthly by W.B. Saunders Co., 6277 Sea Harbor Drive, Orlando, FL 32821-9989.

Perspectives, a journal published quarterly by Health Professions Institute, P.O. Box 801, Modesto, CA 95353.

WORD DIVISION

When typing letters and medical reports, it is preferable to eliminate hyphenation at the end of a line whenever possible. Unhyphenated words are easier to read, and hyphenation is time consuming because the typist must come to a complete stop to decide where to divide the word. Dividing a word incorrectly is the same as misspelling it, and the error is very difficult to correct. Newspapers and magazines divide words in places that do not necessarily conform to spelling rules, so do not use journalistic material for a reference. If a word division is imperative at the end of a typed line, follow the appropriate rule for either English words or medical terms. It is important to know your rules so you do not have to use the dictionary routinely to find the proper place to divide a word.

BASIC RULES FOR DIVISION OF ENGLISH WORDS

■ Rule 8.1 English words may be divided only between syllables and in keeping with proper American pronunciation.

EXAMPLES

dex/ter/ous (not dexte/rous)
cel/lo/phane (not cell/ophane)
nom/i/na/tion (not nomin/ation)

NOTE: If you are unsure of the syllabication of a word despite your understanding of the rules for hyphenation, consult a dictionary. Although it is acceptable to divide a word at any syllable break shown in the dictionary, it is preferable to divide at certain points to obtain a more intelligible grouping of syllables.

■ Rule 8.2 If a one-vowel syllable appears in the middle of a word, divide after, not before, it.

EXAMPLES

organi/zation
regu/late
busi/ness
criti/cal

8

■ Rule 8.3 If two vowels appear together within the word, divide between them.

EXAMPLES

cre/ative
retro/active
valu/able

■ Rule 8.4 Divide a solid compound word between the elements of the compound.

EXAMPLES

time/table
home/owner
sales/person
gall/bladder
child/birth

■ Rule 8.5 Try to avoid dividing dates. If you must, divide dates between the day and the year but not between the month and the day.

EXAMPLE

September 1,/1991 (Not: September/1, 1991 or Sep/tember 1, 1991)

■ Rule 8.6 Divide names before the surname. Names preceded by long titles should be broken between the title and the name. Proper nouns are not divided.

EXAMPLES

Mary Margaret/Smith
Rear Admiral/John Wenworth
John D./Brown

■ Rule 8.7 Divide a hyphenated or compound word at the point of the hyphenation.

EXAMPLES

brother-/in-law
get-/together
cross-/reference

■ Rule 8.8 Divide a word with a prefix between the prefix and the root.

EXAMPLES

ante/natal
post/operative
trans/sacral
non/reactive

■ Rule 8.9 Divide a word between double consonants. Divide a word root that ends with a double consonant between the root and the suffix.

EXAMPLES

salpingo/oophorectomy
admit/ting
misspell/ing

BASIC RULES FOR DIVISION OF MEDICAL TERMS

■ Rule 8.10 Medical terms are *not* divided between syllables but are divided according to their component parts; that is, prefix, suffix, or root of the word. Whenever you have a choice, divide after a prefix or before a suffix rather than within the root word.

EXAMPLES

gono/coccus
ile/ostomy
naso/frontal

REMEMBER: Always refer to your medical or English dictionary when in doubt about hyphenation or division of a word. A misdivided word is a misspelled word.

BASIC RULES FOR AVOIDING DIVISION OF A WORD

These rules are given because the emphasis is to speed transcription by knowing the rules and to keep word sets together. For example, when a physician dictates *25 milligrams,* it should be typed *25 mg* as a word set and not separated if it falls near the end of a line. When using word processing computer software, the word-wrap feature usually moves these unless you give a command to prevent it.

■ Rule 8.11 Avoid dividing words with fewer than six letters.

EXAMPLES

pain
tumor

■ Rule 8.12 Avoid dividing words that leave confusing syllables at the beginning of the next line.

EXAMPLES

ambi-tious (confusing)
am-bitious (better)
coin-cide (confusing)
co-incide (better)
inter-pret (confusing)
in-terpret (better)

■ Rule 8.13 Do not divide one-syllable words.

EXAMPLES

weight
thought
strength

NOTE: Even when "ed" is added to some words, they still remain one syllable and cannot be divided.

EXAMPLES

passed
trimmed
weighed

■ Rule 8.14 Do not set off a one-letter syllable at the beginning or the end of a word.

EXAMPLES

amount (not a-/mount)
bacteria (not bacteri-/a)
ideal (not i-/deal)
piano (not pian-/o)

■ Rule 8.15 Do not divide a word unless you can leave a syllable of at least three characters (the last of which is the hyphen) on the upper line and you can carry a syllable of at least three characters (the last may be a punctuation mark) to the next line.

EXAMPLES

ad-ducent
de-capsulation
bi-lateral
criti-cal
radi-ator
accept-able

■ Rule 8.16 Do not divide names, other proper nouns, abbreviations, numbers, or contractions.

EXAMPLES

William/son (incorrect)
Ph.D.
UNESCO
f.o.b.
CMT
wouldn't
couldn't
200,000

NOTE: Write out the contraction and divide it in that manner.

EXAMPLES

would / not
could / not

■ Rule 8.17 Street addresses may be divided after the name of the street and before the word *street, avenue, circle,* and so on, but not between the number and the street name.

8

EXAMPLES

3821 Ocean / Street
821 East Hazard / Road
or 821 East/Hazard Road

NOTE: Avoid breaking these word groups whenever possible.

■ Rule 8.18 Do not divide identifying information from accompanying numbers. As mentioned, the word-wrap feature of word processing computer software helps you to avoid this problem.

EXAMPLES

2 cm
page 421
8 lb 3 oz
gravida 1 para 1

■ Rule 8.19 Do not divide a word that would change its meaning when hyphenated. If unsure of the meaning of a word that has been dictated, look it up in the English dictionary so you do not make a mistake.

EXAMPLES

Dr. Cho re-treated the inflamed area.	She retreated to Hawaii for a vacation.
I will re-collect the patient daily slips.	He had to recollect the operative procedure.
Meg re-marked the x-ray cassette.	Mrs. Avery remarked to me about the case.
Please re-sort the ledger cards.	She had to resort to turning the patient's account over to a collection agency.

■ Rule 8.20 Do not allow more than two consecutive lines to end in hyphens.

■ Rule 8.21 Do not divide at the end of the first line or the last full line in a paragraph.

■ Rule 8.22 Do not divide the last word on a page. (See also Chapter 6, page 150.)

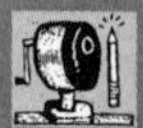

8–4: SELF-STUDY

Directions: Decide if each of the following words and word groups should be divided at the end of a line. If so, indicate the best division point. If necessary, refer to Rules 8.1 through 8.22 to complete this exercise.

8

1. critical criti/cal
2. Medical Assistant Jane Ever ________
3. Marie Carey Collins ________
4. radiator ________
5. 35 mg ________
6. preoperative ________
7. angiectasis ________
8. businessman ________
9. January 2, 1984 ________
10. 5 ft 10 in ________
11. clerk-typist ________
12. rested ________
13. acceptable ________
14. infra-axillary ________
15. president-elect ________

Turn to the end of the chapter for the answers to these problems.

8–5: PRACTICE TEST

Directions: Decide if each of the following words and word groups should be divided at the end of a line. If so, indicate the best division point. If necessary, refer to Rules 8.1 through 8.22 to complete this exercise.

Rule No.

1. eject ________
2. couldn't ________
3. page 590 ________
4. impossible ________
5. scheme ________
6. 7 o'clock ________
7. today ________
8. doesn't ________

9. 2480 Ames Drive ______
10. CHAMPUS ______
11. t.i.d. ______
12. shipped ______
13. around ______
14. 7,201,082,976 ______
15. John Jeffers, M.D. ______
16. 35-year-old ______

The answers to these are in Appendix A.

8-6: PRACTICE TEST

8

Directions: Divide the following medical terms at their most desirable point. Remember that medical words must be divided only where root elements have been combined.

EXAMPLE

pre-mature rather than prema-ture

1. claustrophobia ______
2. infraorbital ______
3. leukopenia ______
4. postoperative ______
5. posterolateral ______
6. tuberosity ______
7. acromion ______
8. metatarsus ______
9. myoplasty ______
10. bursitis ______
11. edema ______
12. viruses ______

The answers to these are in Appendix A.

ENGLISH SPELLING

A prudent transcriptionist must work hard to become a good speller. Although accurate spelling is an invaluable skill in any occupation, it is especially vital in the medical field. Few people feel secure and self-confident about their ability to spell accurately; therefore, unless you are one of those rare persons who remembers when to double a consonant (acco*mm*odate or acco*m*odate, occasion or ocasion), whether to type *ie* or *ei;* whether to use *-able* or *-ible,* and whether to finish a word with *-ance* or *-ence,* you must be continually on the alert for these and other problem-causing syllables. Another difficulty is our inability to recognize that we have a spelling problem. Never accept the spelling of a word given by the dictator or anyone else unless you know it is correct or have checked it in a reference source.

English computer software spell checkers may miss typographical errors, such as *by* for *my* or *of* for *on.* Medical spell checkers may pick the incorrect version of a sound-alike word, such as *ileum* for *ilium* or *plural* for *pleural. Court* and *count* look nearly identical on the screen, as do literally hundreds of other properly spelled words. Never rely totally on spell checkers, and always perform careful proofreading on the screen.

The following is a list of 150 frequently misspelled words. Read this list carefully to become familiar with the words, or ask a friend, co-worker, or instructor to dictate some of these words to you, after you have studied them, to see how you might score. You can develop a similar spelling list for hard-to-spell medical terms and post it near your typing area for quick reference. Be sure that you place both English and medical words that cause you difficulties in your own reference notebook. Every time you misspell a word, concentrate on the area where the problem occurs, and develop and memorize a device to help you remember it in the future. For example, to remember that *irresistible* is spelled *-ible* and not *-able,* you memorize "*I am irresistible.*" If you have difficulty with principle and principal, remember princip*le* is a ru*le* (we follow certain spelling principles) and princip*al* is either an adjective meaning m*a*in or a noun meaning m*a*in person, thing, or amount.

EXAMPLE

The principal diagnosis is pneumonia.

ONE HUNDRED AND FIFTY FREQUENTLY MISSPELLED WORDS

1. accommodate
2. accumulate
3. achievement
4. acknowledgment, acknowledgement
5. acquire
6. affect
7. aftereffect
8. allegedly
9. all right
10. among
11. apparent
12. arguing
13. argument
14. assistance
15. believe
16. beneficial
17. benefited, benefitted
18. canceling
19. cancellation
20. category
21. Caucasian
22. cigarette, cigaret
23. cite (to quote)
24. coming
25. commitment
26. comparative
27. conscientious
28. conscious
29. controversial
30. controversy
31. define
32. definitely
33. definition
34. describe
35. description
36. disastrous
37. effect
38. elicit
39. embarrass
40. enlargement
41. environment
42. exaggerate
43. except
44. existence
45. experience
46. explanation
47. fascinate
48. February
49. forty
50. fulfill
51. gauge
52. government
53. height
54. hindrance
55. hygiene
56. illicit
57. inasmuch
58. incidentally
59. indispensable
60. inflamed
61. inflammation
62. inoculate
63. insistence
64. insofar
65. interfered
66. iridescent
67. irresistible
68. its (it's)
69. judgment, judgement
70. led
71. license
72. likelihood
73. loose
74. lose
75. losing
76. maintenance
77. marriage
78. misspell
79. necessary
80. ninety
81. occasion
82. occur

83. occurred
84. occurrence
85. opinion
86. opportunity
87. particular
88. permissible
89. persistent
90. personal
91. personnel
92. persuade
93. possession
94. possible
95. practical
96. precede
97. preferable
98. prejudice
99. prepare
100. prescription
101. prevalent
102. principal (main or chief officer)
103. principle (rule)
104. privilege
105. probably
106. procedure
107. proceed
108. profession
109. professor
110. prominent
111. publicly
112. pursue
113. questionnaire
114. quiet
115. receive
116. receiving
117. recommend
118. referring
119. repetition
120. resistant
121. rhythm
122. seize
123. separate
124. separation
125. sieve
126. sight (to view)
127. similar
128. sincerity
129. site (a place)
130. studying
131. succeed
132. succession
133. suing
134. surprise
135. technique
136. than (conjunction of comparison)
137. then (at that time)
138. their (belonging to them)
139. there (in that place)
140. they're
141. thorough
142. to, too, two
143. transferable
144. transferred
145. unnecessary
146. usage
147. villain
148. vertical
149. visible
150. weird

8–7: PRACTICE TEST

Directions: Here are some "spelling demons." Each word is spelled here in two ways: the correct way and the commonly misspelled way. See if you can decide which is correct. Write the letter of the correct spelling in the blank provided. Do not consult your references.

1. (a) alright (b) all right __________
2. (a) supersede (b) supercede __________
3. (a) embarassed (b) embarrassed __________
4. (a) drunkeness (b) drunkenness __________
5. (a) irresistible (b) irresistable __________
6. (a) occurrance (b) occurrence __________
7. (a) ecstasy (b) ecstacy __________
8. (a) anoint (b) annoint __________
9. (a) occassion (b) occasion __________
10. (a) disappoint (b) dissapoint __________

11. (a) analize (b) analyze ______
12. (a) tyranny (b) tyrrany ______
13. (a) inoculate (b) inocculate ______
14. (a) cooly (b) coolly ______
15. (a) indispensable (b) indispensible ______
16. (a) superintendent (b) superintendant ______
17. (a) battalion (b) batallion ______
18. (a) perseverance (b) perseverence ______
19. (a) iridescent (b) irridescent ______
20. (a) reccomend (b) recommend ______

8

Scoring: If you are able to select 9 to 13 correct answers, you are far above the average speller. A score of 14 or more is considered superior. Check your answers in Appendix A at the end of this text.

MEDICAL SPELLING

Many medical terms of Greek derivation are difficult to spell. Those that start with a silent letter cause particular problems because we cannot locate them in the dictionary unless we know which phonetic sounds are likely to begin with a silent consonant.

Here is a list of some typical Greek word beginnings, along with their phonetic sounds and an example of a word in which each is used.

Spelling at Beginning of Word	*Phonetic Sound*	*Example*
pn	n	pneumonia (nu-MO-ne-ah)
ps	s	psychiatric (si″ke-AT-rik)
pt	t	ptosis (TO-sis)
ct	t	ctetology (te-TOL-o-je)
cn	n	cnemis (NE-mis)
gn	n	gnathalgia (nath-AL-je-ah)
mn	n	mnemonic (ne-MON-ik)
kn	n	knuckle (NUK-l)
eu	you	euphoria (u-FOR-e-ah)

Medical terms of Greek derivation may also have silent letters in the middle of the word. Notice the silent *g* in *phlegm* (flem) and the silent *h* in *hemorrhoid* (HEM-o-roid).

Furthermore, the *ch* combination makes the sound of *k*, as in *key*, and the *ph* combination makes the sound of *f*, as in *find*.

Two other Greek combinations are *ae* and *oe*. In modern use, they often become simply *e*. For example, *anaesthesia* is now written as *anesthesia* and *orthopaedic* as *orthopedic*. However, when corresponding with the American Academy of Orthopaedic Surgeons (AAOS), use the *ae* spelling. The suffix *-coele* is now written as *-cele*, as in the word "rectocele."

Some combinations of prefixes sound similar in dictation. Watch out for *ante/anti, para/peri, inter/intra, hyper/hypo,* and *super/supra*. Refer to Chapter 10 and Appendix A for help with these troublemakers.

Last, there are six Greek suffixes that cause spelling problems for the beginning transcriptionist. They are *-rrhagia* (RA-je-ah), *-rrhaphy* (RHA-fe), *-rrhexis* (REK-sis), *-rrhea* (RE-ah), *-rrhage* (raj), and *-rrhoid* (royd). You will notice the double *r* but you will hear only one. Memorize these.

REMINDER: Refer to Appendix B, Sound and Word Finder Table, to provide you with some phonetic clues when you encounter the possibility of a silent letter.

8–8: PRACTICE TEST

Directions: Before beginning this practice test, read and review the Sound and Word Finder Table in Appendix B. The left column indicates how certain words would sound when dictated. See if you can spell them correctly by using your medical dictionary as a reference. Refer to the Sound and Word Finder Table for help in looking up the words. Explanation of pronunciation: ā as in *nate*, ă as in *apple*, short stress mark (″), and long stress is noted in capital letters.

Phonetic Sound	Remember the Silent	Spelling
soo″dō-lŭk-SĀ-shŭn	p	pseudoluxation
1. năth″ō-DĬN-ē-ah		
2. tĕ-RĬJ-ē-ŭm		
3. nū-MĂT-ĭk		
4. NĒ-mē-ăl		
5. NŎK-nē		
6. dĭs-mĕn″ō-RĒ-ah		
7. HEM-or-ij		
8. kak-o-JU-se-ah		
9. met-ro-REK-sis		
10. men″o-met-ro-RA-je-ah		

The answers to these are in Appendix A.

8

COMPOUND WORDS

Compounds consist of two or more separate words and/or phrases that are used as a single word, often with the help of a hyphen to join them. A common dilemma confronting the medical transcriptionist is whether certain compound words are written as one or two words and are hyphenated. This problem occurs with English words as well as medical words. Often, there are no specific rules to follow for these compound words other than those applicable to hyphenation and word division. For example, there is no rule to explain why *shin bone* is two words and *cheekbone* is one word.

Combining Forms

Another confusing issue is medical noun-and-adjective combining forms. For example, the physician dictates what sounds like two adjectives: *tracheal bronchial tree.* The transcriptionist types it incorrectly as *tracheal-bronchial tree* and then correctly as *tracheobronchial tree.* An example of a noun is *oral pharynx,* which typed correctly is *oropharynx.* Always consult the dictionary for help when unsure about compound words. The following phrases are written as one word. They may be heard or perceived as a combination of modifier plus noun, but they are combined modifiers.

electric shock therapy	is typed as *electroshock*
cardial esophageal junction	is typed as *cardioesophageal*
gastral intestinal hemorrhage	is typed as *gastrointestinal*
cardial respiratory system	is typed as *cardiorespiratory*
tracheal bronchial tree	is typed as *tracheobronchial*
anterior lateral position	is typed as *anterolateral*
posterior lateral position	is typed as *posterolateral*

The following words may be heard or perceived as compound modifiers, but they are not and are typed as separate words. Never combine the modifier with the noun.

medial rectus muscle	is **not** typed as *mediorectus*
articular cartilage	is **not** typed as *articulocartilage*
palpebral fissue	is **not** typed as *palpebrofissure*

The following are combined because they have a prefix-plus-root combination and should not be separated:

para hilar mass	is typed as *parahilar*
extra ocular movement	is typed as *extraocular*
post operative recovery	is typed as *postoperative*
peri anal skin	is typed as *perianal*

The following word combinations (and many more) are written and understood as one word:

patent *air way* is typed as *airway*
still born infant is typed as *stillborn*
normal *eye sight* is typed as *eyesight*
oral pharynx is typed as *oropharynx*
normal tensive is typed as *normotensive*
electric cautery is typed *electrocautery*
nasal labial is typed *nasolabial*

Try the following self-study to brush up on your compound and combining form word skills.

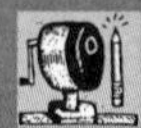 8–9: SELF-STUDY

Directions: Select the proper word choice in the sentences that follow.

1. The *femoral-popliteal/femoropopliteal* pulse was full and bounding.
2. The patient was admitted with a *para-appendicitis/periappendicitis.*
3. Mr. Johnson had a CVA *(cerebral vascular accident/cerebrovascular accident).*
4. The patient was diagnosed with *muscular dystrophy/musculodystrophy.*
5. Please check the *metatarsal-phalangeal/metatarsophalangeal* joint again.
6. She returned for her *bi manual/by manual/bimanual* examination.

The answers are given at the end of the chapter.

8

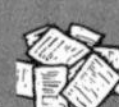 8–10: PRACTICE TEST

Directions: Circle the correct word—or two words—in italics for each of the following sentences.

1. The four hospital visits cost $150 *altogether/all together.*
2. We should learn how to operate the new word processors *altogether/all together.*
3. At this hospital, *anyone/any one* is entitled to incentive pay when doing medical transcription.
4. The laboratory information is outdated, but type it into the chart note *anyway/any way.*
5. Is there *anyway/any way* you can have the history and physical typed by 2 p.m.?
6. *Although/All though* it is Friday, we still have to put in some overtime.
7. Is it *alright/all right* to turn the discharge summary in a day late?
8. The cholecystectomy is planned for *someday/some day* in January.
9. She knows that *someday/some day* she will be given a raise.
10. The medical records and medical transcription supervisors are finally *already/all ready* to announce the new incentive policy.
11. The radiology report was *already/all ready* filed in the medical record when the physician asked for it.
12. Dr. Gordon should be able to see you *anytime/any time* in February.
13. The emergency room services are open for your use *anytime/any time.*
14. He has certain clothes for *everyday/every day* wear and surgical gowns for work.
15. For *sometime/some time* now, he has been dictating his medical reports a day late.
16. The consultation reports were sent *sometime/some time* last week.
17. Her senior medical typists do not get *anymore/any more* pay raises.
18. Is there *anything/any thing* Dr. Avery can get you for your headache?

19. It took her *awhile/a while* to understand what the patient was complaining about.
20. Is there *anywhere/any where* we have not looked for that missing patient's medical record?
21. This new medical position means *everything/every thing* to her.
22. Dr. Champion will take *anybody/any body* who wants to volunteer for this typing task.

The answers to these are in Appendix A.

8–11: SELF-STUDY

Directions: The following self-test includes some frequently encountered compound words in medical letters and reports. Indicate your choice by writing a letter in the blank. First, use your medical dictionary; if you are unable to find the word, check your English dictionary.

8

EXAMPLE

				Answer
	(a) gallbladder	(b) gall-bladder	(c) gall bladder	a
1.	(a) nosedrops	(b) nose drops	(c) nose-drops	______
2.	(a) chickenpox	(b) chicken pox	(c) chicken-pox	______
3.	(a) reexamine	(b) re-examine	(c) re examine	______
4.	(a) herpes virus	(b) herpesvirus	(c) herpes-virus	______
5.	(a) nailplate	(b) nail-plate	(c) nail plate	______
6.	(a) finger nail	(b) finger-nail	(c) fingernail	______
7.	(a) lidlag	(b) lid lag	(c) lid-lag	______
8.	(a) pacemaker	(b) pace maker	(c) pace-maker	______
9.	(a) ear drum	(b) ear-drum	(c) eardrum	______
10.	(a) ear wax	(b) ear-wax	(c) earwax	______

Check your answers at the end of the chapter.

FRENCH MEDICAL WORDS

French words are difficult to pronounce for English-speaking people because different sounds are given to the letters. Furthermore, some physicians do not attempt to use the French pronunciation but instead pronounce the word as if it were English. The following are some commonly used French medical terms with their pronunciation in French, with an occasional English version. Practice these words by repeating them aloud several times as you write them. To further enhance your spelling skills, ask someone to dictate them to you.

ballottement	(bah-LOT-maw) or (bah-LOT-ment)
bougie	(boo-ZHE) or (BOO-zhe, BOO-je)
bougienage	(boo-zhe-NAHZH)
bruit	(brwe) or (broot)
cafe-au-lait	(kah-FAY-o-LAY)
chancre	(SHANG-ker)
contrecoup, contracoup	(kon-tr-KOO)
cul-de-sac	(KUL-de-sahk)
curette, curet	(ku-RET)
debridement	(da-BRED-maw) or (de-BRIDE-ment)
douche	(doosh)
fourchette	(foor-SHET)
gastrogavage	(gas″tro-gah-VAHZH)
gastrolavage	(gas″tro-lah-VAHZH)
grand mal	(grahn MAHL)

lavage	(lah-VAHZH) or (LAV-ij)	poudrage	(poo-DRAHZH)
milieu	(me-LOO)	rale	(rahl)
peau d'orange	(po-do-RAHNJ)	Roux-en-Y	(ROO-en-why)
perleche	(per-LESH)	tic douloureux	(tik doo-loo-ROO)
petit mal	(pe-TE MAHL)	triage	(tre-AHZH)

8–12: SELF-STUDY

Directions: The following words are medical "spelling demons." Each term is spelled two ways: the approved form and the common misspelling. See if you can select the correctly spelled medical word. Write the letter of the correct form in the blank provided.

8

1. (a) sequela (b) sequella ____________
2. (a) accomodation (b) accommodation ____________
3. (a) inoculate (b) innoculate ____________
4. (a) fascia (b) fasia ____________
5. (a) sagittal (b) saggital ____________
6. (a) currettage (b) curettage ____________
7. (a) palliative (b) paliative ____________
8. (a) inflamed (b) inflammed ____________
9. (a) syphillis (b) syphilis ____________
10. (a) flacid (b) flaccid ____________
11. (a) inflamation (b) inflammation ____________
12. (a) diptheria (b) diphtheria ____________
13. (a) opthalmology (b) ophthalmology ____________
14. (a) hemorrhoid (b) hemorroid ____________
15. (a) supuration (b) suppuration ____________
16. (a) arhenoblastoma (b) arrhenoblastoma ____________
17. (a) cirrhosis (b) cirhosis ____________
18. (a) cachexia (b) cacexia ____________
19. (a) tonsilectomy (b) tonsillectomy ____________
20. (a) catarrhal (b) catarhal ____________
21. (a) transacral (b) transsacral ____________
22. (a) sessile (b) sesile ____________
23. (a) splenectomy (b) spleenectomy ____________
24. (a) xiphoid (b) ziphoid ____________
25. (a) menstruation (b) menstration ____________
26. (a) absorbtion (b) absorption ____________

Check your answers at the end of the chapter.

SPELLING THE NAMES OF DRUGS

A drug has three different names: the *chemical name* is the long and often complicated formula for the drug; the *generic* (or nonproprietary) *name* is usually a short, single name; and the *brand name* is the proprietary or trade name of the drug and is copyrighted by the manufacturer. Popular drugs have several brand names because each manufacturer gives the drug a different identity. You can often spot a brand name by the superscript ® before or after it. Brand names begin with a capital letter. When researching the spelling of a drug name, it is difficult to know when drug names are generic or brand unless the reference book used shows both. If a physician dictates a report about a patient using a drug on clinical trial, this also may present a problem. Sometimes the spelling of a drug name used in trials may change by the time the pharmaceutical company announces that the drug is available by prescription.

Look at the following list of everyday items to help you differentiate between the brand name for an item (capitalized) and the generic name for the same item (not capitalized).

Brand Name	*Generic Name*
Scotch tape	cellophane tape
Kleenex	facial tissue
Xerox	photocopy machine
Schwinn	bicycle

Now, look at the brand names and chemical name for a well-known tranquilizer, meprobamate. You will see that the same principles apply to drugs.

Brand Names
SK-Bamate Tablets
Deprol
Equanil
Milpath
Miltown

Chemical Name
2-methyl-2-*n*-propyl-1,3-propanediol dicarbamate

Generic Name
meprobamate

Drug names also include words that describe trademarked forms of how drugs are packaged, dosage form, and delivery systems (e.g., Captabs, Spansule, Wyseal). An excellent reference list appears in Appendix B. Make a copy of this to place in your personal reference notebook.

Notice that *only* the first letter of most brand-name drugs is a capital except for a few unusual exceptions, such as AcroBid, NegGram, and pHiso-Hex. Most hyphenated brand names also have a capital letter after the hyphen, as in Ser-Ap-Es or Slo-Phyllin (alternately pronounced as either "sa-LAW-fa-lin" or "slow-fillin"). A generic term is not capitalized. Some drug names can appear either capitalized or in lower case, such as the word penicillin. However, if the physician dictates a certain type of penicillin, such as Penicillin-VK, the term should always be capitalized. When dictated, the brand name *Kay Ciel* is often mistakenly transcribed as *KCl,* the abbreviation for potassium chloride. Look this up in your PDR to see why it is prescribed. Some similar brand names end in different letters, such as Urispas, Anaspaz, and Cystospaz. Another common spelling mistake occurs when typing the generic drug *phenytoin* because the *y* is not usually pronounced. Physicians commonly pronounce *lozenger* for the word *lozenge*—there is no final *r.*

To refresh your memory of what you learned in Chapter 3, here are some general guidelines on typing medications. When drugs are to be listed in a transcribed document, they should be separated by commas.

EXAMPLE

The patient has been taking Cardizem CD, Mevacor, and Persantine.

When metric units of measure are used with numerals, the metric term is abbreviated and it is not followed by a period.

EXAMPLE

The patient has been taking Lanoxin 0.25 mg, Calan SR 180 mg, and Solu-Medrol 40 mg.

As you learned in Chapter 3, when several drugs are listed with dosages given, the units are separated by semicolons or periods. Instructions on when and how the medication is to be taken are preferably typed in lower case with periods separating the initials.

EXAMPLE

Medications include Tenex 1 mg p.o. q.h.s.; Lasix 20 mg p.o. q.day; Clinoril 200 mg p.o. b.i.d.; and nitroglycerin 1/150 sublingually p.r.n. chest pain.

You may omit hyphens and slashes inserted after prefixes or before appended words, numerals, or abbreviations.

EXAMPLES

Antivert 50 not *Antivert/50*
Percocet 5 not *Percocet-5*

8

When a drug name can be either generic or brand and most of the other medications listed in the dictation are brand names, then capitalize the drug in question, and vice versa.

The fact that brand names for drugs are always capitalized and that generic names are not presents a difficult problem to the beginning transcriptionist. Fortunately, help in the form of word books that specialize in listing only drug terms is available. Some books show whether a drug is generic or brand and what type of drug it is (e.g., narcotic, laxative, diet aid, hormone, and so on). The use of such books speeds location of the term because detailed drug information is not included. However, most physicians who belong to the American Medical Association receive the *Physicians' Desk Reference* (PDR) along with their membership. This reference book lists only those drugs that the pharmaceutical companies pay to have listed, and therefore not all drugs are shown. Because most physicians refer to the PDR and have one in their office, we emphasize how to use the book; any self-study or practice tests in this chapter are based on its use because of its availability.

The PDR is published annually by Medical Economics, Inc., in cooperation with the manufacturers whose products are described in the book. During the year, supplements are published to update the current edition until the next year's edition is released. Beginning with the 1994 edition, the PDR is divided into six different color-coded sections, instead of seven, to facilitate use. However, these sections may vary in color designation with different editions, and the titles may also vary slightly in wording. With the 1994 edition, the PDR no longer features a separate section listing generic and chemical names but instead integrates them alphabetically in Section 2 (pink), the Product Name Index. To distinguish the difference, only the brand names are followed by the manufacturer's name in parentheses. However, as a basis of discussion, the 1996 PDR consists of the following color-coded sections (only those sections preceded by an asterisk are used by the transcriptionist).

Section 1 (white): Manufacturers' Index (alphabetical list that includes names, addresses, telephone numbers, and emergency contacts).

*Section 2 (pink): Product Name Index (alphabetical list of integrated brand and generic names).

*Section 3 (blue): Product Category Index (list of drugs by prescribing category).

Section 4 (gray): Product Identification Section (full-color, actual-size photos of tablets and capsules).

*Section 5 (white): Product Information (provides prescribing information on drugs).

Section 6 (green): Diagnostic Product Information (gives usage guidelines for common diagnostic agents).

Previous editions of the PDR should not be discarded too hastily when a new edition appears because a patient may have used a drug in the past (e.g., C-Quens and Lippes Loop) that cannot be located in the new edition.

In addition to indicating the spellings of drugs, the PDR lists injectable materials used in radiographic procedures and the brand names of products used for laboratory and skin tests. The alphabetical index by manufacturer is helpful when you are writing to a pharmaceutical firm to request drug samples for the physician. It gives current national and regional office addresses for each major drug firm.

When the physician dictates an unfamiliar drug name, refer first to the *Brand and Generic Name Index* to see if you can find the proper spelling and decide whether the word should be capitalized or in lower case. This is a listing of all the brand or generic names of drugs. The horizontal diamond symbol preceding a drug name indicates that a photograph appears in the Product Identification Section (gray).

If using an old PDR and you cannot find the dictated drug name in the *Brand and Generic Name Index,* check next to see if it is in the *Generic and Chemical Name Index* as a heading. If you find it in this section as a heading, you will know it is a generic name and is not capitalized.

Although some generic names have been adopted by drug manufacturers as brand names, use the generic form when transcribing unless the dictator wishes otherwise. At times the physician prescribes a generic drug instead of a brand-name drug because generic drugs are usually less expensive. Furthermore, in some medical writing, the dictator is asked to use generic names rather than to specify the brand. Some drug references use a format whereby brand and generic names appear capitalized. If in doubt about a generic name, check a good medical dictionary, which will list most generic drug names.

If you cannot clearly understand the name of the drug, it may be necessary to look it up under the *Product* (Drug) *Category Index* (see page 214), which lists drugs by their class, such as antihistamines, antibiotics, laxatives, and so on. For example, if the physician dictates that a drug for the patient's arthritis, "FEL-deen," was prescribed, you may look up "arthritis" and check

BRAND AND GENERIC NAME INDEX ECHOTHIOPHATE IODIDE/115

8

Generic and Chemical Name Index 303

Those headings listed in capitals, e.g., AMPICILLIN, are the generic names, and indented beneath them are the brand names of the drugs. Typed correctly, the generic name would be typed in all lower-case letters.

PRODUCT CATEGORY INDEX BIOLOGICALS/**207**

Aralen Phosphate Tablets (Sanofi Winthrop) **333, 2301**
Daraprim Tablets (Burroughs Wellcome/Glaxo Wellcome Inc.) **308, 314, 1090**
Fansidar Tablets (Roche Laboratories) **330, 2114**
Lariam Tablets (Roche Laboratories) **330, 2128**
Plaquenil Sulfate Tablets (Sanofi Winthrop) **333, 2328**

TOXOPLASMA
Daraprim Tablets (Burroughs Wellcome/Glaxo Wellcome Inc.) **308, 314, 1090**

TRICHOMONAS
Protostat Tablets (Ortho Pharmaceutical) **326, 1883**

ANTIPERSPIRANTS
(see DEODORANTS; DERMATOLOGICALS, ANTIPERSPIRANTS)

ANTIPROTOZOAL AGENTS
NebuPent for Inhalation Solution (Fujisawa) **1040**
Pentam 300 Injection (Fujisawa) . . **1041**

ANTIPSYCHOTIC MEDICATIONS
(see PSYCHOTROPICS)

ANTIPYRETICS
Aleve (Procter & Gamble) **328, 1975**
IBU Tablets (Knoll Laboratories) . . . **1342**
Children's Motrin Ibuprofen Oral Suspension (McNeil Consumer) **322, 1546**
Motrin Ibuprofen Suspension, Oral Drops, Chewable Tablets, Caplets (McNeil Consumer) **322, 1546**
Trilisate Liquid (Purdue Frederick) **328, 2000**
Trilisate Tablets (Purdue Frederick) **328, 2000**
Children's TYLENOL acetaminophen Chewable Tablets, Elixir, Suspension Liquid (McNeil Consumer) **322, 323, 1555**
Infants' TYLENOL acetaminophen Drops and Suspension Drops (McNeil Consumer) **323, 1555**
TYLENOL Extended Relief Caplets (McNeil Consumer) **322, 1558**

Betadine Pre-Mixed Medicated Disposable Douche (Purdue Frederick) **1992**
Betadine Skin Cleanser (Purdue Frederick) **1992**
Betadine Solution (Purdue Frederick)**1992**
Betadine Surgical Scrub (Purdue Frederick) **1992**
Betasept Surgical Scrub (Purdue Frederick) **1993**
Furacin Soluble Dressing (Roberts) . **2045**
Furacin Topical Cream (Roberts) . . **2045**
Hibiclens Antimicrobial Skin Cleanser (Zeneca) . . . **342, 2840**
Hibistat Germicidal Hand Rinse (Zeneca) **342, 2841**
Hibistat Towelette (Zeneca) . . **342, 2841**
Impregon Concentrate (Fleming) . . **1005**

ANTISPASMODICS & ANTICHOLINERGICS

GASTROINTESTINAL
Arco-Lase Plus Tablets (Arco) **512**
Bellatal Belladonna with Phenobarbital Alkaloids-Tablets (Richwood) **325, 2036**
Bentyl 10 mg Capsules (Marion Merrell Dow) **321, 1501**
Bentyl 20 mg Tablets (Marion Merrell Dow) **321, 1501**
Bentyl Injection (Marion Merrell Dow) **1501**
Bentyl Syrup (Marion Merrell Dow) . **1501**
Cystospaz (PolyMedica) **1963**
Cystospaz-M (PolyMedica) **1963**
Donnatal Capsules (Robins) . .**329, 2060**
Donnatal Elixir (Robins) **2060**
Donnatal Extentabs (Robins) . **329, 2061**
Donnatal Tablets (Robins) . . . **329, 2060**
Kutrase Capsules (Schwarz) . .**334, 2402**
Levbid Extended-Release Tablets (Schwarz) **334, 2405**
Levsin Drops (Schwarz) **2405**
Levsin Elixir (Schwarz) **2405**
Levsin Injection (Schwarz) **2405**
Levsin Tablets (Schwarz) **2405**
Levsin/SL Tablets (Schwarz) . **334, 2405**
Levsinex Timecaps (Schwarz) **334, 2405**
Librax Capsules (Roche Products) **330, 2176**
Pro-Banthine Tablets (Roberts) . . . **2052**
Quarzan Capsules (Roche Products) **331, 2181**
Robinul Forte Tablets (Robins) **330, 2072**
Robinul Injectable (Robins) . . **330, 2072**
Robinul Tablets (Robins) **330, 2072**

URINARY
(see URINARY TRACT AGENTS)

Dexedrine Spansule Capsules (SmithKline Beecham Pharmaceuticals) . **335, 2474**
Dexedrine Tablets (SmithKline Beecham Pharmaceuticals) **335, 2474**

NON-AMPHETAMINES
Adipex-P Tablets and Capsules (Gate) **312, 1048**
Bontril Slow-Release Capsules (Carnrick) **308, 781**
Didrex Tablets (Upjohn) **338, 2607**
Fastin Capsules (SmithKline Beecham Pharmaceuticals) . **336, 2488**
Ionamin Capsules (Fisons) **990**
Pondimin Tablets (Robins) . . **329, 2066**
Prelu-2 Timed Release Capsules (Boehringer Ingelheim) **306, 681**
Sanorex Tablets (Sandoz Pharmaceuticals) **2294**

ARTHRITIS MEDICATIONS

GOLD COMPOUNDS
Myochrysine Injection (Merck & Co., Inc.) **1711**
Ridaura Capsules (SmithKline Beecham Pharmaceuticals) **336, 2513**
Solganal Suspension (Schering) . . . **2388**

NSAIDS
Aleve (Procter & Gamble) **328, 1975**
Anaprox Tablets (Roche Laboratories) **330, 2110**
Anaprox DS Tablets (Roche Laboratories) **330, 2110**
Ansaid Tablets (Upjohn) **338, 2579**
Cataflam (CibaGeneva) **309, 816**
Clinoril Tablets (Merck & Co., Inc.) **324, 1618**
Daypro Caplets (Searle) **334, 2426**
Dolobid Tablets (Merck & Co., Inc.) **324, 1654**
EC-Naprosyn Delayed-Release Tablets (Roche Laboratories) **330, 2110**
Ecotrin Enteric Coated Aspirin Low Strength Tablets (SmithKline Beecham) **2455**
Ecotrin Enteric Coated Aspirin Maximum Strength Tablets and Caplets (SmithKline Beecham) . . .**2455**
Ecotrin Enteric Coated Aspirin Regular Strength Tablets (SmithKline Beecham) **2455**
Feldene Capsules (Pratt) . . . **328, 1965**
IBU Tablets (Knoll Laboratories) . . . **1342**
Indocin Capsules (Merck & Co., Inc.) **324, 1680**
Indocin Oral Suspension (Merck & Co., Inc.) **1680**

Cortone Acetate Tablets (Merck & Co., Inc.) **324, 1624**
Decadron Elixir (Merck & Co., Inc.) . **1633**
Decadron Phosphate Injection (Merck & Co., Inc.) **1637**
Decadron Phosphate with Xylocaine Injection, Sterile (Merck & Co., Inc.) **1639**
Decadron Tablets (Merck & Co., Inc.) **324, 1635**
Decadron-LA Sterile Suspension (Merck & Co., Inc.) **1646**
Depo-Medrol Single-Dose Vial (Upjohn) **2600**
Depo-Medrol Sterile Aqueous Suspension (Upjohn) **338, 2597**
Hydeltrasol Injection, Sterile (Merck & Co., Inc.) **1665**
Hydeltra-T.B.A. Sterile Suspension (Merck & Co., Inc.) **1667**
Hydrocortone Acetate Sterile Suspension (Merck & Co., Inc.) . . **1669**
Hydrocortone Phosphate Injection, Sterile (Merck & Co., Inc.) **1670**
Hydrocortone Tablets (Merck & Co., Inc.) **324, 1672**
Medrol Dosepak Unit of Use (Upjohn) **338, 2621**
Medrol Tablets (Upjohn) **338, 2621**

OTHERS
Cuprimine Capsules (Merck & Co., Inc.) **324, 1630**
Depen Titratable Tablets (Wallace) . **2662**
Imuran Injection (Burroughs Wellcome/Glaxo Wellcome Inc.) . . **1110**
Imuran Tablets (Burroughs Wellcome/Glaxo Wellcome Inc.) **308, 315, 1110**
Plaquenil Sulfate Tablets (Sanofi Winthrop) **333, 2328**

ARTIFICIAL TEARS PREPARATIONS
(see OPHTHALMIC PREPARATIONS)

ASTHMA PREPARATIONS
(see RESPIRATORY DRUGS)

ATARACTICS
(see PSYCHOTROPICS)

ATHLETE'S FOOT TREATMENT
(see DERMATOLOGICALS, FUNGICIDES)

B

BACKACHE REMEDIES
(see ANALGESICS)

the list to see if you can find a word that sounds like what was said; you will find "Feldene capsules." Notice that this brand-name drug is capitalized.

If you have the brand name for the drug and you wish to find the generic name, you must look in the Product Information Section. Refer to Figure 8–3 and you will see that the generic name of the drug is listed in parentheses below the brand name. This section is awkward to use because the drugs are listed alphabetically *after* the name of the drug company that manufactures them.

If after checking all of these sections you are still uncertain about what drug name was dictated, leave a space on the line and write a note to the dictator, describing how the drug name sounded. When the physician dictates a drug name that does not appear in the PDR, write it in the PDR in the place where it would normally appear, after you determine the correct spelling. Be sure to place it in your reference notebook as well, and be careful to indicate if it is a brand or generic name by using capital or lower-case letters. After looking up and locating a drug that is difficult to spell because it does not follow common phonetic rules, write it in your notebook in two places: the phonetic location as well as in the correct alphabetical location.

EXAMPLE

Eucerin
Ucerin, see *Eucerin*

Another dilemma when researching the spelling of drug names is when prescription medications fall "off patent," which allows a drug to be manufactured by a number of pharmaceutical companies. They may give it slightly different names, but the chemical content remains the same. This situation makes it difficult to find the spelling of new drug names even when using the most current drug reference book.

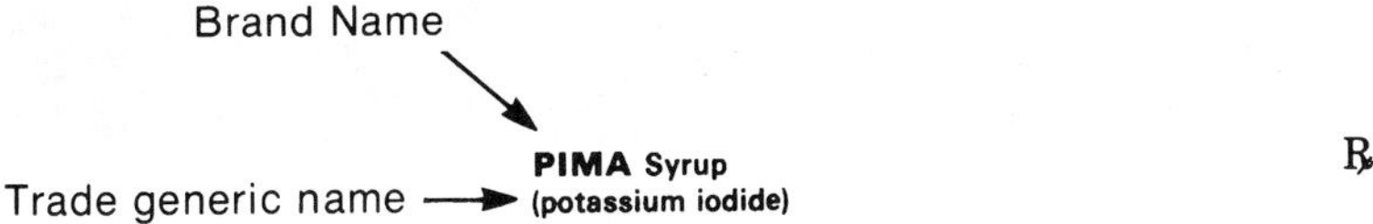

COMPOSITION
Contains KI 5 grs./tsp., in a black raspberry flavored base.

ACTION AND USES
An expectorant in the symptomatic treatment of chronic pulmonary diseases where tenacious mucus complicates the problem, including bronchial asthma, bronchitis and pulmonary emphysema.

ADMINISTRATION AND DOSAGE
Children—one half to one tsp. and adults one or two tsp. every 4-6 hours.

SIDE EFFECTS
May include gastrointestinal upset, metallic taste, minor skin eruptions, nausea, vomiting and epigastric pain. Therapy should be withdrawn.

PRECAUTIONS
In patients sensitive to iodides, in hyperthyroidism, and in rare cases iodine-induced goiter may occur.

HOW SUPPLIED
Plastic pints and gallons.

Information on composition of the drug, its action and uses, administration and dosage, and possible side effects. Precautions are given as well as in what form the drug is available.

Figure 8–3. A typical drug listing from the Product Information Section (white) of the Copyright Physicians' Desk Reference ® 1996, 50th edition, published annually by Medical Economics, Montvale, New Jersey 07645. Reprinted by permission. All rights reserved.

An additional problem that occurs is that some patented and off-patent drugs may be offered as over-the-counter (or OTC) drugs after Federal Drug Administration (FDA) approval. The FDA assesses the potential for abuse, and the drug is usually offered in a lower strength with instructions for less frequent use (e.g., 100 or 200 mg Tagamet for heartburn). However, if the patient has a stomach ulcer, the physician may want the patient to take 800 mg Tagamet, which requires a prescription. Most OTC medications are intended for short-term use to relieve acute symptoms. Conversely, there are some drugs that would never become available as an OTC drug, e.g., cardiac drugs. Because physicians may routinely prescribe OTC drugs for various minor illnesses and these drug names are not listed in the physician's or transcriptionist's drug reference books, it is wise to use a good reference, such as *Physicians' Desk Reference for Nonprescription Drugs* (Medical Economics, Inc., Montvale, NJ; published annually).

The Saunders Pharmaceutical Word Book (E. Drake and R. Drake, W.B. Saunders Co., 6277 Sea Harbor Drive, Orlando, FL 32821-9989) was written specifically for medical transcriptionists. It is a quick, easy, and reliable source for spelling and capitalization of both generic and brand names of drugs. It lists the drug's use and how commonly prescribed. It is updated annually.

Another drug reference is the *American Drug Index* (Facts and Comparisons, 111 West Port Plaza, Suite 400, St. Louis, MO 63146-9976; published annually). In this book, official generic drug names are preceded by a dot. Every trade name has a manufacturer's name in parentheses after the name of the drug. If a manufacturer's name does not appear there, the drug is generic and should be typed in lower case, regardless of whether there is a dot. This is not an easy reference to use.

Some additional medication word books that make it easier and quicker to find the spelling of generic or brand drug terms are:

Guide to Drug Names and Classifications
Springhouse Corporation
P.O. Box 908
Springhouse, PA 19477-0908

Instant Drug Index (Aloisi)
William Kaufmann, Inc.
1200 Hamilton Court
Menlo Park, CA 94024

Quick Look Drug Book
Williams & Wilkins
P.O. Box 1496
Baltimore, MD 21298–9724

Two computer software packages available for locating drug names are *Medical/Pharmaceutical Dictionary* and *Pharmaceutical Dictionary* (Sylvan Software, 5144 North Academy Boulevard, Suite 531, Colorado Springs, CO 80918).

8–13: PRACTICE TEST

Directions: To become better acquainted with the *Physicians' Desk Reference,* complete the following exercises:

1. Give the name of the section in the PDR that can help you to spell a brand-name drug.

   ____

2. The following are generic and brand drug names. Write in all brand name(s) for the generic. Write in the generic name for the brand.
   a. diazepam ____________ ____________ ____________
   b. Tenormin ____________
   c. Zocor ____________
   d. lovastatin ____________
   e. atenolol ____________ ____________ ____________
   f. Coumadin ____________

3. The software spell checker shows two selections (Lincocin and Lanoxin) for the drug dictated. The report is about a patient suffering from heart disease. Write in the correct drug name. ____________

   ____

   However, what would you do if you were unsure of your selection?____________

   ____

The answers are in Appendix A.

8–14: PRACTICE TEST

Directions: Using your *Physicians' Desk Reference,* write in the generic name for each brand given.

Brand Name	*Generic Name*
1. Thorazine	____________
2. Benadryl	____________
3. Hygroton	____________
4. Dilantin	____________
5. Provera	____________
6. Gantrisin	____________
7. Tofranil	____________
8. Lomotil	____________
9. Pyridium	____________
10. Mellaril	____________

The answers to these are in Appendix A.

LABORATORY TERMINOLOGY AND NORMAL VALUES

A beginning medical transcriptionist may have difficulty when the physician dictates laboratory results. The sequence of numbers, metric terms, abbreviations, and development of short-form expressions all sound like a foreign language. Some forms are acceptable and typed as dictated. A list of short forms is shown in Appendix B.

EXAMPLES

bands, basos, blasts, eos, monos, polys, pro time, segs, and stabs

However, other laboratory slang expressions or short forms that are dictated must always be spelled out.

EXAMPLES

bili for *bilirubin*

B strep for *beta-hemolytic streptococcus*

coags for *coagulation studies*

crit for *hematocrit*

diff for *differential* (blood cells seen in smear of a white blood count)

H. flu for *H. influenzae* or *Haemophilus influenzae*

lytes for *electrolytes*

H&H for *hematocrit and hemoglobin*

The word *milliequivalent* is often mispronounced as *millequivalent,* and its abbreviation is unusual and is typed *mEq.*

Dictation of a report from a urine specimen may list the appearance, color, and smell along with the specific gravity, dictated as *ten ten* or *one oh one oh* and typed with a decimal as *1.010.* Urine is examined under the microscope using a *high-power field,* NOT *high-powered field;* findings include bacteria, crystals and urates, blood, white blood cells, ketones, glucose, bile, protein, and uric acid.

8

Normal laboratory values for many tests vary from one laboratory to another depending on the type of equipment used. Appendix B gives additional laboratory terminology information and *approximate* normal values so you will know whether the information dictated is abnormal or within normal limits. A self-study exercise is presented to help you become more familiar with the terminology and numbers and thus overcome difficulty in transcribing such information.

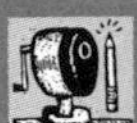

8–15: SELF-STUDY

Directions: The physician has dictated the following sentences in some discharge summaries. Refer to Appendix B, Laboratory Terminology and Normal Values, to help you obtain the answers. Read the statement, list the normal ranges, and then indicate whether the figure is high, low, or within normal limits (WNL).

	Normal Range	*High or Low*
Example: Laboratory data revealed a BUN of 16.	10.0 to 26.0 mg/dL	WNL
1. Glucose 107.	___	___
2. Chloride 110.	___	___
3. White blood count was 16,000,	___	___
4. with 69% polys,	___	___
5. 6% lymphs,	___	___
6. 5% monocytes.	___	___
7. SGPT 44.	___	___
8. SGOT 38.	___	___
9. The triglycerides were 646 mg/dL.	___	___
10. (female) Hemoglobin was 15	HGB ___	___
11. and hematocrit was 42.2,	HCT ___	___

12. with an MCV of 84, ______
13. and MCHC of 35.2. ______
14. Urinalysis was 1.020 for specific gravity with negative dipstick. ______
15. Uric acid 7.7. ______

The answers to this exercise are given at the end of this chapter.

8–16: REVIEW TEST

Directions: The physician has dictated these 10 brand or generic drug names in a research paper. See if you can determine the correct spelling for each by referring to your *Physicians' Desk Reference*. Be sure to begin all brand names with a capital letter and all generic names with a lower-case letter. Type your answers on a separate sheet of paper.

Drug Name Physician Dictated	*Phonetics*
1. ibuprophen	eye-bu-PRO-fen
2. diasapam	die-AS-a-pam
3. nembutal	NEM-bu-tal
4. xylocain	ZY-lo-kane
5. alprasolam	AL-PRA-SO-lam
6. dramamene	DRAM-ah-meen
7. sekanol	SEK-oh-nal
8. bensokain	BEN-zoe-kane
9. klonadene	klo-NA-dene
10. floorandrenolide	floor″an-DREN-o-līd

8–1: COMPUTER EXERCISE

Before proceeding, you may want to do more exercises based on the concepts you have learned. Additional practice material is on your computer diskette.

Directions: Insert the diskette into the computer and follow the instructions on the screen for Computer Exercise 8–1.

SPELLING WORD HUNT

The following article, which appeared as an editorial in *Cutis,* has 25 spelling errors. See if you can spot the incorrectly spelled words and list them on a separate sheet of paper with their correct spelling. Check your answers with those given at the end of this chapter.

PRURITIS

For some years I used to bet new groups of medical students that they could not correctly spell the medical word for itching. Only one lad in over ten years won the bet.

Burrough's solution, a commonly prescribed medium for wet compresses, is often mispelled. Electrodessication and curretage, the ubiquitous twins of dermatologic surgery, seem to confuse many. Innoculation is a medical teaser few seem to spell correctly.

Lichen sclerosis et atrophicus and condyloma lata are derived from Latin and with our de-Latinized educational system, I guess knowledge of their proper spelling is too much to ask.

As you can see your Editor is using his alloted space to ventilate his pet peeve—mispelling. In our youth-oriented culture, many educational leaders feel that spelling is merely a boring detail and that the "grasp of the concept" is all important. "Rap sessions" replace disciplined original essays. I disagree, but in a democracy we must accomodate all views.

There are three ways to avoid mispelling: 1. If you don't know how to spell a word, use an alternate. I personally find this much easier than hauling out the old dictionery; 2. Look it up in the dictionery. This takes time and is certainly an authoritarian method completely foreign to many of our younger set; 3. Who cares! Use it anyway. Someday our youngsters will run the goverment, which will supervise medical journals and mispelling will be so common we can all dispense with dictioneries. Practitioneers will not have to be bored by spelling and will have more time for goverment forms.

This, the 107th CUTIS Editorial, is devoted to spelling, and it is with the greatest personal pride that your Editor has never knowingly mispelled a word on this page. Burrough's is correctly spelled Burrow's; pruritis is puritus, and there are 25 spelling errors in this epistle.

John T. McCarthy, MD

8

A *Answers to* 8–1: SELF-STUDY*

1. muscle — bipennate
2. nerve — pilomotor
3. reflex — myenteric
4. os — peroneum
5. test — Schiller's
6. symptom — labyrinthine
7. syndrome — Horner's
8. paralysis — decubitus
9. tic — douloureux

A *Answers to* 8–4: SELF-STUDY

1. critical — criti/cal
2. Medical Assistant Jane Ever — Medical Assistant/Jane Ever
3. Marie Carey Collins — Marie Carey/Collins
4. radiator — radi/ator
5. 35 mg — do not divide
6. preoperative — pre/operative
7. angiectasis — angi/ectasis
8. businessman — business/man
9. January 2, 1984 — January 2,/1984
10. 5 ft 10 in — do not divide
11. clerk-typist — clerk-/typist
12. rested — do not divide
13. acceptable — accept/able
14. infra-axillary — infra-/axillary
15. president-elect — president-/elect

* This exercise can be used with Dorland's or Taber's Medical Dictionary. If using Stedman's Dictionary, numbers 4, and 6 are not listed under the noun. If using the pocket-size Dorland's Dictionary, numbers 1, 3, and 4 are not listed under the noun.

A *Answers to* **8–9: SELF-STUDY**

1. femoropopliteal
2. para-appendicitis
3. cerebrovascular accident
4. muscular dystrophy
5. metatarsophalangeal
6. bimanual

A *Answers to* **8–11: SELF-STUDY**

1. (b) nose drops
2. (a) chickenpox
3. (a) reexamine
4. (b) herpesvirus
5. (c) nail plate
6. (c) fingernail
7. (b) lid lag
8. (a) pacemaker
9. (c) eardrum
10. (c) earwax

A *Answers to* **8–12: SELF-STUDY**

1. a (sequela)
2. b (accommodation)
3. a (inoculate)
4. a (fascia)
5. a (sagittal)
6. b (curettage)
7. a (palliative)
8. a (inflamed)
9. b (syphilis)
10. b (flaccid)
11. b (inflammation)
12. b (diphtheria)
13. b (ophthalmology)
14. a (hemorrhoid)
15. b (suppuration)
16. b (arrhenoblastoma)
17. a (cirrhosis)
18. a (cachexia)
19. b (tonsillectomy)
20. a (catarrhal)
21. b (transsacral)
22. a (sessile)
23. a (splenectomy)
24. a (xiphoid)
25. a (menstruation)
26. b (absorption)

A *Answers to* **8–15: SELF-STUDY**

1. 60 to 100 mg/dL	High
2. 96 to 106 mEq/L	High
3. 4,200 to 10,000	High

4. 54 to 62%	High
5. 25 to 33%	Low
6. 3 to 7%	WNL
7. 0 to 17 milliunits/mL	High
8. 0 to 19 milliunits/mL	High
9. 40 to 150 mg/dL	High
10. HGB 12.0 to 16.0 gm/dL	WNL
11. HCT 37 to 47 ml/dL	WNL
12. 80 to 105 microns	WNL
13. 32 to 36%	WNL
14. 1.002 to 1.030	WNL
15. 2.2 to 7.7 mg/dL	WNL

A *Answers to Spelling Word Hunt*

1. pruritus
2. Burow's
3. misspelled
4. electrodesiccation
5. curettage
6. inoculation
7. sclerosus
8. atrophicans
9. latum
10. allotted
11. misspelling
12. accommodate
13. misspelling
14. dictionary
15. dictionary
16. government
17. misspelling
18. dictionaries
19. practitioners
20. government
21. misspelled
22. Burow's
23. Burow's
24. pruritus
25. pruritus

CHAPTER

9

Word Endings: Plurals, Nouns, and Adjectives

9

OBJECTIVES

After reading this chapter and working the exercises, you should be able to

1. Explain the rules for making medical and English words plural.
2. Identify adjective and noun endings.
3. Construct plural and adjective endings of medical terms.

INTRODUCTION

Word endings are emphasized in this textbook because they can cause problems for both the beginning and the experienced typist when transcribing medical documents. Some dictators tend to "swallow up" the endings of words as they dictate or may dictate a singular ending when the context of the sentence indicates a plural form should be used. The spelling of plural forms of Latin and Greek words does not follow English rules. Therefore, it is important to become familiar with these differences. You will also learn that some of the Latin and Greek words have been Anglicized to have English plural endings. In addition to Latin and Greek endings, you will learn the difference between noun endings and adjective endings. In the examples and exercises presented, some of the most common words dictated in medical reports will be introduced so you can have experience in working with them.

VOCABULARY

Adjective: Word used to limit or qualify a noun.

EXAMPLE: This is a *well-developed* and *well-nourished young Hispanic* boy.

Noun: Name of a person, place, or thing (see Chapter 4, p. 96).

EXAMPLE: This is a well-developed and well-nourished young Hispanic *boy.*

Plural: Noun that refers to more than one.

EXAMPLE: No *x-rays* are available for review.

Singular: Noun that refers to only one.

EXAMPLE: No *x-ray* is available for review.

Suffix: Letter or group of letters added to the end of a word to give it grammatical function or to form a new word.

EXAMPLE: Diagn*osis:* Cellul*itis,* left arm.

PLURAL ENDINGS

Medical terms, as you know from previous study, stem mainly from Greek and Latin. The rules to make these words plural differ from the rules for forming English plurals. You will have to know these rules and the few variations. If the physician dictates a plural form that is unfamiliar to you, check it in a medical dictionary to be sure of the ending. In current usage, many terms have developed English plural endings, and it is good policy to use an English plural whenever one is available. There is a wide variation among physicians, however, and you will notice that some will dictate Latin or Greek endings even though English ones are acceptable.

FORMING PLURALS OF MEDICAL TERMS

The following are some rules for making medical terms plural.

■ Rule 9.1 When a word ends in *"um,"* change the *"um"* to *"a"* (pronounced ah).

EXAMPLE: *labium* becomes *labia*

9–1: SELF-STUDY

Directions: Read the following sentences and choose the correct singular or plural form. On the blank line type or handwrite the word you choose to reinforce spelling. Use your medical dictionary as a reference, if necessary. Check your answers with those given at the end of this chapter.

1. A culture (medium, media) was prepared. __________
2. The Table of Culture (Medium, Media) had a typographical error in the spelling of "Mycoplasma." __________
3. The right and left (acetabulum, acetabula) showed mild degeneration. __________
4. Mark Evans had four (diverticulum, diverticula) noted during the colonoscopy. __________
5. The (ischium, ischia) on the left showed a fracture line on the x-ray. __________
6. The (bacterium, bacteria) in question were *Escherichia coli.* __________

■ Rule 9.2 When a word ends in *"a,"* form the plural by adding an *"e"* (variably pronounced ī, ē, or ā).*

EXAMPLE: *vertebra* becomes *vertebrae*

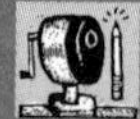

9–2: SELF-STUDY

Directions: Read the following sentences and choose the correct singular or plural form. On the blank line type or handwrite the word you choose to reinforce spelling. Use your medical dictionary as a reference, if necessary. Check your answers with those given at the end of this chapter.

*Dictionaries do not agree on pronunciation.

1. The patient's right shoulder (bursa, bursae) was injected with cortisone. ______________
2. The (pleura, pleurae) of both lungs were filled with fluid. ______________
3. The posterior pleura overlying the (aorta, aortae) was incised. ______________
4. The remaining attachments of the muscle at the base of the (lamina, laminae) were removed. ______________
5. The infant had congenital defects of the right and left (maxilla, maxillae). ______________
6. Eyes: (Conjuctiva, Conjunctivae) clear; (sclera, sclerae) clear. ______________

■ Rule 9.3 When a word ends in *"us,"* change the *"us"* to *"i"* (pronounced ī).

EXAMPLE: *coccus* becomes *cocci*

EXCEPTIONS: *plexus* becomes *plexuses*
corpus becomes *corpora*
meatus stays *meatus* or becomes *meatuses*
syllabus becomes *syllabuses* or *syllabi*
viscus becomes *viscera*

9

9–3: SELF-STUDY

Directions: Read the following sentences and choose the correct singular or plural form. On the blank line type or handwrite the word you choose to reinforce spelling. Use your medical dictionary as a reference, if necessary. Check your answers with those given at the end of this chapter.

1. This patient was diagnosed as having pneumonia, as she has an acute inflammation and infection of the (alveolus, alveoli). ______________
2. The tumor apparently originated at the left main (bronchus, bronchi) and extends peripherally. ______________
3. Specimen consists of an irregular black (calculus, calculi) that measures 5 mm in maximum dimension. ______________
4. A scraping from the skin lesion on the dorsal aspect of the left foot was sent for a test for (fungus, fungi). ______________
5. Leg length was measured from the medial (malleolus, malleoli) to the crest of the (ileum, ilium, ilia). ______________
6. After removal of the dumbbell cyst, the (glomerulus, glomeruli) of the left kidney did not function. ______________

■ Rule 9.4 When a word ends in *"is,"* change the *"is"* to *"es"* (pronounced ēz or ēs).

EXAMPLE: *urinalysis* becomes *urinalyses*

EXCEPTIONS: *iris* becomes *irides*
arthritis becomes *arthritides*
epididymis becomes *epididymides*
femoris becomes *femora*

9–4: SELF-STUDY

Directions: Read the following sentences and choose the correct singular or plural form. On the blank line type or handwrite the word you choose to reinforce spelling. Use your medical dictionary as a reference, if necessary. Check your answers with those given at the end of this chapter.

1. The rectal stump was considered to be quite adequate for (anastomosis, anastomoses). __________
2. (Diagnosis, Diagnoses): 1. Amyotrophic lateral sclerosis. 2. Ventilatory insufficiency. __________
3. An (ecchymosis, ecchymoses) was noted on examination of the right arm. __________
4. The x-ray film revealed an (exostosis, exostoses) on the distal end of the femur. __________
5. The patient's (prognosis, prognoses) is poor. __________
6. The body scan showed one bone and two liver (metastasis, metastases). __________

9

■ Rule 9.5 When a word ends in *"ax"* or *"ix,"* change the *"x"* to *"c"* and add *"es."*

EXAMPLES

thorax becomes *thoraces*
calyx or *calix* becomes *calyces* or *calices*

■ Rule 9.6 When a word ends in *"ex"* or *"ix,"* change the *"ex"* or *"ix"* to *"ices."*

EXAMPLES

appendix becomes *appendices*
apex becomes *apices*

■ Rule 9.7 When a word ends in *"en,"* change the *"en"* to *"ina."*

EXAMPLE

foramen becomes *foramina*

■ Rule 9.8 When a word ends in *"ma,"* change the *"ma"* to *"mata."*

EXAMPLE

carcinoma becomes *carcinomata*

NOTE: With this ending, it is also permissible to add an "s" to the singular.

EXAMPLE

carcinomas

■ Rule 9.9 When a word ends in *"nx,"* change the *"x"* to *"g"* and add *"es."*

EXAMPLE

phalanx becomes *phalanges*

■ Rule 9.10 When a word ends in *"on,"* change the *"on"* to *"a."*

EXAMPLES

criterion becomes *criteria*
zygion becomes *zygia*

9–5: SELF-STUDY

Directions: Read the following sentences and choose the correct singular or plural form. On the blank line type or handwrite the word you choose to reinforce spelling. Use your medical dictionary as a reference, if necessary. Check your answers with those given at the end of the chapter.

1. A Pap smear report stated minimal dysplasia of the (cervix, cervices). __________
2. The patient's blood pressure of 200/100 was a symptom of her tumor of the adrenal (cortex, cortices) of the adrenal gland. __________
3. The (lumen, lumens, lumina) of the catheters had defects, so they were returned to the manufacturer. __________
4. The male anatomy has two (epididymis, epididymides). __________

5. Obstruction of the (larynx, larynges) was caused by a benign growth. ____________

6. There were many (fibroma, fibromata, fibromas) that formed in the soft tissue of the upper thigh. ____________

This summary showing how to form plurals is also in Appendix B and can be torn out and inserted in your personal notebook for quick reference.

PLURAL FORM SYNOPSIS

If the Singular Ending Is	Example	The Plural Ending Is	Example
a	bursa	ae (pronounce ae as i)	bursae
us	alveolus	i	alveoli
um	labium	a	labia
ma	carcinoma	mata	carcinomata
on	criterion	a	criteria
is	anastomosis	es	anastomoses
ix	appendix	ices	appendices
ex	apex	ices	apices
ax	thorax	aces	thoraces
en	foramen	ina	foramina
nx	phalanx	ges	phalanges

Exceptions to Rules for Plural Endings

The words in the following list form plurals in irregular ways:

1. *cornu* becomes *cornua*
2. *femur* becomes *femora*
3. *os*, which has two meanings, becomes *ora* for mouths or *ossa* for bones
4. *paries* becomes *parietes*
5. *pons* becomes *pontes*
6. *vas* becomes *vasa*

NOTE: Add these to your personal notebook.

BASIC PLURAL RULES FOR ENGLISH WORDS

Many medical terms take English plurals by applying the basic rules for forming plurals of English nouns.

■ Rule 9.11 The plural is usually formed by adding "s" to the singular.

EXAMPLES

myelogram myelogram*s* disease disease*s*
bronchoscope bronchoscope*s*

■ Rule 9.12 When a noun ends in "s," "x," "ch," "sh," or "z," add "es" to the singular.

EXAMPLES

stress stress*es* fax fax*es* patch patch*es*
mash mash*es* crutch crutch*es*

EXCEPTION: os ora os ossa

■ Rule 9.13 When a noun ends in "y" preceded by a consonant, change the "y" to "i" and add "es."

EXAMPLES

mammoplasty mammoplast*ies* artery arter*ies*
ovary ovar*ies* therapy therap*ies*

■ Rule 9.14 When a noun ends in "y" preceded by a vowel, add an "s" to the singular word.

EXAMPLES

attorney attorneys

NOTE: There are only a few of these nouns.

■ Rule 9.15 When nouns ending in "o" are preceded by a consonant, in most cases "es" is added to the singular.

EXAMPLES

tomato tomato*es* mulatto mulatto*es*
vertigo vertigo*es* zero zero*es*

NOTE: In regard to this rule, many words are pluralized by simply adding an "s" to the singular.
albino albinos ego egos embryo embryos
impetigo impetigos placebo placebos

EXCEPTIONS: comedo comedones
lentigo lentigines ambo ambones

■ Rule 9.16 Most nouns that end in "f" or "fe" are made plural by changing the "f" or "fe" to "ves."

EXAMPLES

scarf scar*ves* life li*ves*
calf cal*ves* knife kni*ves*

■ Rule 9.17 Compounds are made plural on the main word when there is one. When there is not a main word, the plural is formed at the end.

EXAMPLES

hangers-on mothers-in-law surgeons general
fingerbreadths follow-ups go-betweens

9

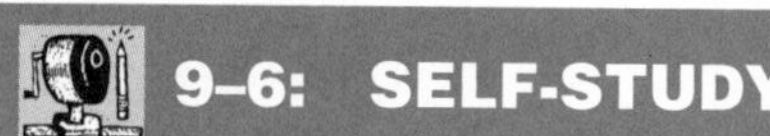

9–6: SELF-STUDY

Directions: Practice these endings by changing the nouns to both foreign and English plurals. Fill in the blanks. Check your answers with those given at the end of this chapter.

1. The head of the femur fits into the *acetabulum.* A human has two ______________ or ______________.
2. An *antrum* is a cavity or chamber. The patient has fluid in three sinus ______________ or ______________.
3. The *aorta* is one of the main arteries of the body. We do not have two ______________ or ______________.
4. Some books have an *appendix.* Many large reference books have several ______________ or ______________.
5. *Axilla* means armpit. He had cysts of both ______________ or ______________.
6. The first skin *biopsy* was taken from Mrs. Aver's arm, but the second and third ______________ were taken from the knee and thigh.
7. She has basal cell *carcinoma,* but previously she had two other types of ______________ or ______________ of the thyroid and kidney.
8. *Comedo* is another word for blackhead. The teenager came in with many ______________ or ______________.
9. The *conjunctiva* protects our eyes from dust and dirt. We have two ______________ or ______________ in our anatomy.
10. The thigh bone is called the *femur.* We have two ______________ or ______________ in our anatomy.
11. *Foramen* means opening or passage. We have numerous ______________ or ______________ throughout our skeletal anatomy.

9

In addition to the English, Latin, and Greek rules for pluralizing words, there are other variances that a beginning medical typist should know. In units of measurement (e.g., inches or pounds), although the plural may sound right, actually the singular is correct.

EXAMPLES

Dictated
"Mrs. Seitz weighs one hundred and twelve *pounds.*"

Transcribe
Mrs. Seitz weighs 112 *lb.*

Dictated
"There *were* two milliliters drawn up in the syringe."

Transcribe
There *was* 2 ml drawn up in the syringe.

Dictated
"Her height is five feet two *inches.*"

Transcribe
Her height is 5 ft 2 *in.*

If the number is one plus a fraction, the sentence should read, "one and a half *inches is* the length of the little finger." Note that the verb must be singular.

Some medical terms are commonly seen as plurals in all dictation. We have two eyes and two ears, but physicians commonly dictate:

EXAMPLES

Dictated
"Conjunctiva clear."

Transcribe
Conjunctivae clear.

Dictated
"Tympanic membrane intact."

Transcribe
Tympanic membranes intact.

Because heart sounds are multiple, physicians commonly dictate the word *bruits,* which is the plural form of *bruit.* The use of the word determines whether it is singular or plural.

EXAMPLES

There is no bruit heard. (singular)

There are no bruits heard. (plural)

Some words can be singular or plural in use, for example, biceps, triceps, data, series, none (means not one or not any). Some words are always plural in use, for example, adnexa, feces, forceps, genitalia, measles, menses, scabies, scissors, tongs, tweezers. Some words are always singular in use, for example, ascites, herpes, lues, news, physics, and so forth.

■ Rule 9.18 To form the plural of French words that end in *eau* and *eu*, add an *x*.

EXAMPLES

milieu (singular) milieux (plural)

rouleau (singular) rouleaux (plural)

■ Rule 9.19 To form the plural of Italian words that end in *o*, change the *o* to an *i*.

EXAMPLE

virtuoso (singular) virtuosi (plural)

NOUN ENDINGS

There are many more noun endings to medical terms than adjective endings. Take as an example the words *microscope, microscopic,* and *microscopy.*

1. The *-scope* on the end of microscope tells us two things about the word:
   a. it is a noun.
   b. it is an instrument.
2. The *-scopic* on the end of the word tells us two things:
   a. it is an adjective.
   b. it means pertaining to an examination.
3. The *-scopy* on the end tells us two things:
   a. it is a noun.
   b. it means the process of examining.

Notice how these endings have changed the meaning of the word. If the dictator slurs the ends of words, you can see how difficult it is to determine which way to spell the word unless you know the meaning of how the word is used in context. Dictated phrases with the term *bilateral* in front of a noun (a procedure) may confuse the transcriptionist in deciding whether to make the noun plural. The noun should be plural, e.g., *bilateral mastectomy* should be typed *bilateral mastectomies.* A list of some of the most frequently used noun endings, their meanings, and an example of how each is used is found on page 230.

9

ADJECTIVE ENDINGS

As you recall from the vocabulary, a word that qualifies or restricts the meaning of a noun is called an adjective. Example: "A *small* cyst was present at the olecranon process." Medical terms can have either English or Latin adjective endings, and in certain instances, this can confuse the transcriptionist. For example, *mucus* is a noun, whereas *mucous* is an adjective. Mucous describes a kind of membrane, and therefore is an adjective, and mucus is the membrane's secretion, and therefore a noun. These words are pronounced exactly alike, so the transcriptionist must see how the word is used in the sentence to determine its spelling.

In many instances, the medical dictionary does not list the adjective form. It is therefore vital to know the noun and be able to convert it to an adjective based on what you hear being dictated. For example, if the dictator says "HI-lar," you look in the dictionary and find the noun "hilum." You then recognize that "ar" has to fit on the root "hil" and come up with "hilar."

See page 230 for a list of the most common adjective endings with their literal translations and examples of how they appear in medical terms. You will notice that a few of these adjective endings are interchangeable with the noun forms (designated by asterisks).

SUFFIX THAT MAKES WORD

Noun	Meaning	Example
-algia	pain	neuralgia
-ase	an enzyme	phosphatase
-asia, asis,	condition or state of	phlegmasia
-esis,		hypophonesis
-osia, -osis,		synarthrosis
-ia,* -iasis		calcemia, cholelithiasis
-ation, -tion, -ion	act of	disarticulation
-ectomy	excision, the process of cutting out	hysterectomy
-emia	condition of the blood	leukemia
-er	agent	ultrasonographer
-gram	record tracing (record)	cardiogram
-graph	instrument to record	cardiograph
-graphy	process or action of recording	cardiography
-ician, -ist	one who specializes in, agent, one who practices	physician, allergist
-ism	condition or theory	mutism
-itis	inflammation	cystitis
-ity	expresses quality	clarity, obesity
-meter	instrument that measures	thermometer
-metry	process of measuring	optometry
-ologist	one who studies, specialist in disease of . . .	endocrinologist
-ology	study of, science of	endocrinology
-oma	tumor, a morbid condition	carcinoma
-or	denoting an agent, doer, a person; a quality or condition	objector error, horror
-pen, -penia	need, deficiency, poverty	leukopenia
-scope	an instrument for visual examination	cytoscope
-scopy	process, action, examination	cytoscopy
-stomy, -stomata, -ostomy	an artificial opening	colostomy, stomata
-tom, -tome	an instrument for cutting	microtome
-tomy, -otomy	a cutting into, incision	meatotomy
-um, -us	pertaining to	diverticulum, digitus
-y	process or action	acromegaly

*Many Greek nouns that end in *-ia* appear in English with *-y* instead of *-ia.*

Adjective Ending	Meaning	Example
-able, -ible	capable of, able to be, fit or likely	friable, digestible
-ac	characteristic of, relating to, affected by or having	cardiac
-al, -alis	of or pertaining to, belonging to	oral, brachialis†
-ar, -ary	pertaining to, belonging to, showing	ocular, elementary
-ate	possessing or characterized by, caused by	quadrate
-ery, -ary*	one who, that which, place where, relating to, engaging in or performing	surgery, capillary
-ic, -icus	dealing with, pertaining to, connected with, resembling	organic, cephalicus†
-id,	signifying state or condition, marked by, giving to showing	viscid
-ive	having power to, have the quality of	palliative
-oid	like or resembling	sphenoid
-ory*	having the nature of	circulatory
-ous, -ose	to be full of, marked by, given to, having the quality of	squamous, adipose

*Many Greek nouns that end in *-ia* appear in English with *-y* instead of *-ia.*
†These are Latin endings and can usually be found in a medical dictionary under the headings of veins, arteries, nerves, ligaments, and so on.

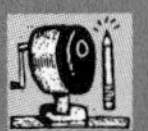 9–7: SELF-STUDY

Directions: Now see if you can identify the following endings by indicating whether the word is an adjective or a noun. State whether the nouns have singular or plural endings. Adjectives are not found in singular or plural forms. Check your answers with those given at the end of this chapter.

	Adjective or Noun	*Singular or Plural*
derm*oid*	adjective	
lymph*omas*	noun	plural
1. sphygmomano*meter*		
2. arthr*algias*		
3. lumbosacr*al*		
4. progno*ses*		
5. cyto*penia*		
6. ento*pic*		
7. rhin*itis*		
8. annul*ar*		
9. gly*cemia*		
10. lapar*otomy*		

9

9–8: REVIEW TEST

Directions: Make these nouns into plurals and then into adjectives. Use your English dictionary to help.

Noun	*Greek or Latin Plural*	*English Plural*	*Adjective*
axilla	axillae	axillas	axillary
1. cranium			
2. focus			
3. caput			
4. pelvimeter			
5. prognosis			
6. lingua			
7. pelvis			
8. phalanx			

Directions: Make these adjectives into nouns by locating the noun in the dictionary. Then spell out the medical term that the physician dictated as an adjective.

The Physician Has Dictated an Adjective That Sounds Like	*The Spelling of the Adjective Is*	*The Noun Is*
AN-u-lar	annular	annulus or anulus or anus
9. VIS-er-al		

9–8: REVIEW TEST *(Continued)*

10. kar″de-o-GRAF-ik ______ ______
11. kil-o-MET-rik ______ ______
12. sis″to-SKOP-ik ______ ______
13. in-FEK-shus ______ ______
14. an″es-THET-ik ______ ______
15. du″-o-DE-nal ______ ______
16. kon″di-LO-mah-toid ______ ______
17. BRONG-ke-al ______ ______
18. FEE-kal ______ ______
19. AB-sessed ______ ______
20. her-PET-ik ______ ______

9–1 COMPUTER EXERCISE

Before proceeding, you may want to do more exercises based on the concepts you have learned. Additional practice material is on your computer diskette.

Directions: Insert the diskette into the computer and follow the instructions on the screen for Computer Exercise 9–1.

A *Answers to* 9–1: SELF-STUDY

1. medium
2. media
3. acetabula
4. diverticula
5. ischium
6. bacteria

A *Answers to* 9–2: SELF-STUDY

1. bursa
2. pleurae
3. aorta
4. lamina
5. maxillae
6. conjunctivae, sclerae. Rationale: Two eyes, so plural must be shown.

A *Answers to* 9–3: SELF-STUDY

1. alveoli. Rationale: Lungs have many clusters of air sacs (alveoli).
2. bronchus
3. calculus
4. fungi. Rationale: Plural since pathologists test for more than one fungus.
5. malleolus, ilium
6. glomeruli. Rationale: A kidney has many filtering units (glomeruli), not just one unit.

A *Answers to* **9–4: SELF-STUDY**

1. anastomosis
2. Diagnoses
3. ecchymosis
4. exostosis
5. prognosis
6. metastases. Rationale: Cancer cells have spread to two locations in the liver.

A *Answers to* **9–5: SELF-STUDY**

1. cervix. Rationale: Patient has a single cervix of the uterus.
2. cortex
3. lumina or lumens
4. epididymides
5. larynx
6. fibromata and fibromas (both are plural forms)

A *Answers to* **9–6: SELF-STUDY**

1. acetabulums or acetabula
2. antra or antrums
3. aortas or aortae
4. appendixes or appendices
5. axillas or axillae
6. biopsies
7. carcinomas or carcinomata
8. comedos or comedones
9. conjunctivas or conjunctivae
10. femurs or femora
11. foramens or foramina

A *Answers to* **9–7: SELF-STUDY**

1. noun singular
2. noun plural
3. adjective
4. noun plural
5. noun singular
6. adjective
7. noun singular
8. adjective
9. noun singular
10. noun singular

CHAPTER

10

Antonyms, Eponyms, and Homonyms

OBJECTIVES

After reading this chapter and working the exercises, you should be able to

1. Identify words that sound alike but have different meanings and different spellings.
2. Define the difference between the terms "antonym," "eponym," and "homonym."
3. Locate eponyms in the medical dictionary.

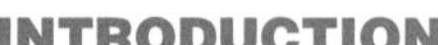

INTRODUCTION

This chapter will introduce the "word demons" of medical language. We will discuss words that sound alike but are spelled differently and have different meanings (homonyms), words that have opposite meanings (antonyms), and words that derive from the name of a place or particular person because of research done in the medical field (eponyms). Distinguishing between these pairs of words can be confusing to the transcriptionist; a good deal of experience may be required to choose the correct term and to spell it properly. Homonyms are the most difficult of the "word demons" for many transcriptionists; hence a large part of the chapter is devoted to them.

Because heteronyms are not as troublesome for the majority of people, they are only briefly touched on in this chapter. Generally, heteronyms are problem words for the foreign-born individual trying to learn the English language. A heteronym is a word that has the same spelling as another but a different meaning and a different pronunciation. For example, let's take the word *tear.* It can mean a drop of water as from the eye, or it can mean to pull or rip something apart. Suppose you hear "the details are so *minute* that it takes more than a *minute* or two to dictate that paragraph in the operative report." Or "The patient stated, 'Several weeks ago I fell into a *slough* and suffered an ulcer on the left arm.' After examination the doctor removed a *slough* of dead tissue from the left arm ulcerated area." Do you know the meaning of minute and slough in these instances? There are literally hundreds of these words in the English language that are accepted daily.

VOCABULARY

Antonym: A word, prefix, or suffix that means the opposite of another word.

Eponym: The place or person for whom something is or is believed to be named; a name (as of a drug or a disease) based on or derived from an eponym.

10

Heteronym: A word that has the same spelling as another but a different meaning and a different pronunciation.

Homonym: A word that is similar in pronunciation but different in meaning and spelling. Also known as homophone.

Homophone: See homonym.

ANTONYMS

An antonym is a whole word, a prefix, or a suffix that means the opposite of another word. To give an example from nonmedical English, *sad* is the antonym of *happy.* Sometimes these antonyms cause spelling trouble because of their similarities in sound. Here is a list of confusing antonyms, their meanings, and some examples. You will notice that the prefixes are shown with a hyphen following the component and that the suffixes have a hyphen preceding the component.

ANTONYM PAIRS

Component	Meaning	Example
ab-	away from	abducent
ad-	to, near, toward	adducent
ecto-	without, outside	ectopic
ento-	within, inner	entopic
-ectomy	excision	cholecystectomy
-tomy	incision	cholecystotomy
hypo-	under, below	hypotension
hyper-	over, above	hypertension
macro-	large, long, great	macroscopic
micro-	small	microscopic

Note: Although not true antonyms, common medical prefixes that also may cause considerable trouble are

Component	Meaning	Example
ante-	preceding or in front of	antecubital
anti-	against	antivenin

EPONYMS

Medical eponyms are adjectives used to describe specific operations, surgical instruments, diseases, and parts of the anatomy. Each of these words is the surname (or an adjective formed from the surname) of an individual who is prominently connected with the development or discovery of the disease, instrument, or surgical procedure. Currently, the American Medical Association recommends that an eponym not be used when a comparable medical term can be substituted for it. It is the dictator's responsibility to dictate the proper term, since in this instance the transcriptionist merely types what was heard.

An example of an eponym is "Buerger disease" (or "Buerger's disease"). The comparable medical term is "thromboangiitis obliterans." It is important to note that more and more writers are making exceptions to the possessive rule by not showing the possessive ('s) with an eponym. In checking dictionaries and other reference books, you will find conflicting styles, one showing the eponym with the possessive and one showing it without. These are alternative acceptable forms. Generally, when surgical and diagnostic instruments, materials, and solutions are dictated, there is no possessive. In summary, one may eliminate the possessive if the dictator does not use it or has no objection to its elimination.

EXAMPLES

Foley catheter

Gigli saw

Mayo scissors

Richard retractors

Anatomic eponyms are written in lower case, such as eustachian tube, fallopian tube, and so forth when used as an adjective. Words derived from eponymic names (parkinsonism, addisonian, cushingoid facies, and so forth) are also not capitalized. See Chapter 4, page 98, for the rule on these words.

To find the medical term or definition that corresponds to an eponym, look up the second term, the *clue word,* as shown in the following italicized examples. These are just a few of the many thousands of medical eponyms. The paragraph on Cross References in Chapter 8 will help you to locate others.

1. Abbe's *anemia*
2. Addison's *anemia*
3. Babinski's *reflex*
4. Bell's *palsy*
5. Bravais-jacksonian *epilepsy*
6. Bright's *disease*
7. Cheyne-Stokes *respiration*
8. Colles' *fracture*
9. Cooper's *ligament*
10. Dupuytren's *contracture*
11. Feleky's *instrument*
12. Hanot's *cirrhosis*
13. Highmore's *antrum*
14. Koch's *bacillus*
15. Laennec's *cirrhosis*
16. Romberg's *sign*
17. Skene's *glands*
18. Stensen's *duct*

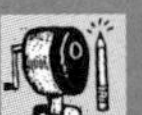

10–1: SELF-STUDY

Directions: Match the following with their correct definitions. Check your answers with those at the end of this chapter.

1. antonyms ______ a. Words that have the same spelling but different meanings and different pronunciations.
2. eponyms ______ b. Words that are opposite to each other in meaning.
3. homonyms ______ c. Words that sound alike but are spelled differently and have different meanings.
4. heteronyms ______ d. Words that have been derived from the surname of a person.

Do you remember what an acronym is, as mentioned in Chapter 4? Define it here. ______

______

ENGLISH HOMONYMS

Homonyms are words that are similar in pronunciation but different in meaning and spelling. Sometimes these are called "phonetic pairs." A few English examples are *hare* and *hair, weak* and *week,* and *too, two,* and *to.* If one of these words were dictated, knowing its meaning would help you decide how to spell it.

ENGLISH TROUBLESOME TWOSOMES

Word	Meaning	Example
advice (n) advise (v)	counsel; recommendation to counsel; to notify	The advice that Dr. Blake gave was excellent. Dr. Blake will advise (influence) her to have surgery.
affect (v)	to influence	The recession affects our business. Our business was affected by the recession. Note: This is almost always used as a verb. Do not use *affect* as a noun in everyday speech. In psychiatry, *affect* is a noun meaning the emotional reactions associated with an experience and generally follows an adjective describing it.
affect (n)	a disposition or mood	The patient had a blunted affect.

ENGLISH TROUBLESOME TWOSOMES *Continued*

Word	Meaning	Example
effect (v)	to bring about or cause	He effected the changes in our department. The treatment did not effect (bring about) any change. Note: In ordinary speech, the verb use of *effect* is not common. It is used most often in the context of power, influence, creation, and administration and usually has a physiological connotation with an intent.
effect (n)	a result	The recession had a bad effect on our business. One effect (result) of physical therapy is more mobility of injured joints.
all ready (adj)	completely ready	The office was all ready to close when an emergency case came in.
already (adv)	by this time, previously	The physician was already gone when the call came in.
all together	in a group, collectively	By typing the same insurance forms all together, fewer errors will occur.
altogether (adv)	entirely, completely	The two medical cases are altogether different.
bare (adj)	uncovered, plain	For ultrasound, the area must be bare.
bear (n or v)	to carry; an animal; to be directed	The physican prefers to bear the good news to the patient.
breath (n)	air taken into the lungs and then expelled; the act of breathing	The patient becomes out of breath when walking up a flight of stairs.
breathe (v)	to inhale and exhale air	The patient was able to breathe again easily.
cite (v)	to quote	You may cite the article as your reference.
sight (n)	vision	His sight was 20/20 on right and left.
site (n)	location	The site of the injury was the left leg.
complement (n or v)	something that completes, harmonize	The office has a full complement of staff members.
compliment (n or v)	praise, congratulate	Maria was complimented several times by her employer.
elicit (v)	to draw forth	The physician tried to elicit the facts about the patient's condition.
illicit (adj)	unlawful	It is illicit to give out information about a patient without his written permission.
imply (v)	to indicate indirectly or by allusion	His silence will imply consent. Note: *Imply* is what you give out when you say or do something a certain way.
infer (v)	to arrive at a conclusion from facts or premises	From your response, I infer that you're angry. Note: *Infer* is what the listener takes in or perceives the speaker to be saying.
The main problem with the following troublesome twosomes is that the past tense of lie (meaning to recline) is the present tense of lay (mean to place).		
lay (v) [lay, laid, laying]	to place	The blame lay on her inability to communicate. Note: *Lay* always takes an object.
lie (v) [lie, lay, lain, lying]	to recline	The patient was told to lie down. Note: *Lie* never takes an object.
lei (n)	Hawaiian flower garland	A beautiful lei was placed around her neck on arrival in Kona.
loose (adj)	not tightly bound	The patient complained of loose stools.
lose (v)	to suffer loss or deprivation	The patient began to lose weight.
principal (adj, n)	chief; main; leader	The patient's principal complaint was pain.
principle (n)	rule	Her knowledge of punctuation principles is questionable.
set (v)	to place	He set the file on the desk. Note: This word takes an object.
sit (v)	to be in a certain position	She will sit tomorrow to have her picture taken. Note: This word has no object.
stationary (adj)	still, not moving	The patient's condition was stationary.
stationery (n)	writing paper	Please purchase some stationery at the store.
than (conj)	conjunction of comparison	A word processor is faster than an electric typewriter.
then (adv)	at that time	Proofread your work; then you can vouch for its accuracy.

ENGLISH TROUBLESOME TWOSOMES *Continued*

Word	Meaning	Example
their (adj)	of, belonging to, made, or done by them	Pat and Jo have done their homework.
there (adv)	at or in that place; toward	There are several laboratory tests to be performed
In the last set of trouble twosomes, focus on the clause where "who" or "whom" is working to identify if it is the subject or object.		
who (pronoun)	what or which person	She was one of the transcriptionists who were introduced. Who was there? Note: *Who* is always the subject of the sentence of clause (the doer of the action).
whom (pronoun)		I need an employee whom I can depend on. Note: *Whom* is always the object of the sentence (the receiver of the action). Substitute "him" for "whom"—I can depend on *him.* Notice that "him" and "whom" end in the letter "M."

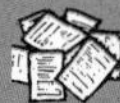 10–2: PRACTICE TEST

10

Directions: Perhaps you are still a bit confused by English words that sound alike. Try this exercise to see how you score. For each of the following sentences, select the word within the parentheses that completes the sentence correctly. Mark through the incorrect word. (If both words are incorrect, mark through both words and write the correct word above them.) Note that some sentences have two sets of selections.

1. He will (advice, advise) anyone on his or her medical problems.
2. Please (lay, lei) the paper down on the examination table.
3. The medical assistant intended the remark as a (compliment, complement).
4. (Whose, Who's) dictionary is this on my desk?
5. (Your, You're) office is (too, two) far from the hospital.
6. The old medical building was (razed, raised) to make room for a new hospital.
7. With a great (serge, surge) the patient leaped (fourth, forth).
8. Tell the patient to (sight, cite) an example for you.
9. Ms. Drake had one (coarse, course) of radiation treatment following her left mastectomy.
10. Sitting (here, hear), I can (here, hear) you clearly.
11. Our stock of office (stationary, stationery) is almost exhausted.
12. The patient's rhinoplasty had a tremendous (affect, effect) on her social relationships.
13. The (affect, effect) of the new surgical procedure gave hope to millions of people.
14. The patient would prefer to come at 8 a.m. if an appointment is available (than, then).
15. Developing x-ray films is much faster (than, then) it was ten years ago.
16. The medical assistant quickly sorted the (correspondence, correspondents) for filing.
17. The surgery on Mr. Salazar lasted nine hours, and Dr. Cho performed another surgery on Mrs. Baker without a (brake, break).
18. The (principle, principal) reason for the trip was to search for a new hospital (sight, site).
19. The physician gave the medical assistant instructions to (accept, except) the subpoena when it was served.
20. A horizontal osteotomy was (affected, effected).

21. On general examination of the abdominal cavity, (they're, their, there) was no abnormality found.
22. (They're, Their, There) bringing in the accident case to the emergency room.
23. The tubes were traced out to the fimbriae to doubly identify (they're, their, there) anatomy.

The answers to these are in Appendix A.

MEDICAL HOMONYMS

Medical homonyms may prove somewhat tougher if you are not thoroughly versed in terminology or if the difficult word pairs have never been pointed out to you. Perhaps even now you are using an incorrect spelling of a word. Mastery of some of the more challenging ones can save you time and possibly embarrassment. A list of common homonyms, showing their pronunciation and meaning and the words that sound similar to them is found in Appendix B.

What if a word is dictated that sounds like pair-ah-NEE-al? Is it spelled p-e-r-o-n-e-a-l or p-e-r-i-n-e-a-l? Do you know their meanings and know which word to select because of how it is used in the sentence dictated? You will be confronted by homonyms throughout your career as a medical transcriptionist.

10–3: SELF-STUDY

Directions: The following components are used daily in dictation. See if you can match them with their definitions.

1. ab-	____________	a. washing
2. ad-	____________	b. small
3. ante-	____________	c. muscle
4. anti-	____________	d. to, near, toward
5. -lysis	____________	e. before
6. -clysis	____________	f. from, away from
7. myo-	____________	g. loosening, destroying
8. myco-	____________	h. fungus
9. myelo-	____________	i. against
10. mio-	____________	j. marrow, spinal cord

Check your answers at the end of this chapter and then tackle the next two assignments encompassing still more medical sound-alikes.

10–4: PRACTICE TEST

Directions: Let's do some vocabulary-building homonym exercises and enrich our mastery of medical terms. The following sentences are arranged in pairs. If you have difficulty completing the exercises, refer to Appendix B, Common Medical Homonyms. Select the word from the left column that is needed to complete correctly each sentence in the right column.

position
apposition
opposition

1. The physician was in ____________ when Sally wanted to make a new policy in the office.
2. Successive layers in the cell walls were in ____________ to each other.

3. Dry, sterile dressings were applied and a modified Jones ______________ utilized, incorporating a dorsal plaster of Paris splint.

aberration
abrasion

4. On examination, Miss Baker had a 1-cm ______________ over the right patella.
5. The patient's illness showed an ______________ in his condition.

dysphagia
dysphasia

6. The patient denies at any time any pain or tenderness in the neck, any ______________, hoarseness, or enlargement of the thyroid gland.
7. After suffering a stroke, Mr. James had ______________ for six months and then regained normal speech.

absorption
adsorption

8. The physician used a collagen suture material so there would be ______________ into the tissues.
9. The bandage showed an ______________ to the surface of the skin.

adherence
adherents

10. There are ______________ to the cause of Martin Luther King.
11. The ______________ of the bandage to the skin caused Mrs. Base to break out in a rash.

The answers to these are in Appendix A.

10

10-5: REVIEW TEST

Directions: The following sentences are arranged in groups. If you have difficulty completing the exercises, refer to Appendix B, Common Medical Homonyms. Select the word from the left column that is needed to correctly complete each sentence in the right column.

aura
aural
ora
oral

1. The ear is concerned with the acoustic or ______________ sense.
2. Betsy Blake complained of having an ______________ before her epileptic attacks.
3. Valium is an ______________ medication.
4. The ______________ serrata is the serrated margin of the retina in the anterior portion of the eyeball.

hypertension
Hypertensin
hypotension

5. Mr. Yoshida's blood pressure was 165/90, indicating ______________.
6. Mrs. Lockhard had a blood pressure reading of 100/60, which is a condition of ______________.
7. ______________ is a drug that produces a rise in blood pressure.

amenorrhea
dysmenorrhea
menorrhea
menorrhagia
metrorrhagia

8. Her chief complaint was ______________, meaning absence of the menses.
9. One of Miss Mason's symptoms was abnormal uterine hemorrhage between periods, and this is called ______________.

antiseptic
asepsis
aseptic
sepsis
septic

10. The surgical instruments must be ______________ at all times.
11. The laboratory report indicated pus-forming microorganisms in the blood, a condition of ______________.

palpation
palpitation

12. She has had no further episodes of ______________ of the heart.
13. The physician examined the area by ______________ and felt a small cyst.

dilation dilatation	14. Because of hemorrhaging, Beth was advised to have a ______________ and curettage.
	15. The process of ______________ is used when examining the eyes.
discrete discreet	16. Breast exam reveals no ______________ masses or abnormalities.
tract track	17. He was seen in consultation by Dr. Friedman, who did an upper ______________ endoscopy with no unusual findings.
regimen regime	18. On this ______________, it was noted his electrolytes remained normal.
introitus enteritis	19. Preliminary pelvic examination showed a parous ______________ .
instillation installation	20. Prior to the ______________ of general anesthesia, a KUB was obtained.

10–1: COMPUTER EXERCISE

Before proceeding, you may want to do more exercises based on the concepts you have learned. Additional practice material is on your computer diskette.

Directions: Insert the diskette into the computer and follow the instructions on the screen for Computer Exercise 10–1.

A *Answers to* 10–1: SELF-STUDY

1. b
2. d
3. c
4. a

An acronym is a word composed from the initial letters of other words.

A *Answers to* 10–3: SELF-STUDY

1. f
2. d
3. e
4. i
5. g
6. a
7. c
8. h
9. j
10. b

Medical Records and Reports

CHAPTER

11

Medical Chart Notes and Progress Notes

11

OBJECTIVES

After reading this chapter and working the exercises, you should be able to

1. Explain the necessity of typing accurate notes on patient progress.
2. Demonstrate the proper procedure and format for transcribing patient medical chart notes.
3. Use the different methods employed in preparing medical chart notes.
4. Recognize and correct any erroneous entry made into the medical record.
5. List the basic information to be found in patient notes in emergency departments and medical offices.

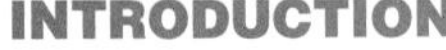

INTRODUCTION

Chart notes (also called progress notes) are the formal or informal notes taken by the physician when he or she meets with or examines a patient in the office, clinic, acute care center, or emergency department. These notes are a part of the patient's permanent medical record; as you recall from Chapter 1, medical records are a vital key in patient care. Although medical records are used mainly to assist the physician with care of the patient, they can be reviewed by attorneys, other physicians, insurance companies, or the court. It is essential that they be neat, accurate, and complete.

"Accurate" means that they are transcribed as dictated, and "complete" requires that they be dated and signed or initialed by the dictator. One can hardly insist that the physician sign or initial the records, but you might overcome the physician's reluctance by making it easier to do so, for example, by typing a line at the end of each chart entry for the signature or initials. Then, at the end of the shift or the day, all of the reports can be stacked on the physician's desk for signing. In a medical office or setting, one suggestion is for the physician to sign the notes when the patient returns for a follow-up visit; this is when the previous notes are usually reviewed.

For a chart to be admissible as evidence in court, the party dictating or writing entries should be able to attest that they were true and correct at the time they were written. The best indication of that is the physician's signature or initials at the end of each typed note. The hospital will insist that the physician sign all dictated material and all entries he or she makes on the patient's record; failure to do so could result in a loss of hospital staff privileges.

Furthermore, before copies of records leave the facility, the originals must be checked for accuracy; if they were not signed before, they must be signed now. Any liability of the transcriptionist personally is of small significance unless there are unusual circumstances, such as negligence, willfulness, or malice. A physician cannot easily shift the blame to another because the faulty records are his or her responsibility as long as the proper procedure for release of information has been established. If a medical transcriptionist is at fault in recording improperly, the physician has the right to discharge him or her for inefficiency, and this is a peril for the careless worker.

Most physicians handwrite daily progress entries into the patient's hospital medical record. In office or clinic situations, some physicians never dictate chart notes, preferring to enter them into the patient's record in longhand. Although it is not essential that medical records be typed, it is best to do so. Obviously, typed notes are easier to read; when more than one physician is involved in patient care, such as in a large office or clinic, it is vital that all notes be easily read with no chance of misinterpretation. In this chapter, we are not concerned with longhand notes but rather with learning the process of taking chart notes from the transcribing equipment and typing them properly into the patient's record.

The physician should try to dictate as soon as he or she is finished seeing a patient and the details are still fresh in his or her mind. Some physicians have also found it helpful to dictate the notes with the patient present. This gives the physician the opportunity to ask for any details that may have been overlooked in the initial history taking; it also gives him or her an opportunity to reinstruct the patient on medication or the purpose of tests and the expected results. An advantage to the patient is the ability to hear the same information repeated into the dictating machine, reinforcing what was previously discussed. The patient will also get another opportunity to ask questions that may have been forgotten, and he or she may even provide additional pieces of information. Last, patients get a better understanding of the amount of time spent in the physician's care. Emergency department chart notes are written or dictated as the patient is being seen. They are usually transcribed on a STAT (immediate) basis. Some emergency departments or urgent care centers place the transcribing station within the facility or in a nearby area so the dictator can have immediate access to the chart note. If the patient is admitted to the hospital for treatment or observation, this initial note or dictation will accompany the patient.

The items dictated into a chart note will vary and may include all or only some of the following: an account of health history of the patient and family, the findings on physical examination, the signs or symptoms occurring while the patient is under observation, and the medication and treatments the patient receives or those recommended. This information may be set off by individual topics, such as the chief complaint (CC), the reason the patient is visiting the doctor or emergency department; the history (Hx) of the complaint; the treatment (Rx) recommended by the physician; and the physician's impression (Imp) or diagnosis (Dx) of the problem. Abbreviations are used very freely in chart notes, and you might like to refer again to the list of abbreviations in Appendix B. In addition, a brief general list is provided for you to refer to as you begin your assignments.

The office transcriptionist will be working with dictated progress notes made when the patient is seen in the office, at home, or in the emergency department, with reference made to admissions and discharges from the hospital or a nursing facility. Telephone conversations made with the patient or with other physicians treating the patient may also be recorded.

GENERAL PRINCIPLES FOR COMPLETE DOCUMENTATION IN MEDICAL RECORDS

You must be aware of the general principles for complete documentation of medical records to ensure that these are written or transcribed into the record, documenting services for which the provider of care expects to be paid. The following is a general outline of the principles through which payments are made. It is important to observe that these components are documented and to alert your employer when they are not mentioned. To do this, you must know what billing codes are used by the facility for the service documented.

The nature and amount of physician work and documentation vary by the type of service performed, the place of the service, and the status of the patient. These general principles are applicable to all types of medical and surgical services in all settings. The billing and diagnosis codes reported on the health insurance claim form should be supported by the documentation in the record.

In addition, the following teaches you about the information that is generally found in these records and helps you set it up in a logical fashion.

1. The records must be complete and legible
2. Each patient encounter should include the following documentation:
   a. date
   b. reason for the encounter
   c. history, physical examination, prior diagnostic test results
   d. diagnosis (assessment, impression)
   e. plan for care
   f. name of the observer
3. Rationale for ordering diagnostic or other services, documented or inferred
4. Health risk factors identified
5. Progress, response to treatment, changes in treatment, and revision of diagnosis documented

Seven components are used when describing the level of services for evaluation and management of the patient. The level of care given will determine how many of these components are used. Therefore, it is important that they are documented when done. These may be listed as separate elements of the history, or they may be included in the history of the present illness.

History

The history includes the chief complaint (CC), the history of present illness (HPI), the review of systems (ROS), and past history, family, and/or social history (PFSH).

The CC describes the symptom, problem, or condition that is the reason for the encounter, and this must be clearly described in the record.

The HPI is the chronological description of the development of the patient's present illness from the first sign and/or symptom or from the previous encounter to the present.

A problem-pertinent ROS inquires about the system directly related to the problems identified in the HPI. The patient's positive responses and pertinent negatives related to the problem are documented. Signs or symptoms the patient might be experiencing or has experienced are identified, including constitutional symptoms (fever, weight loss, fatigue); integumentary (skin and/or breast); eyes, ears, nose, and throat; mouth; cardiovascular; respiratory; gastrointestinal; genitourinary; musculoskeletal; neurologic; psychiatric; endocrine; hematologic/lymphatic; and allergic/immunologic.

The ROS and PFSH may be recorded by an ancillary staff member or on a form completed by the patient. When directly related to the problem identified in the HPI, the PFSH is a review of the patient's past illnesses, operations, injuries, and treatments; a review of medical events in the patient's family, including diseases that may be hereditary; and a review of past and current activities in which the patient was or is engaged. (The time spent with the patient in history taking, care, examination, counseling, coordination of services should also be documented.)

Examination

The extent of the examination performed and documented is dependent on clinical judgment and the nature of the presenting problems. Examinations range from limited to complete. Depending on the level of services performed, there are four types of examinations:

1. Problem focused: a limited examination of the affected body area or system.
2. Expanded: a limited examination of the affected body area or system and other symptomatic related systems.
3. Detailed: an extended examination of the affected body area and other symptomatic or related systems.
4. Comprehensive: a general multisystem examination or a complete examination of a single system.

Medical Decision Making

There are four types of medical decision making, and they are measured by the number of possible diagnoses or management options that must be considered; the complexity of medical records, tests, and other information that must be obtained, reviewed, and analyzed; the risk of significant complications associated with the problem(s), the diagnostic procedures; and/or possible management options. They are as follows:

1. Straightforward: self-limited or minor problem
2. Low complexity:
   a. two or more self-limited or minor problems
   b. stable chronic illness
   c. acute uncomplicated illness or injury

INFORMATION REQUIRED FOR CASE HISTORY FILE

Date..

Patient.. Date of Birth...................... Age................
(Mr., Mrs., Miss, Master) First Name Initial Last Name

Name of Husband, Wife or Parent... Home Phone...................................

Home Address.. If Military, Serial No. Soc. Sec. No.......................................

Patient Employed By:...
City or Town Zip Code

Business Address...

Occupation... Business Phone...............................

Husband or Wife Employed by:..

Business Address...
City or Town Zip Code

Occupation... Business Phone...............................

Name of nearest relative
not named above (indicate relationship)...

Address..

Insured by:..Group No............... Member No......................

Recommended by:... Former Physician...

If patient a minor
Give name of person legally responsible:..

I hereby authorize and request the .... Insurance Company to pay the amount due me in my pending claim for medical expense Benefits directly to ....MD

Date... Signature..

Figure 11–1. Example of a social data sheet.

3. Moderate complexity
   a. one or more chronic illnesses with mild exacerbation, progression, or side effects of treatment
   b. two or more stable chronic illnesses
   c. undiagnosed new problem
   d. acute illness
   e. acute complicated injury
4. High complexity
   a. one or more chronic illnesses with severe exacerbation, progression, or side effects of treatment
   b. acute or chronic illness or injuries that pose a threat to life or bodily function

Counseling and Coordination of Care

When counseling and/or coordination of care involves more than 50% of the physician/patient/family encounter time in the office, outpatient setting, hospital, or nursing facility, the total length of time of the encounter (face-to-face) must be documented, and the record should describe the counseling and/or activities to coordinate care.

NEW PATIENT, OFFICE

When a patient comes into the office for the initial visit, a chart is prepared. These charts will vary, just as physicians and their medical specialties vary. Therefore, we shall examine the broad methods of record preparation; you can easily apply these instructions to the method used where you work. There really is no "best" way to keep medical records other than that they be neat, accurate, complete, and timely (made as soon as possible after the patient is seen).

The patient will complete a social data sheet on the initial visit (Fig. 11–1). These data sheets, again, will vary according to the wishes of the individual physician or staff. This information is then used to prepare the accounting (ledger) file for the patient as well as to supply the initial information for the patient's chart. Some offices will transfer all of this information to the initial page of the medical record; others will take the barest minimum (complete name and birthdate or age). Medical consultants often wish to have the name and telephone number of the referring physician. It will be important for you to learn exactly what information your employer wants transferred from the social data sheet to this initial chart page.

Figures 11–2 to 11–6 illustrate a variety of chart paper styles. You will notice that both lined and unlined paper are used. Some physicians have special paper printed for notes, others purchase

Mary Neidgrinhaus   DOB: 06-11-9x   REF: Yuen Wong, MD

12-18-9x

HX: This 4½-year-old girl has been having URIs beginning in October, 19xx. She has had several of these infections since that time and has been seen by another otolaryngologist who recommended that she have surgery including an adenotonsillectomy and bilateral myringotomies with tubes. The mother desired another opinion and the family doctor referred her to me.

ALLERGIES: AMPICILLIN and SEPTRA

PX: Well-developed, well-nourished girl in no acute distress.

VS: Pulse: 84/min. Resp: 20/min. Temp: 98.8° axillary.

HEENT: Eyes: PERRLA. EOMs normal. Ears: The rt TM was retracted and slightly injected. The left TM was retracted but not injected. Both canals were negative. Nose: The nasal septum was roughly in the midline. Mucous membrane lining somewhat pale and slightly swollen. Throat: Tonsils were +3 and very cryptic. Neck: There were tonsillar nodes palpable in both anterior cervical triangles.

CHEST: Lungs: Clear to auscultation. Heart: Regular rate and rhythm, no murmurs.

IMP: 1. Hypertrophy of tonsils and adenoids.
2. Bilateral recurrent serous otitis media.

RX: Dimetapp elixir, 4 oz, 1 t q.i.d.

mlo

Gene M. Kasten, MD

DEC. 28 199x
Rt ear improved; no change in the left. Mother still does not want surgery.

RX: Actifed syrup, 2 oz, ½ t q.i.d.

mlo

Gene M. Kasten, MD

1-3-9x Mother telephoned Actifed "not helping." Called in Ceclor, 4 oz, 1t qid per Dr. Kasten. mlo

JAN. 14 199x No improvement in left ear. Rt ear significantly the same as when last seen. Mother now approves surgical removal of the tonsils and adenoids and bilateral myringotomies with tube insertions.

mlo

Gene M. Kasten, MD

2-5-9X See Copy of History and Physical dictated for View of the Lakes Memorial. mlo

2-6-9X Pt admitted 3:30PM mlo

2-8-9X See letter to Dr. Wong. mlo

Figure 11–2. Example of typical unlined chart note paper. See note of December 18 to see how the "allergy" is handled.

KARL ROBRECHT, MD
INTERNAL MEDICINE
555 LAKE VIEW DRIVE
BAY VILLAGE, OHIO 44140

Name			Date
Legal Address			Tel. No.
Local Address			Tel. No.
Birthplace	Age	Sex	Marital Status
Occupation	Employer	Address	Tel. No.
Nearest Relative, or Guardian (Relationship)		Address	Tel. No.
Occupation	Employer	Address	Tel. No.
Referred by		Address	Tel. No.
Insurance Company		Address	Policy No./Type

PHYSICAL EXAMINATION

Height ________ Weight ________ T ________ P ________ General Appearance ________

Eyes ________ Vision Recorded on Sight Screener ________

Ears ________ Hearing: rt ________ lt ________

Teeth ________ Nose ________

Throat ________ Thyroid ________

Skin ________ Scars ________

Heart ________ BP ________

Lungs ________

Breasts ________

Abdomen ________

Rectum ________ Hernia ________

Extremities ________

Nervous System ________

Reflexes ________

Personality ________

Hygiene ________

Remarks ________

Figure 11–3. Example of medical office chart paper, initial visit.

EMERGENCY DEPARTMENT RECORD

Holly P. Woodsen

CHART REQUESTED

LOCATION	DATE	TIME REGISTERED	TRIAGE TIME	AM ☐ PM ☐	OUTPT	INPT
202	11/29/95	11:32			☐	☐

ARRIVED ▶ [X] WALKED ☐ WC ☐ AMB ☐ PARA AMB ☐ OTHER

ACCOMPANIED BY ▶ ☐ ALONE ☐ SPOUSE ☐ PARENT ☐ FRIEND ☐ RELATIVE

PATIENT'S ADDRESS

1335 11th Street
Mt. Channel, XX 54321

HOME PHONE 619 278-6489
WORK PHONE 619 278-6489
RELATIVE TO CONTACT / PHONE

PRIMARY CARE CLINIC: 221
PERSONAL PHYSICIAN: W.A. Berry

AGE	SEX	TEMP	BLOOD PRESSURE	PULSE	RESP	WEIGHT (Peds)
027	F	99.9	111/76	87	20	

CURRENT MEDICATIONS: Ø

DRUG SENSITIVITY ☐ NO ☑ YES | IF YES, SPECIFY DRUG: PCN | LMP | LAST TETANUS

CHIEF COMPLAINT (IF INJURY - WHERE AND HOW DID IT OCCUR?) ASSAULTED by boyfriend

	✓
CBC WBC	
CBC H&H	
Lytes	
Bun/Creat	
Glucose/Acet	
Amylase	
U/A	
C&S___	
Preg Test	
CPK	
CXR	
Abd Ser/KUB	
ABG	
Peak Flow	
Pulse Ox	
EKG	

Visual Acuity OD (R)____ OS (L)__

TIME OF INITIAL EXAM | HISTORY AND EXAM

S: 27 y/o female who presents to the ER after an altercation. Pt reports that she was driving her car, her boyfriend was in the front passenger seat. The pt reported to me that she reached across and struck him on the chest, and that he responded by punching her on the right side of her face three times. Pt was driving the car and apparently did not lose consciousness and did not lose control of the car. She denies being struck in the chest or abdomen.

Incident has been reported to the police by nursing staff.

O: She is awake, alert and appropriate. Head and face appear atraumatic, no STS or ecchymosis is noted. The neck is supple. Pupils midposition and reactive, EOMs are intact. Full ROM to the mandible, no malocclusion. No chest wall or bony pelvic tenderness.

A: Facial contusions.

P: Reassurance. Ice. ASA. Tylenol. Soft diet as needed. Re-exam for persistent pain or malocclusion.

DISABILITY ☐ NO ☐ YES | IF YES, GIVE RETURN TO WORK DATE

CONDITION AT DISCHARGE (CHECK ALL THAT APPLY) ☐ UNCHANGED ☐ ALERT/ORIENTED ☐ ON CRUTCHES ☐ DOA ☐ ASYMPTOMATIC ☐ AMBULATORY ☐ EXPIRED ☐ OTHER ▶ SPECIFY | ED PHYSICIAN

INSTRUCTIONS TO PATIENT ☐ WRITTEN ☐ VERBAL ▶ SPECIFY,

DISPOSITION (CHECK ALL THAT APPLY) ☐ RETURN PRN ☐ HOME ☐ WORK ☐ HOLDING ☐ ADMITTED ☐ TRANSFERRED ▶ SERVICE & FLOOR ☐ REFERRED TO ☐ RETURN TO ▶ DOCTOR, DATE, LOCATION, TIME | TIME

Figure 11–4. Example of emergency department chart note illustrating minimum heads and SOAP format.

William A. Berry, MD

PATIENT NAME	AGE	CHART NUMBER
Stoffer, Grace W. (Mrs. William J.)	47	G-96390

JAN 23 199x

CC: Rectal bleeding, intermittent for 2 months.

After BM, bright red blood.

PX: No external hemorrhoids or fissures seen.

Internal hemorrhoids but none ulcerated on anoscopic exam.

Can see no bleeding.

On digital, at finger end, feels like fold or may be mass

above on rt, posterior rectal wall?

Rx: Return tomorrow for sigmoidoscopy and biopsy.

CBC ordered. WAB/ref

JAN 24 199x

CC: Rectal bleeding, intermittent.

Possible mass on posterior rectal wall.

PE: Sigmoidoscopy to 15 cm. Unable to get beyond at 15 cm on

the left posterolateral wall of the rectum because of a

hemorrhagic area. Biopsy taken of this area.

No other areas seen.

Hx: Father had abnormalities of rectum, 1961.

Patient has no history of skin or scalp lesions.

Rx: Barium enema ordered. WAB/ref

Rtn. in 4 days to discuss results of BE and biopsy.

JAN 28 199x

CC: Several more episodes of rectal bleeding, always following

a BM

Biopsy and BE essentially negative for source of bleeding

PE: Anoscopy: moderate hemorrhoidal tags.

Rx: Anusol HC suppositories, 1 morning and evening/ 6 days.

Call or return in 3-4 weeks.

February 15, 199x Telephone call, no symptoms. Will call if

episodes begin again. WAB/ref

Figure 11–5. Example of typed chart notes on lined paper.

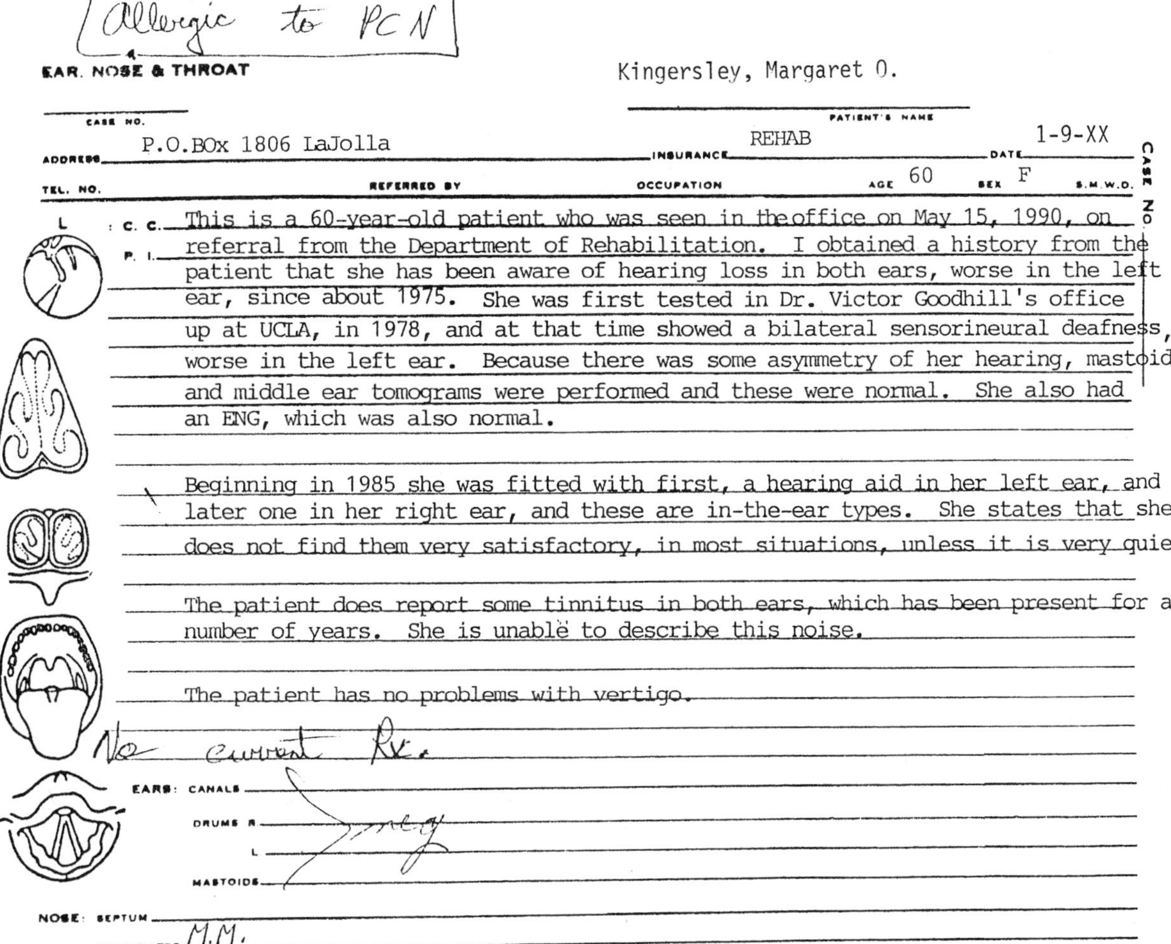

[Allergic to PCN]

EAR, NOSE & THROAT

Kingersley, Margaret O.

CASE NO. | PATIENT'S NAME

ADDRESS P.O.BOx 1806 LaJolla | INSURANCE REHAB | DATE 1-9-XX

TEL. NO. | REFERRED BY | OCCUPATION | AGE 60 | SEX F | S.M.W.D. | CASE NO.

C.C. / P.I. This is a 60-year-old patient who was seen in the office on May 15, 1990, on referral from the Department of Rehabilitation. I obtained a history from the patient that she has been aware of hearing loss in both ears, worse in the left ear, since about 1975. She was first tested in Dr. Victor Goodhill's office up at UCLA, in 1978, and at that time showed a bilateral sensorineural deafness, worse in the left ear. Because there was some asymmetry of her hearing, mastoid and middle ear tomograms were performed and these were normal. She also had an ENG, which was also normal.

Beginning in 1985 she was fitted with first, a hearing aid in her left ear, and later one in her right ear, and these are in-the-ear types. She states that she does not find them very satisfactory, in most situations, unless it is very quiet

The patient does report some tinnitus in both ears, which has been present for a number of years. She is unable to describe this noise.

The patient has no problems with vertigo.

No current Rx.

EARS: CANALS

DRUMS R

L

MASTOIDS

NOSE: SEPTUM

TURBINATES M.M.

Figure 11–6. Example of a chart note from an ear, nose, and throat specialist that shows the use of chart paper with diagramed body parts.

chart paper from medical printing supply houses, and others prefer plain 8 1/2 × 11 inch typing paper. When typing via computer onto a lined sheet, care must be taken to ensure that the paper is aligned in the printer; it takes practice with the computer and printer to do this. Generally, these notes on lined paper are double spaced. This is an awkward arrangement, but it is often used because many handwritten notes are added to the typed notes, and writers find the lined paper more convenient. It is perfectly acceptable to ignore the lines when transcribing onto lined paper. See Figures 11–4 and 11–5 for examples of transcription on lined paper. Also, special paper with small illustrations of body parts printed in the margins is used in the emergency department, private medical offices, dental offices, and specialty offices (e.g., gynecologists, ophthalmologists, orthopedic surgeons, urologists, medicolegal specialists, and so on) (Fig. 11–6). These are then fed into a laser printer.

After the initial information is transferred from the patient's social data sheet, the receptionist or the secretary will then date the chart paper using a date stamp, typewriter, or longhand. The date may be written out, abbreviated, or written in figures. The paper is then placed into a labeled file folder or a clipboard and presented to the physician at the time he or she sees the patient.

After seeing the patient, the physician will write the notes in the chart, dictate them to be transcribed into the chart, or dictate a separate document that will take the place of the chart entry. This document can be a formal history and physical report (which you will learn to prepare in Chapter 12), it may be a formal report to an attorney or workers' compensation company, or it may be a consultation report to the physician who referred the patient to the office (see Fig. 11–2, entry of 2-5-9X). If the dictator prefers not to make a chart entry and dictates a document, as just discussed, to take the place of the entry, you will transcribe the document and make a note of it in the patient's chart where the normal chart entry belongs.

EXAMPLE

February 7, 199x See note to Dr. Normington mlo

(also correct)

Feb. 7, 199x See note to Dr. Normington mlo

You may type this entry or write it in longhand. Always follow *your* personal chart entry with *your* initials written in longhand.

ESTABLISHED PATIENT, OFFICE

Although the initial visit notes are usually lengthy, subsequent or follow-up notes may be as brief as one line, but they will vary according to the patient's complaint and type of visit to the office. For example, an entry for an established patient being seen in the office in follow-up to a hospitalization for a myringotomy could well read as follows *(note the 5-5 and 5-12 entries):*

In some offices, typewriters are used for these brief entries. However, the use of special paper in your printer makes these very easy to handle. Several companies manufacture pressure-sensitive paper for transcribing medical notes. This paper comes in a variety of forms as well as a continuous sheet of paper folded or on a roll. It is placed behind the pin-feed printer where the regular paper is placed or is fed into the laser printer when needed. One simply types the patient's name, date, and dictation, leaving a space at the end for the dictator's signature or initials. Each note is typed without removal of paper from the medical record. Then, when the transcript is finished, the entire sheet is cut off and given to the dictator for signature. The use of this method makes it easier

EXAMPLE

Tammy O. Beckley BD: 02-15-9x

AGE: 3

5-1-9x Sunday, 3 a.m., pt seen in ER complaining of pain, a.d./3 days. PX revealed fluid and pus. Temp. 101.

ADVICE: Myringotomy.

IMPRESSION: Rt otitis media

tat

Jillian Cooke-Dieter

Jillian Cooke-Dieter, MD

5-1-9x Admit Mercy Hospital tat

5-2-9x Rt myringotomy with aspiration tat

5-3-9x Discharged 10:15 a.m. tat

5-5-9x No pain rt ear. Pt progressing. Rtn 1 week. Temp 98.

tat

Jillian Cooke-Dieter

Jillian Cooke-Dieter, MD

5-12-9x Temp normal, no fluid, no pus, no pain. Rtn PRN.

tat

Jillian Cooke-Dieter

Jillian Cooke-Dieter, MD

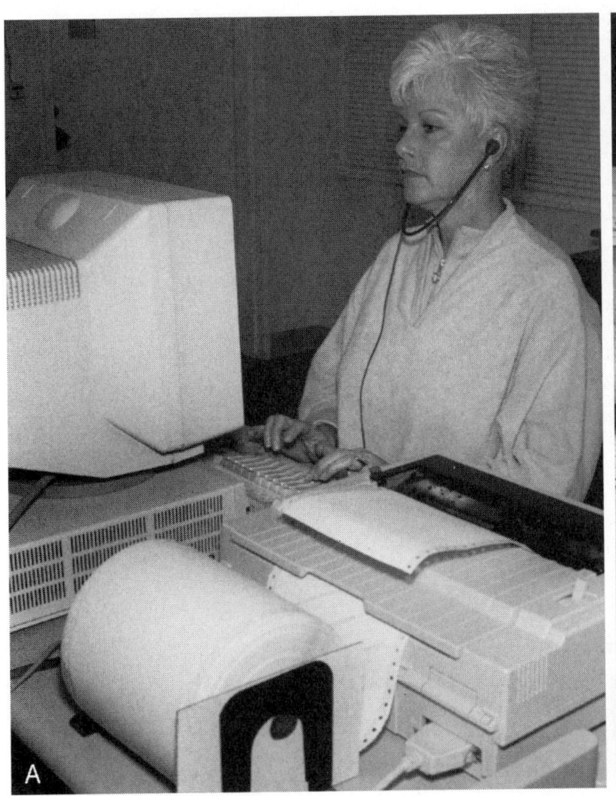

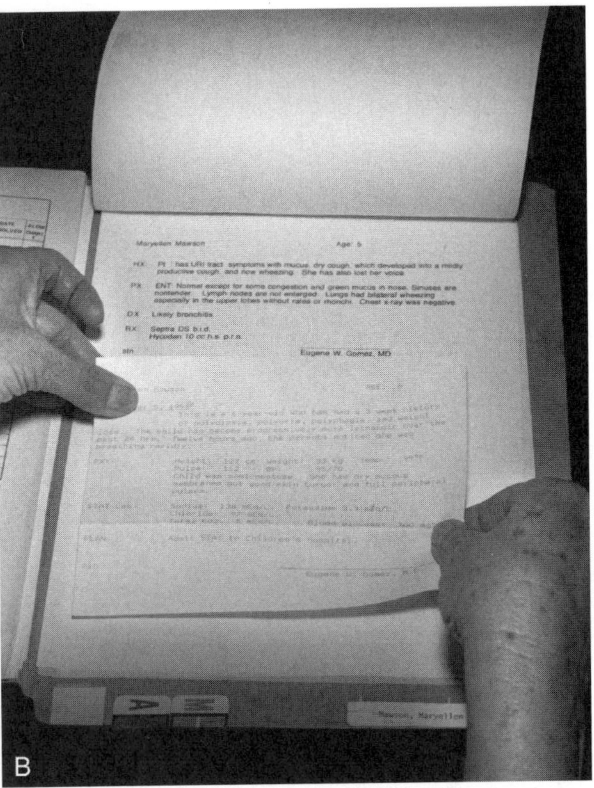

Figure 11–7. *A*, Transcriptionist using PAT Systems pressure-sensitive paper on a roll. *B*, Demonstration of ease of placing the pressure-sensitive paper onto the existing chart note in the medical record. (Paper courtesy of PAT Systems 1-800-543-1911; photograph courtesy of John Dixon, Grossmont College.)

for the physician as well because individual charts do not have to be opened and signed. This is particularly helpful when dictation is sent out of the office and the medical records do not accompany it. After approval, the notes are cut apart with a paper cutter or scissors or separated at the perforations (Fig. 11–7*A*). The backing is peeled off of each one, and the note is then placed on the next blank space of the progress sheet so as not to obliterate the information previously entered (Fig. 11–7*B*). When you have a stack of charts, it can become a nuisance to find the proper page in the chart, unfasten the medical record sheets (if fasteners are used), feed the paper into a typewriter, and type the note. Then, it must be removed, placed in the proper place in the chart, refastened, and returned to the dictator for approval and signature. If you are working on a computer, it is very difficult to allow for items that may already appear on the sheet. For efficiency, you would use the paper made for this purpose.

Again, a follow-up letter may be dictated to a referring physician at this point, rather than making a regular entry note. As new pages are added, be sure that the patient's name is typed on the top of the page. There is no reason why you cannot continue the notes to the back of the chart paper, and many offices do this to prevent the medical record from becoming bulky. Other physicians prefer to use one side of the chart paper only. The second and all subsequent pages of the progress notes are headed up with the patient's name. If you must continue a chart entry to the following page in the middle of an entry, be sure to type *continued* at the bottom of the beginning page and head up the following page with the date of the chart entry and the word *continued* as well as the patient's name.

Figures 11–5, 11–6, and 11–8 through 11–10 show examples of medical office progress notes.

These examples of chart entries that you have just examined are intended not to show *exactly* how to type entries but rather to indicate a variety of methods used by different transcriptionists. At this point, you will not be able to determine exactly how a chart is to be typed because your employer may have definite guidelines for you to follow. For now, and to practice, try to achieve a readable note. Do not combine all the information, but pull out the main topics. In one style, you do not bring the

```
Flanaghan, Michael R.                                AGE:  82

03-17-9x

SUBJECTIVE:     Pt presented complaining of insomnia, weakness and
                shortness of breath.  Described Hx of progressive
dyspnea on exertion over a 2-3 year period.

OBJECTIVE:      BP:  150/110.  Pulse 120 and regular.  Visible neck
                vein distention at 45 degrees elevation; rales at both
lung bases.  Cardiac examination revealed an enlarged heart with PMI
felt at the midclavicular line.  Sounds were distant but a systolic
murmur was described.

     EKG:  Sinus tachycardia, left axis deviation and right bundle
           branch block.

     ECHO: Enlarged left ventricle and calcified and stenotic aortic
           valve.  Left ventricular hypertrophy also demonstrated.

ASSESSMENT:     Calcified aortic stenosis and congestive heart failure.

PLAN:           1.  Admit to hospital.
                2.  Treat with sodium restriction, digitalis and a
                    diuretic.

mlo
                                        ______________________
                                        Joseph D. Becquer, MD
A
```

Figure 11–8. *A* and *B.* Sample chart showing the SOAP (Subjective, Objective, Assessment, Plan) method.

line of typing back to the left margin until the third line so that the date and topics will stand out clearly; the third and subsequent lines may be brought back to the left margin or blocked under the first two lines. (See Figs. 11–8*A* and 11–10 for this method.) Establish a clean, easy-to-read format for progress notes.

The following illustrates an actual chart note that *appears* to have a format, but the format does not contribute to ease of reading or scanning. The patient's name is not appropriately placed. Nothing is gained by having a tab setting after the date in this manner, which leaves a great deal of space that serves no purpose. The use of bold works better when subtopics are found within text.

EXAMPLE OF POOR FORMAT

5-4-9X   Erma Wong returns today, wearing her shoulder immobilizer. She is having difficulty sleeping at night and finds the Vicodin is quite helpful for that.

Examination reveals ecchymosis of the arm, elbow, and forearm as her hematoma is resolving. She has normal neurovascular examination and normal appearance of her right hand.

X-RAYS: AP and lateral x-rays of the right shoulder were obtained. Interpretation: The x-rays show severe osteoporosis. There is impaction of the humeral head fracture. There has been slight change with further impaction since her previous x-rays. There is no displacement of the tuberosity fragment.

IMPRESSION: Satisfactory course with an unstable proximal humerus fracture of the right dominant upper extremity and severe osteoporosis.

RECOMMENDATIONS: The patient will remain in her shoulder immobilizer and will have her use of the

OUTLINE FORMAT PROGRESS NOTES

Patient Name Flanaghan Michael R. AGE: 82

Prob. No. or Letter	DATE	S Subjective	O Objective	A Assess	P Plans	Page 1

3-17-9X Patient presented complaining of insomnia, weakness and shortness of breath. Described Hx of progressive dyspnea on exertion over a 2-3 year period.

BP: 150/110. Pulse 120 and regular. Visible neck vein distention at 45 degrees elevation; rales at both lung bases. Cardiac exam revealed an enlarged heart with PMI felt at the midclavicular line. Sounds were distant but a systolic murmur was described.

EKG: Sinus tachycardia, left axis deviation and right bundle branch block.

ECHO: Enlarged left ventricle and calcified and stenotic aortic valve. Left ventricular hypertrophy also demonstrated.

Calcified aortic stenosis and congestive heart failure.

1. Admit to hospital.
2. Treat with sodium restriction, digitalis, and a diuretic.

JDB/mlo

Start each Progress Note (Subjective, Objective, Assessment and Plans) at the appropriate margin of the page. Write through the intervening columns to the right shaded column to create an outline form.

B ANDRUS/CLINI-REC® PRIMARY CARE CHARTING SYSTEM, FORM NO. 26-7115-01, ©1976 BIBBERO SYSTEMS, INC., PETALUMA, CA.

Figure 11–8 *Continued*

Flanaghan, Michael R. AGE: 82

March 17, 199x

HX: Pt presented complaining of insomnia, weakness and shortness of breath. Described Hx of progressive dyspnea on exertion over a 2-3 year period.

PX: BP: 110. Pulse 120 and regular. Visible neck vein distention at 45 degrees elevation; rales at both lung bases. Cardiac examination revealed an enlarged heart with PMI felt at the midclavicular line. Sounds were distant but a systolic murmur was described.

EKG: Sinus tachycardia, left axis deviation and rt bundle branch block.

ECHO: Enlarged left ventricle and calcified and stenotic aortic valve. Left ventricular hypertrophy also demonstrated.

DX: 1) Calcified aortic stenosis
2) Congestive heart failure

RX: 1) Admit to hospital
2) Treat with sodium restriction, digitalis, diuretic

Joseph D. Becquer, MD/mlo

Figure 11–9. Sample chart entry showing the HX, PX, DX, RX method.

right upper extremity severely limited until such time that more stability is obtained by progressive healing. She will return for follow-up examination and x-rays in ten days. Hopefully, we will be able to start some early pendulum exercises at that time.

RFV: bmg

EXAMPLE OF IMPROVED FORMAT

Erma Wong

5-4-9X Pt returns today, wearing her shoulder immobilizer. She is having difficulty sleeping at night and finds the Vicodin is quite helpful for that.

PX: Ecchymosis of the arm, elbow, and forearm as her hematoma is resolving. She has normal neurovascular examination and normal appearance of her right hand.

X-RAYS: AP and lateral x-rays of the right shoulder were obtained.

Interpretation: The x-rays show **severe osteoporosis.** There is impaction of the humeral head fracture. There has been slight change with further impaction since her previous x-rays. There is no displacement of the tuberosity fragment.

DX: 1. Satisfactory course with an unstable proximal humerus.
2. Fracture of the right dominant upper extremity.
3. Severe osteoporosis.

RX: Pt will remain in her shoulder immobilizer and will have her use of the right upper extremity severely limited until such time that more stability is obtained by progressive healing. Will return for follow-up examination and x-rays in 10 days. Hopefully, we will be able to start some early pendulum exercises at that time.

RFV:bmg

(Master) Norman Brockman AGE: 4

February 22, 199x The patient is a white male, age 4, who came in to see me today with a history of yellow discharge in the right ear, a fever and a sore throat of two days duration. His oral temperature wa 100°. The pharynx was infected, the tonsils inflamed, and there was crusted purulent material seen in the right ear canal. The tympanic membrane was normal.

DIAGNOSIS: Tonsillitis and otitis externa.

Medication: Erythrocin, 400 mg, q4H.

Michael R. Stearn, MD

lr

February ~~22~~ 24 lr, 199x After 24 h of therapy, the pt was afebrile and comfortable. Temperature is 99.6°. The throat is slightly infected. Secretions in the ear canal were dry and both TMs normal.

Michael R. Stearn, MD

lr

February 26, 199x Follow-up exam showed him to be completely asymptomatic and free of unusual physical findings. The drug was stopped at this time.

Michael R. Stearn, MD

lr

July 6, 199x Stepped on a piece of glass. Cleansed wound. Mother said Norman had tetanus booster just six weeks ago in Boyd Hosp.ER after a dog bite. Pt not to return unless problem develops.

Michael R. Stearn, MD

jt

November 11, 199x Pt caught right index finger in car door ~~4~~ 2 MRS days ago; finger became inflamed, red, swollen yesterday. Today there is seropurulent discharge present; no lymphangitis visible. Distal phalanx is involved.

Advice: Hot compress to right hand t.i.d. To return in 24 hours if no change.

DIAGNOSIS: Cellulitis, right index finger, distal phalanx.

Michael R. Stearn, MD

lr

Figure 11–10. Example of a properly corrected chart note.

CHART NOTE, EMERGENCY DEPARTMENT VISIT

When patients are initially seen in the emergency department, the triage nurse determines the sequence in which patients will see a physician. Laboratory, x-rays, and simple tests may be ordered at this time by the triage nurse. At this point, the level of care is determined and may be described as the following:

EMERGENCY DEPARTMENT RECORD **CHART REQUEST**

LOCATION	DATE	TIME REGISTERED	TRIAGE TIME	OUTPT.	INPT.
202	10-08-9X	2:45 ☐AM ☒PM	☐AM ☐PM	☐	☐

NAME: REILLY, RANDA O

ARRIVED ☐ WALKED ☐ WC ☐ AMB ☐ PARA AMB ☐ OTHER

ACCOMPANIED BY ☐ ALONE ☐ SPOUSE ☐ PARENT ☐ FRIEND ☐ RELATIVE

PATIENT'S ADDRESS: 3228 East Main, Century City, XX 12345

MED. REC. NO.:

BIRTHDATE: 11-10-9X

HOME TELEPHONE	WORK TELEPHONE	PRIMARY CARE CLINIC	PERSONAL PHYSICIAN
(800) 654-9863	( )		John Lambert, MD

AGE	SEX	TEMP.	B.P.	PULSE	RESP.	WEIGHT (Peds)	CHIEF COMPLAINT
25	F	98.7	120.70				Head pain, post fall

ALLERGIES:

MEDICATIONS: none

S: This 25 YO pt presents with a HX of falling from a horse into a heavy wooden fence, breaking the fence. Pt complains primarily of head pain, neck pain, right knee pain and some mild coccyx pain. There was a brief loss of consciousness observed by her brother and regaining of consciousness with repetitive questioning. Thereafter she again lost consciousness for a short period of time. Pt has been slow to answer questions and has been noted to have repetitive questions since the accident.

O: Pt in no acute distress. Appears to be stable with C-collar and rigid back board. HEENT: minimal tears in the occipital area. Pupils: equal and reactive. EOMs: Full. EARS: TMs without blood. NECK: C-collar in place, with a tenderness over the mid C-spine bony area without obvious swelling or deformity. (C-collar left in place) CHEST: Nontender to compression. Equal breath sounds. CVA: Regular rhythm. ABDOMEN: soft. Nontender extremities. NM: Moves all fours well. There is mild tenderness on palpitation over the right patella but no instability, no limitation of ROM. Cranial nerves II-VII intact. No meds.

A: Mild concussion.

P: CT of the head after C-spine is clear. Home with head injury instructions. Recheck with private doctor in 1-2 days or return here PRN with any change in mental status.

D: 10-08-9X
T: 10-08-9X
mlo

ED PHYSICIAN: [signature] DATE: 10-08-9X

NS-7672 (9-95)

Figure 11–11. Example of emergency department chart note showing SOAP format and special chart paper for use in the emergency department. See Figure 11–12 for the same note transcribed on plain paper.

Reilly, Randa ER D&T: 10-08-9X DOB: 11-11-XX

CC: Head pain, post fall.
S: This 25 YO pt presents with a HX of falling from a horse into a heavy wooden fence, breaking the fence. Pt complains primarily of head pain, neck pain, right knee pain and some mild coccyx pain. There was a brief loss of consciousness observed by her brother and regaining of consciousness with repetitive questioning. Thereafter she again lost consciousness for a short period of time. Pt has been slow to answer questions and has been noted to have repetitive questions since the accident.
O: Pt in no acute distress. Appears to be stable with C-collar and rigid back board.
HEENT: Minimal tears in the occipital area; pupils: equal and reactive.
EOMs: Full.
EARS: TMs without blood.
NECK: C-collar in place, with a tenderness over the mid C-spine bony area without obvious swelling or deformity. (C-collar left in place.)
CHEST: Nontender to compression. Equal breath sounds.
CVA: Regular rhythm.
ABDOMEN: Soft. Nontender extremities.
NM: Moves all fours well. There is mild tenderness on palpation over the right patella but no instability, no limitation of ROM. Cranial nerves II-VII intact. No meds.
A: Mild concussion.
P: CT of the head after C-spine is clear. Home with head injury instructions. Recheck with private doctor in 1-2 days or return here PRN with any change in mental status.

Kip I. Praycroft, MD/ref

Figure 11–12. Example of emergency department chart note showing SOAP format. See Figure 11–11 for the same note transcribed on an emergency department form.

- Nonurgent: Involves routine care that could have taken place in a physician's office during office hours, or patients who have no physician. Problems include mild flu symptoms, earache, and prescription refills. Admission to the hospital is unlikely.
- Urgent: Involves care requiring basic emergency services. Problems include lacerations, acute flu symptoms, mild shortness of breath, broken bones, threatened abortion, and rectal bleeding. Admission to the hospital is possible.
- Emergent: Involves care requiring immediate attention of the physician. Problems include chest pain, stroke, acute trauma, acute shortness of breath, respiratory arrest, and conditions requiring cardiopulmonary resuscitation. Admission to the hospital is likely.

The patient, family member, or person bringing the patient to the department completes the social data information sheet. If the patient is brought in via emergency vehicle, those personnel generally provide some of the necessary information. Care is not withheld during the gathering of this information; often, care is begun while other personnel interview family or friends for the social history. Initial caregivers will handwrite notes as history is taken from the patient or individuals with the patient. A nurse or technician initially assesses the patient and handwrites notes or inputs data via computer. When the physician sees the patient, he or she will usually handwrite a brief initial impression and orders to be carried out (i.e., medications, laboratory tests, x-rays, and treatment). At this point, dictation may begin. The dictator will indicate whether the dictation is STAT (to be transcribed immediately). This may be done with a handheld recorder and the completed tape placed directly on the chart. Dictation for patients requiring admission or transfer is delivered directly to the transcriptionist. (See Figs. 11–4, 11–11, and 11–12 for examples of notes dictated from the emergency department.)

After the release of the patient, the physician will write (or dictate) a formal diagnosis and update, append, or complete the dictation. These notes are generally brief, and format may vary with the dictator. Some dictators ask for bold headings for each section, whereas others may prefer the condensed story format. The following hints will give you ideas for both office and emergency department chart notes.

TRANSCRIPTION HINTS

1. Be sure the patient's complete name is entered.
2. Date every entry with the month, day, and year. These may be spelled out, abbreviated, or made with a date stamp.
3. Single space and keep the margins narrow (not less than 1/2 inch, however). Double space between topics or major headings.
4. Condense the note to conserve space. Use phrases rather than complete sentences and utilize abbreviations.

EXAMPLE

Dictated: Today's date is November 11, 199X, and this is a chart note on Nancy Marques a 32-year-old female who came in today in follow up to an upper respiratory tract infection either viral or secondary to mycoplasma. She is much better except that she has had a chronic cough now for about ten days. The ears, nose, and throat are normal, and the sinus is nontender. The lymph nodes are normal and the lungs are clear. The diagnosis is postviral cough. I have given her a prescription for Hycodan five to ten milliliters for up to ten days and then observation. If the cough is still present in two weeks I will consider steroid trial.

Transcribed:

Nancy Marques Age: 32

November 11, 199X

HPI: F/Up URI either viral or secondary to mycoplasma. She is much better except for chronic cough X 10 days.

PX: ENT: Normal. Sinus: Nontender. Lymph nodes: Normal. Lungs: Clear.

DX: Postviral cough.

RX: Hycodan 5-10 mL for 10 days and then observation. If cough present in 2 weeks I will consider steroid trial.

ntw

Mary Laudenslayer, MD

This is sharp looking and easy to read, and specific data can be immediately located. However, it is not that quick and simple for the transcriptionist, because you cannot type exactly what is heard; instead, you must stop and analyze.

5. Make outline headings on all but very brief entries. These headings will vary according to the physician's style. Some use the *SOAP* method or variations (see Figs. 11–8*A* and 11–8*B*):
   a. S: This signifies *subjective. Subjective* means from the patient's point of view. This is the reason the patient is seeking care. It is the main problem requiring care (also called chief complaint).
   b. O: This refers to *objective* or the physician's point of view and what is found on physical examination, x-ray film, or laboratory work: the clinical evidence.
   c. A: This refers to *assessment* or what the examiner thinks may be or is wrong with the patient based on the information gathered above: the diagnosis.
   d. P: This refers to *plan* or what the physician plans to do or advises the patient to do: laboratory tests, surgery, medications, referral to another practitioner, treatment, management, and so forth.

There are variations on this style. Some dictators begin with the chief complaint (CC), and others may leave out one or more of the headings. It is very important that the note be explicit and complete. Because the encounter with the patient is the basis for reimbursement from insurance companies, some physicians may want to include additional entries to reflect the *nature* of the presenting problem (N); the *counseling* or *coordination of care* that is involved (C), particularly when these two areas make up more than half of the time of the visit; and the *medical decision making* (M). These items are often difficult for the coder or reviewer to find in the note, and this kind of information is vital in determining the level of service performed during a patient encounter as described earlier.

Another format choice could include

a. CC: This refers to the *chief complaint* (the same as *subjective* above).
b. Px: This refers to the *physical examination,* also PE (the same as *objective* above).
c. Dx: This refers to the *diagnosis, impression* (IMP), or *assessment* (the same as *assessment* above).
d. Rx: This abbreviation for *prescription* is used for the advice or plans for the patient (the same as *Plan* above). See Figure 11–5.

Other titles such as LAB or X-RAY may be used as headings. Multiple-physician practices, clinics, and hospitals often use the Problem-Oriented Medical Record (POMR) format, which is a problem list with corresponding numbered progress notes. Briefly this includes the following areas:

a. Data base: The chief complaint, the history of this complaint, a review of the body systems, physical examination, and laboratory work.
b. Problem list: A numbered list of every problem that the patient has that requires further investigation.
c. Treatment plan: Numbered list to correspond with each item on the problem list.
d. Notes: Numbered progress notes to correspond with each item on the problem list.

6. Use abbreviations and symbols freely as the dictator wishes, but be sure that the abbreviations are standard. (Remember that the records could be viewed by persons outside the office or hospital.) Abbreviations save space, and notes should be as concise as possible.
7. Insert indentations to make topics stand out. Type the main topics in full caps. Use bold when it is helpful or requested by the dictator.
8. Underline and type drug allergies in full caps.
9. Initial the entry just as you initial any other document that you type or transcribe. Initials may be placed at the left margin or following the dictator's name or initials.
10. Type a signature line or leave sufficient space for the dictator's signature or initials.
11. In the medical office, check daily about the previous day's house calls, emergency department calls, and hospital admissions or discharges, so that the charts can be pulled and these entries made.

Examine all the figures again for typing format.

These are some common abbreviations found frequently in office chart notes. You may use these as well as those found in Appendix B as you complete the following assignments.

11

pt	patient
Hx	history
Px	physical or physical exam
PE	physical or physical exam
CC	chief complaint
Dx	diagnosis
Tx	treatment
Rx	prescription or plan
STAT	immediate
BP	blood pressure
VS	vital signs
IMP	impression
PH	past history
R/O	rule out
PO	postoperative
pre	preoperative or prepartum
FUO	fever of unknown origin
H&P	history and physical
TPR	temperature, pulse, respiration
inj	injection
anPX	annual exam
CPX	complete physical exam
DKA	did not keep appointment
DNS	did not show (keep appointment)
pre-op	preoperative
consult	consultation
PG?	question of being pregnant

11-1: SELF-STUDY

Directions: Retype the following material into chart note format, as illustrated in Figure 11–9.

The date is October 10, 199X. The patient is Anthony Frishman. Tony is now 12 1/2 years old. He underwent bilateral triple arthrodesis in August 199X. He is out of his splints and doing well. His foot rests are a bit long and his feet are not touching them. He has no major complaints as far as his feet are concerned. Exam: He has a long c-curve to the right, which may be slightly increased clinically since last x-rayed in June 199X when it was twenty-five degrees. His feet are in neutral position as far as equinus. There is a slight varus inclination. X-rays: multiple views of his feet demonstrate fusion bilaterally of the triple staples. Diagnosis is limb girdle dystrophy. The plan is to return to clinic in one to two months for sitting SP spine x-ray. Also we will obtain pulmonary function test at that time. Karl T. Robrecht, MD. (After you have completed this assignment, turn to the end of the chapter for a possible transcript.)

11-2: PRACTICE TEST

Directions: Retype the following information as an emergency department report for Eugene W. Gomez, MD. Use the current date, minimum chart note heading, and plain (unlined) 8 1/2 × 11 inch paper.

The patient's name is Maryellen Mawson.

Note: this is a six year old who has had a three week history of polydipsia polyuria polyphagia and weight loss. the child has become progressively more lethargic over the past twenty four hours and twelve hours ago the parents noticed she was breathing rapidly. physical examination reveals height one hundred twenty seven centimeters weight thirty three kilograms temperature ninety nine degrees fahrenheit pulse one hundred twelve and blood pressure ninety five over seventy. the child was semicomatose. she has dry mucous membranes but good skin turgor and full peripheral pulses. a stat lab report shows: sodium one hundred thirty eight milliequivalents per liter, potassium three point three milliequivalents per liter chloride ninety seven milliequivalents per liter and a total carbon dioxide of five milliequivalents per liter. blood glucose is seven hundred milligrams percent. plan is to admit stat to childrens hospital. (After you complete this, see Appendix A for a possible transcript.)

11-3: REVIEW TEST

Directions: Carefully examine the examples of chart notes that have been illustrated and retype the following information as office chart notes for your employer, Laurel R. Denison, MD. You may use the minimum chart note heading, plain (unlined) 8 1/2 × 11 inch paper, format of your choice, and standard abbreviations where applicable. Use today's date. Please notice that these are notes about several patients; therefore, each patient will have a separate sheet of paper.

1. *Gustavo deVargas.* Birthdate 3-3-34. Patient had onset of persistent vomiting five days ago. He does not appear seriously ill. The abdomen remains flat and there is no tenderness or rigidity; no masses are palpable; bowel sounds are scarce. X-ray of the abdomen yesterday revealed a four centimeter, ill-defined, round mass in the right upper quadrant and loops of small bowel containing air. Subsequent x-rays, including some taken today, revealed that this rounded mass persists, is quite well outlined on some of the x-rays, and is now in the left lower quadrant. There is small bowel distention in relation to the mass, which suggests that the mass is a loop of small bowel with gaseous distention proximal to it. It is questionable whether there is any gas in the colon. Rectal examination is negative. Impression: intestinal obstruction due to ingested foreign body. Advice: laparotomy.
2. *Mrs. Esther Conway.* Age 33. Patient complains of constant dribbling, wetting at night, uses fifteen pads a day. Urinalysis: specific gravity one point zero, few bacteria, few urates. Diagnosis: urinary incontinence. Patient is to return in four days for diagnostic testing.
3. *Robin Vincenti.* Age 27. Patient complains of having had the flu and headache, and of being tired. Unable to go to work today. Exam shows weakness of left hand. Hyperreflexia on the left. X-ray shows cardiomegaly and slight pulmonary congestion. Impression: post flu syndrome, transient ischemic attack; possible CVA. Patient to return in four days and may return to work in approximately one week.
4. *Marissa Weeks.* Age 17. CC: thrown from a horse. Px: numerous contusions, tenderness in thoracic region, x-ray ordered. Dx: compression fracture of "tee twelve." Rx: patient referred to Edward Harrison, orthopedic specialist.
5. *Bobby West.* Age 1 month. Make your entry showing a letter was dictated, rather than a chart entry made. (See Typing Assignment 6–1, page 152, for the actual letter that was dictated and transcribed.)

11

11–4: REVIEW TEST

Directions: Using the instructions you have just received, type the following information into the patients' charts that you previously prepared. Use a date four days from the date you used for Review Test 11–3.

1. *Gustavo deVargas.* Patient telephoned office today and agreed to laparotomy. He is to be admitted to Valley Presbyterian Hospital tomorrow afternoon at 3 for surgery the following day.
2. Secretary: Please make your own entry into the chart showing that Mr. deVargas was admitted to the hospital on the appropriate day.
3. *Robin Vincenti.* Chest clear to P&A. X-ray is clear and shows normal heart silhouette. Full use of left hand, no residual pain or weakness. Plans to return to work tomorrow.
4. *Mrs. Esther Conway.* Intravenous pyelogram and cystoscopy revealed multiple fistulae of bladder with two openings into urinary bladder and copious leakage into vagina. Continued to work. Diagnosis: multiple vesicovaginal fistulae. To be admitted to the hospital for repair.
5. Secretary: Please make your own entry into the chart for day of admission, four days from her last visit, into University Hospital for Mrs. Conway.

MAKING CORRECTIONS

Errors in handwritten chart notes are corrected as follows. Draw a line through the error, being careful not to obliterate it; make the correct notation either above or below the error, wherever there is room, and date and initial the entry. Do not write over your error, do not erase the error, do not try to "fix" the error, and do not attempt to blot it out with heavy applications of ink or self-adhesive typing strips.

Errors that are made while the entry is being typed are corrected just as you would correct any other typewritten material. Errors found subsequently are corrected in longhand following the above procedures. However, it is not necessary to date errors when they are made or discovered on the same day as they are entered; just correct and initial the error.

See Figure 11–10 for an example of chart notes with entry errors properly corrected. You will notice that these corrections are not dated, which indicates that they were made on the day of the entry.

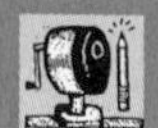

11-5: SELF-STUDY

Directions: In the following chart note, the entry of "left thoracotomy" should read "right thoracotomy." You discover the error on February 1, 199X. Please correct it.

Please look at the end of the chapter for the proper correction technique.

```
Brad Philman                                               Age 47

1-13-9X  Pt admitted to Good Sam for bronchoscopy and possible left
         thoracotomy and pleural poudrage. ren
```

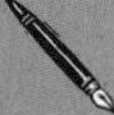

11-6: REVIEW TEST

Directions: Pretend that you are typing the following notes on pressure-sensitive paper. Do not forget to leave a little space between the notes so they can be cut apart, but do not cut your notes apart. Use today's date. Use the SOAP format for chart note #5. Your employer is Catherine R. Schultz, MD.

11

1. *Lupe Morales.* Lump, right breast. Patient found this lump four weeks ago. It has increased in size rapidly, she says. She also has a lump under her right arm. Ordered mammograms. Diagnosis: Possible carcinoma of the breast.
2. *Adeline Pierson.* CC: pain and swelling over the right wrist. Hx: The patient states that while she was working as a waitress she was lifting and carrying a tray of dishes and it slipped, resulting in pain and swelling over the radial side of the distal radius of her right wrist. This was found to be a ganglion and was aspirated by another physician. However, it has recurred and is larger than before. She wishes this surgically removed. Her past general health has been good. She has had no serious illnesses and no surgeries. She takes no medications. Allergies: None known.
3. *Peter Barton.* PO follow-up. Incision looks good, some slight swelling and tenderness.
4. *Kellis McNeil.* CC: Right inguinal hernia. Hx: Patient first noticed that he had a right inguinal hernia because of pain there approximately one week ago. He presents with a very tender right inguinal ring. The hernia was reduced but readily protruded. PH: The patient had an umbilical hernia repair eight years ago. He had a hemorrhoidectomy four years ago. Drugs: Valium, 5 mg, t.i.d. Advise: Right herniorrhaphy.
5. *Arnott B. Weeks.* stiff finger joints. pt says more severe after sleeping or nonuse. general fatigue stopped, occurred again in last 2 weeks. stopped drinking, some weight loss. on exam there is swelling and pain around joints of fingers. symmetrical involvement. bp is one hundred forty four over eighty five pulse is sixty seven weight is one hundred seventy eight. x-ray: narrowed joint space, osteoporosis at joint. uric acid: four point two. rheumatoid arthritis. aspirin ten grains qid, phenylbutazone one hundred milligrams qid, number twenty eight. return one month.

11-7: REVIEW TEST

Directions: Transcribe the following notes for the emergency department. Use the SOAP format or any variation that is appropriate and easy to read. The dictator is Marc Nielsen, MD. The date is May 1, 199X.

Colleen Lynkins is a 33-year-old female whose chief complaint is upper mid back pain. The patient woke up tonight with upper mid back pain. Patient states that she has a new mattress. There is no history of trauma or other insults. She had spontaneous pneumothorax twice in the past year. Had tubal ligation ten years ago. She states that she cannot be pregnant. Physical examination: NKA. Temperature is 98.

Blood pressure is one hundred ten over eighty. The chest is clear. The heart is in regular rhythm. The abdomen is soft. Extremities were non neurological. Central nervous system is intact. Head and neck are benign. Plan. Chest x-ray and proceed.

11-7: REVIEW TEST B

See 11–3 Review Test, Project 1, Gustavo deVargas chart note. Use the SOAP method and prepare the chart note for Dr. Denison.

11-1: COMPUTER EXERCISE

Before proceeding, you may want to do more exercises based on the concepts you have learned. Additional practice material is on your computer diskette.

Directions: Insert the diskette into the computer and follow the instructions on the screen for Computer Exercise 11–1.

A *Answers to* 11-1: SELF-STUDY

Anthony Frishman AGE: 12½

October 10, 199x

HX: Pt underwent bilateral triple arthrodesis in August, 199x . He is out of splints and doing well. His foot rests are a bit long and his feet are not touching them. He has no major complaints as far as his feet are concerned.

PX: He has a long C-curve to the right which may be slightly increased clinically since last x-rayed in June, 199x , when it was 25°. His feet are in neutral position as far as equinus. There is a slight varus inclination.

X-RAY: Multiple views of his feet demonstrate fusion bilaterally of the triple staples.

DX: Limb girdle dystrophy.

RX
1. Return to Clinic in one-two months for sitting SP spine x-ray.
2. Obtain pulmonary function test.

ref

Karl T. Robrecht, MD

A *Answers to* 11-5: SELF-STUDY

Brad Philman Age 47

1-13-9X Pt admitted to Good Sam for bronchoscopy and possible ~~left~~ right thoracotomy and pleural poudrage. ren

2-1-9X ren

CHAPTER

12

Preparation of a History and Physical

OBJECTIVES

After reading this chapter and working the exercises, you should be able to

1. Identify the various mechanical formats used to prepare a history and physical.
2. Explain why certain information is obtained from the patient and recorded.
3. Describe the many different ways of gathering and dictating vital medical data.
4. Prepare a formal history and physical using a variety of acceptable styles.
5. Make a template for a standard history and physical.

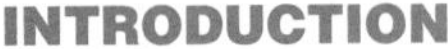

INTRODUCTION

The history and physical (H&P) is the first in a set of documents referred to as "The Big Four," which are the four main documents transcribed in a hospital setting: the H&P, operative report, discharge summary, and consultation report. Furthermore, the H&P is the document that takes priority in transcription because it must be on the patient's chart/record before certain other procedures can be carried out. In the previous chapter, you learned how an H&P is set up in its condensed form: the chart note. The SOAP format is a miniature H&P with the S (subjective) taking the place of the history; O (objective), physical examination (PX or PE); A (assessment), diagnostic portion of the examination; and P (plan), outlined future treatment. In fact, the guidelines presented to you entitled "General Principles for Complete Documentation in Medical Records" on page 244 apply to the H&P as well. Some physicians will dictate an H&P in lieu of an initial chart note. Because the hospital requires this document to be in the patient's hospital record before surgery, surgeons carry out an H&P on the preoperative visit with a patient, and some trauma surgeons likewise prefer a more complete H&P to the SOAP chart note in the emergency department.

The primary purpose of the H&P is to assist the physician in making a diagnosis on which he or she will base the patient's care and treatment. There are no precise rules for exactly how a history is taken down or a PX carried out, nor is there an exact format for recording the data gathered. These will vary just as the personalities of the dictators vary. However, most physicians, regardless of medical specialty, approach the evaluation of the patient in a similar fashion.

All patients, when initially seen, need to give the physician a complete history of their problems and be examined. How many questions they are asked, the types of questions, and the body area emphasized are determined both by the patient's problem and by the medical specialty involved. For example, a patient with chest pain seeing a cardiologist will have far more attention paid to the chest than to the bladder and bowels. The patient with a hearing problem does not expect an extensive examination of the abdomen or extremities. However, when a patient is scheduled for a major operative procedure or has symptoms that suggest a complex systemic illness, all body systems are examined to some extent.

You will need to know how to transcribe an H&P if you work in the word processing unit of a hospital or clinic. If you work in a private medical office for a surgical or medical specialist, you will also be required to type H&Ps. As with chart notes, some physicians will write their H&Ps in longhand. There is certainly no requirement that they be typed. However, because they are part of the patient's medical record, it is important that they be neat, readable, complete, and accurate.

The H&P performs an important function as a diary of what has happened to the patient in the past, a plan for care in the present, and an outline of how the patient may be helped in the future.

THE FORMATS AND STYLES

Several formats are used for typing an H&P. There is no "best" style or method, but each hospital, clinic, or medical office should adopt a standard outline. The responsibility for designing the format for the hospital belongs to the hospital forms committee. The hospital will generally accept the H&P prepared by the medical office assistant as long as it falls within the general guidelines of the styles that follow.

Most transcriptionists who transcribe H&Ps on a regular basis make a template, macro, or boilerplate of a typical H&P. In doing so, when the transcriptionist is ready to transcribe the H&P, the outline is in place, narrow one-half inch to three-quarter inch margins are set, tab stops are set up, and any required bolding or underlining is done; all that is necessary is to "fill in the blanks." Parts of the outline that are not needed are simply deleted during transcription. A new topic may be given, and it is added at this time. A copy of this macro or template also acts as a prompt for the dictator so that he or she will remember to obtain and dictate vital data.

EXAMPLE

Patient name

HISTORY

CHIEF COMPLAINT:

PRESENT ILLNESS:

PAST HISTORY:

OPERATIONS:

MEDICATIONS:

HABITS:

ALLERGIES:

SOCIAL:

FAMILY HISTORY:

REVIEW OF SYSTEMS:

SKIN:

HEENT:

CR:

GI:

GU:

GYN:

NM:

William A. Berry, MD

initials
D:
T:

When you fill in the outline during transcription, you may leave in the prompt for patient's name and type the name after it, but usually you simply type over the prompt and insert the patient's name. You may add any other social demographics needed, e.g., hospital number, name of referring physician, and so on. You place your reference initials at the prompt indicated with "initials." What you do not see on the template are the commands for narrow margins, tab stops, and pause commands (which is where the cursor would position itself to permit you to type in the necessary data). If you have not yet learned to make a macro, start with something less complicated for practice.

Just as we examined the three formats for letter set-up, we will now discuss the four formats, with variations, for H&P set-up. The actual wording of the outline itself may vary, too, but we will discuss that and the data that go into the report later. Keeping the facts in the proper sequence, spacing them properly, and typing them accurately make the work of transcribing interesting and challenging.

Usually the data for the history are obtained first. The following four examples and guides for typing histories are observed when you are typing the PX as well. Always check with your employer for the preferred style.

12

FULL BLOCK FORMAT REPORT STYLE (Fig. 12–1)

Statistical Data: As determined by the medical facility.

Title: *History* or *Personal History* centered on the page.
Typed in all capital letters.

Main Topics: Typed in all capitals, followed by a colon.
Underlined.
On a line by itself.
Begun on edge of left border.

Subtopics: Capitalized, followed by a colon.

Data: Begun on the *same* line as subtopic.
Single spaced.
All lines return to the left margin.
Double space between the last line of one heading and the next heading.

Margins: Narrow (one-half inch to three-quarter inch is appropriate).

Close: Typed line for signature.
Dictator's typed name.
Transcriptionist's initials.
Date of dictation (D).
Date of transcription (T).

Variations:

1. No space below main topic.
2. Subtopics grouped after main heading in paragraph format. Subtopic title typed in full capitals or both upper and lower case.
3. Main topics not underlined.

Comment: This is a very easy format and requires no tab stops.

12

de Mars, Verna Marie
76-83-06
Cortland M. Struthers, MD

HISTORY

CHIEF COMPLAINT:

Prolapse and bleeding after each bowel movement for the past 3-4 months.

PRESENT ILLNESS:

This 68-year-old white female says she usually has three bowel movements a day in small amounts, and there has been a recent change in the frequency, size and type of bowel movement she has been having. She is also having some pain and irritation in this area. She has had no previous anorectal surgery or rectal infection. She denies any blood in the stool itself.

PAST HISTORY:

ILLNESSES: The patient had polio at age 8 from which she has made a remarkable recovery. Apparently, she was paralyzed in both lower extremities and now has adequate use of these. She has no other serious illnesses.

ALLERGIES: ALLERGIC TO PENICILLIN. She denies any other drug or food allergies.

MEDICATIONS: None.

OPERATIONS: Herniorrhaphy, 25 years ago.

SOCIAL: She does not smoke or drink. She lives with her husband who is an invalid and for whom she cares. She is a retired former municipal court judge.

FAMILY HISTORY:

One brother died of cancer of the throat, another has cancer of the kidney.

REVIEW OF SYSTEMS:

SKIN: No rashes or jaundice.

HEENT: Unremarkable.

CR: No history of chest pain, shortness of breath, or pedal edema. She has had some mild hypertension in the past but is not under any medical supervision nor is she taking any medication for this.

GI: Weight is stable. See Present Illness.

OB-GYN: Gravida II Para II. Climacteric at age 46, no sequelae.

EXTREMITIES: No edema.

NEUROLOGIC: Unremarkable.

Cortland M. Struthers, MD

jrt
D: 5-17-9x
T: 5-20-9x

Figure 12–1. Example of a history done in full block format.

Modified Block Format Report Style (Fig. 12–2)

Statistical Data: As determined by the medical facility.

Title: *History* or *Personal History* centered on the page.
Typed in all capital letters.

Main Topics: Typed in all capitals, followed by a colon.
Underlined.
Begun on edge of left border.

Subtopics: Indented one tab stop (five spaces) under main topics.
Typed in full capitals, followed by a colon.

Data: Begun on the same line as the topic or subtopic.

Data input begun two tab stops after the heading. (Tabbing and blocking are determined by the length of the first line, the longest line in the history: "Chief Complaint" plus the colon plus the two tab stops after the colon. All other data are tabbed and blocked to this same point under the previous line. The initial tab at this place is adequate so that all data are evenly blocked. The "Block Indent" feature of software programs is very helpful in this format.) Begin typing on the same line as the topic or subtopic after the appropriate tab or indentation setting is reached.
Single spaced.
Double space between the last line of a topic and the next heading.

Margins: Narrow (one-half inch to three-quarter inch).

Close: Typed line for signature.
Dictator's typed name.
Transcriptionist's initials.
Date of dictation (D).
Date of transcription (T).

Variations:
1. No underlining.
2. Single space between subtopics.

Comment: This is clean and easy to read, but there is quite a bit of wasted space and much use of the tab or indent key.

12

de Mars, Verna Marie

Cortland M. Struthers, MD

Hospital Number: 76-83-06

HISTORY

CHIEF COMPLAINT: Prolapse and bleeding after each bowel movement for the past 3-4 months.

PRESENT ILLNESS: This 68-year-old white female says she usually has three bowel movements a day in small amounts, and there has been a recent change in frequency, size and type of bowel movement she has been having. She is also having some pain and irritation in this area. She has had no previous anorectal surgery or rectal infection. She denies any blood in the stool itself.

PAST HISTORY:

ILLNESSES: The patient had polio at age 8 from which she has made a remarkable recovery. Apparently, she was paralyzed in both lower extremities and now has adequate use of these. She has no other serious illnesses.

ALLERGIES: ALLERGIC TO PENICILLIN. She denies any other drug or food allergies.

MEDICATIONS: None.

OPERATIONS: Herniorrhaphy, 25 years ago.

SOCIAL: She does not smoke or drink. She lives with her husband who is an invalid and for whom she cares. She is a retired former municipal court judge.

FAMILY HISTORY: One brother died of cancer of the throat, another has cancer of the kidney.

REVIEW OF SYSTEMS:

SKIN: No rashes or jaundice.

HEENT: Unremarkable.

CR: No history of chest pain, shortness of breath, or pedal edema. She has had some mild hypertension in the past but is not under any medical supervision nor is she taking any medication for this.

GI: Weight is stable. See Present Illness.

OB-GYN: Gravida II Para II. Climacteric at age 46, no sequelae.

EXTREMITIES: No edema.

NEUROLOGIC: Unremarkable.

Cortland M. Struthers, MD

jrt
D: 5-17-9x
T: 5-20-9x

Figure 12–2. Example of a history done in modified block format.

12

Indented Format Report Style (Fig. 12–3)

Statistical Data: As determined by the medical facility.

Title: *History* or *Personal History* centered on the page.
Typed in all capital letters.

Main Topics: Typed in all capitals, followed by a colon.
Underlined.
Begun flush with the left margin.

Subtopics: Typed in all capitals, followed by a colon.
Indented one tab stop (or five spaces) under main topics.

Data: Begun on the *same* line as topic or subtopic.

First *and* second lines tabulated to an indentation of 25 characters or spaces, which is the 2.5 tab stop. To prepare the tab stops for this format, clear all tabs and set the first tab stop at 0.5, the second at 2.5, and the third at 4.0. These will clear the outline when you are ready to tabulate.
Third and *subsequent* lines brought back to the left margin (as long as they clear the outline—if too brief, block under first two lines). See Figure 12–3, data after "Social."
Single spaced.
Double space between topics.

Margins: Narrow (one-half inch to three-quarter inch).

Close: Typed line for signature at the tab stop of 4.0.
Dictator's typed name.
Transcriptionist's initials.
Date of dictation (D).
Date of transcription (T).

Variations:
1. No underlining.
2. Do not indent subtopics.

Comment: This style is popular because it is clean and easy to read without using a lot of "white space." Tab stops are minimal but do require you to be alert for them.

de Mars, Verna Marie
76-83-06
Cortland M. Struthers, MD

HISTORY

CHIEF COMPLAINT: Prolapse and bleeding after each bowel movement for the past 3-4 months.

PRESENT ILLNESS: This 68-year-old white female says she usually has three bowel movements a day in small amounts, and there has been a recent change in the frequency, size and type of bowel movement she has been having. She is also having some pain and irritation in this area. She has had no previous anorectal surgery or rectal infection. She denies any blood in the stool itself.

PAST HISTORY:

ILLNESSES: The patient had polio at age 8 from which she has made a remarkable recovery. Apparently, she was paralyzed in both lower extremities and now has adequate use of these. She has had no other serious illnesses.

ALLERGIES: ALLERGIC TO PENICILLIN. She denies any other drug or food allergies.

MEDICATIONS: None.

OPERATIONS: Herniorrhaphy, 25 years ago.

SOCIAL: She does not smoke or drink. She lives with her husband who is an invalid and for whom she cares. She is a retired former municipal court judge.

FAMILY HISTORY: One brother died of cancer of the throat, another has cancer of the kidney.

REVIEW OF SYSTEMS:

SKIN: No rashes or jaundice.

HEENT: Unremarkable.

CR: No history of chest pain, shortness of breath, or pedal edema. She has had some mild hypertension in the past but is not under any medical supervision nor is she taking any medication for this.

GI: Weight is stable. See Present Illness.

OB-GYN: Gravida II Para II. Climacteric at age 46, no sequelae.

EXTREMITIES: No edema.

NEUROLOGIC: Unremarkable.

Cortland M. Struthers, MD

jrt
D: 5-17-9x
T: 5-20-9x

Figure 12–3. Example of a history done in indented format.

12

12

Run-On Format Report Style (Fig. 12–4)

Statistical Data: As determined by the medical facility.

Title: *History* or *Personal History* centered on the page.
Typed in all capital letters.

Main Topics: Full capitals, followed by a colon.
Begun flush with the left margin.

Subtopics: Upper and lower case, followed by a colon.
Data continued within the paragraph.

Data: Begun on the same line as the outline, a double space after the colon.
Single spaced.
Double space between topics.

Margins: Narrow (one-half inch to three-quarter inch).

Close: Typed line for signature.
Dictator's typed name.
Transcriptionist's initials.
Date of dictation (D).
Date of transcription (T).

Variations:
1. Single space between topics.
2. Subtopics begun on a separate line and typed in caps.
3. Main topic underlined and in full caps.

Comment: Run-on format uses much less space on the paper and takes less time to prepare because tabulations, underlining, and double spacing are lessened or eliminated. It takes time to feed such information in and play it out again on automated equipment. Production and speed must not be sacrificed for format in this case. However, if you have made a boilerplate or macro for your report, it is not necessary to run all of your data together in this fashion. Production and speed are maintained at a high level.

de Mars, Verna Marie
76-83-06
Cortland M. Struthers, MD

HISTORY

CHIEF COMPLAINT: Prolapse and bleeding after each bowel movement for the past 3-4 months.

PRESENT ILLNESS: This 68-year-old white female says she usually has three bowel movements a day in small amounts, and there has been a recent change in the frequency, size and type of bowel movement she has been having. She is also having some pain and irritation in this area. She has had no previous anorectal surgery or rectal infection. She denies any blood in the stool itself.

PAST HISTORY: Illnesses: The patient had polio at age 8 from which she has made a remarkable recovery. Apparently, she was paralyzed in both lower extremities and now has adequate use of these. She has had no other serious illnesses. Allergies: ALLERGIC TO PENICILLIN. She denies any other drug or food allergies. Medications: None. Operations: Herniorrhaphy, 25 years ago. Social: She does not smoke or drink. She lives with her husband who is an invalid and for whom she cares. She is a retired former municipal court judge.

FAMILY HISTORY: One brother died of cancer of the throat, another has cancer of the kidney.

REVIEW OF SYSTEMS: Skin: No rashes or jaundice. HEENT: Unremarkable. CR: No history of chest pain, shortness of breath, or pedal edema. She has had some mild hypertension in the past but is not under any medical supervision nor is she taking any medication for this. GI: Weight is stable. See Present Illness. OB-GYN: Gravida II Para II. Climacteric at age 46, no sequelae. Extremities: No edema. Nuerologic: Unremarkable.

jrt
D: 5-17-9x
T: 5-20-9x

Cortland M. Struthers, MD

Figure 12–4. Example of a history done in run-on format.

THE HISTORY

The physician obtains information for the history by questioning the patient or the family or persons accompanying the patient when the patient is unable to provide the history. A carefully taken history will direct the focus of the PX and assist with making the final diagnosis.

Now we will briefly examine each part of the outline. You can look at the examples and see how it develops.

Statistical Data. These always include the name of the patient and any other means of identification that the hospital, office, or clinic uses. It may include the patient's record number, age, room number, date of admission, referring physician, dictator's name, and names of anyone who is to receive a copy of the dictation. This material may be preimprinted on forms at the time of admission.

Chief Complaint. (This is abbreviated *CC.*) Most facilities prefer spelled out main headings and abbreviated subtopics. The SOAP format is an exception. This is a description of what symptom or sign brought the patient to the physician, emergency department, or hospital. It is usually brief, may be specific or vague, and may be dictated in the patient's own words. The nature of the patient's complaints gives focus and direction to the H&P. If there is a list of complaints, they are usually dictated in the order of importance.

Present Illness. (Abbreviated *PI.*) This is also called *History of Chief Complaint* or *History of Present Illness* (abbreviated *HPI*). The patient's problem is now discussed in detail with emphasis on duration and severity. The patient will relate the details he or she feels are significant, and the physician will inquire if they are related to other symptoms or events. If the patient has been treated by another physician for the same or a similar problem, this will be discussed, along with the possible diagnosis and treatment prescribed.

Past History. (Abbreviated *PH.*) This section begins with the patient's childhood and includes all past medical history with reference to chronic diseases and conditions not directly related to the present condition; past injuries, including fractures, wounds, burns, trauma, and injuries from falls or accidents (including industrial accidents and injuries); illnesses; and surgical procedures. This main topic is generally broken down into subtopics as follows:

Habits This includes information about the patient's usual lifestyle, including exercise, recreation, and the use of alcohol, tobacco, and drugs, both prescription and recreational. The dictator may use a separate topic for drugs the patient has taken recently or is currently taking and call this subtopic *Medications.*

Diseases This includes both childhood and adult diseases and any complications that arose as a result.

Operations All surgical procedures, dates, and sequelae are recorded. This subtopic may also be called *Surgeries.*

Allergies This includes any reactions the patient may have to drugs, food, or the environment. (Many physicians direct the transcriptionist to bold, underline [or type in all capital letters] a positive reply to a query regarding a drug allergy.)

Social The socioeconomic status of the patient, including his or her occupation, profession, or trade; recreational interests; home environment; and marital status.

Gynecologic (when the patient is a female) The number of pregnancies, deliveries, complications, living children, and abortions and sexual activity. The times of menarche and menopause are noted, along with any problems associated with the menses.

Prolonged investigation of any one or more of these topics is made, depending on the patient's chief complaint. Some dictators use some or all of the topics listed; others group all of these data into a brief paragraph entitled *Past History.* You will also notice that physicians list many negative replies to some of these items; for example, "the patient denies any allergies or drug sensitivities"; "there is no history of familial disease"; or "the patient does not use drugs or alcohol." These expressions are recorded after the listed topic. This last sentence would read as follows on your transcript:

EXAMPLE

MEDICATIONS: No use of drugs or alcohol.

Dictated: The patient denies allergies to drugs.
Transcribed: ALLERGIES: Denies allergies to drugs.

Family History. The state of health of the patient's parents, siblings, and grandparents is discussed. If they are deceased, the age and cause of death are recorded. Inquiry is made concerning certain diseases that tend to be familial, such as tuberculosis, diabetes, epilepsy, carcinoma, and heart disease. The place and circumstances of the patient's birth might also be noteworthy.

Review of Systems. This is also called *Systemic Review, Functional Inquiry,* or *Inventory by Systems.* This is an oral review conducted in question-and-answer style with the patient, as stated, of all the body systems to ensure that nothing has been overlooked. The absence or presence of problems is noted. Again, a variety of methods are used for typing this information. Generally, the physician will review by starting at the top of the body and going through the body systems, ending with the nervous or musculoskeletal system. He or she may dictate the data as a single paragraph with no headings or break them down into subtopics. The subtopics used are as follows, along with the abbreviations commonly used and accepted:

Skin Includes eruptions, rashes, itches, discolorations, dryness, and scaling. Sometimes the dictator will dictate quotes around a response from the patient. This indicates that the patient has made a decision about the problem that may or may not be correct, particularly when the dictator has asked whether another physician had treated the patient for this condition and whether the patient had treated himself or herself.

12

EXAMPLE

Dictated: No rashes or scaling, but the patient says that he has had *quote* psoriasis in the past *unquote.*
Transcribed: SKIN: No rashes or scaling; "psoriasis" in the past.

Hair Includes changes in its texture or distribution, loss of hair, and excessive hair.

HEENT This pertains to the *h*ead, *e*yes, *e*ars, *n*ose, and *t*hroat. Additional subtopics may be added, or a single, all-inclusive paragraph may be used.

Eyes Includes vision problems such as glaucoma, scotoma, conjunctivitis, trachoma, pain, discharge, redness, fields, use of glasses, blurring, double vision, seeing spots or rings around lights, watering, itching, and abnormal sensitivity to light.

Ears Includes hearing loss, discharge, dizziness, syncope, tinnitus, pain, and condition of the tympanic membranes.

Nose Includes discharges, sense of smell, colds, allergies, and epistaxis.

Mouth and Throat Includes condition of teeth, dental hygiene, dentures, gums, difficulty in swallowing, hoarseness, thyroid, movement of the neck, position of the trachea, sore throat, postnasal drip, and choking.

CR (Cardiorespiratory) Refers to both the cardiovascular and respiratory systems. The cardiovascular problems may include chest pain and its severity, tachycardia, bradycardia, heart murmurs, heart attacks, palpitations, high blood pressure, and varicose veins. Closely related respiratory problems include the sequelae of heart problems, dyspnea, orthopnea, shortness of breath, edema, hemoptysis, and pneumonia.

GI (Gastrointestinal) Includes abdominal pain of any type or severity, appetite, indigestion, dysphagia, anorexia, vomiting, hematemesis, change in weight or diet, change in bowel habits, melena, flatus, diarrhea, constipation, and jaundice.

GU (Genitourinary) Includes dysuria, nocturia, hematuria, urgency, frequency, pyuria, oliguria, venereal disease, incontinence, hesitancy, dribbling, discharge, lumbar pain, stones, and sexually transmitted diseases.

GYN (Gynecologic) Includes menarche, flow, dysmenorrhea, menorrhagia, metrorrhagia, dyspareunia, leukorrhea, use of contraceptives, obstetric history, pregnancies, deliveries, and abortions. *Gravida* followed by a number (either arabic or roman) refers to the number of pregnancies, including ectopics, hydatidiform moles, abortions, and normal pregnancies. *Para* followed by a number (either arabic or roman) refers to the number of deliveries after the 20th week of gestation (live or stillbirth, single or multiple, vaginal or cesarean) and does not correspond to the number of infants born.

NP (Neuropsychiatric) Includes syncope, headache, vertigo, pain, scotomata, paralysis, ataxia, convulsion, and emotional state.

MS (Musculoskeletal) Includes pain, stiffness, limitation of movement, and fractures.

Sometimes there is nothing noteworthy to add to the history in the systemic review (it was covered adequately in the history as related), so the dictator says, "systemic review is essentially negative." This expression is typed after the outline topic.

The actual structuring of the paragraphs is the responsibility of the transcriptionist, and therefore this basic understanding of a history will aid you. The physician may not dictate the outline, and you must be able to recognize each body part he or she is discussing so you can choose the appropriate topic or subtopic.

If the history continues to a second page, type the word *continued* in parentheses after the last typed line on the first page. On the second page, beginning at the left margin, repeat the statistical data from the first page and add the heading *History, page 2.* This is often difficult to carry out correctly, and you should use the Print Preview on your computer to ensure that these headings appear in the correct place. If your work is printed off-site, you may be asked not to type *continued* on the bottom of your page.

Before you begin your first assignment, briefly review the illustrated histories.

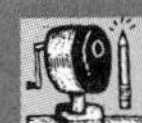

12–1: SELF-STUDY

Directions: Retype the following data into history outline using the indented format and no variations.

- Begin each exercise by setting the right and left margins at 0.5, which means a change from the default setting of 1.0. Be sure that the right margin is not justified.
- Clear all tabs and set new tab stops at 0.5, 2.0, and 4.0.
- Hint: You will be using the underline key a lot. It is important to remember to get it off and on at the correct time. Try to remember to remove the underline and then insert the colon. If you have used the caps lock key, you will have a semicolon instead of a colon if you forget to turn it off, so remember this sequence: underline on, caps lock, type word, caps lock off, underline off, colon.
- Try using the indent key after you type the outline word. Be sure to press enter at the end of the second line to come back to the left margin. Some people find it easier to type the entire document and then go back and use the tab in front of the second line to shift it over. You should try it both ways to see which one works the best for you.
- Another suggestion to try is to use the flush right feature to put in the typed signature line and dictator's name. If you do this, you do not need the 4.0 tab setting in any of the exercises.
- The patient's name and other statistical data can be set up as you desire. Be alert to topic changes and proper mechanics.

12

The patient is Geoffrey Paul Hawkins. The dictating physician is Paul R. Elsner, MD. The tape was dictated yesterday. The patient's hospital ID number is 54-98-10. His chief complaint is abdominal pains and vomiting since 3 a.m. Present illness: This 11 1/2 year old white male, who was perfectly well yesterday and last evening, awoke from his sleep with vomiting at 3 a.m. today. This was followed by nausea, which has been severe, together with a little bile coming up, but no great amount of continued vomiting. There is severe, recurrent, doubling-up type cramping to time of admission at 10 o'clock. There has been no recent upper respiratory tract infection, no prior similar episode, no history of recurrent constipation or diarrhea. Patient's last bowel movement was yesterday and of normal quality. His mother reports that he eats sunflower seeds to excess and may have done so yesterday. Past history: Patient was born at home with midwife delivery, uncomplicated. He has had the usual immunizations for childhood. There has been no prior hospitalization, no tonsillectomy, no surgery, no fracture. He has had stitches a couple of times in the office. Family History: Mother is 35 and at the present time is under treatment for cancer of the breast. She reports that she had surgery and is on chemotherapy at the present time. She has not been given radiation. Father is age 40, living and well. There are two sisters, both older than the patient, both living and well. They both had appendectomies, one of which had ruptured. There are a maternal great niece, uncle and paternal grandmother who have had diabetes. There is no diabetes in the immediate family and no other history of familial disorders such as bleeding, anemia, tuberculosis, heart disease. Personal history: The patient has no known drug allergies, has not been on any medication at the present time. Grade six, but does poorly. Seems to be the class clown according to his mother. He has no hobbies. Systemic review: HEENT: There has been a muscle in one eye which has been off for years; Dr. McMannis is following this. His vision is good, hearing is normal. CR: No known murmurs. No chronic cough, no recent cough, no dyspnea. GI: no prior GI difficulty. No food allergies. No chronic or recurrent constipation. GU: No nocturia, no enuresis, no GU infection. NM: No history of head injury, no history of polio, paralysis, meningitis, or numbness.

Turn to the end of the chapter to check your work. Pay close attention to format.

12-2: PRACTICE TEST

Directions: Retype the following data into a history outline using modified block format. Be alert to topic changes. Remember that the dictator might not follow the exact wording or format seen in the sample outlines.

- Change left and right margin settings to 0.5.
- Clear all tabs and set new tab stops at 0.5, 2.0, and 4.0.
- Hint: The indent feature works perfectly for this format because the indent goes off each time you push enter to return to the left margin for your outline. The indent will be at the tab setting for 2.0.
- Try using the flush right features to put in the typed signature line and dictator's name.

The patient is Joseph R. Balentine. The report was dictated on 11-16-9X and transcribed the same day. The dictating physician is Benjamin B. Abboud. He requests that a copy be sent to Stuart L. Paulson, MD. The patient's ID number is 423-12-22. His chief complaint: the patient is a 25 year old male complaining of recurring epistaxis. Present illness: the patient reports that yesterday he had onset of epistaxis in the left side of his nose. This was intermittent throughout the day and at 4:30 this morning, he came to the ER. Past History: Allergies: None. Illnesses: The patient had a collapsed lung about five years ago and subsequently had surgery, but does not know the exact etiology of the problem or the exact name of the surgery. There is no bleeding history except for PI. Medications: None. Family History: Essentially unremarkable. Father, mother, siblings are all well and healthy. Review of Systems: Skin: no rashes or jaundice. HEENT: See PI. CR: See past history. No history of pneumonia, tuberculosis, chronic cough, or hemoptysis. No history of pedal edema. GI: Weight is stable. He denies any nausea, vomiting, diarrhea, or food intolerance. GU: no history of GU tract infections, dysuria, hematuria, pyuria. Endocrine: no polyuria or polydipsia. Neurologic: no history of psychiatric disorder.

A transcript for this appears in Appendix A.

THE PHYSICAL EXAMINATION

A thorough *physical examination (PX or PE)* comprises an examination and complete assessment of all body systems. It is usually done after the history is taken and includes an inspection of the body, beginning with the head and concluding with the feet: cephalocaudal. An analysis of the subjective findings that were taken down during the history and review of systems indicates the extent of the PX of different body parts that is required. For example, extensive complaints regarding the cardiovascular system will result in intensive examination of the lungs and heart.

Four basic procedures are included in the complete PX:

1. Inspection: looking at the body.
2. Palpation: feeling various parts and organs.
3. Percussion: listening to the sounds produced when a particular region is tapped (percussed).
4. Auscultation: listening to body sounds.

The style and format for the PX are identical to those for the history. Be consistent and follow the same style you use for the history when typing the PX. The PX is typed on a separate sheet of paper with full headings but, again, in run-on format you simply continue on the same sheet. The first example is run-on format, showing you both a history and a PX.

Follow the same guidelines as illustrated in the history section for typing the PX.

Morris G. Heslop

March 7, 199x

527-98-6540

Room 631-A

HISTORY

CHIEF COMPLAINT: Acute onset, severe abdominal pain and indigestion.

PRESENT ILLNESS: This 41-year-old male patient presented to Fletcher Hills Memorial Emergency Room at approximately 12 o'clock on Friday, March 6, 199x, complaining of a gaseous feeling in his upper abdomen, radiating to the right side, and down to the right lower quadrant of the abdomen. The patient is a pilot for Atlantic-Pacific Airlines. Last night, approximately 6 p.m., he had a spaghetti dinner in Denver, Colorado, and was restless approximately 5-6 hours later, and while he did not have diarrhea, he felt bloating and indigestion, which was relieved to a very small extent by Maalox. He continued to have increasing discomfort in his upper abdomen with radiation to the back, between the shoulder blades, but there was no vomiting, diarrhea, or fever. He became quite sweaty and pale while flying and had the co-pilot take over.

PAST HISTORY:
Operations: The patient had a herniorrhaphy two years ago at Fletcher Memorial and an appendectomy as a teenager.
Allergies: None.
Habits: He does not smoke. The only alcohol intake is occasional wine with meals. No current drugs or medications.

FAMILY HISTORY: There is no family history of importance.

REVIEW OF SYSTEMS:
EENT: No double vision, no ringing of the ears. No headache.
GI: No weight change, no change in bowel habits or any blood in the bowel movements.
GU: No difficulty urinating, no blood in the urine.
CR: Denies any chest pain or radiation of any type of pain into his left hand or arm over to the shoulders.

PHYSICAL EXAMINATION

GENERAL: The patient is an alert, cooperative male, clutching at the right lower portion of his abdomen at times during the interview. He says that this is still uncomfortable. Pulse: 78 and regular. BP: 116/80. Temperature: 98.6. Afebrile.

HEENT: React to L&A, no AV nicking. Ears are normal. Pharynx is normal. No thyroid enlargement or bruit noted.

CHEST: Heart tones are normal.

ABDOMEN: On pressure in the epigastrium, he complains of little discomfort more to the right side of the abdomen and on pressure in the right lower quadrant he does wince. Bowel sounds are

(continued)

Figure 12–5. Example of a history and physical examination done in run-on format, first page.

Morris G. Heslop
527-98-6540
Room 631-A
Physical Examination, Page 2

hypoactive, and there is no palpable liver, kidney, spleen. There is no rebound on percussion. There is no inguinal hernia.

GENITALIA: Testicles are normal.

RECTAL: No heat and there is no blood in the bowel movements on gross examination. There is no diarrhea present.

NEUROMUSCULAR: Biceps, triceps, Achilles, patellar reflexes are normal. Range of motion of all extremities is normal. There is no pedal edema and pedal pulses are normal.

DIAGNOSIS:
1. Possible acute cholecystitis.
2. Possible food poisoning.
3. Possible early, penetrating ulcer.
4. Rule out pancreatitis.

PLAN OF DIRECTION: X-rays, ulcer-type diet, EKG, two-hour urine amylase.

Frank O. Bodner, MD

cjt
D: 3-7-9x
T: 3-9-9x

Figure 12–5 *Continued* Page 2 of a physical examination done in run-on format.

History and Physical, Run-On Format

Examples of a combined H&P in run-on format are shown in Figures 12–5 and 12–6. Note the preferred line-up when there is more than one diagnosis.

Text continued on page 285

Morris G. Heslop March 7, 199x
527-98-6540

Room 631

HISTORY

CHIEF COMPLAINT: Acute onset, severe abdominal pain and indigestion.
PRESENT ILLNESS: This 41-year-old male patient presented to Fletcher Hills Memorial Emergency Room at approximately 12 o'clock on Friday, March 6, 199x, complaining of a gaseous feeling in his upper abdomen, radiating to the right side, and down to the right lower quadrant of the abdomen. The patient is a pilot for Atlantic-Pacific Airlines. Last night, approximately 6 p.m., he had a spaghetti dinner in Denver, Colorado, and was restless approximately 5-6 hours later, and while he did not have diarrhea, he felt bloating and indigestion, which was relieved to a very small extent by Maalox. He continued to have increasing discomfort in his upper abdomen with radiation to the back, between the shoulder blades, but there was no vomiting, diarrhea, or fever. He became quite sweaty and pale while flying and had the co-pilot take over.
PAST HISTORY:
Operations: The patient had a herniorrhaphy two years ago at Fletcher Memorial and an appendectomy as a teenager.
Allergies: None.
Habits: He does not smoke. The only alcohol intake is occasional wine with meals. No current drugs or medications.
FAMILY HISTORY: There is no family history of importance.
REVIEW OF SYSTEMS:
EENT: No double vision, no ringing of the ears. No headache.
GI: No weight change, no change in bowel habits or any blood in the bowel movements.
GU: No difficulty urinating, no blood in the urine.
CR: Denies any chest pain or radiation of any type of pain into his left hand or arm over to the shoulders.

PHYSICAL EXAMINATION

GENERAL: The patient is an alert, cooperative male, clutching at the right lower portion of his abdomen at times during the interview. He says that this is still uncomfortable. Pulse: 78 and regular.
BP: 116/80. Temperature: 98.6. Afebrile.
HEENT: React to L&A, no AV nicking. Ears are normal. Pharynx is normal. No thyroid enlargement or bruit noted.
CHEST: Heart tones are normal.
ABDOMEN: On pressure in the epigastrium, he complains of little discomfort more to the right side of the abdomen and on pressure in the right lower quadrant he does wince. Bowel sounds are hypoactive, and there is no palpable liver, kidney, spleen. There is no rebound on percussion. There is no inguinal hernia.
GENITALIA: Testicles are normal.
RECTAL: No heat and there is no blood in the bowel movements on gross examination. There is no diarrhea present.
NEUROMUSCULAR: Biceps, triceps, Achilles, patellar reflexes are normal. Range of motion of all extremities is normal. There is no pedal edema and pedal pulses are normal.
DIAGNOSIS: 1) Possible acute cholecystitis 2) Possible food poisoning 3) Possible early, penetrating ulcer. 4) Rule out pancreatitis.
PLAN OF DIRECTION: X-rays, ulcer-type diet, EKG, two-hour urine amylase.

ref D: 3-7-9x T: 3-9-9x Frank O. Bodner, MD

Figure 12–6. Example of a history and physical examination done in run-on format.

de Mars, Verna Marie
76-83-06
Cortland M. Struthers, MD

PHYSICAL EXAMINATION

GENERAL:

This is a 68-year-old, well-developed, well-nourished, slightly obese white woman in no acute distress. She is alert and oriented to time, place, and person.

VITAL SIGNS:

PULSE: 76/min. BP: 130/80. RESP: 12. TEMPERATURE: 99°.

HEENT:

EYES: Pupils equal and react to light and accommodation. EOMs intact. Sclerae white. Fundi not visualized.

EARS: Hearing and drums are normal.

MOUTH: The teeth are in poor repair. Several bridges are present. The tongue protrudes in the midline with some questionable deviation to the right. Uvula projects upward on elicitation of the gag reflex. No lesions of the mucous membranes.

NECK:

Supple with some limitation of motion to the right. No masses present. The carotid pulsations are equal with no bruit. There is no neck vein distention and no thyromegaly. The trachea is deviated slightly to the right.

CHEST:

No increase in AP diameter.

LUNGS: Clear to P&A.

HEART: Quiet precordium. Normal sinus rhythm without murmurs, rubs or gallops. Heart sounds appear normal and to split physiologically. No S-4 heard.

ABDOMEN:

Flat without scars. No organomegaly. Liver, kidneys, and spleen not palpable. Tympanic to percussion. The bowel sounds are normoactive.

PELVIC:

Deferred.

RECTAL:

On anoscopy, there is an exophytic, soft, easily movable mass encompassing one-half the circumference of the rectum directly at the dentate line. Full sigmoidoscopic examination to 25 cm was unremarkable.

EXTREMITIES:

Range of motion is within normal limits. No pedal edema. All pulses appear equal and full bilaterally. No evidence of chronic arterial or venous disease.

NEUROLOGICAL:

Cranial nerves II-XII appear grossly intact. There are no pathological reflexes demonstrated. Reflexes within normal limits.

IMPRESSION:

Rectal tumor.

jrt
D: 5-17-9x
T: 5-20-9x

Cortland M. Struthers, MD

Figure 12–7. Example of a physical examination done in full block format.

Physical Examination, Full Block Format

Follow the same format as illustrated for you in typing the history. The statistical data are repeated on the new page, and the title *Physical Examination* is centered on the page, typed in full capital letters.

Figure 12–7, page 285, is an example of a PX typed in full block format. Note: The line-and-a-half spacing on this illustration was done to save space on the page.

de Mars, Verna Marie Hospital number: 76-83-06

Cortland M. Struthers, MD

PHYSICAL EXAMINATION

GENERAL: This is a 68-year-old, well-developed, well-nourished, slightly obese white woman in no acute distress. She is alert and oriented to time, place, and person.

VITAL SIGNS: PULSE: 76/min. BP: 130/80. RESP: 12. TEMPERATURE: 99°.

HEENT:

EYES: Pupils equal and react to light and accommodation. EOMs intact. Sclerae white. Fundi not visualized.

EARS: Hearing and drums are normal.

MOUTH: The teeth are in poor repair. Several bridges are present. The tongue protrudes in the midline with some questionable deviation to the right. Uvula projects upward on elicitation of the gag reflex. No lesions of the mucous membranes.

NECK: Supple with some limitation of motion to the right. No masses present. The carotid pulsations are equal with no bruit. There is no neck vein distention and no thyromegaly. The trachea is deviated slightly to the right.

CHEST: No increase in AP diameter.

LUNGS: Clear to P&A.

HEART: Quiet precordium. Normal sinus rhythm without murmurs, rubs or gallops. Heart sounds appear normal and to split physiologically. No S-4 heard.

ABDOMEN: Flat without scars. No organomegaly. Liver, kidneys, and spleen not palpable. Tympanic to percussion. The bowel sounds are normoactive.

PELVIC: Deferred.

RECTAL: On anoscopy, there is an exophytic, soft, easily movable mass encompassing one-half the circumference of the rectum directly at the dentate line. Full sigmoidoscopic examination to 25 cm was unremarkable.

EXTREMITIES: Range of motion is within normal limits. No pedal edema. All pulses appear equal and full bilaterally. No evidence of chronic arterial or venous disease.

NEUROLOGICAL: Cranial nerves II-XII appear grossly intact. There are no pathological reflexes demonstrated. Reflexes within normal limits.

IMPRESSION: Rectal tumor.

jrt
D: 5-17-9x
T: 5-20-9x

Cortland M. Struthers, MD

Figure 12–8. Example of a physical examination done in modified block format.

12

Physical Examination, Modified Block Format

Follow the same method that was illustrated for the history typed in this style. The statistical information is repeated on the new page, and the title *Physical Examination* is centered on the page, typed in full capital letters. Set your tabs at 0.5 and 1.5 (rather than 2.0, as you did for the history).

Figure 12–8 is an example of a physical examination typed in modified block format.

de Mars, Verna Marie
76-83-06
Cortland M. Struthers, MD

PHYSICAL EXAMINATION

GENERAL: This is a 68-year-old, well-developed, well-nourished, slightly obese white woman in no acute distress. She is alert and oriented to time, place, and person.

VITAL SIGNS: PULSE: 76/min. BP: 130/80. RESP: 12. TEMPERATURE: 99^{0}.

HEENT:

EYES: Pupils equal and react to light and accommodation. EOMs intact. Sclerae white. Fundi not visualized.

EARS: Hearing and drums are normal.

MOUTH: The teeth are in poor repair. Several bridges are present. The tongue protrudes in the midline with some questionable deviation to the right. Uvula projects upward on elicitation of the gag reflex. No lesions of the mucous membranes.

NECK: Supple with some limitation of motion to the right. No masses present. The carotid pulsations are equal with no bruit. There is no neck vein distention and no thyromegaly. The trachea is deviated slightly to the right.

CHEST: No increase in AP diameter.

LUNGS: Clear to P&A.

HEART: Quiet precordium. Normal sinus rhythm without murmurs, rubs or gallops. Heart sounds appear normal and to split physiologically. No S-4 heard.

ABDOMEN: Flat without scars. No organomegaly. Liver, kidneys, and spleen not palpable. Tympanic to percussion. The bowel sounds are normoactive.

PELVIC: Deferred.

RECTAL: On anoscopy, there is an exophytic, soft, easily movable mass encompassing one-half the circumference of the rectum directly at the dentate line. Full sigmoidoscopic examination to 25 cm was unremarkable.

EXTREMITIES: Range of motion is within normal limits. No pedal edema. All pulses appear equal and full bilaterally. No evidence of chronic arterial or venous disease.

NEUROLOGICAL: Cranial nerves II-XII appear grossly intact. There are no pathological reflexes demonstrated. Reflexes within normal limits.

IMPRESSION: Rectal tumor.

jrt
D: 5-17-9x
T: 5-20-9x

Cortland M. Struthers, MD

Figure 12–9. Example of a physical examination done in indented format.

Physical Examination, Indented Format

Follow the same format that was illustrated for the history typed in this style. The statistical data are repeated on the new page, and the title *Physical Examination* is centered on the page, typed in full capital letters. Set the tabs at 0.5, 1.5, and 4.0.

Note the subtopics under "HEENT" in Figure 12–9. Some medical transcriptionists group these as a single paragraph after the main heading "HEENT." This illustrated style shows you, however, that the subtopic format is more attractive and easier to read. The subtopics under "Chest" could also have been typed in paragraph form. In both cases, type the outline title or topic in full caps. Also notice that the third line under the topic "Extremities" is not brought back to the left margin but is blocked under the previous two lines. This is done to avoid a few words dangling in the margin.

THE OUTLINE

The physical examination (PX or PE) is the examiner's objective (O) observations of abnormalities or signs of the illness or injury. Part of this observation was taking place while the history was being taken from the patient but is recorded now.

As we did with the history, we will briefly examine each part of the outline used in the PX. You will type the statistical data just as you did for this history and the heading *Physical Examination.* Now begin with the topics:

General. This includes the general appearance and nutritional state of the patient, body build, alertness, personal hygiene, general state of health, age, height, weight, and race. It may include the emotional condition (euphoric, lethargic, distracted, well-oriented, agitated).

Vital Signs. Includes the temperature, pulse, respiration, and blood pressure. Most often, however, this information is included with the previous topic.

12

HEENT (or Head and Neck). This includes the head, eyes, ears, nose, and throat. After the main heading abbreviation, the individual subtopics are pulled out and typed in either outline or paragraph form, depending on the emphasis placed on all or each. The personal wishes of either the dictator or the transcriptionist will also determine which method is used; both methods were illustrated for you in the previous examples. These subtopics include the following:

Head Includes shape, and color and texture of the skin and hair.

Eyes Includes the sclerae, corneas, conjunctivae, fundi, reaction of the pupils to light and accommodation (PERLA or PERRLA), extraocular movements (EOMs), and visual acuity and fields.

Ears Includes canals, ossicles, tympanic membranes (TMs), hearing, and discharge.

Nose Includes airway, septum, and sinuses.

Mouth and Throat Includes teeth, gums, lips, tongue, salivary glands, tonsils, dentures, palate, uvula, and mucosa.

Neck Includes contour, mobility, lymph nodes, thyroid size and shape, position of trachea, carotid pulses, and neck vein distention. "Neck" is often used as a main topic. If the dictator just dictates "HEENT" and then "Neck," use "Neck" as a main topic. If "Head and Neck" are dictated, then "Neck" is a subtopic.

The next main topic is the chest, which is often divided into the subtopics of heart and lungs.

Chest. Includes the shape, symmetry, expansion, and breasts.

Lungs Includes breath sounds, expansion, fields, resonance, and adventitious sounds (rales, rhonchi, wheeze, rubs, stridor).

Heart Includes rhythm (sinus rhythm), borders, silhouette, rate, murmurs, rubs, gallops, heaves, lifts, thrills, and palpitation.

Abdomen. Includes the symmetry, shape, contour, bowel sounds, tenderness, rigidity, guarding, herniation, and palpation of the liver, spleen, and kidneys.

Genitalia (or Pelvic or Genitourinary). In the female, includes external genitalia (vulva), Skene's and Bartholin's glands, introitus, vagina, cervix, uterus, adnexa, discharge, escutcheon, urethral meatus, perineum, and anus. In the male, includes prostate, testes, epididymis, penis, lesions, and discharge.

Rectal. Includes anus, sphincter tone, perineum, and hemorrhoids.

Extremities. Includes bones, joints, movement, color, temperature, edema, and varicosities.

Neurologic. Includes reflexes, cranial nerves, orientation in all three spheres (time, place, person), signs (Babinski, Brudzinski, Hoffmann, Kernig, Romberg, Strunsky), station, and gait.

Diagnosis (Impression, Assessment, or Conclusion). Includes a provisional or final diagnosis, which is the conclusion the examiner has reached based on the history he or she has taken down and the examination just concluded. It may be an explanation for the patient's problem, the identification or explanation of a disease process, or the actual name of a disease. Diagnostic studies may be ordered (such as x-rays, electrocardiogram, blood work-up) before making a final diagnosis. These are generally typed in lined-up format when there is more than one diagnosis. See Figures 12–5 and 12–6.

NOTE: Do not use abbreviations in the diagnosis portion of this part of the medical record.

Treatment (or Recommendation). Includes the plan of treatment and may indicate surgery or some of the diagnostic studies mentioned above.

THE DATA

The physician may dictate the data in narrative form without topics or subtopics, or he or she may dictate the topics and subtopics for you. You will use the proper topic as soon as reference is made to it, no matter how it is dictated. For instance, the dictator may say: "The abdomen is scaphoid. There are no masses or rigidity." You will type:

ABDOMEN: Scaphoid, no masses or rigidity.

On the other hand, some records departments require everything in sentence form. In this case you would type:

ABDOMEN: The abdomen is scaphoid; there are no masses or rigidity.

Always ask your employer for preferred format and style.

In transcribing PXs, you should be prepared to write a tactful note to the physician or your supervisor if the dictator leaves out a vital part of the examination; for example, a hysterectomy is the contemplated procedure and the pelvic examination was not dictated. Be alert to laboratory values so that you recognize where a decimal point belongs when it is not dictated. (Laboratory values are given in Appendix B.)

12-3: REVIEW TEST

12

Directions: Retype the following data into physical examination outline using the indented format.

- Change right and left margin settings to 0.5.
- Clear all tabs and set new tab stops at 0.5, 1.5, and 4.0. This is a little different from the tabs you needed for the history that was done in this format.
- Try to use the indent and flush right features to facilitate ease in using this format.
- This is the physical examination for the patient in Self-Study 12–1, Geoffrey Paul Hawkins.

The patient is a well-developed, well-nourished, white male who appears his age of eleven and a half. He is of moderately small stature but is well tanned from being in the sun. He appears to be in no acute distress but is quite apprehensive. The skin is warm and dry, well-tanned, no jaundice, no lesions. The pupils are round, regular and equal; react to light and accommodation. No icterus seen. Conjunctivae normal. Nose: septum straight. No lesions. The mouth and throat are benign. The tonsils are small and the teeth are in good repair. The neck is supple. The thyroid is not enlarged. There is no remarkable lymphadenopathy. Trachea is in the midline with no tug. Ears: drums pearly, hearing is good to spoken voice. The lungs are clear to percussion and auscultation. Heart: regular sinus rhythm, no murmurs heard. A-2 is louder than P-2. The abdomen is scaphoid with no scars. Patient indicates midepigastric tenderness. Peristalsis is audible and possibly slightly hyperactive but very close to average in intensity. There is some tenderness, mainly in the right upper quadrant. Both left and right lower quadrants appear to be soft with no rebound present. Equivocal Murphy punch tenderness is present. No CVA tenderness. Genitalia: testes down, no penile lesions. Rectal: There is stool in the ampulla. Sphincter tone is good. Patient complains of some tenderness in both vaults, but no masses found. Skeletal: No gross bone or joint anomalies. Neurologic: no motor or sensory loss found. Deep tendon reflexes active and equal. Toe signs down. Pedal pulses palpable. Impression: Abdominal pain, etiology unproved, but probable gastroenteritis. Rule out early appendicitis.

12–4: REVIEW TEST

Directions: Retype the following data into PX outline using modified block format. This is the patient you had for Practice Test 12–2, Joseph R. Balentine.

The patient is a well-developed, muscular, slightly pale, young man in somewhat acute distress, secondary to the apprehension and bleeding. Blood pressure is one hundred ten over seventy. Pulse is seventy four. Respirations are sixteen. HEENT: Head is normocephalic. Eyes are round, regular and equal and bilaterally react to light and accommodation. There is bilateral cerumen in the ears, TMs are normal. The right nasal cavity was somewhat congested to the nasopharynx. There is active bleeding from the left nasal cavity. There are no palpable nodes in the neck and the thyroid is in the midline. The chest is symmetrical; normal male breasts. The lungs are clear bilaterally, no rales or wheezes. There is a pneumonectomy scar, left anterolateral chest. The heart is normal in size. There is normal sinus rhythm, no murmurs, thrills or rubs. The abdomen is soft, no tenderness. The rectal exam is deferred. The extremities are symmetrical, no cyanosis, edema or deformities. There is normal range of motion. Reflexes are physiological. Pulses are two plus and equal bilaterally. There is no cranial or neurological deficit. The impression is left posterior epistaxis, recurrent.

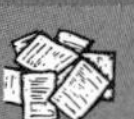 12-5: PRACTICE TEST

Directions: Retype the following data into correct H&P form. The patient is Lily Mae Jenkins and the dictator is Philip D. Quince. He wants copies sent to Dr. Willow Moran and Dr. Gordon Bender. The patient's clinic number is 5980-A. Please use run-on format and today's date.

The chief complaint is rectal bleeding, one day. Present illness: This ninety-year-old lady has been looking after her own personal affairs and living with her daughter for the last three years. Last night, she had a bowel movement that had some bright rectal blood mixed in with it. This morning, she had another bowel movement, and it consisted mostly of bright-red blood. She has a history of gallbladder disease, dating back over 50 years. She refused to have her gallbladder taken out but has been on a low fat diet ever since that time. Her daughter describes numerous gallbladder attacks, lasting for several days, consisting of severe, right upper quadrant pain. She has had occasional, intermittent right lower quadrant pain that does not seem similar to the gallbladder attacks. Past History: Operations: In 1977 she had enucleation of the left eye. She had surgery in 1986 for glaucoma in the right eye. Medical: 1976, Colles' fracture, right wrist. 1980s severe arthritis of her spine. Medications: patient is presently taking Peritrate, one capsule, b.i.d. Reserpine-A, one tablet every morning. Indocin, one tablet, t.i.d. She takes Bufferin p.r.n. for pain. She takes nitroglycerin, 2-3 tablets a week for chest pain and has done so for five years. Both of her parents lived until their nineties. She had six children: one died at age three as the result of injuries sustained in an automobile accident, one died at age 56 of carcinoma of the breast. Otherwise, the family history is unremarkable. There are four children who are alive and well. Functional inquiry: HEENT: Hearing in her right ear is absent. Hearing in her left ear is decreased. There is an artificial eye in the left and there is only slight vision in her right eye if one comes exactly in the middle of her visual field. Patient has been edentulous for several years. Chest: Nonsmoker. CV: Patient has had angina for over five years and abnormal cardiograms for the last three. She is cold all of the time and is constantly bundling herself up in an effort to keep warm. GI: Her bowel movements have been normal. See history of present illness. GU: She has no history of any bladder or kidney infections, despite the fact that she had a

12

history of kidney failure last year. NM: Patient has shooting, severe pains up her spine, which are relatively incapacitating, but she manages to keep going by just taking Bufferin. Physical examination: This is a ninety year old black woman in no obvious distress, who is hard of hearing, but can answer questions. HEENT: The ears: There is wax in both ears. The drums, beyond the wax, appear within normal limits. There is no hearing in the right ear and only slight hearing in the left. The left eye is artificial. The right eye is pinpoint. There is no scarring in the right eye, consistent with an iridectomy. She has a cataract in the right eye, as well. Nose is unremarkable. Mouth is edentulous. Neck: There are no carotid bruits. No jugular venous distention. Thyroid is palpable and unremarkable. Range of motion of the neck is generally slightly restricted. Chest is clear to percussion and auscultation. Heart: The apical beat is not palpable. There is some tenderness over the costochondral cartilages on the left side. The heart size is not enlarged to percussion. There is muffled heart sound. There is no third or fourth heart sound. There are no murmurs heard in the supine position. Breasts are palpable and there are no masses noted. Abdomen is soft. There are marked senile keratoses over the abdominal wall. There is some diffuse tenderness on deep palpation over the cecum in the right lower quadrant. There is no other tenderness noted or abnormal bowel sounds noted in the abdomen. Bowel sounds are within normal limits. Pelvic: Not done. Rectal: Full sigmoidoscopic examination to 25 cm revealed fresh blood in the sigmoid area with no obvious bleeding source noted. Extremities: There is essentially no motion in the back. Range of motion of the hips is within normal limits and painless. There is only a +1 dorsalis pedis on the right; otherwise, there are no peripheral pulses present. There is marked coldness of both feet. Central nervous system: The patient's strength is within normal limits. The reflexes are within normal limits. Coordination is not tested. There is an involuntary shaking, consistent with the diagnosis of old Parkinson's disease. Impression: Acute gastrointestinal hemorrhage, etiology not yet diagnosed. Chronic cholecystitis. Severe osteoarthritis of spine. Arteriosclerotic heart disease with angina pectoris.

See Appendix A at the end of the book for the proper response to this assignment.

12-6: SELF-STUDY

Directions: Please answer the following questions by referring to the figures in this chapter. Answer here or on a separate sheet of paper.

USING FIGURE 12-1

1. Under the subtopic "Allergies": why is "allergic to penicillin" typed in capital letters and underlined?
2. Under the subtopic "Neurologic": what does "unremarkable" mean?
3. Under "GI": why is "Present Illness" capitalized?
4. Under "OB-GYN": what does "climacteric" mean?

USING FIGURE 12-6

5. Under "Present Illness": why is "between the shoulder blades" enclosed in commas?
6. Under "General": what does "afebrile" mean?
7. Under "Family History": what does it mean when it is said that "there is no family history of importance"?
8. Under "HEENT": what does "L&A" mean?
9. Under "Neuromuscular": why did the transcriptionist not abbreviate that as "NM"?

12

USING FIGURE 12-8

10. Under "Eyes": why is "sclerae" not written as "sclera," "fundi" not written as "fundus," and EOMs not written as "EOM" or "eom"?
11. Under "Neurological": why are the roman numerals used to describe the cranial nerves two through twelve?

USING FIGURE 12-10

12. Under "Recommendation": why not use the standard abbreviation "T&A" instead of "tonsillectomy and adenoidectomy"?

USING FIGURES 12-7, 12-8, AND 12-9: ALL HAVE IDENTICAL MATERIAL

13. Which one is the most attractive?
14. Which one is easiest to read?
15. Which one was the easiest to type? (You have typed all three formats, so you should have an opinion on this one, too.)

See the end of the chapter, page 298, for the answers to these questions.

12-7: REVIEW TEST

Directions: Retype the following data into correct H&P form. The patient is J. J. "Kip" Siegler. The physician is Felix Rios, MD. Use today's date and full block format.

The chief complaint is right sided, abdominal pain, eight hours duration. The present illness is as follows: this is the first Brookside Hospital admission for this twenty-four year old unemployed carpenter who was in his usual state of excellent health until approximately eight hours prior to admission when he developed some high, transverse midepigastric abdominal pain following completion of a Chinese meal. The pain became progressively more intense and gradually, over the following four hours, localized in the right lower quadrant. One hour prior to admission, while preparing to come to the hospital, the patient had one episode of emesis. The patient denies any subsequent nausea and diarrhea but has been "constipated" for the past two days. The past medical history: Serious injuries: None. Surgery: None. Illnesses: None. Allergies: Assorted pollens, undetermined. Medications: None. Smoke: None. Alcohol: Very infrequently. Immunizations: None in the past four years. The father is deceased, age 21, apparent suicide. The mother is living and well, age 41. One sister, age 22, living and well. The patient is married and has one child and has been unemployed for the past six months. He spends most of his time refurbishing an old sailboat. Systemic review is unremarkable. On physical examination there is an alert, oriented, Caucasian male, in very mild abdominal distress, lying supine, with his right hip flexed. His temperature is one hundred one point two degrees, pulse is eighty eight, respirations twenty, blood pressure is one hundred thirty over seventy eight. The skin is warm and moist without pallor, icterus, or cyanosis. There are no acute lesions or petechiae. Tympanic membranes are clear. Pupils are equal and reactive to light. Conjunctivae are mildly injected. Nares, likewise mildly injected. Pharynx and mouth, likewise, very minimally injected, without evidence of purulent debris. The neck is supple without cervical adenopathy. The lungs are clear to auscultation and percussion. The heart rhythm is regular without murmurs or enlargement. The abdomen is somewhat protuberant with absent bowel sounds, with moderate tenderness and guarding in the right lower quadrant without rebound. There is also very mild tenderness in the right "See vee a" area. There are no apparent herniae determined in the supine position. Rectal: Prostate is normal. There is moderate to exquisite tenderness in the right quadrant. Stool is brown, and hematest is negative. Genitalia: Patient is circumcised. Testicles are bilaterally descended, appear normal in size and shape. Extremities: No deformities or edema. Neurologic: Two plus deep tendon reflexes, bilaterally. Diagnosis: Acute appendicitis.

SHORT-STAY RECORD

When the patient is being admitted for 48 hours or less or being sent to an outpatient surgical or diagnostic center, a shortened form of the H&P record is acceptable in most facilities. This form is appropriate for many diagnostic procedures and minor operative procedures. The statistical data would be the same as those required on the longer forms, but the description of the patient's condition and the PX would be considerably condensed.

Figure 12–10 is an example of a short-stay record set up in modified block format.

Roland, Jamie T.
543098

June 8, 199x

Copy: Robert R. Shoemaker, MD

SHORT-STAY RECORD

HISTORY: Patient is a 6-year-old male complaining of frequent episodes of tonsillitis. He has missed several weeks of school this spring because of infections. He is a constant mouth breather. He snores loudly at night. He has constant nasal obstruction. There is no history of earaches.

PAST HISTORY: There are no allergies. Bleeding history: None. Operations: None. Illnesses: None Medications: Vitamins, iron. Has been on Penicillin for resolution of symptoms. Family History: Noncontributory.

PHYSICAL EXAMINATION: Skin: No rashes. EENT: Ears: TM and canals appeared normal. Nose: Congested posteriorly but not anteriorly. Throat: Very large cryptic tonsils meeting in the midline. Neck: Numerous palpable nodes.

CHEST: Lungs: Clear to percussion and auscultation. Heart: Not enlarged, normal sinus rhythm, no murmurs.

ABDOMEN: Soft, nontender.

EXTREMITIES: Full range of motion.

NEUROLOGICAL: Completely normal.

IMPRESSION: Chronic hypertrophic tonsils and adenoids with recurrent infections.

RECOMMENDATION: Tonsillectomy and adenoidectomy.

Peter Anthony Nelson, MD

sd
D: 6-8-9x
T: 6-8-9x

Figure 12–10. Example of a short-stay record done in modified block format.

INTERVAL HISTORY

If the patient returns to the hospital within a month of being discharged and has the same complaint, a complete H&P does not have to be written on the patient. However, an interval history (or interval note) is completed to describe what has happened to the patient since discharge. The complete statistical data are used, but the medical information is considerably briefer, with emphasis on the present complaint and interval history. The PX would include any new findings since the last examination and may also include a brief check on vital body systems. A more extensive examination would be done in the area prompting the readmission to the hospital.

Figure 12–11 is an example of an interval history note.

Benita L. Martinez　　　　March 17, 199x

09-74-12　　　　William B. Dixon, MD

INTERVAL HISTORY

PRESENT COMPLAINT: This is a 45-year-old female who the first of March had a Roux-en-Y gastrojejunostomy done for a reflux bile gastritis. Postoperatively, she did moderately well; however, she began to evidence signs of anastomotic obstruction which got persistently worse. Upper GI series was done 4 days ago which showed an almost complete obstruction of the anastomosis. Patient is now being admitted for decompression of her stomach and revision of the gastrojejunostomy.

PAST HISTORY: Regional family, see old chart.

PHYSICAL EXAMINATION: Well-developed, well-nourished, but nervous, white female in no acute distress.

HEENT: Eyes: React to L&A. Ears: Canals and membranes normal. Nose: Negative. Neck: Supple with no masses, no enlargement of glands. Thyroid: Not palpable.

LUNGS: Clear to percussion and auscultation.

HEART: Rhythm and rate normal. No murmurs. No enlargements.

ABDOMEN: Recent bilateral, subcostal incision, well-healed. No other abdominal masses.

PELVIC: Not done.

EXTREMITIES: Negative.

IMPRESSION: Gastrojejunal anastomotic obstruction.

ADVICE:
1. Decompression by Levin tube.
2. Re-resection and anastomose tomorrow.

William B. Dixon, MD

mlo
D: 3-17-9x
T: 3-20-9x

Figure 12–11. Example of an interval history done in modified block style.

12-1 COMPUTER EXERCISE

Before proceeding, you may want to do more exercises based on the concepts you have learned. Additional practice material is on your computer diskette.

Directions: Insert the diskette into the computer and follow the instructions on the screen for Computer Exercise 12–1.

TRANSCRIPTION EXERCISE

For transcribing histories and physicals, documents 32 through 38 are on *Sound Tapes to Accompany Medical Keyboarding, Typing, and Transcribing Techniques and Procedures,* Cassette 2, Side C.

A *Answers to* 12-1: SELF-STUDY

Geoffrey Paul Hawkins
54-98-10

HISTORY

CHIEF COMPLAINT: Abdominal pains and vomiting since 3 a.m.

PRESENT ILLNESS: This 11 1/2-year-old white male, who was perfectly well yesterday and last evening, awoke from his sleep with vomiting at 3 a.m. today. This was followed by nausea, which has been severe, together with a little bile coming up, but no great amount of continued vomiting. There is severe, recurrent, doubling-up type cramping to time of admission at 10 o'clock. There has been no recent upper respiratory tract infection, no prior similar episode, no history of recurrent constipation or diarrhea. Patient's last bowel movement was yesterday and of normal quality. His mother reports that he eats sunflower seeds to excess and may have done so yesterday.

PAST HISTORY: Patient was born at home with midwife delivery, uncomplicated. He has had the usual immunizations for childhood. There has been no prior hospitalization, no tonsillectomy, no surgery, no fracture. He has had stitches a couple of times in the office.

FAMILY HISTORY: Mother is 35 and at the present time is under treatment for cancer of the breast. She reports that she has had surgery and is on chemotherapy at the present time. She has not been given radiation. Father is age 40, living and well. There are two sisters, both older than the patient, both living and well. They both had appendectomies, one of which had ruptured. There are a maternal great niece, uncle and paternal grandmother who have had diabetes. There is no diabetes in the immediate family and no other history of familial disorders such as bleeding, anemia, tuberculosis, heart disease.

PERSONAL HISTORY: The patient has no known drug allergies, has not been on any medication at the present time. Grade six, but does poorly. Seems to be the class clown according to his mother. He has no hobbies.

SYSTEMIC REVIEW:

HEENT: There has been a muscle in one eye which has been off for years; Dr. McMannis is following this. His vision is good, hearing is normal.

CR: No known murmurs. No chronic cough, no recent cough, no dyspnea.

GI: No prior GI difficulty. No food allergies. No chronic or recurrent constipation.

GU: No nocturia, no enuresis, no GU infection.

NM: No history of head injury, no history of polio, paralysis, meningitis, or numbness.

mlo
D: (yesterday's date)
T: (today's date)

Paul R. Elsner, MD

NOTE: Check to be sure that the format followed is that illustrated, that the outline is typed in full capital letters and underlined, that all first and second lines are blocked evenly and that third and subsequent lines are brought back to the left margin, and that subtopics are indented a single tab from the left margin. Also check the signature line. The assignment should be neat and attractive, with narrow margins.

12

A *Answers to* **12–6: SELF-STUDY**

1. To call attention to it.
2. There were no abnormal findings.
3. Because it refers back to that major topic in the outline.
4. The "menopause," or end of her regular menstrual cycles.
5. It is a nonessential phrase.
6. The patient did not have a fever or elevated body temperature.
7. No one suffers from or has died of any diseases or conditions that are considered hereditary.
8. How the pupils react to light and accommodation.
9. It was not in keeping with the rest of the format, where topics were spelled out in full. Also, one must presume that if the outline were dictated, the dictator did not say "NM" but "neuromuscular."
10. It is clear from the transcript that the dictator is referring to both eyes; therefore, the plural form is necessary. English abbreviations are written in capital letters, not lower case letters, as are Latin abbreviations.
11. This is the custom; one could call it tradition.
12. One must presume that the dictator did not say "T&A"; furthermore, it is not a good idea to abbreviate items of this importance.
13. This is up to you.
14. All three are pretty easy, certainly easier than the run-on format. It is up to you.
15. This is up to you and what you enjoy doing.

CHAPTER

13

Preparation of Miscellaneous Medical Reports

13

OBJECTIVES

After reading this chapter and working the exercises, you should be able to

1. Identify the kind of information that appears in various medical reports.
2. Prepare a discharge summary, operative report, pathology report, radiology report, consultation report, autopsy protocol, and medicolegal report.
3. List the kind of information that appears in a medicolegal report.
4. Explain the differences in typing a medical report versus an autopsy protocol.

INTRODUCTION

This chapter continues the instruction for the preparation of "The Big Four": the history and physical (see Chap. 12), operative report, consultation report, and discharge summary. These and a variety of other medical reports concerning patients may be transcribed by medical transcriptionists in the word processing department or medical records department of a hospital. On a few occasions, a physician may want his or her private secretary to transcribe some of these reports; in some medical facilities, the department secretary will transcribe. For example, the pathology department may have laboratory reports and autopsy reports transcribed in the department. Consultation reports may be transcribed in the hospital or physician's office, and medicolegal reports are usually done in the private medical office. Private transcription agencies are prepared to do a variety of medical typing and transcribing. Because you do not know where you will seek employment, it is necessary for you to be prepared to type the different parts of the medical record.

Reports are sent to consultants who participated in the management of the patient, to insurance companies who want background information on patients, to third-party carriers to justify bills, to referring physicians, and to the Social Security Administration to assess a patient for total disability.

Accuracy and readability are the most important factors emphasized in reference to format. All headings and subheadings must follow the same format, so it is important to determine how you will set up the report before you begin typing. Topics of equal importance are given equal emphasis through the use of capital letters, lowercase letters, spacing, underlining, centering, and so on. The figures in this chapter give you a glimpse of possible headings; each physician/dictator will choose different words to emphasize. The sequence of the topic words may also be reversed in some dictations. The general guideline to follow is to transcribe exactly the sequence that is dictated and to determine the words requiring the most emphasis for major headings and those requiring less emphasis for subheadings. In some institutions, forms with preprinted headings require that you reformat the dictation so that it is typed in the sequence given on the forms.

DISCHARGE SUMMARIES

A discharge summary (clinical resume or final progress note) is required for each patient who is discharged from a hospital. It contains the same information that is found in the patient's history and physical with the addition of the admitting

Silverman, Elaine J.
97-32-11
July 16, 199X

DISCHARGE SUMMARY

ADMISSION DATE: June 14, 199x DISCHARGE DATE: July 15, 199x

HISTORY OF PRESENT ILLNESS:
This 19-year-old black female, nulligravida, was admitted to the hospital on June 14, 199x with fever of 102,° left lower quadrant pain, vaginal discharge, constipation, and a tender left adnexal mass. Her past history and family history were unremarkable. Present pain had started two to three weeks prior to admission. Her periods were irregular, with the latest period starting on May 30, 199x and lasting for six days. She had taken contraceptive pills in the past, but had stopped because she was not sexually active.

PHYSICAL EXAMINATION:
She appeared well developed and well nourished, and in mild distress. The only positive physical findings were limited to the abdomen and pelvis. Her abdomen was mildly distended, and it was tender, especially in the left lower quadrant. At pelvic examination her cervix was tender on motion, and the uterus was of normal size, retroverted, and somewhat fixed. There was a tender cystic mass about 4-5 cm in the left adnexa. Rectal examination was negative.

ADMITTING DIAGNOSIS:
1. Probable pelvic inflammatory disease (PID).
2. Rule out ectopic pregnancy.

LABORATORY DATA ON ADMISSION:
Hgb 8.8, Hct 26.5, WBC 8,100 with 80 segs and 18 lymphs. Sedimentation rate 100 mm in one hour. Sickle cell prep + (turned out to be a trait). Urinalysis normal. Electrolytes normal. SMA-12 normal. Chest x-ray negative, 2-hour UCG negative.

HOSPITAL COURSE AND TREATMENT:
Initially, she was given cephalothin 2 gm IV q6h, and kanamycin 0.5 gm IM b.i.d. Over the next 2 days the patient's condition improved. Her pain decreased and her temperature came down to normal in the morning and spiked to 101° in the evening. Repeat CBC showed Hb 7.8, Hct 23.5. The pregnancy test was negative. On the second night following admission she spiked to 104.° The patient was started on anti-tuberculosis treatment, consisting of isoniazid 300 mg/day, ethambutol 600 mg b.i.d. and rifampin 600 mg daily. She became afebrile on the sixth postoperative day and was discharged on July 15, 199x in good condition. She will be seen in the office in one week.

SURGICAL PROCEDURES:
Biopsy of omentum for frozen section; culture specimens.

DISCHARGE DIAGNOSIS:
Genital tuberculosis.

____
Harold B. Cooper, MD

mtf
d: 7-15-9x
t: 7-16-9x

Figure 13–1. Discharge summary, report form, typed in full-block format. The absence of a letterhead and the final two notations on the left side of the page indicate that this report was prepared by a hospital transcriptionist. In paragraph four, "PID" was dictated, and the transcriptionist spelled out the diagnosis and put the abbreviation in parentheses. In paragraph five, "UCG" means urinary chorionic gonadotropin.

and discharge diagnoses, operations performed, laboratory and x-ray studies, consultations, hospital course, and the condition of the patient at the time of discharge including medications on discharge, instructions for continuing care, therapy, and possibly a follow-up postoperative office visit date. The condition of the patient on discharge should be stated in terms that permit a specific measurable comparison with the condition on admission, avoiding the use of vague terminology such as "improved." Many medical transcriptionists have the documentation available and skill to assemble a discharge summary and are being asked to do so. If a resident or intern (house staff physician) dictates the discharge summary, it is usually approved by the attending physician (attending staff physician). If authorized in writing by the patient or a legally qualified representative, a copy of the discharge summary should be sent to any known medical practitioner or medical facility responsible for follow-up care of the patient. Often, discharge summaries for patients being transferred are transcribed on a STAT basis. If STAT material is processed at an off-site location, a facsimile is placed with the medical record and replaced with the original report when it is delivered to the facility.

In the case of a patient's death, a summary statement should be added to the record either as a final progress note or as a separate resume. This final note should give the reason for admission, the findings and course in the hospital, and the events leading to death.

Because the previous chapter discussed the history and physical in detail, we will not repeat the entire contents. However, Figures 13–1 and 13–2 give examples of complete discharge summaries showing appearance, formats, and content. The formats discussed follow the four illustrated in Chapter 12.

COLLEGE MEDICAL CENTER
1000 North Main Street •College Town, XY 12345-0001 •PHONE: (013) 123-4567 FAX: (013) 130-4599

DISCHARGE SUMMARY

DATE OF ADMISSION: July 9, 199x DATE OF DISCHARGE: July 15, 199x

ADMITTING DIAGNOSIS:
1) Pneumonia.
2) Hypertension.
3) History of congestive heart failure.
4) Menopause.

BRIEF HISTORY:
A 67-year-old female with a complaint of chest tightness and who was seen at Smith-Davis Urgent Care, found to have bilateral pneumonia and hypoxemia. The patient was subsequently transferred to St. Charles for admission.

HOSPITAL COURSE:
The patient was admitted and placed on antibiotics and oxygen supplement. The patient improved, showing gradual resolution of hypoxemia. The patient was discharged in stable condition.

DISCHARGE DIAGNOSIS:
1) Pneumonia.
2) Hypertension.
3) History of congestive heart failure.
4) Menopause.

PROGNOSIS:
Good. Discharged on medications. Ceftin 100 mg b.i.d. for seven days. The patient is to follow up with Dr. Doe in one week.

____
Raul Garcia, MD

RG:mtf
D: 7/15/9x
T: 7/15/9x

DISCHARGE SUMMARY	PT. NAME:	MONTEZ, MARIA B.
	ID NO:	JT-890480
	ROOM NO:	598
	ATT. PHYS.	RAUL GARCIA, MD

Figure 13–2. Discharge summary, report form, typed in full-block format. The bottom of the report illustrates the method used at some hospitals to insert the patient's identifying data.

13–1: SELF-STUDY

Directions: Retype the following data into discharge summary outline using the full-block format. Set margins at 0.5 and one tab stop at 4.5. Pay careful attention to punctuation and capitalization. The patient's name and other statistical data may be set up as you desire. Note topic changes and proper mechanics. The location of the headings, admitting diagnosis and discharge diagnosis, may vary—occurring at the beginning of the report, in the natural order of dictation (as seen in Fig. 13–1), or at the end of the report—as specified by the individual facility. See page 270 for the full-block format report style.

The patient is Marcia M. Bacon. The dictating physician is Henry R. Knowles, MD. The summary was dictated on May 10 and transcribed on May 11. The patient's hospital ID number is 52-01-96. The patient's room number is 248-C. The date of hospital admission is May 7, 199X, and she was discharged on May 9, 199X. Admission diagnosis: Torn medial meniscus, left knee. Discharge diagnosis: Torn medial meniscus, left knee; chondromalacia of the medial femoral condyle. History of present illness: The patient injured her left knee on April 11, 199X, while playing tennis. She subsequently had difficulty with persistent effusion and pain in the left knee. An arthrogram prior to admission revealed a tear of the medial meniscus. Physical examination: absence of tenderness to palpation of any of the joint structures. There was approximately 30-55 cc of fluid within the joint. Range of motion was full. Laboratory data: admission hemoglobin was 15.9, hematocrit 47% with a white count of 7,400 with normal differential. Urinalysis was within normal limits. Chem panel 19 showed an elevated cholesterol of 379 mg%. Chest x-ray was reported as negative. Treatment and hospital courses: The patient was taken to the Operating Room on the same day as admission, at which time she underwent arthroscopy. This revealed that she had a tear of the medial meniscus. Arthrotomy was performed, with medial meniscectomy. A chondral fracture was noted in the medial femoral condyle, measuring approximately 5 mm in greatest diameter. The edges of this were sheathed. Postoperatively, the patient's course was benign. There was no significant temperature elevation. She became ambulatory with crutches on the first postoperative day with no difficulty with straight leg raising. Disposition: The patient is being discharged home ambulatory with crutches and an exercise program. She is to be seen in the office in one week for suture removal. Condition at the time of discharge: Improved. Complications: None. Medications: None.

See the end of the chapter for a possible transcript of this assignment.

OPERATIVE REPORTS

Whenever a surgical procedure is done in the hospital, an outpatient surgical center, or a clinic, an operative report should be dictated or written in the medical record immediately after surgery. It should contain a description of the findings, the technical procedures used, the specimens removed, the preoperative and postoperative diagnosis or diagnoses, the type of operation performed, and the name of the primary surgeon and any assistants. If the postoperative diagnosis is the same as the preoperative diagnosis, repeat it exactly. The body of the report is a narrative of the procedure and findings and contains the type of anesthetic, incision, instruments used, drains, packs, closure, sponge count, tissue removed or altered, materials removed or inserted, blood loss and replacement, wound status, complications or unusual events, and condition of patient on leaving the surgical area. The completed operative report should be authenticated by the surgeon and filed in the medical record as soon as possible after surgery. When there is a transcription or filing delay, a comprehensive operative progress note should be entered in the medical record immediately after surgery to provide pertinent information for other physicians who may be attending the patient. If a patient requires additional surgery after the initial surgery has been completed, the report may be transcribed on a STAT basis.

See Figure 13–3 for an example of an operative report. Notice that the first paragraph is one long

13

COLLEGE HOSPITAL
4567 BROAD AVENUE
WOODLAND HILLS, XY 12345

Patient: Elaine J. Silverman   Date: June 20, 199x

Hospital No.: 84-32-11   Room No.: 1308

OPERATIVE REPORT

PREOPERATIVE DIAGNOSIS:
1. Menorrhagia.
2. Chronic pelvic inflammatory disease.
3. Perineal relaxation.

POSTOPERATIVE DIAGNOSIS:
1. Menorrhagia.
2. Chronic pelvic inflammatory disease.
3. Perineal relaxation.

OPERATION:
1. Total abdominal hysterectomy.
2. Lysis of pelvic adhesions.
3. Bilateral salpingo-oophorectomy.
4. Appendectomy.
5. Posterior colpoplasty.

(continued)

Figure 13–3. Operative report, report form, typed in indented format with the body of the report done in one or two large paragraphs.

Illustration continued on following page

Elaine J. Silverman Page 2 June 20, 199x

PROCEDURE: Under general anesthesia, the patient was prepared and draped for abdominal operation. The abdomen was opened through a Pfannenstiel incision, and examination of the upper abdomen was entirely normal. Examination of the pelvis revealed an enlarged uterus. The uterus was three degrees retroverted and adhered to the cul-de-sac. Both tubes and ovaries were involved in an inflammatory mass, with extensive adhesions to the lateral pelvic wall on both sides. The tubes revealed evidence of chronic pelvic inflammatory disease. The omentum was also attached to the fundus and to the left adnexa. The omentum was dissected by means of blunt and sharp dissection; the dissection was carried to each adnexa, freeing both tubes and ovaries by means of blunt and sharp dissection. The uterus was found to be approximately two times enlarged, after freeing all the adhesions. The uterovesical fold of peritoneum was then incised in an elliptical manner, bladder was dissected off the lower uterine segment. The round ligament, infundibulopelvic ligament on each side was identified, clamped, cut, and ligated. The uterine artery on each side, was clamped, cut and doubly ligated. Paracervical fascia was developed. Heaney clamps were placed on the cardinal ligaments, the cardinal ligaments cut, and pedicles ligated. The vagina was circumscribed; the uterus, both tubes and ovaries were removed from the operative field. The cardinal ligaments were then sutured into the lateral angles of the vagina by means of interrupted sutures; the vagina was then closed with continuous over-and-over stitch. The paracervical fascia was sutured into place with interrupted figure-of-eight suture; the lateral suture incorporated the stumps of the uterine arteries; the pelvis was then reperitonealized with continuous length of GI 2-0 atraumatic suture. Appendix was identified, and appendectomy was done in the usual manner. The appendiceal stump was cauterized with phenol and neutralized with alcohol. Re-examination at this time of the pelvis revealed all bleeding well controlled. The abdominal wall was then closed in layers, and the skin was approximated with camelback clips. During the procedure, the patient received one unit of blood. Patient was then prepared for vaginal surgery.
Patient was placed in lithotomy position, prepared and draped. Posterior colpoplasty was begun, for repair of rectocele and perineal relaxation. The posterior vaginal mucosa was dissected from the perirectal fascia; the excess posterior vaginal mucosa was excised and perirectal fascia was brought together with continuous interlocking suture of 0 chromic. The posterior vaginal mucosa was closed with continuous interlocking suture of 0 chromic. Perineal body was closed with subcutaneous, subcuticular stitch. There was a correct sponge count. The patient withstood the operation well. Patient left the operating room in good condition.

Surgeon ______________
Harold B. Cooper, MD

mtf
D: 6-20-9x
T: 6-22-9x

Figure 13–3 *Continued*

13

paragraph. Although this may seem awkward to you, this is how many surgeons dictate their operative records. However, some hospitals require that surgeons separate the report into subheadings, such as anesthesia, incision, findings, procedure, closure, and so on. In designating suture material size, see Chapter 5, Rule 5.18. Figure 13–4 illustrates another format for an operative report.

TUFTS MEDICAL CENTER OUTPATIENT CARE

PATIENT: Ouddy, Busaba
DATE: 11/15/9X
SURGEON: Henry D. Sousa, DPM
ANESTHESIOLOGIST: Jeffrey B. Morgan, MD
ANESTHESIA: 10 cc of equally mixed 2% Xylocaine plain and 0.5% Marcaine plain.
PROCEDURE TIME: The operation began at 7:30 and ended at 8:15.

OPERATIVE REPORT

PREOPERATIVE DIAGNOSIS: Hallux limitus, right foot.

POSTOPERATIVE DIAGNOSIS: Hallus limitus, right foot.

OPERATION PERFORMED: Cheilectomy first metatarsal phalangeal joint, right foot.

OPERATIVE TECHNIQUE IN DETAIL: The patient was brought to the operating room and placed in the supine position. Anesthesia was achieved with the use of the aforementioned anesthesia distributed in a Mayo block to the right foot. Following sterile preparation, application of Betadine solution, and sterile draping with hemostasis obtained by the placement of a tourniquet to the level of the ankle and inflated to 250 mgHg, the following surgical procedures were performed:

RIGHT FOOT: A linear incision was placed on the dorsal aspect of the foot medial to the extensor hallucis longus tendon. This incision began proximally at the midshaft of the first metatarsal and extended distally to the midshaft of the first proximal phalanx. The wound edges were underscored and all vital structures were retracted. Superficial bleeders were coagulated with the use of a Bovie unit. The incision was deepened via anatomical dissection to the level of the capsule and periosteal structures about the first metatarsal phalangeal joint. Using an incision that paralleled the initial skin incision, the capsule and periosteal structures were dissected free, delivering the dorsal exostosis that was located on the first metatarsal and proximal phalanx into the surgical site. The first metatarsal phalangeal joint at this time was inspected, and there were free floating ossicles that were excised from the wound sites. The cartilage was noted to have central erosions located on both the head of the first metatarsal and base of the proximal phalanx. The bony exostosis that was present on the medial dorsal lateral aspect of the first metatarsal head and base of the proximal phalanx were resected in total. The surgical site was then flushed with copious amounts of sterile saline, inspected, and found to be free of debris. The hypertropic synovium was then excised. The surgical site was then freed further with the use of a McGlamery scoop. The surgical site was then flushed again with copious amounts of sterile saline, inspected, and found to be free of debris. The surgical site was then remodeled to make a more normal appearing metatarsal head and base of the proximal phalanx. The surgical site was then again flushed with copious amounts of sterile saline, inspected, and found to be free of debris. The patient was then placed through a range of motion and was noted to have 70 degrees of motion at the time of the surgery procedure. This was in comparison to 40 degrees preoperatively, with the last 15 degrees of that 40 degrees being painful. The surgical site was then reapposed with the periosteum and capsular structures closed via 3-0 PDS. The subcutaneous tissues were closed in layers using simple interrupted sutures of 4-0 Vicryl. The skin edges were reapposed using subcutaneous stitching of 4-0 Prolene. The surgical site was then further maintained using tincture of benzoin and Steri-Strips. The surgical site was then covered with a dry, sterile dressing consisting of Adaptic, 3 x 3 Fluffs, and a 3-inch roll of Kling. Tourniquet was released. Capillary filling time was noted to return to digits one through five on the right foot within normal limits. Prior to application of the dressing, 1.0 cc of Celestone Soluspan was injected into the surgical site. Dressing was further maintained using 3-inch Coban.

Patient tolerated surgical procedure well and left the operating room with vital signs stable.

____
HENRY D. SOUSA, DPM

HDS:mtf D: 11/15/9x T: 11/15/9x

Figure 13–4. Operative report, report form, dictated by a podiatrist. It is typed with no tabulations or indentations and in a run-on format to conserve space and save paper.

 13–2: PRACTICE TEST

Directions: Retype the following data into an operative report using the indented format and no variations. Set a 0.5 margin on right and left. Clear the tab stops and set a tab at 3.0 and 5.0. The patient's name and other statistical data may be set up as you desire. Pay attention to proper mechanics and capitalization. Date the report January 4, 199X. See page 274 for the indented format.

The patient's name is John P. Dwight, and his hospital ID number is 86-30-21. The surgeon is Felix A. Konig. The patient's room number is 582-B. The preoperative and postoperative diagnosis is: otosclerosis, left ear. The operation is a left stapedectomy. The findings, otosclerosis, footplate. Under local anesthesia, the ear was prepared and draped in the usual manner. The ear was injected with two percent lidocaine and one to six thousand epinephrine. A stapes-type flap was elevated from the posterosuperior canal wall, and the bony overhang was removed with the stapes curet. The chorda tympani nerve was removed from the field. The incudostapedial joint was separated. The stapes tendon was cut. The superstructure was removed. The mucous membrane was reflected from the ear, stapes, and facial nerve promontory. The footplate was then reamed with small picks and hooks. A flattened piece of Gelfoam was placed over the oval window and a five millimeter wire loop prosthesis was inserted and crimped in the incus. The drum was reflected, and a small umbilical tape was placed in the ear canal. The patient tolerated the procedure well.

13

See Appendix A for a possible transcript of this test.

PATHOLOGY REPORTS

As a medical transcriptionist, you can specialize by typing pathology or radiology reports. Pathology transcriptionists work in laboratories, hospital medical laboratories, and coroners' offices. There is a wide variety of job duties other than transcription, and these can consist of giving reports via the telephone; filing; retrieving diagnoses from *Systematized Nomenclature of Human and Veterinary Medicine (SNOMED International), Current Procedural Terminology* (CPT), and *International Classification of Diseases, Ninth Revision, Clinical Modification* (ICD-9-CM) coding; keeping tumor and autopsy logs; typing statistical reports; delivering reports; sorting and delivering mail; labeling and filing specimens; maintaining cross files; preparing procedure manuals throughout the laboratory; and other miscellaneous laboratory tasks depending on the size of the workplace and the number of pathologists on the staff. Some of the departments in the laboratory include histology, chemistry, hematology, microbiology/bacteriology, immunology, and blood bank. Pathology consists of two divisions: anatomic (surgical and autopsy) and clinical (blood bank, microbiology, hematology, and chemistry).

When a surgical procedure is done to remove tissue or fluid from the body, these specimens may be examined by the pathologist to determine the nature and extent of the disease. In some instances, a pathologist may render his or her opinion before the patient is sutured, as in the event of a malignancy, in which case more extensive surgery may be required. This tissue examination, or biopsy report, is called a pathology report or tissue report

College Hospital
4567 Broad Avenue
Woodland Hills, XY 12345

PATHOLOGY REPORT

Date:	June 20, 199x	Pathology No.	430211
Patient:	Elaine J. Silverman	Room No.	1308
Physician:	Harold B. Cooper, MD		
Specimen Submitted:	Tumor, right axilla		

GROSS DESCRIPTION: Specimen A consists of an oval mass of yellow fibroadipose tissue measuring 4 x 3 x 2 cm. On cut section, there are some small, soft, pliable areas of gray apparent lymph node alternating with adipose tissue. A frozen section consultation at time of surgery was delivered as NO EVIDENCE OF MALIGNANCY on frozen section, to await permanent section for final diagnosis. Majority of the specimen will be submitted for microscopic examination.

Specimen B consists of an oval mass of yellow soft tissue measuring 2.5 x 2.5 x 1.5 cm. On cut section, there is a thin rim of pink to tan-brown lymphatic tissue and the mid portion appears to be adipose tissue. A pathological consultation at time of surgery was delivered as no suspicious areas noted and to await permanent sections for final diagnosis. The entire specimen will be submitted for microscopic examination.

RFW:mtf

MICROSCOPIC DESCRIPTION: Specimen A sections show fibroadipose tissue and nine fragments of lymph nodes. The lymph nodes show areas with prominent germinal centers and moderate sinus histiocytosis. There appears to be some increased vascularity and reactive endothelial cells seen. There is no evidence of malignancy.

Specimen B sections show adipose tissue and 5 lymph node fragments. These 5 portions of lymph nodes show reactive changes including sinus histiocytosis. There is no evidence of malignancy.

DIAGNOSIS: A & B: TUMOR, RIGHT AXILLA: SHOWING 14 LYMPH NODE FRAGMENTS WITH REACTIVE CHANGES AND NO EVIDENCE OF MALIGNANCY.

Stanley T. Nason, MD

STN:mtf
D: 6-18-9x
T: 6-18-9x

Figure 13–5. Pathology report, report form, typed in modified-block format with no variations.

(Fig. 13–5). It consists of a *gross description* of the specimen submitted, which means the way the specimen looks with the naked eye before it is prepared for microscopic study. The *microscopic description* is the description of the tissue after it has been prepared and carefully examined under the microscope. The *diagnosis* is then given. Often, the gross descriptions *(grosses)* of all of the surgical specimens are dictated, transcribed, and given to the pathologist, who then dictates the microscopic descriptions *(micros)*. These are transcribed, and the completed pathology reports are given to the pathologist for signature. A copy of the report is given to each physician involved in the case, and a copy is retained in the laboratory. The original is placed in the patient's medical record. In addition to tissue and tumor reports, a pathology transcriptionist may type second-opinion reports, fine-needle aspiration reports, muscle biopsy reports, renal biopsy reports, bone marrow examinations, autopsy reports, forensic reports, and coroner reports. Pathology reports must be completed within 24 hours. Pathologists usually dictate in the present tense because they interpret the pathologic findings as they look at the specimen. The history is in past tense, and the findings are in present tense. Each dictation may include certain headings, but the headings are not always used and are not always in the same sequence.

In dictation involving pathology, it is often the nonmedical term that puzzles the novice transcriptionist because it may be difficult to understand the mechanics behind the dictated words. A common phrase encountered and typed incorrectly is "The specimen is submitted in toto." This means that all of the specimen is submitted by the pathologist for further processing. Because many pathologic terms cannot be found in standard references, always obtain a good word reference book or pathology/laboratory medicine dictionary if you do a great deal of transcription dealing with pathology.

13-3: PRACTICE TEST

Directions: Retype the following data into a pathology report using the modified-block format and no variations. Set narrow, 0.5, margins and clear tabs. Set new tabs at 1.5, 3.0, and 5.0. Remember to double space between topics. Date the report June 6, 199X. See page 272 for modified-block format.

13

The patient's name is Joan Alice Jayne, and her hospital ID number is 72-11-03. The referring physician is John A. Myhre, MD, and the pathologist is James T. Rodgers, MD. The date the specimen was removed was June 6, 199X. The patient's room number is 453-A. Pathology number is 532009. Specimen(s): The specimen consists of a four point five centimeter in diameter nodule of fibro-fatty tissue removed from the right breast at biopsy and enclosing a central, firm, sharply demarcated nodule one centimeter in diameter. Surrounding breast parenchyma reveals dilated ductules (microcystic disease). Frozen section impression: Myxoid fibroadenoma of breast. Microscopic and diagnosis: Myxoid fibroadenoma of breast. Microscopic and diagnosis: Myxoid fibroadenoma occurring in right parenchyma, the site of microcystic disease of right breast.

See Appendix A for a possible transcript of this test.

TRANSCRIPTION EXERCISE

For transcribing discharge summaries, operative reports, and pathology reports, documents 39 through 46 are on *Sound Tapes to Accompany Medical Keyboarding, Typing, and Transcribing Techniques and Procedures,* Cassette 2, Side D.

RADIOLOGY REPORTS

As mentioned previously, another way of specializing is to become a radiology transcriptionist for a group of radiologists or for the radiology department of a hospital.

An x-ray report is a description of the findings and interpretations of the radiologist who reviews

College Hospital
4567 Broad Avenue
Woodland Hills, XY 12345

RADIOLOGY REPORT

Examination Date:	June 14, 199x	Patient:	Elaine J. Silverman
Date Reported:	June 14, 199x	X-ray No.:	43200
Physician:	Harold B. Cooper, MD	Age:	19
Examination:	PA Chest, Abdomen	Hospital No.:	80-32-11

Findings:

PA CHEST: Upright PA view of chest shows the lung fields are clear, without evidence of an active process. Heart size is normal.

There is no evidence of pneumoperitoneum.

IMPRESSION: NEGATIVE CHEST.

ABDOMEN: Flat and upright views of the abdomen show a normal gas pattern without evidence of obstruction or ileus. There are no calcifications or abnormal masses noted.

IMPRESSION: NEGATIVE STUDY.

Radiologist______________________
Marian B. Skinner, MD

mtf
D: 6-14-9x
T: 6-14-9x

Figure 13–6. Radiology report, report form, typed in modified-block format with no variations.

the x-ray films taken of a patient (Fig. 13–6). These can be bone and joint films, soft tissue films, or special studies of the internal organs that require the patient to take contrast media (dyes) orally or by injection. These contrast media may be radiolucent (permitting the passage of some roentgen rays) or radiopaque (not permitting the passage of roentgen rays). For assistance in spelling the types of contrast media, refer to the back of the current *Physicians' Desk Reference (PDR),* which has a comprehensive reference list. When an examination of an organ with radioactive isotopes is done, it is called a *scan.* Radiologists may change from present to past tense within the body of a report. As a rule, the procedure was performed (past tense), and the findings are given in the present tense. At some facilities, each physician has a set of normal phrases or paragraphs logged into computer memory. The physician may choose to dictate the radiologic examination and say, "add note N1," to access one of these phrases; if necessary, the phrase may be edited depending on the case dictated.

Technology has produced methods to view structures in dimension (stereoscopy) or in layers (tomography). Through the use of x-rays with computers, a specific slice of the abdomen, chest, or head can be seen; this is called computed tomography (CT scan). A process for measuring temperature by photographically recording infrared radiations emanating from the surface of the body is called thermography. Use of high-frequency sound waves without the use of x-ray can give a composite picture of an area; this is called a sonogram or an echogram. A system that produces sectional images of the body without the use of x-rays is magnetic resonance imaging (MRI), also called nuclear magnetic resonance (NMR) imaging (Fig. 13–7). It uses a band of radio frequencies and a range of magnetic field strengths,

13

XYZ Magnetic Imaging Center
4500 College Road
Woodland Hills, XY 12345
(013) 647-0980

INTERPRETATION

PATIENT: Jeffrey Clauson   AGE: 27
NUMBER: 4309x   DATE: August 30, 199x

MAGNETIC RESONANCE IMAGING, CERVICAL SPINE:

HISTORY: Cervical radiculopathy

TECHNIQUE: Sag. G.E. 600/30/23. M.R., 43 Nex, 5 mm., C.C.
Sag. S.E. 500/24, M.R., 4 Nex, 5mm., C.C.
Ax. S.E. 1000/30, H.R., 2 Nex, 5 mm., C.C.

FINDINGS:

The sagittal sequences cover from the lower posterior fossa to approximately T4-5. The axial sequence covered from the upper odontoid process through mid T1.

There is mild reversal of the normal lordotic curve of the cervical spine.

The C2-3 and C3-4 interspaces are normal.

There is posterior osteophyte formation projecting broadly across the anterior aspect of the spinal canal at C4-5 level. On the sagittal sequences this appears to contact the cord. There is no deformity identified with the cord to indicate compression. The foramina are patent.

The C5-6 level is unremarkable aside from some narrowing of the anterior subarachnoid space, probably a result of mild spurring and the effect of the reversal of the normal lordotic curve.

At C6-7 there are degenerative disk changes with disk space narrowing and osteophyte formation. There is no cord compression, although there is moderate left foraminal stenosis.

The C7-T1 level demonstrates moderate left foraminal stenosis.

There is either spur or disk bulge at the T1-2 level. This was only seen on the sagittal sequences. The abnormality appears to contact the cord but does not appear to cause any compression. There are no additional extradural abnormalities. There are no intradural extramedullary lesions. The cord is normal without abnormal intensity to indicate the presence of infarction or mass, and there is no evidence of a syrinx. This is mentioned in that the cerebellar tonsils project somewhat below the foramen magnum indicating the possibility of a Chiari II malformation.

IMPRESSION: CEREBRAL SPONDYLOSIS AS DESCRIBED ABOVE.

PROBABLE CHIARI I MALFORMATION. NO CORD SYRINX.

Jason B. Iverson, MD

rmt

Figure 13–7. Magnetic resonance imaging (MRI) report, report form, typed in full-block format with no variations.

so information is obtained simultaneously from a large number of points in a volume. The information is processed by a computer with the use of mathematical techniques similar to those used to form CT images.

Some facilities provide radiotherapy for treatment or palliation of malignancy, so radiotherapy summaries become part of the patient's medical record. Nuclear medicine diagnostic and therapeutic procedures require reports stating the interpretations, consultation, and therapy (e.g., specific preparation of the patient, identity, date, and amount of radiopharmaceutical used) (Fig. 13–8).

College Hospital
4567 Broad Avenue
Woodland Hills, XY 12345

RADIATION THERAPY CONSULTATION

Name: Theodore V. Valdez   Requested by: John L. Morris, MD

MR# 380780   Rm # 499   Date: 6/15/9x

HISTORY OF PRESENT MEDICAL ILLNESS: This is a 72-year-old who underwent decompressive laminectomy and Harrington rod placement in 1986 for angiosarcoma. Postoperative radiation therapy at Midway Hospital (Camarillo): 4025 cGy[1] in 23 fractions (175 cGy), 4 treatments per week, 2 to 1 PA to AP portals measuring 13 × 9 cm at 100 SSD on 8 Mv Linac, 5 HVL cord block at 3000 cGy. Dr. Davis estimates coverage T2 to T8. Myelogram and CT scan negative two years ago. However, developed cough and hemoptysis in past month. Chest x-ray and CT: right perihilar mass extending into mediastinum with multiple central and one anterior mediastinal mass with postobstructive infiltrate, bilateral pleural effusion. Bronchoscopy: 75% narrowing right upper lobe orifice to subsegments, 50% narrowing right lower lobe orifice. Bleeding at right upper lobe orifice. Draining right pleural effusion and sclerodesis with negative cytology. However, preliminary tissue diagnosis from right paratracheal area and mediastinoscopy: probable angiosarcoma.

PAST MEDICAL HISTORY: Hypertension.

SOCIAL HISTORY: 50 year tobacco habit.

PHYSICAL EXAMINATION: General: Well-developed male in no acute distress. No palpable adenopathy. Lungs: Clear. Heart: Regular rate and rhythm. Abdomen: Unremarkable. Extremities: Without circulatory collapse and edema. Neurologic: Without focal deficit.

ASSESSMENT: Recurrent metastatic angiosarcoma with postobstructive pneumonitis and hemoptysis.

PLAN: 4000 cGy[1] to symptom producing mediastinal disease. Initial 1000 cGy at 200 cGy fractions then oblique off previously irradiated spinal cord and boost with 250 cGy fractions. No plans for chemotherapy. Discussed radiation therapy procedures, risks, and alternatives with patient, emphasizing possible long-term risks to spinal cord, lung, and heart as well as increased potential for morbidity resulting from prior irradiation. He agrees with treatment as outlined.

Sincerely,

Barry T. Goldstein, MD
Radiology Medical Group, Inc.

mtf
D: 6-15-9X
T: 6-16-9x

Figure 13–8. Radiotherapy report generated from a hospital, typed in report form and run-on format. (From Fordney, M.T., and Diehl, M.O.: Medical Transcription Guide. Do's and Don'ts. W. B. Saunders Company, Philadelphia, 1990.)

13

The radiology report provides preliminary information and the type of x-ray films taken or the x-ray examination performed, e.g., "Chest x-ray, PA and lateral," at the top of the report. To avoid confusion, the date in the heading should reflect the date of service rather than the date of dictation. Dictation and transcription dates are best placed at the end of the report. The date in the heading is followed by the number and type of views taken and any special circumstances that may affect the examination, e.g., whether the patient is fasting for a bowel study. Views when performed in addition to what is usual for a given study should be noted. Documentation should also include the quality of the study (*clear* or *blurry*), positive findings (*abnormal*), negative findings (*normal*), incidental findings in other areas of the film, radiologist's impression or interpretation and diagnosis, recommendations for additional studies or treatment, and signature of the radiologist. Several x-ray examinations may be included in the same report. Radiology reports should be incorporated into the patient's medical record for use if the physician needs to prove that the study was medically necessary. Radiology examinations must be documented in sufficient detail to justify reimbursement.

Some of the types of radiology reports dictated are the following:

- aortogram
- arteriogram
- arthrogram
- barium enema
- bronchogram
- cardioangiogram
- cholangiogram
- cholecystogram
- cineradiogram
- computed tomogram (CT scan)
- cystogram
- echogram
- encephalogram
- esophagram
- fluoroscopy (chest, colon, gallbladder, and stomach)
- hysterosalpingogram
- intravenous cholangiogram (IVC)
- intravenous pyelogram (IVP)
- laminagram
- lymphangiogram
- magnetic resonance imaging (MRI)
- myelogram, spinal
- nephrotomogram
- nuclear magnetic resonance (NMR)
- pneumoencephalogram
- retrograde pyelogram (RP)
- scan (blood and heart, bone, full body, brain, liver, lung, spleen, and thyroid)
- Single-photon emission computed tomography (SPECT) (heart and brain)
- sonogram
- sialogram
- stereoscopy
- thermogram
- tomogram
- upper and lower gastrointestinal (GI) series
- ultrasonogram (bile ducts, gallbladder, kidneys, liver, ovaries, and uterus)
- venogram
- ventriculogram

13

13–4: SELF-STUDY

Directions: Retype the following data into a radiology report using the modified-block format and no variations. Set narrow, 0.5 margins; clear tabs, and set tabs at 2.0, 2.5, and 5.0. Remember to double space between topics as done in full-block format. Date the report June 8, current year. See page 270 for full-block format.

The patient's name is Donna Mae Weeser. Her x-ray number is 16-A2 and her hospital number is 52-80-44. This patient is age 46. The referring physician is George B. Bancroft, MD, and the radiologist is Clayton M. Markham, MD. The examination is mammography, right and left breasts. There are retromammary prosthetic devices in position. The anterior parenchyma is somewhat compressed. There is no evidence of neoplastic calcification or skin thickening demonstrated. No dominant masses are noted within the anteriorly displaced parenchyma. No increased vascularity is evident. Impression: mammography right and left breasts shows the presence of retromammary prosthetic devices in position. The demonstrated tissue appears within normal limits.

See the end of the chapter for a possible transcript of this assignment.

TRANSCRIPTION EXERCISE

For more transcribing of pathology and radiology reports, documents 47 through 57 are on *Sound Tapes to Accompany Medical Keyboarding, Typing, and Transcribing Techniques and Procedures,* Cassette 3, Side E.

CONSULTATION REPORTS

Often, the attending physician will seek the advice and opinions of a consulting physician. The consultant will dictate a report that will be incorporated into the patient's hospital record (Fig. 13–9). The physician may see the patient in consultation in the office, emergency room, or hospital; then a report is dictated and sent to the referring physician. Sometimes, a consultation associated with decisions relating to surgical intervention may be transcribed STAT. The report may contain the present history, past history, x-ray and laboratory studies, physical examination, impression and comments on findings, prognosis, and future course of treatment recommended. It may be dictated in letter form or report form, with content and headings similar to a history and physical medical report.

HAROLD B. COOPER, MD
6000 MAIN STREET
VENTURA, CALIFORNIA 93003

June 15, 199x

John F. Millstone, MD
5302 Main Street
Ventura, CA 93003

Dear Dr. Millstone:

RE: Elaine J. Silverman

This 19-year-old woman was seen at your request. The patient was admitted to the hospital yesterday because of chills, fever, and abdominal and back pain.

The history has been reviewed. A prominent feature of the history is the presence of intermittent, severe, shaking chills for four days with associated left lower back pain, left lower quadrant abdominal pain and fever to as high as 103 or 104 degrees. The patient has had hypertension for a number of years and has been managed quite well with Aldomet 250 mg twice a day.

On examination her temperature at this time is 100.6 degrees. The pulse is 110 and regular. Blood pressure is 190/100. The patient has partial bilateral iridectomies, the result of previous cataract surgery. Otherwise, the head and neck are not remarkable. Lung fields are clear throughout. The heart reveals a regular tachycardia, heart sounds are of good quality. No murmurs heard and there is no gallop rhythm present. The abdomen is soft. There is no spasm or guarding. A well-healed surgical scar is present in the right flank area. There is considerable tenderness in the left lower quadrant of the left mid abdomen, but as noted, there is no spasm or guarding present. Bowel sounds are present. Peristaltic rushes are noted and the bowel sounds are slightly high pitched in character. The extremities are unremarkable.

Diagnosis: I believe the patient has acute diverticulitis. She may have some irritation of the left ureter in view of the findings on the urinalyses. She appears to be responding to therapy at this time in that her temperature is coming down and also there has been a slight reduction in the leukocytosis from yesterday.

I agree with the present program of therapy and the only suggestion would be to possibly increase the dose of gentamicin to 60 mg every eight hours, rather than the 40 mg q8h which she is now receiving.

Thank you for asking me to see this patient in consultation.

Sincerely,

Harold B. Cooper, MD

mtf

Figure 13–9. Consultation report generated from a medical office, letter form, typed in modified-block format with indented paragraphs and mixed punctuation.

13

 13–5: PRACTICE TEST

Directions: Retype the following material into letter form. Use modified-block format with indented paragraphs, mixed punctuation, and the current date. See page 141 for modified-block format.

Watch for proper paragraphing, placement, and mechanics.

The letter is from Margo A. Wilkins, MD and is to Glen M. Hiranuma, MD, 2501 Main Street, Ventura, California 93003 and is in reference to Mrs. Hazel R. Plunkett.

Dear Dr. Hiranuma ¶ Thank you for referring your patient Mrs. Hazel R. Plunkett for neurological consultation, evaluation, and treatment of chronic and recurrent headaches. ¶ In the past, the patient has had episodes of probably typical migraine occurring perhaps six or eight times in her life. She remembers that her mother had a similar complaint. This would begin with loss in the field of vision; and then, approximately fifteen minutes thereafter, she would have a relatively typical, unilateral throbbing pain of a significant degree which would often incapacitate her. These headaches disappeared many years ago and have never returned. ¶ However, for the last eight years approximately, the patient has had recurrent daily headaches, always right-sided, with associated pain beginning in the back of the neck with stiffness of the right side of the neck, radiating forward over the vertex to the right orbit, the nose, and the jaw. She also notes some pain in the right trapezius area. The pain tends to appear from 10 a.m. to noon, when she will take a Fiorinal, and often after she goes to sleep at night (at about 12:30 a.m.). She controls this pain by taking Fiorinal, one to four a day, and Elavil, 75 mg at bedtime. She estimates that the headaches occur approximately twice daily, are relatively short-lived but occasionally last a full day. The pain is dull and heavy, not throbbing, and worse at some times than at others. ¶ On examination she was a quiet woman, not in acute distress, and somewhat dour; but she gave a careful and concise history. Her gait and station were normal. The head functions were basically intact. The fundi showed only modest arteriosclerotic changes. The temporal arteries were normal. Facial motility and sensation was normal. There was a significant right carotid bruit present which was persistent and which could be heard all along the course of the right carotid artery. It was not transmitted from the neck. There was moderate pain and tenderness at the insertion of the great muscles of the neck and the occiput, and palpation over this area consistently reproduced the patient's symptoms. She also had a persistent area of tenderness in the right trapezius muscle. Otherwise, power, size, and symmetry of the arms and legs were essentially normal. The deep tendon reflexes were brisk. There were no long tract or focal signs, and sensation was intact.

Impression: 1. Muscle contraction headaches, chronic. 2. Localized myositis, right side of neck, right shoulder girdle. 3. Right carotid bruit, silent, asymptomatic. ¶ Comment: The findings were discussed in detail with the patient but no neurological studies were done. I suggested simple measures of physical therapy to the neck including the use of heat, hot packs, and massage and advised also that she purchase a cervical pillow on which to rest during the day. Motrin, 400 mg twice daily and Maolate, 400 mg at night were suggested in an attempt to provide anti-inflammatory and muscle relaxant properties. It may also be necessary to inject these tender areas which are quite well localized. This can be determined after thirty to sixty days on the treatment regimen outlined above. ¶ The patient also has what seems to be a silent right carotid bruit. Certainly she is without symptoms. This should be brought to the attention of those who are caring for her, so that if transient ischemic attacks appear in the future, appropriate steps can be taken. I do not think that the right carotid bruit has anything to do with the patient's headaches, which are not vascular, and certainly there is no sign of cranial arteritis. ¶ She was referred back to you for continuing medical service. Thank you for the opportunity of seeing this patient. Sincerely,

See Appendix A for a possible transcript of this test.

AUTOPSY PROTOCOLS

When a patient dies while in the hospital, permission may be requested from the next of kin to perform an autopsy or postmortem examination of the body to determine the exact cause of death. The complete protocol should be made part of the record within 90 days from death. Through autopsies, much knowledge has been gained that assists in the diagnosis and treatment of disease. Visual and microscopic examinations are done on every organ and related structure. When an organ is removed from a cadaver for the purpose of donation, there should be an autopsy report that includes a description of the technique used to remove and prepare or preserve the donated organ. All states have laws that govern autopsies. When someone dies unattended or there is suspicion of a crime (e.g., violent death, unusual death, child abuse, self-induced or criminal abortion, homicide, suicide, poisoning, drowning, fire, hanging, stabbing, exposure, starvation, and so on), an autopsy may be ordered by the court, or it may become the responsibility of the coroner's office to determine the cause of death. The professionals associated with the coroner's office include the following: pathologist, forensic pathologist, forensic dentist, chemist, toxicologist, anesthesiologist, radiologist, odontologist, psychiatrist, and psychologist.

The written record of an autopsy is generally referred to as an *autopsy protocol.* In pathology, there are five forms: the narrative (in story form), the numerical (by the numbers), the pictorial (hand drawings or anatomic forms), protocols based on sentence completion and multiple-choice selection, and problem-oriented protocols (a supplement to the Problem-Oriented Medical Record System). A numerical format is an orderly description of all autopsy findings and tends to prevent omission of minor details that can be forgotten during narration. Numerical format is usually a longer protocol due to this fact and requires more time to complete.

Frequently, a hospital autopsy protocol (Fig. 13–10) will contain the clinical history, which is a brief resume of the patient's medical history and course in the hospital before death. It will include the pathologic diagnosis made at autopsy, a report of the final summary, and the gross anatomy findings (visual examination of the organs of the body before any tissues are removed for preparation and examination). There will also be a microscopic examination (an examination of the particular organs through the microscope). An epicrisis or final pathologic diagnosis is given at the end of the protocol. This is a critical analysis (actual finding) or discussion of the cause of disease after its termination.

In forensic pathology, an autopsy protocol may be organized under the following general guidelines:

1. External description
2. Evidence of injury
   a. External
   b. Internal
3. Systems and organs (cavities and organs)
4. Special dissections and examinations
5. Brain (and other organs) after fixation
6. Microscopic examination
7. Findings (diagnoses), factual and interpretative
8. Opinion or summary (conclusion), interpretative and opinion
9. Signature

Some autopsy protocol typing procedures are not necessarily seen in other types of medical dictation and transcription. Because autopsy records may be entered into a court of law to relate information about the cause of death, clarity is essential so that interpretation of the typed material is accurately understood. Because of this, more words tend to be spelled out and abbreviations are kept to a minimum. Many states require that military time be used when documenting the time a body is brought in for autopsy (e.g., 1400 hours). If a person was last seen before midnight, the pathologist dictates "found over the date of January 1, 199X." If the person was last seen after midnight, the pathologist stated "found over the hour of 9:00 a.m. or 0900." Note that ciphers are used in stating the nonmilitary time. Units of measurement may be spelled out, such as pounds, inches, and grams. Quote marks (") are never used to indicate inches but are used when indicating a marking on the body (e.g., tattoo device of the words "J. J. Tramp"). Temperature is typed ("88 degrees Fahrenheit"). Numbers may be typed as "2 fresh punctures" or "two (2) stab wounds."

Numbers may be typed numerically and then spelled out in parentheses when clarity is emphasized. Metric terms are given as abbreviations (e.g., 0.5 cm, 200 ml, 3 × 3 mm).

Forensic dentists work closely with forensic pathologists. They describe bite marks by size, shape, and location. They swab for saliva to determine blood type. They make impressions or molds of the mark and photograph and make impressions of the suspect's dentition. When two medical examiners are involved, both reference initials at the closing of the protocol must be shown (e.g., MB:DVW:mtf). Only general guidelines for typing protocols are stated here. Each county has different practices and must meet various legal requirements.

COLLEGE HOSPITAL
4567 BROAD AVENUE
WOODLAND HILLS, XY 12345-0001

AUTOPSY PROTOCOL

Silverman, Patricia M.

June 21, 199x

This is an autopsy on a prematurely born female infant weighing 2 lb 12 oz. The body measures 15.25 inches in length. The body has not been embalmed prior to this examination.

EXTERNAL EXAMINATION: The head, neck and chest are symmetrical. The abdomen is soft. The external genitalia are normal female. The extremities are symmetrical and show no evidence of developmental abnormality.

INTERNAL EXAMINATION:

ABDOMINAL CAVITY: The abdominal cavity is opened and the liver is enlarged extending 4.0 cm below the costal margin in the right midclavicular line. The spleen appears enlarged. The intestinal coils are freely dispersed and contain gaseous fluid. All other organs are in normal position.

PLEURAL CAVITIES: The pleural cavities are opened revealing the left lung to be collapsed and lying in the left pleural cavity. The right lung is partially expanded and the pleura is smooth and glistening in both pleural cavities.

MEDIASTINUM: The mediastinum contains a moderate amount of thymic tissue.

PERICARDIAL SAC: The pericardial sac is opened containing a few cubic centimeters of serous fluid. The heart is normal in position and appears to be average in size.

HEART: The heart weighs approximately 10 gm. Thorough search of the heart fails to show any evidence of congenital abnormality. The foramen ovale has a thin membrane over the surface. The ductus arteriosus is noted and patent. There is no septal ventricular defect. All valves are competent. There is no rotation of the heart. The pulmonary artery is noted and appears normal. A few subendocardial and subepicardial petechiae and ecchymoses are noted.

LUNGS: The lungs weigh together 33 gm. The left lung and the right lung sink in water, then slowly rise to the surface. The lungs are subcrepitant and atelectatic. This is particularly noted in the left lung. The bronchi contain a small amount of frothy mucus. The cut surfaces of the lungs are beefy and atelectatic. There are no cysts or tumors. The findings are consistent with hyaline membrane disease and pulmonary atelectasis.

LIVER: The liver weighs approximately 75 gm. The liver appears enlarged and is reddish-brown and soft. The cut surface is reddish-brown and soft. There is no gross evidence of bile duct blockage. The gallbladder, cystic duct and common bile duct are not remarkable. (continued)

13

Figure 13–10. Hospital autopsy protocol, report form, typed in indented format with no variations.

Illustration continued on following page

Patricia M. Silverman
Autopsy Protocol, Page 2
June 21, 199x

PANCREAS: The pancreas appears average in size weighing approximately 1.5 grams. The pancreas is yellowish-white and soft on the cut surface. There is no gross evidence of cystic disease.

SPLEEN: The spleen weighs approximately 4 gm and is bluish-purple. The spleen on cut surface is reddish-brown and soft.

ADRENAL GLANDS: The adrenal glands weigh together approximately 4.5 gm. The adrenal glands are soft and tan and the cortical portion is distinct from the medullary portion. There is no gross evidence of hemorrhage, cysts or tumors. Both adrenals are similar.

KIDNEYS: The kidneys weigh together approximately 13 gm. The capsule strips with ease leaving a faint fetal lobulation and a reddish-brown soft surface. The cut surface shows the cortex and medulla, both of which are distinct and in average proportions. The parenchyma is reddish-brown, moist and soft. Both kidneys are similar in appearance and consistency. The ureters are not remarkable.

URINARY BLADDER, UTERUS, TUBES AND OVARIES: These organs are grossly not remarkable.

GASTROINTESTINAL TRACT: The esophagus is examined as well as the stomach. There is no evidence of reduplication, ulcer or tumor. The small and large bowel are not remarkable.

BRAIN: The brain weighs approximately 230 gm. The brain is slightly edematous. A few petechiae are observed. On sectioning the brain anterior to posterior, the brain tissue is soft and somewhat edematous. The fluid in the ventricles is clear and watery. The cerebellum and cerebrum are symmetrical and grossly not remarkable. There is no gross evidence of hemorrhage or tumor.

SKELETAL SYSTEM Not remarkable.

GROSS ANATOMICAL DIAGNOSIS:
1) Prematurity, 2 lb 12 oz.
2) Pulmonary atelectasis.
3) Hyaline membrane disease.

Chief Pathologist__________________________
Stephen M. Choi, MD

mtf
D: 6-20-9x
T: 6-21-9x

Figure 13–10 *Continued*

13

13-6: REVIEW TEST

Directions: Retype the following material into a hospital autopsy protocol using the full-block format with variation number one. The patient's name and other statistical data may be set up as you desire. Use a current date and correct punctuation. The dictator is Dr. Susan R. Foster, chief pathologist. See page 270 for full-block format. Note that the main topic and subtopics vary from those shown in Figure 13–10.

I performed an autopsy on the body of Phyllis B. Dexter, Patient No. 65-43-90, at the College Hospital. ¶ Clinical Diagnosis: Congenital heart defect.

General Examination: The body is that of a well developed and well nourished newborn female infant, having been embalmed prior to examination through a thoracic incision and cannulization of the heart. The recorded birth weight is 7 lb 2 oz. ¶ Thorax opened: Considerable blood is present around the heart incident to the embalming procedure, and two incisions in the cardiac muscle are evident but the valves and great vessels do not appear to have been injured by the embalming procedure. Examination discloses a massive heart lying transversely in the midanterior thorax, the distended right ventricle exceeding in volume the ventricular mass. Examination discloses no enlargement of the ductus arteriosus or any significant deviation of the size of the great vessels. On exploration of the heart there is found to be a completely imperforate pulmonary artery at the level of the pulmonary valve, all three cusps of which appear to be adequately formed but fused by scar tissue slightly proximal to the free margins of the cusps. It is impossible to probe the existence of any opening in this area. The right heart is markedly hypertrophic, approximating three times the muscle mass of the normal infant heart. There is no evidence of an interventricular defect. There is a sacculation adjacent to the valve of the inferior vena cava as it enters the inferior right auricle and in the dome of this sacculated area the foramen ovale is demonstrated. The foramen is unusually small in diameter (estimated to be no more than 4 mm in diameter) and this is covered by a plica. It would appear that the pressure of the distended right auricle would further compromise the capacity of the foramen to transmit blood. In the absence of any interventricular defect, this would be the only way that blood could get from the right to the left side of the heart. The lungs are heavy and poorly serrated and the bronchial tree contains some yellowish fluid which, in the absence of feeding by mouth, must be assumed to be aspirated vernix. ¶ Abdomen Opened: The stomach contains some bloody mucus but no evidence of formula. The liver and abdominal viscera appear entirely negative throughout. ¶ Head: Not opened. ¶ Cause of Death on Gross Findings: Massive chylous pericardial effusion, etiology not established but presumptively related to defect in formation of thoracic duct tissue. ¶ Microscopic: Sections of the thymus gland revealed a generally normal histological architecture for the thymus of the newborn, epithelial elements still being distributed through the lymphoid tissues. Certainly no tumor is present in the thymic tissue. The pulmonary tissues are poorly expanded although the bronchi appear open. There is a general vascular congestion of pulmonary tissue and some apparent extravasation of blood into the poorly expanded alveoli. In addition, there are deposits of hyaline material on the surfaces of some of the air spaces that would indicate the existence of hyaline membrane disease. The liver shows marked congestion and a rather active hematopoiesis. The heart muscle is not remarkable and the epicardial surface does not appear thickened or unusual. The kidney tissue exhibits some punctate hemorrhages in the parenchyma consistent with anoxia. ¶ Microscopic Diagnosis: Renal hemorrhages incident to anoxia.

MEDICOLEGAL REPORTS

Medicolegal reports originate from medical offices and hospitals. When they originate from the latter, they usually come from the medical records department, in which personnel make copies or abstracts of record entries rather than transcribing them (Fig. 13–11). The prudent physician responds to a request for medical information with a prompt and complete report and, in doing so, assists his or her patient in supporting claims for damages (probably including the physician's bill), facilitates the attorney's representation of a client, and can often spare himself or herself a trip to court. Usually, a report of this type involves an accident case or workers' compensation case. The report is a legal document and is admissible as evidence in a court of law. Sometimes, the attorney will abstract data from the report and incorporate the information into a formal document presented to the physician for signature and subsequent notarization. Accuracy is essential.

The properly prepared medicolegal report follows a familiar format and is typed on the physician's letterhead stationery.

Patient Identification. The patient must be identified in the first paragraph. Include the patient's name; age, date of birth, or both; and address. If the patient is a child, he or she should be identified as the son or daughter of his or her parents, whose names should also be included.

Date of Accident or Work-Related Injury. The date of the accident or injury must be noted, including the time of day, if known. (The physician should check the date of the accident given by the patient's attorney against that in the medical record. If they fail to agree, telephone the patient to clarify the discrepancy.)

CLARENCE F. STONES, MD
3700 OCEAN DRIVE
OXNARD, CALIFORNIA 93030

October 20, 199x

Aetna Casualty and Surety Company
3200 Roosevelt Boulevard
Oxnard, CA 93030

Dear Madam or Sir:

Re: Injured - Howard P. Winston
Date of Injury - July 27, 199x
Employer - College Chemistry Company
Case No. - 450-33-0821

EXAMINATION AND REPORT

HISTORY: This 43-year-old white male was working with a chemical pump. It slipped and fell forward. He over-corrected and fell. The pump fell on the patient, striking him in the occiput area. The approximate weight of the pump was 325 lb and was rolled off by a friend. He was knocked unconscious. He attended a meeting the following day in San Mateo. The pain occurred a day later in San Mateo. Three days later the pain was intense in the right shoulder and elbow. He went to Dr. John Garrett for physiotherapy. The left side then began to give him trouble also. He had a pressure type of pain in the left elbow which was relieved by codeine. He entered the College Hospital in Oxnard under Dr. Garrett's service. The right leg, and later the right thigh, began getting numb. A myelogram was followed by fusion at C 5-6 and C 6-7. He wore a brace for six months. He still has right shoulder pain, neck pain with radiation into the right thumb and right mastoid. In June, 199x, he was admitted to the Community Hospital in Ventura, California. The left eye began drooping and there was no pupil dilatation. He was improved one week later. A myelogram and brain scan were performed. There was pain on the left side, with pain into the rectum with spasms. He states that he fell several times. The surgery was postponed because of the eyes and the sudden loss of equilibrium.

FAMILY HISTORY: The father died of burns in a fire in 1940. The mother died of kidney disease at age 82. He has two brothers and one sister, living and well. He is widowed. His wife had cancer of the uterus. He has four children, alive and well. There is no history of diabetes and no accidents.

ALLERGIES: Penicillin and tetanus.

PHYSICAL EXAMINATION: Blood pressure 122/78; pulse 84 and regular.

GENERAL: The patient is cooperative and oriented to time and place.

HEENT: Head: Normal size and shape; no facial asymmetry. He shows no evidence of elevated intra-cranial pressure. Extraocular muscles intact. Pupils are equal and react briskly to light. At first one gets the impression that there might be a Horner's syndrome on the left side because of inconstant ptosis of the right eyelid, but this is not truly present. (continued)

13

Figure 13–11. Medicolegal report, report form, typed in indented format with no underlining and mixed punctuation.

Illustration continued on following page

Howard P. Winston
Page 2
October 20, 199x

NEUROLOGICAL EXAM: The patient walks with sparing of the left leg. There is no true paralysis present.

REFLEXES: The right biceps and triceps are slightly reduced on the left side, but present.

SENSORY: There is evidence of patchy hyperesthesia in the right upper extremity but following no particular dermatomal pattern.

CEREBELLAR FUNCTION: Intact. Lower cranial nerves within normal limits. There were no pathological reflexes elicited.

The remaining exam was deferred.

OPINION AND COMMENT: The patient continues to have slight dysfunction principally in the left lower extremity and right upper extremity. It would seem to me that the pupillary abnormality, which he experienced in June of 199x, merits some investigation including arteriography. For his cervical disk problems, I would think that conservative treatment is warranted.

Very truly yours,

Clarence F. Stones, MD

13

mtf

Figure 13–11 *Continued*

History. The history of the accident, injury, or work-related illness is described. Use the patient's own words, including quotes whenever possible. Be as detailed and complete as possible, listing all the facts.

Present Complaints. The patient's present complaints at the time of the first visit are recorded. (Sometimes these are referred to as subjective complaints.)

Past History. The past history should be described, along with any pre-existing defects or injuries that might affect the present accident.

Physical Findings. The physical findings on examination are recorded in detail. (These are sometimes referred to as objective findings.)

Laboratory or X-ray Findings. Laboratory or x-ray findings should be included in the report. In some instances, photocopies of x-ray, electrocardiograph, or operative reports should be made available. Consultation notes should also be photocopied and submitted with the medicolegal report.

Diagnosis. The diagnosis (or diagnoses in the case of multiple injuries) should be detailed.

Prescribed Therapy. The prescribed therapy must be described in detail. Each visit to the office should be listed, including any physical therapy treatments or medications prescribed.

Patient's Disability. The patient's disability should be outlined, describing work restrictions and including the dates of total or partial disability. The date the patient will be permitted to return to work is given.

Prognosis. The prognosis is of paramount importance to the attorney and thus to the patient. The settlement may depend on the physician's estimate of continued pain and whether there will be future permanent disability.

Physician's Statement. The physician's statement of fees for services rendered is an integral part of the report to an attorney. The statement should be itemized by date and service, making sure the statement correlates in detail with the dates of treatment mentioned in the report. The preparation of a report for an attorney is time consuming, and the physician is entitled to charge a fee. Documents requiring extensive research of hospital records and consultants' reports merit higher fees.

Although many cases are settled out of court, the few that go to trial justify painstaking care in preparation of the medical report. Remember that the value of a detailed document cannot be overemphasized when the physician is asked to testify in a trial three or four years after an injury.

13–7: REVIEW TEST

Directions: Retype the following data into an industrial accident report form and prepare an envelope. Use letterhead stationery. Use full-block format with no underlining, mixed punctuation, and the current date. Watch for proper paragraphing, placement, punctuation, and mechanics.

The letter concerns the patient George R. Champion and was dictated by Dr. James C. Taylor of 4320 Main Street, Ventura, California 93003. It is to be sent to an attorney, Ralph J. Claborne of 165 Cedar Street, Ventura, California 93003. Use a current date.

Dear Mr. Claborne. My patient Mr. George R. Champion was seen on September 14, 199X. History of injury: Mr. Champion was hit on the back of the head by a lettuce crate in April of 199X. He saw stars but was not knocked unconscious. Present complaints: The patient says he can see for an instant then the left eye blurs and also itches. He has had this problem since his accident in April, 199X. When he is working and turns to the left he cannot see things out of that side since they are fuzzy. He can look at an object to the left and five seconds later it is gone. Physical examination: Visual acuity uncorrected: right eye, 20/80; left eye, 20/40. Manifest refraction: right eye, +1.75D = 20/30 Jaeger 1; left eye, +2.50 = 20/30 Jaeger 1–. Visual field: full centrally. Motility: Near point of convergence = 8 cm; Near point of accommodation = 3.5D. Prism cover test: Distance = no shift; Near = 8 prism diopters exophoria. Cycloplegic refraction: right eye = +2.50 + 0.50 x 30 = 20/25 – 2; left eye = +3.25 + 0.75 x 125 = 20/20 – 1. Slit-lamp examination revealed abnormal cornea, conjunctiva, iris and lens. Ocular tension was 11 mm Hg both eyes by applanation. Retinal examination revealed a normal optic disc, macula, vessels and periphery with direct and indirect ophthalmoscopy. Diagnosis: Compound hyperopic astigmatism with early presbyopia. Comments: I feel that this patient's focusing reserve was suddenly decreased by his accident when he was hit on the head. His basic problem of farsightedness coupled with a general weakness after the accident overcame his focusing reserve and caused his symptoms. I feel that glasses of the proper strength will enable him to see and focus. His problem of poor convergence and exophoria at near were also brought into prominence by the weakness he had after the accident. His age (38) means that he would have had symptoms within the next five or seven years due to his farsightedness. Recommended treatment: Glasses to be worn all the time. Eye exercises for convergence problem if the glasses do not relieve his symptoms. Disability: The condition is now stationary and permanent; and with the proper glasses, he should be able to resume his normal work load. Very truly yours.

PSYCHIATRIC REPORTS

Psychiatry is one of the specialties of clinical medicine. It is a diverse field, and the language involves abnormal psychology, human behavior, and treatment terminology. Patients are referred to as clients. In a hospital setting, clients include the mentally deficient (MD) and developmentally disabled (DD), formerly referred to as mentally retarded.

For the mentally deficient client, an admission note might include a presentation of the problem stating the vital signs, current medications, allergies, medication taken in the past four hours, present illness, psychologic history, mental status examination, physical status examination, and a provisional diagnosis. Additional reports on the mentally disabled client might include a psychiatric evaluation, psychologic evaluation, social history evaluation, rehabilitation therapy evaluation, discharge summary, and treatment planning conference. The conference is a program to establish the goals of treatment and track the progress the client is making while under the treatment, with the ultimate goal of being placed back into society as a fully functional person.

The reports for a developmentally disabled client might include a medical history, review of systems, release summary, and clinical record documentation system, which is equivalent to a treatment planning conference for a mentally deficient client. The reports are more detailed because these clients can be so low functioning that even the most basic self-care skills cannot be performed on admission. The facility staff attempts to teach these skills, with attainment of the highest potential of each client as a goal.

A report dictated by a clinical psychologist would not necessarily contain a physical examination of the body systems or a list of the medications but might describe motor skill problems. The main heading might be Psychologic Evaluation, and subheadings might be given as follows: Purpose of the Report, Psychosocial History, Results of the Psychologic Assessment, Mental Status Examination, Test Results, Impressions, Diagnosis, and Recommendations.

Because so many clients have legal problems (divorce, marriage, adoption procedures, negligence, physical abuse, disability, and so on), legal terminology is widely used. Some clients may be seen for chemical abuse, and drugs could be referred to by slang or street terms; often, these terms are unknown by the novice transcriptionist. These terms change from day to day, and the list is constantly enlarging. Most transcriptionists prepare lists of these slang terms for reference to assist in typing up the reports. Many of the words encountered in psychiatric reports do not appear in the standard English dictionary or medical dictionary, so the use of special reference books will assist you. The *Diagnostic and Statistical Manual of Mental Disorders, Fourth Edition, Revised* (DSM-IV) is used for psychiatric diagnoses for the mentally disabled. This is an excellent reference book for the transcriptionist since all mental diagnoses are given with their code numbers. However, for developmentally disabled clients, the *International Classification of Diseases, 9th Edition, Clinical Modification* (ICD-9-CM) is used followed by the etiology. If the psychiatrist wishes, the DSM-V is also used for the diagnosis. Refer to the last paragraph in Figure 13–12 to see how the diagnoses and code numbers might be typed.

Reports that contain information about a per-

State of California—Health and Welfare Agency | Department of Mental Health

GUIDELINES	Date of Report: 11-9-9x Date Dictated: 11-14-9x Date Typed: 11-15-9x PSYCHIATRIC EVALUATION Unit 99

A. PSYCHIATRIC HISTORY
1. Identification data
2. Source of information
3. Chief complaint
4. History of present illness (focus on recent illness, and include emotional behavior)
5. History of past psychiatric episodes
6. Relevant medical/surgical/trauma/medication history
7. Developmental history (if applicable)
8. Educational/Vocational
9. Relevant family history
10. Relevant social history

B. MENTAL STATUS EXAM
11. Attitude/Cooperation
12. General appearance (include speech)
13. Motor activity
14. Orientation
15. Mood and affect
16. Mental content
17. Memory
18. Fund of general knowledge
19. Cognition and comprehension
20. Abstraction ability
21. Counting and calculating
22. Judgement
23. Insight regarding illness
24. Patient strengths
25. Suicide, homicide, dangerousness

C. SUMMARY OF PSYCHIATRIC ASSESSMENT
26. Narrative summary (including Risk Potential)
27. Diagnosis (DSM III R)
28. Preliminary Treatment Plan
29. Prognosis
30. Signature and Title

PSYCHIATRIC HISTORY:

1. This 17-year-old, single, Hispanic male patient was admitted to XYZ Hospital on 11-8-9x on a temporary conservatorship 5353 from XYZ County. His birth date is 9-24-xx. There is no religious preference. His mother is Mary Sanchez. Her address is 300 East Date Street, Woodland Hills, XY 12345, (013) 999-9999.
2. Information obtained by interviewing the patient and reviewing the accompanying papers from XYZ Medical Center. The patient speaks only Spanish. The interview had to be done through an interpreter. His information is not very reliable.
3. "I don't know why they sent me here."
4. Pedro was admitted to XYZ Medical Center on August 26, 199x because of bizarre behavior for five days. According to the report five days prior to admission, he smoked marijuana dipped in PCP. He also smoked cocaine. He demonstrated bizarre behavior such as running nude in the streets, sticking his fingers into light sockets and receiving electric shocks, crawling under a car and trying to set it on fire. He was not sleeping. He laughed and cried inappropriately. He broke a restraint in the hospital. The drug screening test on August 26, 199x showed a positive cocaine and negative for PCP and other drugs. Peabody test in Spanish revealed his IQ was about 76. Beery developmental test of visual motor integration did not suggest organicity. He was treated with Haldol and discharged to his mother on 9-22-9x; however, he was readmitted to XYZ Medical Center on 9-24-9x on a 5150. His mother stated that after discharge from the hospital he was fearful and childish. He presented bizarre behavior such as collecting household articles, painting the walls, attempting to play with medicine bottles, refusing to eat or sleep, walking around the house nude, collecting piles of objects in his room, attempting suicide by jumping off an apartment building. He laughed and cried inappropriately. His mother stated that he did not take street drugs and he took only Haldol and Cogentin. However, on one occasion he went to the store without supervision. At the XYZ Medical Center he was confused, disorganized and disoriented. It was difficult for him to attend to a conversation or to concentrate. He was not able to function in school. He needs close supervision and care. He had been in physical restraints many times because of assaultive behavior. He also banged the walls and screamed. He was treated with Haldol 10 mg t.i.d. A long-term hospitalization was

SANCHEZ, Pedro J. 999999-9 U. 99

☐ Continued

EVALUATION REPORT
PSYCHIATRIC
Confidential Client/Patient Information
See W & I Code Section 5328

MH 5702 (Revised 7/87)
CRDM Reference 2410

Figure 13–12. Pages 1 and 4 of a psychiatric evaluation on a developmentally disabled client, typed in full-block format with no variations. At the end of the report, note the typing of the diagnoses and the code numbers. GAF means Global Assessment of Functioning Scale.

Illustration continued on following page

13

State of California—Health and Welfare Agency | Department of Mental Health

Date of Report: 11-9-9x
Date Dictated: 11-14-9x
Date Typed: 11-15-9x

Unit 99—PSYCHIATRIC EVALUATION

SUMMARY OF PSYCHIATRIC ASSESSMENT: (Continued)

26. Pedro's father deserted the family when Pedro was 11 years old. Around that time he stopped going to school after finishing sixth grade. The reason for that was not clear, but it is well known that people with mild mental retardation cannot go further than the sixth grade. He lived with his grandmother after his mother left Honduras four years ago. About eight months ago, he came to the United States to live with his mother because his grandmother was unable to handle him. He had been using cocaine and PCP for six or seven months. It was felt that his first hospitalization at XYZ Medical Center was due to PCP, Organic Mental Disorder. At this time, he appears retarded with residual symptoms of psychosis such as flat and inappropriate affect, loose associations, poverty of thoughts, no intention to go to school and he needs constant supervision for daily living activities.

27.

Axis I:	298.9	Psychotic Disorder, NOS. (Rule out 292.90 PCP, Organic Mental Disorder)
	305.90	Psychoactive Substance Abuse, NOS.
Axis II:	V71.09	No diagnosis. (Rule out Mental Retardation)
Axis III:		No somatic disorder.
Axis IV:		Discord with classmates.
Axis V:		GAF on admission 25; highest GAF last year unknown.

28. Structured environment, special educational program, unit milieu, individual therapy, group therapy, and chemotherapy.
29. Guarded.
30.

______________________________, MD
Dan W. Stewart, MD

mtf

Page 4 SANCHEZ, Pedro J. 999999-9 U. 99 ☐ Continued Page ________

CONTINUATION PAGE

☒ Assessment (Specify: Psychiatric)
☐ Team Conference (Specify: ________)
☐ Consultation (Specify: ________)
☐ Other (Specify ________)

Confidential Client/Patient Information
See W & I Code Section 5378

MH 5705

Figure 13–12 *Continued*

13

son's mental stability are very confidential. In fact, sometimes the information contained in the report is not divulged to the client. To obtain medical information, the signatures of the physician and the client are required on a special release of information form. If the client is developmentally disabled, the signatures of the physician and the guardian are needed. If authorized in writing by the client or his or her legally qualified representative and the psychiatrist in charge of the case, a copy of the report is sent to the referring medical practitioner or medical facility responsible for follow-up care of the patient. Psychiatric information can be sent to a placement facility if a client is to live in the community in a residential facility. This gives the receiving facility information regarding treatment and medication. At times, the court system may subpoena the medical records.

13-8: OPTIONAL TEST

Directions: Retype the following data into a psychiatric report form. Use letterhead stationery. Use full-block format with variation number one, mixed punctuation, and the current date. Watch for proper paragraphing, punctuation, placement, and mechanics.

The letter concerns the patient Tu Anh Dao and was dictated by Dr. Stephen B. Salazar of 5028 South Broadway, Woodland Hills, CA 90217. It is to be sent to Department of Social Services Disability Evaluation Unit, 15 Kenneth Street, Woodland Hills, CA 90217.

Head this report Psychiatric Social Survey. Presenting Problem: This 29 year old Vietnamese male was seen today at the request of the Department of Social Services Disability Evaluation Unit. Questions regarding mental status appearance simple repetitive tasks interests and daily activities and ability to relate and interact with public and co-workers were raised. The interview was conducted in the living room of the home in which he lives and has lived for the last three or four years. The claimant resides in this home with his mother and his 11 year old younger sister. His mother and an interpreter were present in the room during the interview. The interview lasted one hour. The claimant was very quiet and at some points hardly audible. He declined to answer questions quite often during the interview. Several times during the interview the mother interrupted and gave answers to him. He seemed to show some pressure of speech and memory difficulties during the interview. History: The history revealed that Mr. Dao was born in Hanoi Vietnam where he went to school up to the eighth grade. At the eighth grade he dropped out and began to farm doing rice farming. At age 26 he moved to Santa Monica. After arriving in Santa Monica he worked in a restaurant which he cannot name as a dishwasher for two or three months but he quit because the job in the first place was part time and temporary. He then worked for two years as a gardener and quit this job because of health problems he was always feeling sick. He also worked for one or two months as a carpenter but he quit because he did not have the money to buy the tools. In 1990 he was admitted to College Hospital where he had surgery and was in the hospital for one or two months during the winter of the year. He claims that the surgery was neurological although it could have been rather than on the brain an inner ear surgery due to vertigo and tinnitus problems. There is no history of any other hospitalizations. The claimant is the oldest son of five children he has two sisters and two brothers they are all living in the United States. Environment: The claimant has lived in his present house for one and a half years with his mother and his 10 year old sister. He states that he wakes at 8 or 9 am. He walks around in the yard for awhile and then he eats breakfast he does not eat lunch but does eat dinner. He said that during this time his appetite is good and he eats because he is hungry. Once a week he leaves the house to see a doctor who checks for the surgery and his neurological problems. He states that he had a ringing in the left ear which was partially a result of the surgery. He has not done any kind of work since the head surgery and he has not done anything around the house. He reports difficulty with memory. He rarely does anything with friends except when they come over to visit him and only leaves the house to walk around the yard or go to the doctor appointments. He is able to dress himself and bathe himself but does not do any chores of any kind around the house. He states that his mother cooks for him and he has never cooked for himself and he does not do anything around the yard either. His grooming showed him to be wearing a shirt slacks with no shoes or socks and he was clean shaven his hair styled and neatly brushed. He reports going to bed around 1 or 2 am. Most of his day is spent listening to the radio and watching television. While showing that he could ambulate he had significant difficulty walking on his toes; he was unable to do this but he was able to walk on his heels and his gait appeared to be normal. There was no significant psychomotor retardation noted. Mental status: The mental status reveals a 29 year old Vietnamese male who appears to be of average height and weight. He denied any paranoid ideations or auditory or visual hallucinations. He was oriented to time place and date and he was able to do 1 to 20 forward and backwards without any difficulty. He refused to do serial 7's although he was able to subtract 7 from 10 correctly. He showed difficulty with memory although he could remember that he had lived in the house that he lives in now for the last year and a half. He denied any headaches or visual difficulties or aura that might indicate seizure activity. He did have an affect of sadness and depression. When asked what he would change about himself he stated that he would change his bad health to good health. He has no goals at the present time. He is on no medication at the present time and he does not have a history of drug or alcohol use or abuse. He denied sleep or appetite problems or crying. There does appear to be some anhedonia. Medications: The claimant is taking no medications at the present time. Provisional Diagnosis: Axis I. Transient situational depression due to surgery mild to moderate. Axis II. Rule out organic brain syndrome. Observations and recommendations: Because there were no medical reports sent with this individual it would be recommended that there be a review to see if there actually was a surgery at College Hospital and what was the purpose of the surgery and what an update may be on his neurological function. In fact I would recommend a neurological evaluation to see if the depression emanates from the surgery itself or from some emotional disturbance. There is no indication that Mr. Dao could handle his own funds and it is recommended that a payee be appointed if he is approved for disability. Thank you for the consultation. Very truly yours

TRANSCRIPTION EXERCISE

For transcribing complex medical correspondence, documents 58 through 60 are on *Sound Tapes to Accompany Medical Keyboarding, Typing, and Transcribing Techniques and Procedures*, Cassette 3, Side F.

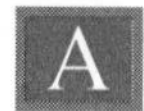

Answer to **13–1: SELF-STUDY**

Bacon, Marcia M.
52-01-96
Room No. 248-C

DISCHARGE SUMMARY

ADMISSION DATE: May 7, 199X DISCHARGE DATE: May 9, 199X

ADMISSION DIAGNOSIS:
Torn medial meniscus, left knee.

HISTORY OF PRESENT ILLNESS:
The patient injured her left knee on April 11, 199X, while playing tennis. She subsequently had difficulty with persistent effusion and pain in the left knee. An arthrogram prior to admission revealed a tear of the medial meniscus.

PHYSICAL EXAMINATION:
Absence of tenderness to palpation of any of the joint structures. There was approximately 30-55 cc of fluid within the joint. Range of motion was full.

LABORATORY DATA:
Admission hemoglobin was 15.9, hematocrit 47% with a white count of 7400 with normal differential. Urinalysis was within normal limits. Chem panel 19 showed an elevated cholesterol of 379 mg%. Chest x-ray was reported as negative.

TREATMENT AND HOSPITAL COURSE:
The patient was taken to the operating room on the same day as admission, at which time she underwent arthroscopy. This revealed that she had a tear of the medial meniscus. Arthrotomy was performed, with medial meniscectomy. A chondral fracture was noted in the medial femoral condyle, measuring approximately 5 mm in greatest diameter. The edges of this were sheathed. Postoperatively, the patient's course was benign. There was no significant temperature elevation. She became ambulatory with crutches on the first postoperative day with no difficulty with straight leg raising.

13

DISPOSITION:
The patient is being discharged home, ambulatory, with crutches, and an exercise program. She is to be seen in the office in one week for suture removal.

CONDITION AT THE TIME OF DISCHARGE:
Improved.

COMPLICATIONS:
None.

MEDICATIONS:
None.

DISCHARGE DIAGNOSIS:
Torn medial meniscus, left knee; chondromalacia of the medial femoral condyle.

Surgeon ___________________________

Henry R. Knowles, MD

(student's initials)
D: 5-10-*year*
T: 5-11-*year*

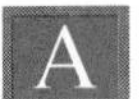

Answer to **13–4: SELF-STUDY**

This assignment is to be set up using modified block format and no variations.

RADIOLOGY REPORT

Examination Date:	June 8, 199X	Patient:	Donna Mae Weeser
Date Reported:	June 8, 199X	X-ray No.:	16-A2
Physician:	George B. Bancroft, MD	Age:	46
Examination:	Mammography, right and left breasts	Hospital No.:	52-80-44

MAMMOGRAPHY, RIGHT AND LEFT BREASTS: There are retromammary prosthetic devices in position. The anterior parenchyma is somewhat compressed. There is no evidence of neoplastic calcification or skin thickening demonstrated. No dominant masses are noted within the anteriorly displaced parenchyma. No increased vascularity is evident.

IMPRESSION: Mammography, right and left breasts, shows the presence of retromammary prosthetic devices in position. The demonstrated tissue appears within normal limits.

Radiologist ______________________________
Clayton M. Markham, MD

(student's initials)
D: 6-8-year
T: *(current date)*

13

Correspondence and Business Documents

CHAPTER

14

Composing Business Letters and Making Travel Arrangements

14

OBJECTIVES

After reading this chapter and working the exercises, you should be able to

1. Discuss the importance of the ability to compose a good business letter.
2. Identify the various types of letters that a secretary in a private office should be able to write.
3. Compose a letter for your employer's signature.
4. Compose letters for your signature under a variety of circumstances.
5. Recognize and use the rules for writing effective business letters.
6. Test the various aids available to writers of business letters.
7. Make travel arrangements, including hotel accommodations, transportation, and itineraries.

INTRODUCTION

This chapter is for the medical office assistant who wants to perform some executive secretarial tasks for an employer. Many assistants are unable, unskilled, or reluctant to perform duties other than those that they are specifically directed to undertake. This chapter is not for the reluctant. It *is* for you if you are willing to shoulder some extra responsibility.

In the business world, an executive secretary can share much of an employer's work load; in contrast, the medical secretary may find the scope somewhat limited. After all, one cannot help practice medicine. But you *can* relieve your physician-employer of many nonmedical business chores.

The area of responsibility that you can assume in a private physician's office is that of handling the office correspondence. As an office secretary, you probably will be responsible for opening, marking, and routing the mail that arrives in the office. Under your employer's direction, some of this mail can be returned to you for reply, either over the physician's signature or over yours. The mail that you will handle over your own signature may be collection letters to patients about overdue accounts, orders for supplies and instruments, the making or confirmation of appointments or hospital admissions, requests for information, inquiries to insurance companies, and the making of travel arrangements for your employer.

The type of mail that you might compose for your employer's signature can range from letters requiring very limited responsibility, such as acknowledgment of professional announcements, to those of great responsibility, such as replying to an insurance company's request for patient data, writing certificates of return to work, making reports about treatment to compensation carriers, and transmitting medical or laboratory results to a patient or another physician. There is no limit concerning the types of letters that you may be asked to write, provided that you can demonstrate the skill to do the work competently. As you can readily see, you will enhance your value to a prospective employer if you have a good command of English and the ability to express yourself well on paper.

14

THE ART OF LETTER WRITING

Entire texts are written about the art of letter writing, and business students spend semesters or years devoted to acquiring this skill. Assuming you already have some skill in letter writing, this chapter will try to redirect and enhance your skills. If you find that you are not an effective correspondent, you might consider a special course in business writing. Many community colleges offer this course in the evening because of the special needs of employed persons.

WRITING BETTER SENTENCES

Good business writing depends on clarity. If the basic element used to convey meaning—the sentence—is unclear, the entire message may be difficult to understand. Good sentence structure requires the application of all the rules of English grammar and the avoidance of certain particularly common errors.

Let us examine some of the common problem areas.

Sentence Fragments

A sentence is a group of words that expresses a complete thought and must contain a subject (usually a noun) and predicate (usually a verb). Any combination of words that does not fulfill these conditions is not a sentence and should be avoided in good business English.

EXAMPLES

Accommodations are required for Dr. Varney so please advise me about.

I want to bring to your attention.

Run-On Sentences

When two sentences are run together without any connecting word (e.g., *although, therefore,* or *and*) or punctuation (a semicolon, dash, or colon) to divide them, they may be difficult to understand.

EXAMPLE

Dr. Broughton is out of town, therefore I am replying to your letter.

Each phrase could stand alone as a separate sentence. Therefore, the phrases should be separated by a word or by some form of punctuation stronger than a comma. The example could be corrected in any of the following ways:

Dr. Broughton is out of town; therefore, I am replying to your letter.

Dr. Broughton is out of town. Therefore, I am replying to your letter.

Because Dr. Broughton is out of town, I am replying to your letter.

Parallel Structure

Always express coordinate elements within a sentence or within a list in similar grammatical forms. Match nouns with nouns, infinitives with infinitives, verbs with verbs, adjectives with adjectives, and so on.

EXAMPLE

Learning to write is a challenge and interesting.

Here, writing is described with an adjective *(interesting)* and a noun *(challenge).* It would be better to use two adjectives and change the sentence to read as follows:

Learning to write is challenging and interesting.

Examine the lack of coordinate elements in the following example:

EXAMPLE

The purpose of this study:

To enhance communication between members of the team.

So that we can provide a retrospective study of care.

To be able to strengthen the transcriptionist's role.

IMPROVED

The following are examples of the purpose of this study:

To enhance communication between members of the team.

To provide a retrospective study of care.

To strengthen the transcriptionist's role.

Dangling Construction

The most awkward and sometimes embarrassing errors in writing often result from poor sentence construction. Sometimes, certain kinds of phrases and clauses, usually occurring at the beginning of a sentence, do not agree logically with the subject. These constructions are referred to as "dangling."

To correct a dangling construction, make the subject of the sentence the doer of the action expressed in the troublesome phrase or clause. If that is not at all feasible, rework your sentence completely to make it logical. Examine these "danglers" and a possible restructure of the sentence.

EXAMPLE

She has protruding eyes which have been present all her life.

IMPROVED

All her life she has had protruding eyes.

EXAMPLE

Having met his wife's aunt, a family dinner was planned.

IMPROVED

A family dinner was planned to celebrate meeting his wife's aunt.

EXAMPLE

Upon leaving the building, the door caught my coat.

IMPROVED

The door caught my coat as I left the building.

Unnecessary or Repetitious Words

Eliminate unnecessary phrases and useless words from your sentences.

Wordy	*Concise*
I have taken the liberty of writing at the present time	I am writing now
In view of the fact that	Since
Additional reports will be issued from time to time in the future	Additional reports will be issued periodically
It is the hope of the undersigned	I hope

Notice the unnecessary phrases and useless words italicized in the following examples:

1. Give this your prompt *and speedy* attention
2. Your letter arrived *in this office*
3. We will have an opening *coming up*
4. The device was circular *in shape*
5. We will convert *over* to
6. My *personal* opinion
7. My *actual* experience

Substitute the words in the second list below for those in the first list:

Avoid	*Use*
converse	talk
fully cognizant of	know
the writer	I
relative to	about
in regard to	about
in connection with	about
will you be so kind as to	please
are in need of	need
in the amount of	for
in the event that	if
under date of	on
in the near future	soon
a substantial segment	many
interrogate	question
due to the circumstance	because

14

14–1: SELF-STUDY

Directions: Restructure the following sentences to avoid run-on structure. Type your answers on a separate piece of paper.

1. Please retype this, it is your responsibility.
2. Remodeling is taking place in the Emergency Room, therefore reroute all patient traffic to Ward B until further notice.
3. The new chief-of-staff will take over the first of next month, furthermore there will be many new physicians added to the active staff roster.

Rewrite the following to maintain parallel structure:

4. To be accurate and meet your production level is important here.
5. Pull the patient's record, notifying the doctor of the emergency, then give the record to the doctor and be sure to relate any information you have received.
6. Please observe the following:
   a. Enter your department number on each requisition.
   b. Use the preprinted requisitions.
   c. If the preprinted requisition is not available for the products you require, refer to the Inventory Stock Catalogue and enter the appropriate stock number.
7. Duties of the custodian of records:
   a. to keep accurate records
   b. correcting must be made in the proper way
   c. be sure the records are signed or initialed
   d. don't let unauthorized persons see the records without a release
8. Rules for taking telephone calls:
   a. If the person is talking, don't interrupt him/her
   b. Remember to pick up the telephone as soon as it rings
   c. Ask the name of the person calling
   d. In transferring calls, be sure to get the right extension
   e. Be sure to answer with your name and the department's name

14

Eliminate the dangling construction in the following sentences:

9. I saw many new flowers jogging through the parking lot.
10. While on vacation, my dog stayed at my mother's house.
11. Her first and only child was born at age 44.
12. The record was finally returned floating through the department.

Strike through the unnecessary words that take up space and add nothing to the ideas expressed. (You may write directly on the page.)

13. Mrs. Benson just recovered from an attack of pneumonia.
14. Your letter arrived at a time when we were on vacation.
15. The water is for drinking purposes only.
16. The consultation fee is the sum of twenty dollars.
17. The color of the new transcriber is beige.
18. We will return the equipment at a later date.
19. The file is made out of steel.
20. We are now engaged in building a new medical wing.

21. The report describes the patient's medical records during the period from May 1995 to May 1996.
22. The operative procedure lasted up to eight hours in duration.
23. The new printer is smaller in size.
24. The patient's disability will last a period of eight weeks.
25. The physician is actively providing professional services to many government employees.

Correct the grammar in the final sentences by adding, eliminating, or changing words.

26. I feel the nursing personnel as well as pulmonary medicine staff will benefit from the information and instructions.
27. The Advisory Committee and Management Department would like to express their thanks for the time you gave to present the material to us.
28. When operating a postage meter, you should remember the following:
    a. The date should be changed daily.
    b. The amount of postage set on the meter should be checked before the envelope is stamped.
    c. The meter should be reset to zero.
    d. All unused postage metered tapes and envelopes should be saved for refund with application for the refund made within a year.
    e. Mail should be deposited on the date shown or postage may be forfeited.
    f. If an error is made by the meter (poor ink, incorrect postage amount) a request for a full refund should be made and no further postage should be imprinted until the problem has been corrected.
    g. *Hand Stamp* should be written in large red letters on both the front and back of a bulky envelope.
29. For this reason, that the medical record might be the physician's only witness in court, that record must be absolutely correct.
30. By writing one, learns to write.

Check the end of this chapter for possible ways to correct these problems.

GETTING STARTED

One of the major hurdles in writing is getting through the agonizing stage of deciding what to say and getting started. Some people, expecting to produce simultaneously a well-planned, well-written, polished, and finely typed letter, try in vain to organize their thoughts and compose while word processing.

Be realistic. Organize your thoughts on scratch paper before you begin. Plan carefully. The extra steps you take to make a rough draft of your thoughts are not wasted because you will have the letter more than half-written before you actually start to compose it.

Make an outline to cover the following points:

1. WHY: Formulate a clear idea of the reason for the message. Clearly state your purpose for writing.
2. WHO: Know the audience to whom you are writing and how that audience should be approached.
3. WHAT: List all information to be conveyed. List the secondary or supporting topics that go with the central idea. Be careful about details.
4. REACTION: Describe how you expect the recipient to react, your desired action, attitude or result.

Using your outline, list exactly what you want to say; be concise and specific. Remember that you want to convey a particular message without confusion or excess verbiage. A concise letter avoids anything that the reader already knows. However, sometimes it is necessary to "remind" the reader of certain things before continuing with new information. If you are writing to order an item, jot down all of the pertinent information to describe it, and add any questions you have concerning its operation, warranty, cost, or delivery. If you are making an appointment for a patient, state the exact day of the week, date, and time that you expect the patient, including any directions to explain specifically how the arrangements may be changed if the patient is dissatisfied with them.

COMPOSING

When you know exactly what you need to say, you must organize your material in an orderly fashion and learn how to express yourself well. Let us see how this plan works with the following outline:

1. WHY: The patient wants an appointment.
2. WHO: An established office patient.
3. WHAT: The exact time, day, and date.
4. PLUS (details): Notification to bring his x-ray films with him; we will change the date if it is not convenient.
5. REACTION: The patient will arrive on the proper date with the x-ray films or reply that the arrangements are not satisfactory.

Here is a letter following our outline:

> Dear Mr. Johnson: [1]An appointment has been reserved [2]for you with [3]Dr. Beem on Friday, May 11, 199X, at 3:30 p.m. [4]Please bring your x-ray films from Dr. Bowers' office with you. I hope these arrangements are convenient for you; if not, [5]please telephone the office. Sincerely,

Because Mr. Johnson is an established patient in our office, we probably have built a friendly rapport with him. Therefore, this rather cold, formal letter may be made more personal without sacrificing our basic plan.

> Dear Mr. Johnson: We are looking forward to seeing you again on Friday, May 11, 199X, at 3:30 p.m. Dr. Beem would like you to bring your x-ray films from Dr. Bowers' office with you for this appointment. I hope these arrangements are convenient; if not, please telephone me. Sincerely,

Finally, reread the letter and see if it covers clearly and exactly what you wish to say. Make sure you have followed your outline and have omitted nothing. Read your document as if you were the person receiving it. Do you have any questions? No. (Good!) Yes. (Rewrite!) Be sure you have written clear, correctly worded sentences. Use proper letter mechanics and prepare the document attractively.

14–2: PRACTICE TEST

14

Directions: Write an outline for a letter using the following information. Do not write the letter, only the outline.

Dr. Berry has received a request from one of his patients who wishes to have a copy of her medical record. He has agreed to make an abstract of this record and meet with the patient to discuss the abstract and answer any questions. He has set a fee of $80 for the conference and the abstract. You are to let the patient know how he is going to respond to her request and make a tentative appointment for the conference.

See Appendix A for a possible outline.

Planning and Writing Paragraphs

A good way to form paragraphs is to use the technique of striving for a two- or three-paragraph letter because most letters require only three paragraphs. If a letter has more than three paragraphs, it might not be poorly constructed, but it probably does need to be tightened up. However, check the letter to see if anything is lacking. (Quite often, the missing element is the personal touch—the extra something that communicates feeling to the reader.)

Therefore, the letter should have three characteristics:

1. One subject
2. Two aspects: feeling and thinking
3. Two or three paragraphs, including a beginning, a middle, and an end

Start by taking out the excess verbiage. One fault of poor letters is complexity. Often this is caused by burying the main point, the main idea, deep in dates of prior correspondence, invoice numbers, identification numbers, and so on. The cure for this is simple: Use a subject line. This lets you get right down to business in the main part of the letter. It allows you to make your point early, clearly, and concisely.

Another frequent cause of complexity is trying to cover more than one subject in one letter. The remedy for this is to write two letters. If this is inconvenient, write one letter as if it were two and use the final paragraph to sum up the substance of both subjects.

Your paragraphs should be concise and courteous. Try this method: Write an opening paragraph that states the problem or makes the point; use a second paragraph that elaborates or provides detail; and sum up or state in the final paragraph what has to be done. Of course, very brief paragraphs may be joined.

Opening Paragraph

Write a topic sentence that states the main idea to be developed. Place the topic sentence at or near the beginning of the letter.

Transitions

Use connective phrases such as *however, therefore, nevertheless, for this reason, in fact, in contrast,* and so on to achieve transitions within or between paragraphs. You do not want an abrupt change in shifting to the next sentence or next paragraph.

Second Paragraph

Give details in sequence (chronological or locational) or use enumerations such as first, second, third, and so on. Remember that this paragraph elaborates and provides all the necessary details for the reader.

Final Paragraph

State clearly the results, reaction, action, or desired attitude. If you followed your plan for outlining your letter, this will coincide with that plan.

The Beginning

1. Get right in and say what you want to say. Be concise, yet complete and courteous.
2. Avoid beginning a letter with *I* or *We*.

NOT: I would like to order a #14 Jackson bronchoscope.
BUT: Please send a #14 Jackson bronchoscope, catalog number . . .

3. Avoid trite openings.

NOT: In reference to your correspondence of July 14 inviting me . . .
BUT: Thank you for the invitation to attend . . .

4. In writing for another person, use an impersonal tone or place the other's name foremost.

NOT: I am glad to inform you that the results of your tests . . .
BUT: This letter is to inform you that the results of your tests . . .

NOT: I want to make reservations for Dr. and Mrs. Kirsch . . .
BUT: Dr. and Mrs. Kirsch would like reservations for . . .

NOT: I submitted the report on . . .
BUT: The report was submitted on . . .

NOTE: In general, avoid using the passive voice verb construction, as illustrated in the last example, because it is wordy and sometimes unclear. Exception: The reason outlined in item 4.

A good balance of active and passive voice can be pleasant but will depend on where you wish to place your emphasis in writing.

NOT: The surgery was performed by Dr. Augustus. (passive)
BUT: Dr. Augustus performed the surgery. (active)

NOT: He was released for return to his regular employment by Dr. Berry. (passive)
BUT: Dr. Berry released him for regular employment. (active)

Notice in the last example of passive voice that it not only takes longer to say what you want to say but also might appear that Dr. Berry is the employer.

14

5. Use a positive approach. Discuss what can be done instead of what cannot.

NOT: We are unable to give you an appointment on the date you requested.
BUT: Dr. Elsner will be pleased to see you at 10:30 a.m. on . . .

6. Avoid words that antagonize, such as *overlooked, failure, neglected, forgot, careless,* and *mistake.*

NOT: We do not understand your failure to pay this bill.
BUT: We are certain that your nonpayment of this bill is an oversight.

7. Use a subject line when appropriate. This device lets you get right down to business in the main part of the letter.

EXAMPLES

Re: Frich pacemaker model Z-141

Subject: Final notice

The Body of the Letter

8. Use simple, natural language similar to your everyday conversation. Avoid unnecessary words and phrases. (See page 335.)

NOT: Enclosed herewith please find my check in the amount of $25 for payment . . .
BUT: Enclosed is my $25 payment.

9. Be sure you tell the reader all he or she needs to know to act or respond. You must remember to support your theme, and any secondary ideas should be related to the main one. Point the recipient toward a required action or attitude.
10. Use courteous language: *please, thank you, I appreciate.*
11. Use short and interesting sentences; vary the construction of your sentences.
12. Avoid favorite words or expressions, and be sure that you are not "cute" or flip.

NOT: It *certainly* was nice to hear from you last week, and I *certainly* appreciate . . .
BUT: It was nice to hear from you last week, and I appreciate . . .

13. Do not confuse the reader with abrupt moves from one idea to the next.
14. Use words your reader will understand, and avoid using technical terms when writing to patients or to other people outside of your profession.

NOT: Dr. Berry wants you to come in for your test NPO, midnight.
BUT: Please do not eat or drink anything after midnight.

14

Closing

15. Acknowledge a favor if there was one.

EXAMPLE

Thank you for the invitation to participate.

16. Make an appropriate apology if necessary.

EXAMPLE

We are sorry for any inconvenience this delay may have caused.

However, do not "overapologize" or pass the blame to someone else.

NOT: I don't know how I could have made such an awful mistake, and I promise I will never let it happen again.
BUT: I am sorry that my negligence inconvenienced you.

17. Create a feeling of cooperation and good will.

We are looking forward to seeing you in the office on Friday, May 19, at 3:30 p.m.

18. Avoid the "ing" endings.

NOT: Hoping to hear from you, Trusting this will give you time, Thanking you in advance, Looking forward to payment,
BUT: We look forward . . .

19. Thank only after the fact. Do not thank in advance.

NOT: Thank you for taking care of this immediately.
BUT: Your cooperation in attending to this will be appreciated.

Review the Final Product

20. Be sure that your grammar, spelling, and punctuation are accurate.
21. Scrutinize for clarity, content, and tone.
22. Review your plan and check that it is complete.
23. Be prepared to revise, rewrite, and eliminate redundant phrases; change the positions of sentences; correct the grammar.
24. Seek criticism and accept it gracefully.
25. Check for attractiveness. The way that the letter looks is almost as important as the message that it carries.

The following are examples of some of the letters the secretary may write for his or her signature.

A letter of apology
Dear Mrs. Steiner: ¶ Thank you for returning the letter which I inadvertently sent to you. ¶ I appreciate its prompt return, and I hope that I did not inconvenience you. ¶ Your letter is enclosed. Sincerely,

A letter of acknowledgment
(When your employer is away from the office for several days, you are expected to acknowledge the mail that would ordinarily receive the employer's prompt attention.)

Dear Dr. Knape: ¶ Dr. Berry is out of the city and is not expected in the office for ten more days. ¶ Your letter will be brought to his attention immediately upon his return to work. Sincerely.

Canceling an appointment
Dear Professor Steele: ¶ Dr. Berry asked me to

cancel all his appointments for Monday, September 8, 199X, because of an unexpected surgery scheduled. ¶ Therefore, it is necessary to cancel your three o'clock appointment that day. I am sorry for the inconvenience. ¶ Please telephone the office so that I can arrange a new appointment for you. Sincerely,

Requesting a fee from an insurance company
Dear Mr. Tomlinson: ¶ Thank you for your check for $25 as payment toward the completion of the Request for Medical Information on Mr. Silas Trotter. ¶ The fee in this office for these medical reports is $50. We will be happy to complete the form and return it to you as soon as we receive the full fee. Sincerely,

NOTE: If you often have to write letters of this kind, it is a good idea to type a form letter with blanks in appropriate places. You can save your original and fill in the blanks to meet the circumstances or use the "merge" feature on the word processor.

Gentle collection letter
(Precise instruction regarding payment is a very important part of collection letters.) Dear Mrs. Lincoln: ¶ Your attention is specifically directed to the enclosed statement for $36. This amount represents the balance due on your account for professional services rendered by Dr. Berry in February of this year. ¶ No further payments can be anticipated from your insurance company and this balance, therefore, remains your personal responsibility. ¶ We would greatly appreciate payment in full within the next ten days. Sincerely,

Less gentle collection letter
Dear Mrs. Dobe: ¶ Your attention is invited to the balance of $85 that is due for professional services rendered you by Dr. Berry in August, 199X. ¶ Although five months have elapsed since these services were rendered, no payment has been received on this account nor have you communicated with the office regarding your plans for payment. ¶ We feel that we have been very patient and lenient in handling this account but now must insist that some arrangements be made to take care of the balance. Unless this account is paid in full prior to February 5, 199X, it will be necessary for us to initiate other means to secure collection. Sincerely,

NOTE: Even though you may copy these collection letters and personalize them to match the circumstances, do not turn them into form letters, since a more personal note may result in better cash flow.

Letter to an insurance company
Dear Sir or Madam: RE: Edna Mae Wright, Policy #782-A. ¶ On March 29, 199X, Dr. Berry submitted to your firm a medical report on the above-named patient. This claim of $175 was for services rendered by Dr. Berry on March 15 and 16, 199X. ¶ Neither Mrs. Wright nor Dr. Berry has heard from you regarding this matter. A photocopy of the original claim form is enclosed. ¶ Please send us a check as soon as possible. Sincerely,

14

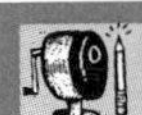

14–3: SELF-STUDY

Directions: Your employer, William A. Berry, MD, has asked you to write the following letter for your signature. Make your outline first. Then compose your letter following the appropriate rules. You will use Dr. Berry's letterhead stationery and identify yourself properly as his secretary. (See Chapter 6, page 147.) Use today's date, modified-block format, and mixed punctuation.

Dr. Berry has made arrangements for one of his patients, Mr. Ray Littlefield, to see another physician, Paul R. Vecchione, in consultation. You may invent the necessary information to write Mr. Littlefield who knows that these arrangements were to be made.

See the end of the chapter for a possible outline and letter.

14–4: REVIEW TEST

Directions: Follow the directions given with Self-Study 14–3 and compose letters for your signature for the following situations. When each individual letter is complete, ask yourself the following questions:

1. Is it attractive? Check it quickly for appearance.
2. Have you used proper letter mechanics for modified-block format with mixed punctuation?
3. Did you need or use a reference line?
4. Did you use a pleasant opening or closing paragraph?
5. Is your main point quickly introduced?
6. Are any details missing? Will the recipient know exactly how to respond?
7. Did you notice any misspelled words or improper use of grammar or punctuation marks?
8. Was the letter precise or could fewer words have been used to say what was said?

After you have thoroughly checked your letter, retype it if necessary.

1. Dr. Berry has agreed to address the high school PTA in his community concerning the increased use of alcohol by young adults. Write the program chairman, inventing the necessary data. Part of Dr. Berry's presentation will be the screening of a film entitled "More Than a Few Beers," and he will be prepared for a question-and-answer period.
2. Dr. Berry's engraved stationery is ordered from a neighboring community. You need to order paper and envelopes. Invent all the necessary information to complete this assignment. Be sure to be precise; cover all details. You may wish to review Chapter 6, page 142, Item 1 and Item 2 concerning the details of office and hospital stationery.
3. Dr. Berry received a letter from a surgeon's office indicating that an operative report was enclosed. You carefully checked the contents of the envelope and discovered that the report had not been included. Write a letter to the surgeon's office concerning this oversight. Invent the necessary information to complete this assignment.
4. A former patient, Mrs. Bertha Wilson, has written that she will be in town next month and would like to see Dr. Berry for an examination and an ECG. Please write to give her an appointment, inventing the necessary data.

Sample Letters

The following are examples of some types of letters that the secretary may compose for his or her employer's signature:

Unable to attend a staff meeting
Dear Dr. Benson: ¶ Please excuse me from attending the Round Valley Hospital Medical Staff Meeting next Wednesday evening. ¶ I am taking a postgraduate class at the university, and the final examination is scheduled for the same evening. Respectfully, William A. Berry, MD

Letter concerning laboratory test results
Dear Mr. Swan: ¶ Enclosed are copies of the results of the urinalysis and biochemical survey that I ordered at Community Hospital. These values are entirely normal. ¶ I will look forward to seeing you again if you have any further problems. Sincerely, William A. Berry, MD

Excuse from physical education class
TO WHOM IT MAY CONCERN: ¶ Since March 18, Angela Marsi has been a patient in this office with an upper respiratory infection requiring the use of antibiotics. ¶ Today I released her to return to school, but I would like her to be excused from physical education classes for one more week. Sincerely, William A. Berry, MD

Letter to compensation carrier
Dear Mr. Thompson: RE: Toni Wilden, File 0713. ¶ An exploration of the right shoulder has been scheduled on Ms. Wilden at Center City Hospital next Wednesday at 7:30 a.m. ¶ Her convalescence will require 2-3 days in the hospital and absence from work for about three weeks. ¶ Thank you for allowing me to continue with her care. Sincerely, William A. Berry, MD

Return to work

Dear Mr. Girard: ¶ Mr. Samuel Gordon was seen today in final examination after his surgery of May 17, 199X. ¶ His wound is well healed; he has no complaints referable to his cardiorespiratory system; he seems in excellent physical condition. ¶ In my opinion, he should be able to resume his normal work load, with no restrictions, on June 10, 199X. Sincerely, William A. Berry, MD

Letter of congratulations

Dear Dr. Kirkham: ¶ My staff and I would like to express our sincere congratulations to you on your new partnership with Dr. John Champe in the practice of thoracic surgery. ¶ We wish you success and happiness in your new association. Sincerely, William A. Berry, MD

Dismissal of a patient who does not pay his medical bill

Dear Mr. Shamkne: ¶ The records in our office indicate a long-overdue balance on your account totaling $278. ¶ My staff assures me that every reasonable effort to arrange some mutually agreeable plan of payment has failed to prompt any sign of cooperation on your part. ¶ Thus I am forced to conclude that the best interests both of this office and of you will be served by the adoption of the following conditions:

1. Unless your debt is paid in full by April 6, 199X, you will be discharged finally and fully as a patient.
2. Your clinical records will be closed for forwarding by our staff to any physician of your choice. Failure on your part to name a new physician or to advise us of your selection in writing will be your responsibility, not ours. Yours very truly, William A. Berry, MD

14-5: REVIEW TEST

Directions: Your employer, Dr. Berry, hands you some mail and asks you to reply to it for his signature; on some letters, he may have made a brief suggestion to guide you. Attempt to make these letters sound as though he dictated them. The relationship between your employer and the recipient will determine the salutation and tone. Use letterhead stationery. Here are the letters and notes for your reply and his signature. Use the current date, full-block format, and mixed punctuation.

1. He received a letter from a physician friend who has a cabin on the lake. The friend has invited him to spend the following three-day weekend there, fishing. Dr. Berry asks you to send his regrets because he is on call that weekend and has a patient entering the hospital Sunday afternoon. Invent the necessary information to complete the assignment.
2. Dr. Berry receives a formal announcement from Frank R. Curtis, MD, a new physician opening his office in the same medical complex, for the practice of family medicine. Dr. Berry asks you to send a note of congratulations. Invent the address.
3. There is a note to you that reads: "I referred Mrs. Dorothy Winters to Dr. John Briton for consultation about three weeks ago, and I have not received a consultation report from him about her. She had a lump in her right breast. Please write him to inquire about her progress." Invent any necessary information to complete this assignment.

ABSTRACTING FROM PATIENTS' CHARTS

Many routine requests for medical information on patients can be handled by the secretary. The physician may review the record first, noting that there is nothing unusual, and then ask you to reply for his or her signature. This request from another physician, hospital, insurance company, lawyer, employer, or compensation carrier must always be accompanied by a signed release from the patient authorizing the physician to release this information (Fig. 14–1 and Figs. 1–6 and 1–7).

Examine the chart note on Mr. Dow (Fig. 14–2). Then read the letter and see how the secretary has included all the pertinent information in the reply (Fig. 14–3).

RECORDS RELEASE

Date 1-25-9x

To William A. Berry, MD
DOCTOR OR HOSPITAL

3933 Navajo Road, San Diego, CA 92119
ADDRESS

I hereby authorize and request you to release

To Quality Life Assurance Society

Box 2187, New York, NY 10001
ADDRESS

The complete medical records in your possession concerning my illness and/or treatment during the period from 9-1-9x to 1-15-9x

Signed Michael T. Dow
PATIENT OR NEAREST RELATIVE

Maryellen Dow
WITNESS

Relationship spouse

Figure 14–1. Authorization to release medical information.

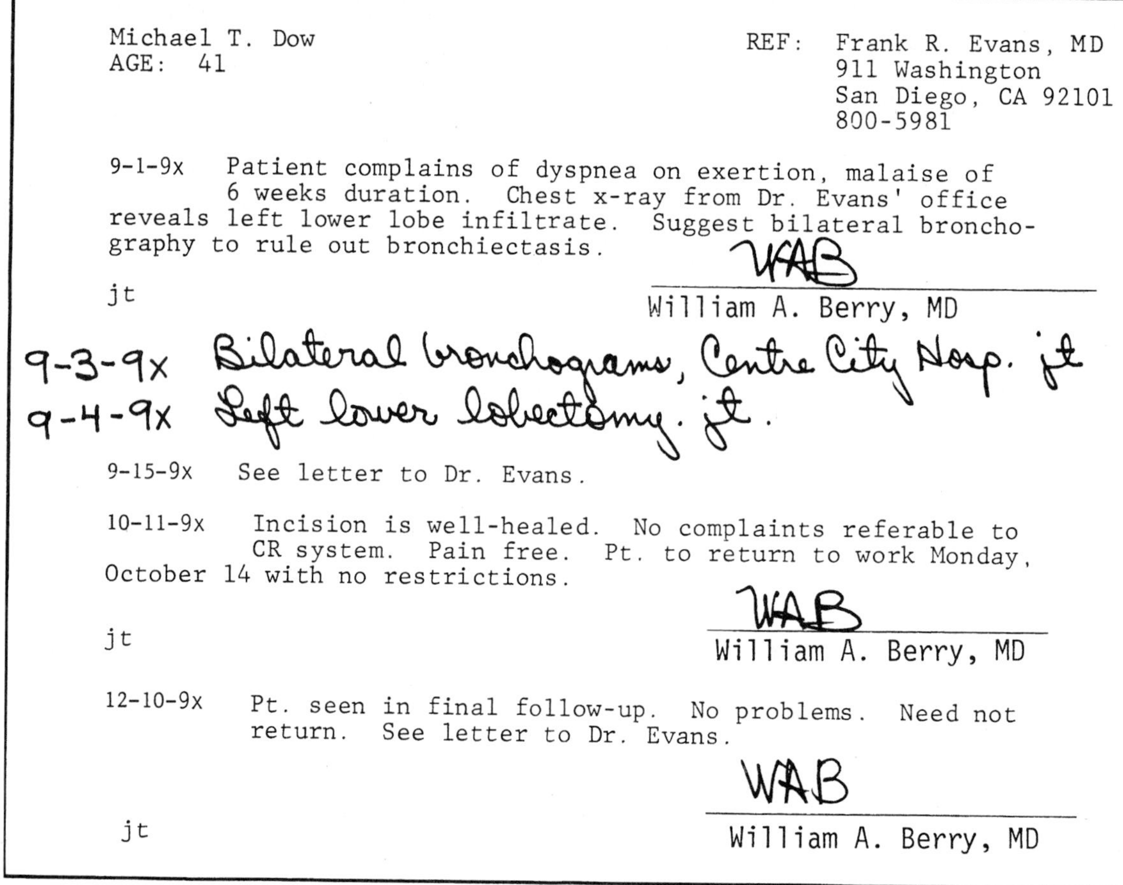

Michael T. Dow
AGE: 41

REF: Frank R. Evans, MD
911 Washington
San Diego, CA 92101
800-5981

9-1-9x Patient complains of dyspnea on exertion, malaise of 6 weeks duration. Chest x-ray from Dr. Evans' office reveals left lower lobe infiltrate. Suggest bilateral bronchography to rule out bronchiectasis.

jt WAB
William A. Berry, MD

9-3-9x Bilateral bronchograms, Centre City Hosp. jt
9-4-9x Left lower lobectomy. jt.

9-15-9x See letter to Dr. Evans.

10-11-9x Incision is well-healed. No complaints referable to CR system. Pain free. Pt. to return to work Monday, October 14 with no restrictions.

jt WAB
William A. Berry, MD

12-10-9x Pt. seen in final follow-up. No problems. Need not return. See letter to Dr. Evans.

jt WAB
William A. Berry, MD

Figure 14–2. Patient's chart note.

William A. Berry, MD
3933 Navajo Road
San Diego California 92119

463-0000

January 28, 199X

Quality Life Assurance Society
Medical Department
Box 2187
New York, NY 10001

Gentlemen:

RE: Michael T. Dow

Mr. Dow was first seen on September 1, 199X, complaining of dyspnea on exertion and malaise of six weeks' duration. A chest x-ray revealed a left lower lobe infiltrate.

After bilateral bronchograms on September 3, 199X, the diagnosis of bronchiectasis was confirmed, and a left lower lobectomy was performed on September 4, 199X.

The patient was released to return to work on October 14, 199X, and was last seen in the office on December 10, 199X, and released from further care.

A copy of the operative report and pathology report are enclosed.

Sincerely yours,

William A. Berry, MD

jt

Enclosures

Figure 14–3. Letter composed by a secretary for his or her employer's signature, based on information in the patient's chart (see Fig. 14–2).

14

REFERENCE MATERIALS

Although there are many kinds of reference materials to assist you in writing letters, you should start your own file of sample letters that you have written, to be adapted or combined to meet individual situations.

A good dictionary, a punctuation and grammar book, a style manual, and a thesaurus should be in your desk library. Because we have discussed all of these except the thesaurus in previous chapters, we will discuss it now.

Thesaurus means *treasury* in Greek, and it can be a real treasure for you. A dictionary is used to find the meaning of a word, and a thesaurus is used to find an alternative word to express the same idea (synonym). Or you may have a negative idea that you wish to make positive; the thesaurus also contains antonyms.

Every synonym listed is not an exact substitute

for the word you might want, however, and care must be taken to see that the word not only fits the context of the sentence but also is a word that you could use comfortably.

For example, if you decide that you want to use another word for *stolen* in the sentence *My dress was stolen,* you look for *steal* in the thesaurus. There you find that many synonyms are given but not all are applicable to *stolen* as expressed in the sentence: The dress could not have been *robbed, abducted, embezzled, purloined, plundered, swindled,* or *plagiarized.* Furthermore, the slang expressions *pinched, carried off,* and *ripped off* might even carry an additional meaning that you do not intend. However, you also find the word *taken; taken* fits what you want to say and you are comfortable with it.

A thesaurus may be arranged alphabetically, like a dictionary, or you may have to look up the "idea" of the word and use cross references. Definitions usually are not given. You will need to explore your thesaurus to see how it is organized. There are computer software programs that contain a thesaurus. (Often these are in combination with a spelling-check program.) When composing a document, you may instantly bring up a list of substitute words for the particular word for which you need a choice. Actually, a book list is frequently faster and more helpful.

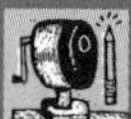

14–6: SELF-STUDY

Directions: You will need a thesaurus for the following assignment. This assignment is to help you become familiar with using a thesaurus as a reference source for achieving variety in word usage.

Using a thesaurus as a reference, type three to five words that can be substituted for the following overworked words:

1. know
2. awful
3. tell
4. nice
5. think

See the end of the chapter for possible responses.

14–7: REVIEW TEST

Directions: As you can see from Self-Study 14–6, the word choices are very broad but become very limiting when they are to be substituted into the context of a complete thought. In the following exercises, there will be more than one word that needs a substitute, and you will need to be sure that each substitute word fits the context of what you wish to say. Often, it is necessary to change other words in the sentence to make the new word fit properly. Retype each of the following sentences, substituting your alternate word or words for those underlined. *You should write two complete sentences for each target sentence.* You may adjust the sentence to fit your needs.

EXAMPLE

How much did you <u>get</u> from that <u>game</u> you played?
Possible rewrites:
How much did you <u>obtain</u> from that <u>contest</u> you *entered?*
How much did you <u>receive</u> from that <u>match</u> you *made?*

1. She <u>needs</u> to <u>ask</u> her boss for a raise.

See the end of the chapter for some possible changes to this statement. Continue with the rest of the exercise without assistance other than your thesaurus.

2. It is <u>difficult</u> to <u>know</u> how to complete <u>certain</u> office tasks.

3. Please arrange for your group to be on time.
4. Please excuse my delay in answering your request.
5. It gives me great pleasure to welcome you.
6. We, as a rule, do not employ inexperienced transcriptionists.

TRAVEL ARRANGEMENTS

The secretary may be asked by the physician to formulate and expedite arrangements for a vacation or travel to a medical convention held in the United States or abroad. A worry-free trip depends on systematic and prudent planning to eliminate the frustrating problems that haphazard arrangements can bring. Regardless of the distance or duration of the trip, the secretary should be able to set it up when the physician announces his or her plans.

The secretary must ensure that applications for attendance at out-of-town seminars or continuing medical education (CME) courses are made as soon as the location is announced. On receiving written confirmation, the secretary should make travel and hotel arrangements. Any delay or procrastination in initiating reservations may mean the physician will be unable to stay at the hotel at which the convention is being held, and it might affect the chance of securing the most direct transportation.

General information on the physician's travel preferences can be accumulated in a permanent travel file folder to help you plan any trip. This would include the following:

1. Name of a reputable travel agent
2. Employer's credit card numbers
3. Car rental preference
4. Travel:
   a. Preferred method of travel (air, rail, or car) to specific destinations
   b. Class of travel
   c. Airline seating choice (window or aisle)
5. Hotel:
   a. Exactly for whom the reservations are to be made
   b. Type of accommodations required: specific features desired, such as bed size; suite; studio; connecting rooms; views of garden, pool, terrace, or ocean; and so on.
   c. Price rate range desired
6. Shuttle: The physician may request door-to-door shuttle service to eliminate driving to and from the airport or having to park a car at the airport.

To the general information, the secretary can then add the more specific information, such as:

1. Destination
2. Preferred route. Any side trips or tours?
3. Date and time for departure and arrival
4. Number in party
5. Approximate hotel arrival and departure time
6. Date and time preferred for arrival. (Which is more important—at destination or departure from homes?)

When you have gathered all of your information, your next step is to call your travel agent, primarily a central source of information for tours, carriers, and accommodations. A travel agent can sell tickets or make reservations, but the service to you is free because the commission is paid by the tour operator, by the hotel, or by the carrier. Most travel agencies have computers providing current information on airline fares and schedules, both domestic and international, and on hotel availability with addresses and telephone numbers. The computer gives information on weather conditions in all parts of the world, train reservation information, special tour packages featuring discounts, and money rates of exchange. In addition to figuring out schedules, making reservations, and centralizing ticket purchases, a travel agent can help you with many small details: arrange for visas, insurance, car rentals, special meals or dietary preferences, airline aisle or window seating choice, and tickets to special events. A valuable agent will usually be familiar with the area your employer is visiting.

To make plane or rail reservations, your travel agent can select from all possible lines out of the city. You provide the specific details; the agent will make and confirm the reservations and mail or deliver the tickets. Tickets may be charged on a credit card. If airline tickets are mailed to the office, the secretary promptly checks arrival and departure dates and times against the information he or she has on the itinerary work sheet to see that they have been made as requested. If your employer wishes to rent a car on arrival at the destination, the travel agent can reserve one. (Note that it is necessary to have a valid driver's license as well as a nationally recognized credit card—for example, VISA, MasterCard, Carte Blanche, or American Express—to rent a car.)

The agent will give you the details concerning arrangements for picking the car up at the airport or rail terminal. If your employer does not want a rental car, you need to know about other available means of transportation. The travel agent can tell you if there is hotel limousine, bus, or taxi service and the methods for obtaining these vehicles.

Hotel reservations can also be made by the travel agent, but many secretaries prefer to write or telephone for these themselves, particularly for a business trip. As a convenience to travelers, most hotel/motel chains have toll-free 800 numbers that can be used to make reservations and check on them. If arrival time is to be after 6 p.m., it is necessary to tell this to the reservation clerk. Sometimes a deposit must be made to ensure that the room will be reserved. If the physician is attending a convention, the assistant needs to convey this to the hotel reservation clerk to obtain special group rates because rooms are held specifically for people attending the convention. In fact, you may be turned down for reservations if you fail to mention the fact that your employer is attending a convention. Provide the following additional information in your letter to the hotel for accommodations: the names of all persons staying in the room, the type of accommodations desired, the date and approximate time of arrival, and the date of departure. Request a room with fax or voice mail equipment when necessary. Send a deposit or credit card number, and ask for written confirmation.

When you have completed all the arrangements, the travel agent may computer-generate an itinerary, which you may use to prepare a complete travel itinerary and present it and a copy to your employer (keep a copy for yourself) with the tickets and hotel confirmation. The itinerary will include:

1. Departure date, time, airlines, class, flight number, including connecting flights. This may also include seating arrangements when you are able to obtain them in advance.

```
                         ITINERARY
                            for
                 Dr. and Mrs. William A. Berry
                        June 1-5, 199x

DEPARTURE:    Buttergold Airlines, Flight 792, Non-stop
              Leaves:    7:05 a.m. Breakfast will be served on board
              Arrives:   11:45 a.m. (their time).
                         (Flying time: 3 hours, 40 minutes)

CAR RENTAL:   Lo-Rate Cars. Booth located near baggage pickup.
              199x Odyssey is reserved. $28/day, unlimited mileage.
              Confirmation attached.

HOTEL:        Saint Ann's Inn, 321 Main Street.
              Phone 222-500-8438
              Confirmation attached.

RETURN:       Buttergold Airlines, Flight 251, Non-stop
              Leaves:     3:15 p.m.  Supper will be served on board
              Arrives:    6:00 p.m. (our time)

Have a good time!

Arrangements: Fiesta International Travel Service. 231-2548.
```

Figure 14–4. Sample itinerary.

Travel Arrangements:

_____ Call covering physician's office to be sure he or she will be available to take calls from the doctor's patients.
_____ Cross off the time in the appointment book.
_____ Call for airline reservations. Airlines preferred _____
_____ Write the hotel.
_____ Arrange for car rental. Agency preferred _____
Credit card # _____
_____ Check driver's license. Expiration date _____
_____ Purchase traveler's checks. Numbers _____
_____ Notify answering service of dates and name of covering physician.
_____ Type itinerary. Copies to _____
_____ Confirm airline reservation.
_____ Confirm hotel reservation.
_____ Confirm car rental.
_____ Obtain names and phone number of anyone the doctor may be visiting while out of the city _____

Figure 14–5. Sample checklist for travel arrangements.

2. Arrival time (if in another time zone, indicate the time zone). You can give approximate air time, information concerning meals, inflight movies when available.
3. Transportation arrangements: bus, taxi, rental car.
4. Hotel arrangement, including address and telephone number.
5. Return date, time, airlines, class of travel, flight number.

This information should be attractively prepared so that it is easy to read (Fig. 14–4).

Your copy of the itinerary is put in the travel folder for future reference. Some secretaries make a check-off sheet to be sure that they have not overlooked any detail of the travel plans (Fig. 14–5).

14

14–8: REVIEW TEST

Directions: Your employer, Dr. Claire Duennes, is flying to Mexico City for the International Congress of Family Physicians. She will have five days in Mexico City, including the arrival day, and three of them will be taken up with the meeting.

1. Please write a letter to make hotel reservations for Dr. Duennes. The convention is being held in the Pan Americas Hotel, 387 Avenida Juarez, Mexico City, Mexico, D.F., and she would like to stay there. She plans to arrive as early in the day as possible (so she can do some sightseeing before the meeting begins). Invent any other data you need to do the assignment properly.
2. Prepare a travel itinerary for Dr. Duennes, inventing all the data you need to complete it properly so you will not have to consult a local travel agent. She is not concerned about the actual return time or arrival to her home city.

WE HOPE YOU HAVEN'T BEEN USING THESE RULES!*

1. Make sure each pronoun agrees with their antecedent.
2. Just between you and I, case is important.
3. Verbs has to agree with their subjects.
4. Watch out for irregular verbs which have crope into English.
5. Don't use no double negatives.
6. A writer must not shift your point of view.

* With permission of THE READER'S DIGEST, March 1963, "Pardon, Your Slip Is Showing."

7. When dangling, don't use participles.
8. Join clauses good like a conjunction should.
9. Don't write a run-on sentence you got to punctuate it.
10. About sentence fragments.
11. In letters reports and articles use commas to separate items in a series.
12. Don't use commas, which are not necessary.
13. Its important to use apostrophe's correctly.
14. Check to see if you have any words out.
15. Don't abbrev.
16. In the case of a letter, check it in terms of jargon.
17. As far as incomplete constructions, they are wrong.
18. About repetition, the repetition of a word might be real effective repetition—take, for instance, the repetition of words in Lincoln's Gettysburg Address.
19. In my opinion, I think that an author when he is writing should not get into the habit of making use of too many unnecessary words that he does not really need in order to put his message across.
20. Last but not least, lay off clichés.

A *Answers to* **14–1: SELF-STUDY**

1. Please retype this; it is your responsibility.
2. Remodeling is taking place in the Emergency Room; therefore, reroute all patient traffic to Ward B until further notice.
   Remodeling is taking place in the Emergency Room, so reroute all patient traffic to Ward B until further notice.
3. The new chief-of-staff will take over the first of next month; furthermore, there will be many new physicians added to the active staff roster.
   The new chief-of-staff will take over the first of next month, and there will be many new physicians added to the active staff roster. (Or write two separate sentences.)

14

4. To be accurate and to meet your production levels are important here.
   It is important here to be accurate and to meet your production levels.
5. Pull the patient's record; notify the doctor of the emergency; give the record to the doctor; relate any information you have received.
6. (Change the final line only.) (3) Refer to the Inventory Stock Catalogue and enter the appropriate stock number if the preprinted requisition is not available for the products you require.
7. The following is a list of the duties of the custodian of records:
   a. to keep accurate records
   b. to make corrections in the proper way
   c. to be sure that records are signed or initialed
   d. to obtain a release before you permit unauthorized persons to see the records.
8. (The order on this one needs changing too.)
   Rules for taking telephone calls:
   a. Pick up the telephone as soon as it rings
   b. Answer with your name and that of the department
   c. Ask for the name of the person calling
   d. Refrain from interrupting the caller
   e. Transfer to the right extension.
9. Jogging through the parking lot I saw many new flowers.
10. My dog stayed at my mother's house while I was on vacation.

11. She was 44 when her first and only child was born.
12. The record, which has been circulated throughout the department, finally was returned.
13. an attack of
14. at a time
15. purposes
16. the sum of/change the twenty dollars to $20
17. color of the
18. at a/date
19. made out of
20. engaged in
21. during the period
22. in duration
23. in size
24. a period of
25. actively
26. I feel *that* the nursing personnel as well as *the* pulmonary medicine staff will benefit from the information and instructions.
27. The *members of the* Advisory Committee and Management Department would like to express their thanks for the time you gave to present the material to us.
28. (In this one, we need to eliminate several "shoulds" as well as rewrite using parallel construction.) When operating a postage meter, remember the following:
    a. Change the date daily.
    b. Check the amount of postage set before stamping the envelope.
    c. Reset the meter to zero.
    d. Save all unused postage metered tapes and envelopes for a refund.
    e. Make application for the refund within a year.
    f. Deposit the mail on the date shown or postage may be forfeited.
    g. Make a request for a full refund if an error is made by the meter (poor ink, incorrect postage amount). A request for a full refund should be made and no further postage imprinted until the problem has been corrected.
    h. Write "HAND STAMP" in large red letters on both the front and back of a bulky envelope.

29. The medical record may be the physician's only witness in court. For this reason, the medical record must be completely accurate.
30. By writing, one learns to write. (Just put the comma in the right place!)

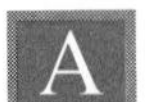

Answers to **14–3: SELF-STUDY**

WHO: Obtain patient's complete name and address.
WHY: Dr. Berry asked me to arrange for a consultation for patient with Dr. Paul Vecchione.
WHAT/WHEN: Give patient complete date, time, place, and reason for visit.
REACTION: Patient will call me to make any changes if necessary.

Today's date, 199X

Mr. Ray Littlefield
1234 Songbird Lane
Cradle Valley, CA 90000

Dear Mr. Littlefield:

Dr. Berry asked me to let you know that your consultation with Paul R. Vecchione, MD, has been arranged. His office is in the same medical complex as Dr. Berry's office, Suite 210. Dr. Vecchione will be pleased to see you:

Monday, July 1
10 a.m.
Suite 210
476-8974

Please let me know if you have any questions or if this appointment is not suitable. I will be happy to make any adjustment to fit your schedule.

Sincerely yours,

(Ms.) Your name, Receptionist

There are many acceptable variations on this assignment. The important areas to consider are as follows:

- *does the patient know why he is seeing another physician*
- *who is this doctor*
- *where is he located*
- *exactly when is this appointment*
- *what does he do if he can't make it then*
- *whom does he call if he has a problem about this*
- *does the letter look attractive*
- *is the letter error free*

A *Answers to* **14–6: SELF-STUDY**

Here are some possible word choices:

1. KNOW: perceive, discern, recognize, see, comprehend, understand, realize, appreciate, experience, be aware of.
2. AWFUL: terrific, tremendous, horrible, dreadful, fearful.
3. TELL: describe, narrate, explain, inform, advise, state.

4. NICE: delicate, fine, pleasing, attractive, accurate.
5. THINK: presume, understand, reason, reflect, speculate.

A *Answer to First Question on* **14–7: REVIEW TEST**

1. She wants to propose that her boss give her a raise.
2. She finds it necessary to request a raise from her boss.

Notice that there are many substitute words for "needs" and "ask." However, one would *not* say: It is a *requirement* to *implore* her boss for a raise.

CHAPTER

15

Typing Reports, Memos, Minutes, and Agenda

OBJECTIVES

After reading this chapter and working the exercises, you should be able to

1. Explain proper report format.
2. Type an agenda for a meeting.
3. Record, prepare, and type minutes for a meeting in correct format.
4. Prepare an intraoffice memo for your employer's signature.

15

INTRODUCTION

This chapter explains in detail the format for reports other than medical reports regarding patient care. Refer to Chapter 12 for information on preparing a history and physical and Chapter 13 for preparing miscellaneous medical reports. Here we discuss how to type hospital protocols and memos as well as how to prepare and type an agenda and how to record and type minutes for a meeting. Formats enhance written communication; however, we cannot overlook the most important aspect of composing such documents: readability, or communication effectiveness.

TYPING HOSPITAL PROTOCOLS

Hospital protocols are also known as hospital reports or hospital policies. Each section of a hospital has department policies and procedures. Because each institution has variances, only general guidelines on format, headings, and subheadings will be given. Hospital protocols have individual headings for the topics and titles. These will vary just as the nature of the report will vary. The originator of a report may or may not formulate the title for the transcriptionist, so he or she should be able to extract the title from the paragraph by pulling out the main idea and composing a brief

MR-1

XYZ Medical Center
30 South Main Street
Woodland Hills, XY 12345

MEDICAL RECORD PROCEDURES

SUBPOENAS
Medical records shall only be removed from the hospital jurisdiction in accordance with court order, subpoena, statute, or upon the approval of the Hospital Administrator.

Only those individuals specifically authorized by the Director of Medical Records may accept subpoenas for medical records.

No subpoena will be accepted by medical record personnel for cases in which the hospital is a party to the action unless specifically authorized to do so by the Administrator. These subpoenas must be served upon the Administrator, or his or her designee in the case of his or her absence. The subpoenaed medical records will be given to the Administrator to be placed in a controlled environment.

If it appears necessary to remove medical records from the hospital's jurisdiction as under court order, subpoena, or statute, an effort will be made to ascertain if it would be acceptable to send copies of the record as opposed to removing the original medical record.

CONTINUING EDUCATION AND INSERVICE
Medical Record Department personnel shall be encouraged to participate in educational programs, professional associations, organizational meetings and pertinent correspondence courses related to their duties. Educational achievement shall be documented.

FILING OF INCOMPLETE MEDICAL RECORDS
No medical record shall be filed until it is complete except on order of the Medical Record Committee.

LIST OF COMMONLY USED ABBREVIATIONS, ACRONYMS, AND SYMBOLS
A list of approved abbreviations, acronyms, and symbols for use in the medical record will be maintained in the Medical Record Department. The list shall be approved by the medical staff.

MICROFILMING MEDICAL RECORDS
Charts will be microfilmed after a reasonable period of time depending upon the filing space available for completed medical records. The process of microfilming will be performed by the Medical Record Microfilm Clerk. Records will be screened to ensure accurate patient identification prior to microfilming. Each processed microfilm roll will be reviewed to assure readability of the film prior to the destruction of the original records.

Approved ____________________	Policy Number 90-100
Effective date: June 1, 199x	Revised:
Reviewed:	Revised:

Figure 15–1. An example of a page from a hospital policy and procedure manual illustrating full-block format. Wording and content of hospital policies and procedures vary from institution to institution.

heading for that section. The hospital or institution will usually have a special format, and often special paper, for typing these documents.

Headings and Format

The format will follow outline form using the full-block, modified-block, or indented style. If there is more than one paragraph under a specific title, paragraph just as you would in a full-block letter: double space and begin the new paragraph flush with the left margin. A policy (protocol) should be headed with the title of the policy and its identifying number. Headings should be consistent throughout the report and follow simple guidelines:

1. Title: centered on the page and typed in full capital letters. It may be underlined if you desire.
2. Main topics: full capital letters underlined.
3. Subtopics: full capital letters not underlined.
4. Minor topics: uppercase and lowercase letters underlined.
5. Page one: If the protocol is for a department in the hospital, e.g., emergency room, the page might be shown as ER-1; radiology department may be shown as RD-1, and so on.

Listing

The following rules apply to listing in memos, reports, minutes, or policies.

1. Lists may be introduced with serial numbers or letters of the alphabet followed by a period or parentheses. Bullets (•) are also appropriate substitutes for numbers or letters.
2. Lists are typed in block format under the beginning of each line, and typing is not brought back under the number, letter, or bullet.
3. Lists do not need to be complete sentences but should be terminated with periods.
4. Lists should have parallel construction and be grammatically consistent, e.g., each line beginning with a verb: *type, list, spell, space;* each line beginning with a noun or pronoun: *who, what, when, where;* or each line being a complete sentence.

Multipage Reports

If a hospital protocol, policy, or report continues past one page, the word *continued* may be typed at the bottom of the completed page. The subsequent page or pages begin 1 inch from the top of the page with the title of the document, the page number (the second page might be shown as ER-2 for emergency room, RD-2 for radiology department, and so on), and any other important data (e.g., the policy number).

Closing Format

Figures 15–1 and 15–2 illustrate a simple report or policy closing format typed with the full-block format. The typist should identify every report or policy she or he prepares with a two- or three-letter identification (i.e., initials). Hospital protocols or policies are approved by hospital committees and revised from time to time.

ALVARADO HOSPITAL MEDICAL CENTER

DEPARTMENT OF NURSING SERVICES

Date:

Approved:

Page: 1 of

PROCEDURE:

Reviewed/ Revised by:								
Date:								

Figure 15–2. Sample format for a hospital procedure or policy. (From Fordney, M. T., and Diehl, M. O.: Medical Transcription Guide: Do's and Don'ts. W. B. Saunders Company, Philadelphia, 1990.)

15

MEMORANDA

The purpose of the memo *(memorandum;* plural, memos or *memoranda)* is to quickly and economically send communication to one or more people within the office, company, department, or hospital. A memo may convey a very formal, a casual or informal, or an impersonal impression. Usually, courtesy titles are not used for the addressees or the writer; the use of first names or initials is acceptable. Decide whether the memo dictates a formal or informal approach, and treat the use of names accordingly. Memos can be of one type or a combination of several types: *informative,* providing facts and explanations; *directive,* containing step-by-step instructions with explanations; or *administrative,* stating policy or official opinion or judgment on a topic. Memos provide permanent or temporary records. Never write memos about a confidential matter or delicate subject, to express delicate feelings, or when emotionally upset or angry.

A special format is used for writing memos, and composing a memo is very much like composing a letter. First, identify what you want to say and why you are saying it. Second, think of your reader. Design the memo in such a way that the information you want to communicate is easy to absorb and in such a form that the reader will be able to make use of the information easily. As in all business writing, the message should be clear, concise, correct, and complete.

15

Format

Preprinted Forms

Some businesses prefer to have preprinted forms available for short memos, which may be handwritten or typed. Care must be taken to match the bottom of each line of typing with the bottom of each line of printing. A variable line spacer can be used to achieve this alignment. The distance between each printed line may determine the spacing of the remainder of the memo. Memos are usually single spaced.

Typed Format

When using plain paper, type out the appropriate headings. Set tabulation stops two or three spaces after the longest guide word in each column so that the information is vertically aligned. This format is preferred when additional space is required for the list of the persons receiving the memo.

The following elements are used in setting up the format for the memo, with an explanation for each. The first four headings are typed on the actual memorandum. (See Fig. 15–3 for the memo format.) Preprinted forms, made of less expensive paper than letter stationery, are usually available, but if not, use plain paper and type in the headings.

Date: Date of origination.

To: A list of the names of the persons or departments for routing of the memo. When sending a memo to individuals who are on the same level (medical transcriptionists), list the names in alphabetical order. If a memo is being sent to individuals on various professional levels, list the names by rank. Indicate distribution by writing *please route* on a single copy of the memo with names listed or by making a copy for each person or department.

From: Writer or dictator. The originator usually does not sign the memo but may initial it next to his or her name or at the bottom of the memo.

Subject: The subject line appears in the heading and tells the reader what the memo is about; thus, the reader can get right to the main point. The accuracy of the subject line is extremely important.

The headings may be vertical or horizontal depending on the employer's or typist's preference.

VERTICAL:

DATE:
TO:
FROM:
SUBJECT:

The headings are typed flush with the left margin, in full capital letters followed by a colon. Begin typing the headings 2 inches from the top of the paper, and double space between headings. Set a tab 12 spaces in from the left margin, and tab over to fill in the headings.

Triple space and then begin the body of the memo.

The body of the memo is single spaced, with a double space between paragraphs. Use full-block format.

Figure 15–3 provides a sample of the vertical-style memo.

```
                         MEMORANDUM

DATE:    September 22, 199x
TO:      Joan M. Abbott
         Shirley N. Andrews
         Marilyn P. Dorley

FROM:    Michael Jones, MD     mj

SUBJECT: Office Procedure Manual

It has come to my attention that when someone is sick or leaves on
vacation, it is difficult to know how to complete certain tasks in
the office.  Therefore, I would like each of you to work on a pro-
cedure manual for your specific job in this office outlining from
A to Z exactly what tasks you perform and how to carry them out.

The following activities should be listed.
     1.  Daily duties.
     2.  Weekly duties.
     3.  Monthly duties.
     4.  Quarterly duties.
     5.  Yearly duties.
     6.  Stat duties.

Please have this ready by November 22.
sna
```

Figure 15–3. Sample memorandum, vertical style.

HORIZONTAL:

TO:	DATE:
FROM:	SUBJECT:

Type the first two headings flush with the left margin, and double space between the headings. Tab over eight spaces from the left margin to fill in the name or names of the recipient or recipients of the memo, and repeat to fill in the name of the author. Type DATE and SUBJECT to the right of the center of the page. From the first letter of DATE, tab over 12 spaces to begin typing the date, and repeat to fill in the name of the subject. You can see that this format is not as easy to do as the more popular vertical style and could be inappropriate if the subject line is lengthy. Triple space down to the body of the memo, and complete as described for the vertical style.

It is simple to prepare a macro on your computer that you can recall anytime you need to compose or transcribe a memo. If you use plain paper and prepare memos often, it is worth the time to make a macro.

HINT: When preparing these macros, do not forget to insert the "pause" feature after each heading so you are able to insert the variables when you play it out. If you frequently use E-mail to send memos, you need only to insert the names of the recipients, with their E-mail addresses and the subject, because the date and your name will appear as a regular part of the E-mail message.

Closing Elements: The memo is completed with the typist's initials a double space after the last line of the body of the memo. It is not necessary to type the author's initials, but one should do so if it is the custom in the organization. A typed signature line is not used, nor does the author/dictator sign the memo. (There is a trend toward omitting the FROM line in favor of a typed signature at the close of the memo. If you choose this less formal approach, the author may initial or sign the memo here.) Even though the memo is not signed by the author, it should always be submitted to him or her for approval before being distributed. Some writers will initial their memo after their name on the FROM line. Reference initials, enclosures, and copy notations should be handled exactly as

15

they are in a letter: reference initials are typed two line spaces below the closing, then the enclosure line, followed by the copy notation, followed by the postscript, in that order, one or two line spaces below one another.

Continuations: If the memo continues to an additional page or pages, begin typing 1 inch from the top of the page and type in your headings: name of the addressee, date, and page number. Triple space and continue with the body of the memo.

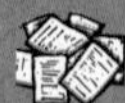 15–1: PRACTICE TEST

Directions: The following is a handwritten note from your employer. Complete the memo with his name as the originator. Your employer is William A. Berry, MD, and the other employees in the office are Mary Connors, CMT, Sue Marcos, RN, and Joan Taylor, CMA-A. Your name and title (office manager) should also be listed as one of the recipients.

5-7-9X
please compose a memo
for my segnature to be distrebuted
to all the staff concerning use
of the new photocopy machine.
I want everyone to receive a copy
of the operation manual +
upkeep of the machine. Each
staff member should be
thoroughly familiar with
operation. The machine is
to be used only for reproducing
billing statements, making copies
of insurance forms, copies of
chart documents when
required + office correspondence.
There will be no personal use of
the machine without my
permission WAB

15

AGENDA

The agenda is prepared before a meeting and establishes the order of business of the meeting and the items to be discussed or the plan of activities. It may be mailed to the membership before the meeting or distributed as the meeting begins. The secretary will be able to use a copy to assist in taking notes and preparing the minutes.

The format of the agenda should be functional and easy to read. These goals are achieved by using layout techniques such as centered headings, columnar lists for agenda items, and white space between items. The agenda should be typed and double spaced and kept to one page if possible. Roman numerals are often used to number the items. The following information may be included in a formal agenda:

1. Name, date, and time of the meeting (centered on the page).
2. Location of the meeting.
3. Call to order.
4. Roll call and/or introduction of members and/or board of directors.
5. Introduction of guests and/or new members.
6. Reading and approval of the minutes of the previous meeting.
7. Officers' reports. This is the main topic, and the individual reports are listed as subtopics.
8. Committee reports. This is the main topic, and the individual committee reports are listed as subtopics.
9. Old business. Unfinished business from the previous meeting is included. This is the main topic, and the individual topics constituting old business are listed as subtopics.
10. New business. This is the main heading, and the individual topics (when known) constituting new business are listed as subtopics. Additional space is allowed at this point so that new topics can be added shortly before the meeting (at the president's discretion) or during the meeting.
11. Announcements. Often includes when and where the next meeting will be held.
12. Adjournment.

Figure 15–4 provides a sample informal agenda, and Figure 15–5 provides a sample formal agenda.

Team Medical Management Program Agenda

May 9, 199X

☐ Call to order
☐ Roll call
☐ Approval of minutes of last meeting
☐ Reports of officers
☐ Reports of committees
☐ Old Business
- Attendance
- Changes in meeting time/day
- Special project funding

☐ New Business
- Health Fair
- Treadmill
- Vacation schedules

☐ Announcements
☐ Adjournment

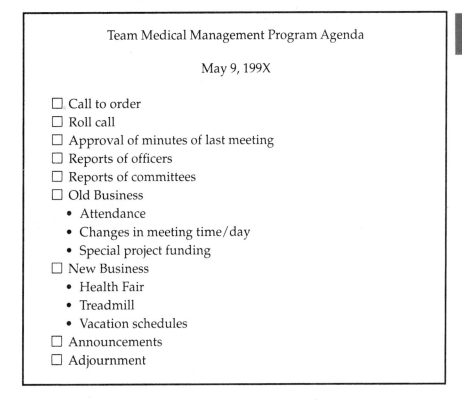

Figure 15–4. Sample of an informal agenda with squares introducing main headings and bullets introducing subheadings. (From Fordney, M. T., and Diehl, M. O.: Medical Transcription Guide: Do's and Don'ts. W. B. Saunders Company, Philadelphia, 1990.)

AGENDA

TEAM MEDICAL MANAGEMENT PROGRAM

May 9, 199X

I. Call to Order

II. Roll Call and introduction of guests

James Morgan, MD, representative from
Bayville Hospital

III. Approval of Minutes of April 14, 199X

IV. Officers' Reports

Treasurer's report

V. Committees

1. Bylaws Committee
2. Membership Committee
3. Nominating Committee
4. Credentials Committee

VI. Old Business

1. Attendance
2. Proposed changes in meeting time or day
3. Special project funding

VII. New Business

1. Health Fair (Dr. Dunn)
2. Evaluation of treadmill (Dr. Patton)
3. Discussion of 199X vacation schedules (Dr. Majur)

VIII. Announcements

Position open at Desert View Community. See Ron Miller.

Next meeting: Wednesday, June 18, 3 p.m., Board Room
(subject to approval today)

IX. Adjournment

Figure 15–5. Sample of a formal agenda. (From Fordney, M. T., and Diehl, M. O.: Medical Transcription Guide: Do's and Don'ts. W. B. Saunders Company, Philadelphia, 1990.)

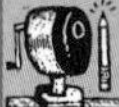

15–2: SELF-STUDY

Directions: Referring to Figure 15–6, use that format, with Roman numerals, and type an agenda that might have been prepared before this meeting took place. See the end of the chapter for a possible agenda after you have completed the exercise.

MINUTES

Minutes are the notes taken or a brief summary of a meeting. They become the official documentation when approved by the members of the organization. A standardized form can be used to fill in information as the meeting is conducted. Basically, it follows the items in the agenda for the meeting.

Minutes are usually taken by the recording secretary, although anyone attending the meeting may take minutes. It is helpful to have the minutes of the previous meeting, a list of the membership, committee lists and their descriptions, a copy of bylaws that the organization has adopted to govern its meetings, and the agenda for the meeting. The detail with which the notes are taken (or tape recorded) is determined by the organization and the business conducted. Depending on the policy of the organization, discussions are summarized and speakers are cited. With experience, you will learn what to record verbatim, what to paraphrase, and what to omit from the record. Format is flexible but can be done as follows:

Title. The heading is usually centered on the page and typed in full capital letters. Underlining is optional.

Date, Time, and Place. Date, time, and place of the meeting may be part of the heading or part of the report itself. The presiding officer is identified with the *call to order* or adjournment notation.

Names of the Members. Names of the members present as well as members absent are listed in the minutes. If roll is taken, that sheet may be attached to the minutes. The names are usually listed in alphabetical order. List the names and include appropriate titles and other identifying information of any ex officio members or guests in attendance.

Format. The format should be consistent from meeting to meeting and secretary to secretary. The events should be reported in the order in which they occurred during the meeting. Outline format should be followed using the full-block, modified-block, or indented style. The titles of the sections follow those of the agenda used at the meeting itself. Roman numerals are often used to introduce the titles of each section. Generally, headings (with or without numbers) should be typed flush with the left margin. Single space the material under the headings and double space between headings. The headings are typed either in full capital letters and underlined or with just the initial letter of the main words capitalized and the entire heading underlined.

The following items should be included: approval of minutes of the previous meeting; records of all officer and committee reports; records of all motions, seconds, and so on; action on any unfinished business; record of new business; announcements, including the date, time, and place of the next meeting; and the time of adjournment.

If the minutes are more than one page, the word *continued* may be typed at the bottom of each completed page. The subsequent page or pages begin 1 inch from the top of the page with the title of the minutes, the page number, and any other important data.

Listing. See *Listing* under Typing Hospital Protocols at the beginning of this chapter.

Closing. The salutation *Respectfully submitted* followed by a triple space and the originator's name closes the minutes. The typist identifies the preparation of the document with a two- or three-letter identification (i.e., initials) and a double space at the end, flush with the left margin.

Distribution. The minutes should be typed as soon as possible after the meeting and a copy distributed to all members (those present at the meeting and those absent) unless it is the custom to read the minutes at the following meeting. Some committees or organizations have a special distribution list that will include anyone who needs to be aware of the proceedings. At the next meeting, the minutes are read aloud and amended if necessary either on the page or, if lengthy, typed and attached as an addendum. See Figure 15–6 for a sample of minutes.

15

OUTLINES

Outlines are traditionally set up as shown in Figure 15–7. Remember that you must have at least two divisions or subdivisions in each set or a set cannot be made. Roman numerals, arabic numerals, and letters of the alphabet are combined to identify different heading levels. A period and a double space follow each number or letter of the alphabet except at the levels where the parentheses are used, at which point you double space after the closing parenthesis. The outlines are indented so that successive levels are obvious. Leave space to backspace from the main topics to accommodate the width of the roman numerals. It is helpful to use the decimal tab set to align these numerals properly.

Desert View Hospital Mirage, Arizona

SAFETY COMMITTEE

MINUTES

DATE:

A meeting of the Safety Committee was called to order at 2:05 p.m. on August 22, 199x, in the Board Room.

MEMBERS PRESENT:

Jack Herzog, Terri Peters, Bobbi Lee, Rita Hardin, Bob Duncan, Roland Wolf, Joan Yubetta, Carolyn Rath, Pam Hollingsworth, and Dave Leithoff.

MEMBERS ABSENT:

Absent and excused were Peter Hulbert, Mary Harreld, and Carolyn Germano.

MINUTES:

The minutes of the previous meeting were read. Bobbie Lee's name was added to the list of members present for the July 26 Safety Committee Meeting. The minutes were then approved as corrected.

ROTATION OF MEMBERSHIP:

A discussion was held concerning rotation of membership. It was suggested that Doreen Black be admitted as a member of the committee. It was also suggested that each member take turns inviting one guest with Bob Duncan bringing the first guest. Jack Herzog will contact the departments not represented at the Safety Committee.

ELECTRICAL SAFETY PROGRAM:

Joan Yubetta suggested that an electrical safety program be started. Rita Hardin reported that electrical cords are not being taped down.

FIRE DRILLS:

Dave Leithoff reported that there had been no fire drill in a month and suggested that there should be one by the end of September.

FIRST AID:

15

Terri Peters reported a total of 36 injuries for the month of August. Back injuries were down to five for August. There were seven falls, three cuts, and one foreign body.

It was suggested by Bob Duncan and Terri Peters that a form be designed for reporting scratches, puncture wounds, etc.

BEVERAGE SPILLING:

It was suggested that Bobbi Lee put an article in the Capsule on the spilling of beverages. It was further suggested that spill stations be set up in key places in the hospital. Bob Duncan will bring this up in the cabinet meeting.

ADJOURNMENT:

There being no further business, the meeting was adjourned at 4:15 p.m. by Bob Duncan, Chairperson.

Respectfully submitted,

Dave Leithoff, Recording Secretary

lro

Figure 15–6. Sample of minutes typed in full-block format.

TITLE CENTERED AND TYPED IN FULL CAPS

I. Main Topic (first item) (Capitalize the first letter of each important word.)
    A. Secondary heading (Capitalize the first letter and any proper nouns here and at all other levels.)
    B. . . .
    C. . . .
    D. . . .
        1. Third level heading
        2. . .
        3. . .
        4. . .
            a. Fourth level heading
            b. . . .
                (1) Fifth level heading
                (2). . . .
                (3). . . .
                    (a) Sixth level heading
                    (b). . . .

II. Main Topic (second item) (You will have to backspace once to allow for the roman numeral — for balance.)
    A. . . .
    B. . . .
    C. . . .
        1. . . .
        2. . . .
    D. . . .
        1. . . .
        2. . . .
        3. . . .

III. Main Topic (third item) (You will have to backspace twice on this line for balance.)

The major headings and subdivisions may be a single word or phrase; long phrases or clauses; complete sentences; or any combination of sentences, phrases, and single words.

Between-line spacing is as follows:
After title: triple-space.
Main topic: double-space before and after each one.
Subdivision items: single-space.
Very brief outline: double-space all.

Indenting is as follows:
Roman numerals: align to the left margin
Division under each topic: set tab stops for four-space indent
Second line: begin the second line of an item directly under the first letter of that line

Figure 15–7. Outline mechanics. (From Fordney, M. T., and Diehl, M. O.: Medical Transcription Guide: Do's and Don'ts. W. B. Saunders Company, Philadelphia, 1990.)

15

 15–3: PRACTICE TEST

Directions: The following is from a section of the hospital's cardiovascular laboratory procedure manual. Type it in correct full-block format with careful attention to main headings, subheadings, and additional heading levels. Refer to Figure 15–1. You will begin by typing page CV-15, and the second page will be CV-16. It will be entitled Holter Monitor. At the end of the procedure, put in the approved signature line; the effective date will be the current date. The policy number is 90-202.

Objective: To obtain a magnetic tape record of a patient's electrocardiographic activity over a 24-hour period. Equipment: 1. Holter monitor. 2. Battery. 3. Tape. 4. Patient cable. 5. Universal cable. 6. ECG machine. 7. ECG electrodes. 8. 2 × 2 pads, alcohol, and Redux paste. 9. Transpore tape. 10. Patient diary. 11. Shaving prep kit. Procedure: 1. Verify the physician's order by checking the medical chart. 2. Assemble all equipment and bring to the patient's bedside. 3. Introduce yourself to the patient and thoroughly explain what you are about to do. 4. Verify the patient's identity by checking the patient's I.D. bracelet. 5. Have the patient remove all clothing covering his or her chest. 6. Locate the necessary anatomical landmarks and prepare the five areas as follows: a. Shave all hair. b. Cleanse the area with alcohol. c. Scrub the cleansed area with Redux paste. d. Remove the Redux paste with alcohol. 7. Attach the electrodes to the patient's chest: a. 2nd rib space on the right side of the sternum. b. 2nd rib space on the left side of the sternum. c. over the xiphoid process. d. Right V4—Right mid-clavicular at the 5th intercostal space. e. Left V4—Left mid-clavicular at the 5th intercostal space. 8. Attach the electrode cables to the patient: a. White—right arm. b. Brown—left arm. c. Black—V1. d. Green—right leg. e. Red—left leg. 9. Tape the electrode cables in a loop on the patient's abdomen allowing the cable to hang free. 10. Place a tape in the Holter monitor unit. 11. Place a battery in the Holter monitor unit. 12. Attach the recorder to the belt or shoulder strap (patient's preference). 13. Plug Universal cable into recorder. 14. Connect RA, LA, RL, LL, and V1 from ECG machine to Universal cable. 15. Connect patient cable to recorder. 16. Run a short strip on the ECG machine to verify the quality of the tracing (L1, L2, L3, AVR, AVL, AVF, and V1). 17. Disconnect Universal cable from recorder unit. 18. Set time on recorder and start Holter monitor. 19. Record starting time in the patient diary and explain the importance of the diary to the patient. 20. If an outpatient, remind the patient of the importance of returning in 24 hours. 21. After 24 hours, record ending time in the patient's diary. 22. Remove the cable from the recorder. 23. Remove the cable and electrodes from the patient. 24. Prepare the tape for scanning. Care of Equipment: 1. Exercise caution when handling unit to avoid dropping. 2. Instruct patient not to bathe, shower, or go swimming while attached to the unit. 3. Clean recording heads and capstan with alcohol after each patient use. Important Points: 1. Proper preparation of the patient's chest is important to a good recording. 2. Run a short strip with the ECG machine to insure that the electrodes are placed correctly. 3. Make sure the patient thoroughly understands the importance of the diary.

A *Answers to* **15–2: SELF-STUDY**

AGENDA
SAFETY COMMITTEE MEETING
August 22, 199X

I. Call to Order
II. Roll Call and Introduction of Guests
III. Approval of Minutes of July 26, 199X
IV. Rotation of Membership
V. Electrical Safety Program
VI. Fire Drills
VII. First Aid
VIII. Beverage Spilling
IX. New Business (This might be included on the agenda in the event someone at the meeting might want to discuss some new problem to work on.)
X. Adjournment

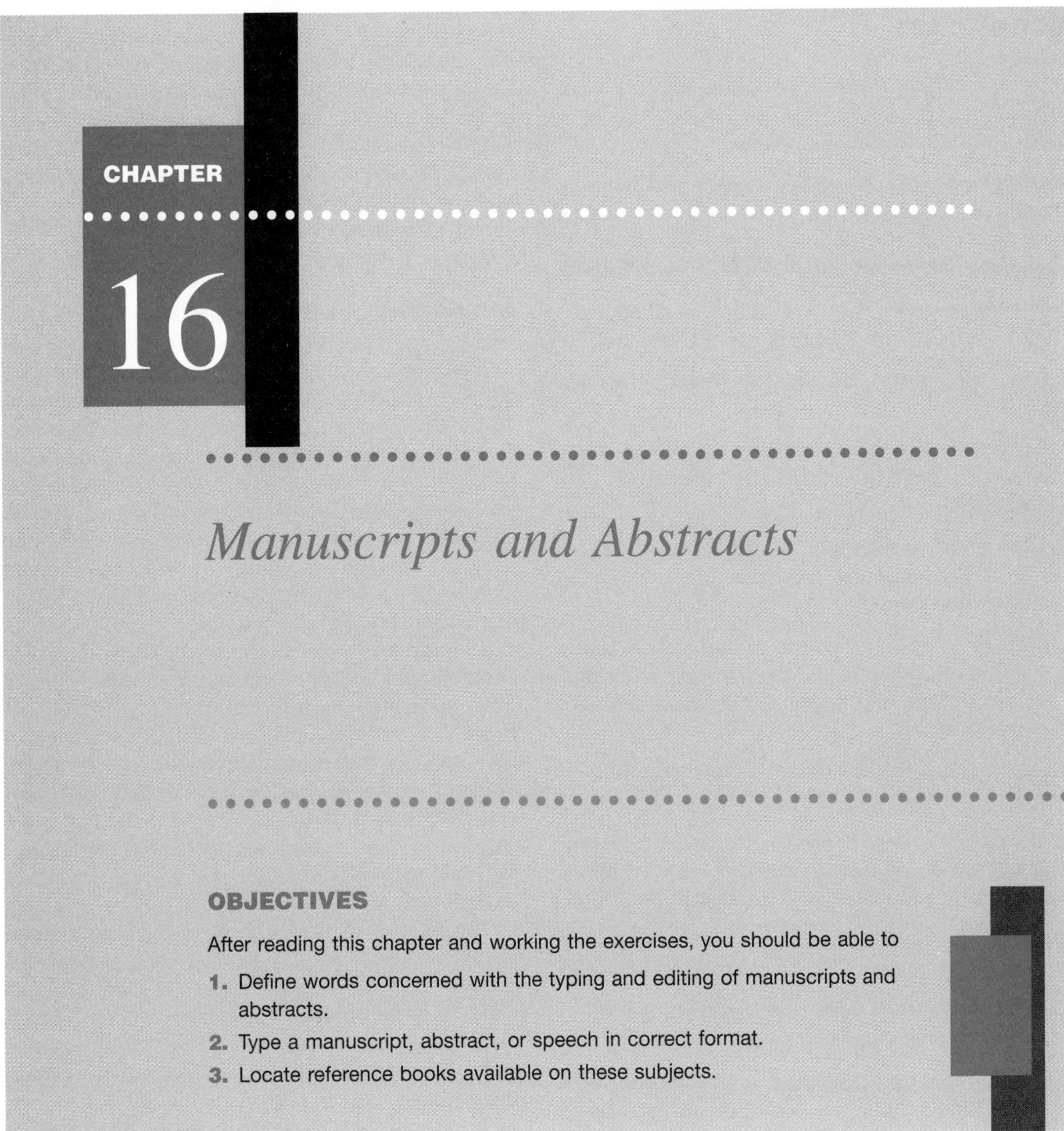

CHAPTER

16

Manuscripts and Abstracts

OBJECTIVES

After reading this chapter and working the exercises, you should be able to

1. Define words concerned with the typing and editing of manuscripts and abstracts.
2. Type a manuscript, abstract, or speech in correct format.
3. Locate reference books available on these subjects.

16

INTRODUCTION

Because of ever-changing surgical techniques, new drugs, and modern equipment, a physician must continue his or her education. Physicians share the information they gain in their practice, in research, and in study by writing and lecturing about their discoveries and observations. The transcriptionist may be asked to assist the physician in the preparation of these articles and speeches by helping to assemble the material and by typing and editing the manuscript. If the article is published, the transcriptionist may help with corrections by checking the galley proofs.

In this chapter, you will learn how to help the physician with his or her research and how to type the manuscript properly. Each medical journal or magazine has different guidelines for the preparation of an abstract or a manuscript. Therefore, it is important for you to have these instructions on hand before attempting to do the final typing. Many times, these instructions are sent to an author after an abstract has been submitted and accepted. These guidelines also appear in journals and magazines, so you can clip these out of a current issue of any journal in question. Because proofreading has been discussed in Chapter 7, we occasionally make reference to that chapter.

VOCABULARY

Abstract: A brief statement of each part of a book, article, speech, court record, or case record as it leads up to the conclusion.

Bibliography: A list of the books, articles, and literary works used or referred to by an author. Each entry includes the name of the author, the title, the publisher, and the date of publication.

Book Review: A critical report and evaluation, as in a newspaper or magazine, of a current book.

Epitome: A short statement of the main points of a book, report, incident, and so on.

Footnote: A note of reference at the bottom of the manuscript page or within the context of the manuscript.

Galley proof: Printer's proof sent in uncut sheets to permit correction of errors before the type is made up into pages.

Heading: A word or words set above or at the beginning of the text to identify text divisions, paragraphs, and so on; usually set in a different typeface in books.

Legend: A description or key to explain an illustration or photograph.

Manuscript: A handwritten or typewritten document or paper, such as an author's copy or his or her work, as submitted to a publisher or printer.

Margin: The blank space around the typed area on a manuscript page.

16

Proofread: To read and mark corrections on a manuscript, galley proof, or page proof.

Reprint: An edition (booklet or pamphlet) of a printed work that is a verbatim copy of the original.

Summary: A statement that abbreviates the contents of the article as a whole.

Synopsis: A statement giving a brief, general review or condensation; a summary.

RESEARCH OF A PROFESSIONAL REPORT

One of the important steps in writing a paper is thorough research of the subject; a medical transcriptionist can help an employer in this if he or she knows where to go for help and what to look for. The reference librarian of your local library can help you locate articles in the *Cumulative Index Medicus,* the *Current List of Medical Literature,* and the *Hospital and Health Information Index,* or you can obtain information from computer systems, such as MEDLARS (Medical Literature Analysis and Retrieval Systems). You can use software termed GRATEFUL MED with a feature called LOANSOME DOC. This MEDLINE software was developed by the National Library of Medicine and provides immediate access to abstracts and journals.

PREPARING A MANUSCRIPT

The proper format of a typed manuscript is shown on the following pages. The manuscript begins with a title page and a table of contents. These may be optional, depending on whether the paper is to be given as a lecture or submitted to a publisher. A professional report also contains a list of acknowledgments, a body, illustrations or figures with legends, and a bibliography. You will notice that on pages 371 to 379, the margins and positions of each typed line are given to you.

The first (or rough) draft may be triple spaced to allow space for corrections and revisions. Paper of different colors may be used to distinguish between first, second, and final drafts. If you make a photocopy of the manuscript, the physician can cut out and rearrange paragraphs or sentences, and you will be spared much extra retyping. If using a word processor or computer, the edited manuscript can then be easily manipulated into a final draft with the cut and paste features.

The final draft is double spaced in manuscript format on white 8 1/2 × 11 inch bond paper. This enables the editor who receives the manuscript to make any additional corrections and to insert instructions to the printer. Type or print on one side of the paper only, and make a photocopy of the original.

If the manuscript is submitted to a journal for publication, the letter of transmittal should contain a statement of its estimated length. Most word processing computer software programs contain a feature that gives you the number of pages in a document, word count, character count, number of paragraphs, and line count. However, if you do not have this feature, you can determine these measurements. To determine the length of a manuscript, add the number of words in six lines. Divide this number by six, to get the average number for one line. Then multiply the average by the number of lines on the page but disregard the lines that have no more than two or three words. The result is the average number of words on one page. To obtain the estimated length for the whole manuscript, multiply the average number of words per page by the total number of pages.

The pages of the body of the manuscript should be numbered. Generally, the first page is not numbered. Beginning with page 2, the numbers should be in the top right corner of the sheet approximately 1/2 inch from the top and 1 inch from the right margin, or they can be centered at the top of the page and typed with a hyphen on each side (-2-). Word processing computer software programs have a feature for placing page numbers automatically and customizing them in your document. When using a word processor, the margins may be less than 1 inch because of the "headers" in the software program.

FIGURES AND ILLUSTRATIONS

If photographs or illustrations are used in the manuscript, these should be attached to separate sheets. It is important to cite these in the body of the manuscript by stating, for example, "see Figure 16–1," meaning the first illustration in the sixteenth chapter. Permission must be obtained for the use of a photograph from the person photographed or, if the illustration is borrowed from another source, from the publisher of the original picture.

Text continued on page 378

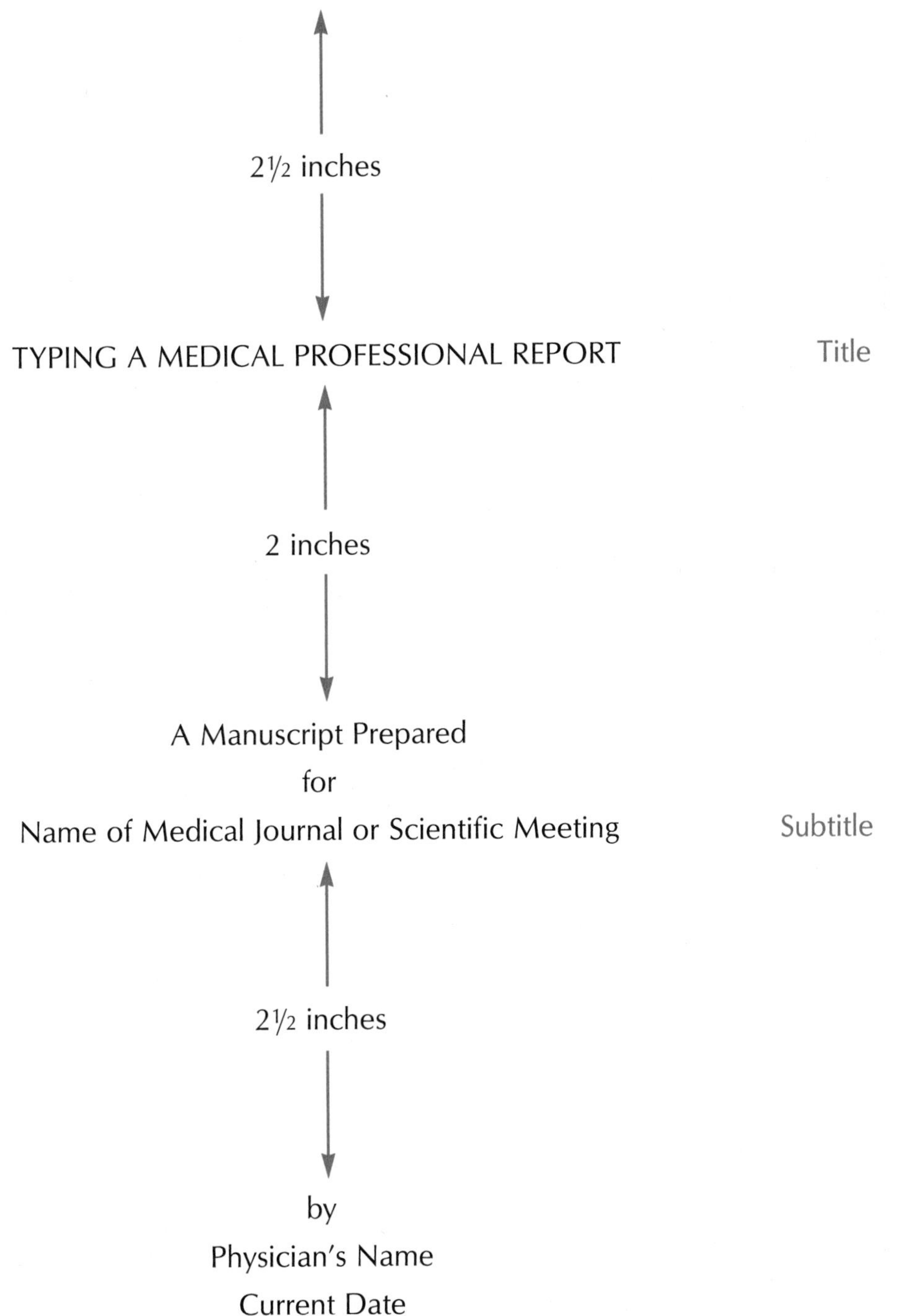

16

Center the Table of Contents on the page.

TABLE OF CONTENTS

← Triple space

Page

↑ 3 spaces

16

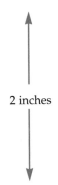

2 inches

Main Heading

TYPING A MEDICAL PROFESSIONAL REPORT

Triple space

Double Space

1- or $1^1/_2$-inch margin

This is your manuscript typing guide. It will help you prepare a manuscript for your physician. Always double space the body of the manuscript and indent five or ten spaces at the beginning of each paragraph. Make a photocopy of each page and retain it for your records. The left margin should be 1 or $1^1/_2$ inches, and the right margin should be 1 inch.

Triple space

1-inch margin

Underline or all caps and no underline

Title Page

A title page is not necessary for most manuscripts submitted for publication. If you need to type a title page, refer to page 371 for proper format.

Underline or all caps and no underline

Table of Contents

The table of contents is a list of headings of the major parts of the manuscript. It is required by some, but not all, publishers. When required, it is composed after the entire manuscript has been completed so that correct page numbers can be inserted. Notice that the entire table of contents has been centered vertically on page 372.

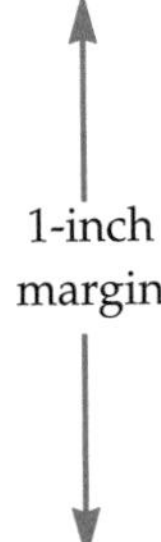

16

—2— ← Page Number

underline → Margins

The body of the manuscript is typed double spaced on 8½ x 11 inch paper. It should have 1-inch top, bottom, and side margins, except for a 2-inch top margin on the first page. If a manuscript is bound, it requires extra space on the left for the binding; therefore you would leave a 1½-inch margin. Direct quotations of four or more lines are single-spaced and indented, without quotation marks, five spaces from each margin. Numbered items are listed numerically and indented five spaces from each margin, single spaced with double spacing between each item.

Try to keep the right margin as even as possible and divide words according to proper word division guidelines. Do not have two consecutive end-of-line hyphenations and do not end a page with a hyphenated word. You may type two or three spaces beyond the desired right margin to avoid word division.

Headings

The titles of the main divisions of the body of the manuscript are called headings. These headings should appear in the table of contents. Main headings are usually centered on the page and typed in all capital letters. There are two kinds of subheadings: side headings and paragraph headings.

Side Heading → Side Headings

These indicate major divisions of the main topic. Type them even with the left margin, with the main words starting with a capital letter.

Underline them and follow with double spacing. Triple space before a side heading and double space after it.

Paragraph Headings. It the paragraph needs to be divided further, paragraph headings may be used. The main words of the heading are begun with a capital letter, indented, underlined, and followed by a period. Do not underline the period.

Footnotes

When original material has been used in a manuscript, credit must be given in a footnote. It is not necessary that it be a direct quotation. Footnotes may be typed in any of the following ways: 1) Typed at the bottom of the page on which the reference has been made, 2) typed in the copy directly below the statement referred to and separated by two solid lines, or 3) typed on a separate sheet listed together at the end of the chapter or report. The format for footnotes is usually determined by the publisher. Footnotes are numbered consecutively throughout the report. If a footnote is to be included at the bottom of the typed page, allowance of space must be made. Allow 1/2 inch (three lines) for each 2-line footnote. A footnote should never be continued on another page. Here is an example of a direct quotation that illustrates how the footnote would appear if typed directly below the statement.

A manuscript submitted to an editor, publisher, or printer should be carefully and attractively typed.[1]

---

1. Sarah Augusta Taintor and Kate M. Monro, *The Secretary's Handbook,* The Macmillan Company, New York, New York, 1969, p. 435.

Look below to see how a footnote would appear if credit is given at the bottom of the typed page. Footnotes placed on the page should be set off from the last line of the text by a 1½- to 2-inch underline. The underline is preceded by a single space and is followed by a double space. Each footnote is single spaced (with the first line indented); a double space is left between footnotes. If the article was presented at a scientific meeting, the information regarding the name of the medical society and the date of the meeting should be included in a footnote. You can also place a light pencil mark about ½ inch above the bottom margin for each footnote that should appear on the bottom of the page. The pencil mark will remind you to type the footnotes. Adjust the left margin for a bound manuscript.

---

1. Sarah Augusta Taintor and Kate M. Munro, *The Secretary's Handbook,* The Macmillan Company, New York, New York, 1969, p. 435.

Any one of a number of special expressions may be used in referring to a previously cited work to avoid repeating the original footnote in its entirety. Here is a key to these and to other special terms used in manuscript preparation.

16

Term	*Meaning*
c., cir.	about
ca., circa	about

cf.	compare
do.	ditto
e.g.	for example
et al.	and elsewhere, or and others
et seq.	and the following
f. or ff.	following. Used after a page number to indicate that the next page or pages are also referred to.
ibid.	in the same place. Refers to a book, article, etc., cited in a reference immediately preceding.
i.e.	that is
l.	line
ll.	lines
loc. cit.	in the place cited. Refers to exactly the same place in a book, article, etc., cited in an earlier reference, but not the one immediately preceding. (For the latter reference you would use "ibid.")
n.b.	note well
op. cit.	in the work cited. Refers to a book, article, etc., cited in a reference not immediately preceding.
sic	thus. Used to emphasize that an unlikely looking expression or spelling is really the one meant.
q.v.	which see
viz.	namely

Bibliography

A bibliography is a list of sources of information related to the topic discussed in the manuscript. It can be a list of the words of an author or of the literature pertaining to a particular subject. Bibliographical entries differ from footnotes in that they are arranged in alphabetical order by the surnames of the authors. If the author is not known, the title of the reference is used. The following page is an example of a typed bibliography, which shows format and spacing. It also gives ten different bibliographic examples.

A legend is written for each of the figures, and these are typed on a separate sheet of paper, double spaced and numbered to correspond to each figure. Place the author's name, the title of the manuscript, and the number of the figure on the back of each photograph or illustration. Black-and-white glossy photographs reproduce best. Some journals will accept color photographs. Charts and line drawings should be done in india ink on heavy white bond paper.

Items Illustrated

1. Unpublished manuscript
2. One-author book
3. Two-author book
4. A book written by a number of authors
5. Book with subtitle and a four-author book
6. Encyclopedia
7. Bound volume of a periodical with page reference
8. Newspaper
9. Bound volume of a professional journal citing volume and page
10. Public document

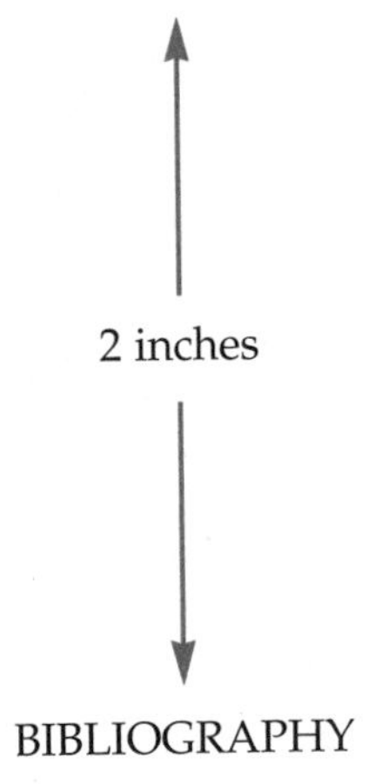

BIBLIOGRAPHY

← Triple space

Item

1 Follis, Joan L., and Marilyn T. Fordney, Medical Office Procedures Worktext, Syllabus, Ventura College, Ventura, California, 1977.

2 Franks, Richard, Simplified Medical Dictionary, Medical Economics/Delmar Publishers, Albany, New York, 1977.

3 Frederick, Portia M., and Mary E. Kinn, The Medical Office Assistant, Administrative and Clinical, W.B. Saunders Company, Philadelphia, Pennsylvania, 1988.

4 Lessenberry, D. D. et al., College Typewriting, South-Western Publishing Company, Cincinnati, Ohio, 1975.

5 Lessenberry, D. D., S. J. Wanousc, C. H. Duncan, and S. E. Warner, College Typewriting, Self-Paced Activities—An Individualized Approach, 9th edition, South-Western Publishing Company, Cincinnati, Ohio, 1976.

6 "Manuscript," The World Book Encyclopedia, 1970, XIII, p. 130.

7 Murphy, Lucie Spence, "Techniques On Writing The Medical Article," Medical Record News, American Medical Record Association, Chicago, Illinois, LIV, No. 6 (April, 1970), pp. 38–43.

8 Oxnard Press Courier, May 23, 1985, p. 15.

9 Swindle, Robert E., "Individualized Instruction in Business Communication," Journal of Business Education, Volume XL (May, 1973), pp. 335–336.

10 United States Government Printing Office Style Manual, Washington, D.C., U.S. Government Printing Office, 1984.

16

EDITING AND PROOFREADING

The entire manuscript should be proofread several times to check for clarity of meaning, spelling, punctuation, grammar, and other mechanics before it is submitted for publication. If the manuscript has been accepted by the publisher, it will be typeset into galley proofs. These are sent to the author for final corrections, deletions, and additions. The galley proof is carefully matched with the original manuscript to be sure that nothing has been omitted and then returned to the publisher to be made into page proofs. Formal proofreading signs and symbols are used on manuscript, galley proof, and page proof. You learned to use these in Chapter 7.

16–1: PRACTICE TEST

Directions: A rough draft of a manuscript page appears below. Retype this draft as it would appear in final manuscript form. You will notice formal proofreading corrections and errors in spelling and punctuation. The title of the manuscript is "Cocktails Can Cause Cardiac Complications."[1] The author is Roger Balor, MD, Mount Sinai Hospital and Mount Sinai School of Medicine of the City University of New York, New York City. Dr. Balor wishes to submit this manuscript to *Modern Medicine* in Chicago, Illinois, for publication. Prepare a title page.

At the bottom of your typed page, place a footnote to indicate that some of the material for this paper came from an abstract that appeared in the *Quarterly Journal for the Study of Alcoholism,* volume 34, pages 774–785, 199X. The paper was written by George J. Sanna, MD, University Hospital, Boston, Massachusetts.

¶ Prolonged, heavy ingestion of alcohol by certain individuals ~~people~~, even though they are well # nourished, may result in cardiac abnormalities that are clinically evident or electrocardiographically, or both. Electrocardiographic abnormalities in these patients may indicate the ~~early~~ stet developmental stages of cardimyopathy, a process that may be reversed if the patient abstrains from ingestion ~~drinking~~ of alcohol. ¶ Cardiac abnormalities in well nourished alcoholics may include resting tachycardia sinus tachycardia or bradycardia premature ventricular contractions premature atrial contractions paroxysmal atrial fibrillation or a rhythm varying between sinus rhythm with frequent premature beats and atrioventricular dissociation. First-degree atriventricular block may be also found. ¶ Notched or tall P waves may be present on the electrocardiogram. In addition, the QRS complex may show some abnormality, as may the S-T segment and T wave. T-wave abnormalities may consist of deminished wave amplitudes, diphasix waves, or frank wave inversion. Some patients may have enlarged hearts. ¶ The electrocardiograms of 50 randomly chosen well nourished alcoholics were studied and compared with those from 50 nonalcholic controls. No subject in either group had any known heart disease. ¶ The electrocardigram was considered to be within normal limits in 36 alcoholic patients but was clearly abnormal

Sp in ④ others. Only one control patient had an abnormal electrocardigram.

ABSTRACT PREPARATION

An abstract is a brief statement of each major part of a report. It shows the reader how the various items in the report lead up to the conclusion. An abstract may also be called a summary or an epitome. Abstracts give the information contained in the article in as brief a fashion as possible.

Many medical and scientific journals include an abstract at the beginning of each major article that they publish. The abstracts may be collected and reissued on a regular basis. Some journals reissue abstracts of articles that originally appeared in other publications; others publish only abstracts of their own articles. See Figure 16–1 for an example of an abstract.

2633

SERUM INTERFERON INHIBITOR FACTOR MODULATES LEVEL OF INTERFERON IN CANCER PATIENTS. R. Medenica, S. Mukerjee*, R. Hankenson*, D. Powell*, T. Huschart*, W. Corbitt*. Cancer Immuno-Biology Laboratory, Hilton Head Island, S.C.

A minimum of 2 regulatory factors of interferon (IFN) were discovered. We previously reported presence of interferon inhibitor factor (IIF) in some immunological disorders. We also reported that patients (pts) suffering from malignant diseases contain IIF in their serum when relapsing; in those pts, serum interferon levels (SIL) were low or non-detectable. In 20 cancer (ca) pts (5-lung non-small cell ca; 5-breast ca; 5-melanoma; 5-colon ca) relapsing after surgery for whom we obtained complete remission (CR) with our combined chemotherapy (CT) and IFN regimen, we evaluated the relationship between serum IIF, SIL and therapy response. Pharmacosensitivity-guided CT and IFN was given for 3 consecutive days/month x 6. The dosage of IFN was adapted for each cycle according to the IIF and SIL. SIL were determined by capability of the pts' sera to protect WISH cells against the viruses if pts' sera contained IFN. These values were compared with standard IFN for testing. Pts' sera containing IIF will neutralize activity of the IFN; therefore, WISH cells will be destroyed by the viruses. The IFN mixture was coupled to the CNBr activated Sepharose-4B and IIF was purified from the pts' sera. Native gel electrophoresis of IIF indicated a single protein band which, when further evaluated on SDS/PAGE, 2 bands were found (200 and 21 Kd range). ELISA and Western blotting analysis failed to show presence of an anti-IFN antibody. With the decrease of the volume of the tumor, IIF decreased in the pts' serum and simultaneously, IFN level increased. In those pts, the IFN to be given needs to be reduced as the pts become sensitive to the IFN (range of decrease was 30-80% dosage given initially). When in remission, repeated tests of IIF confirmed that the pts became free of those factors.

Figure 16–1. Example of an abstract (From Blood 84(suppl 1):662a, 1994).

Some physicians routinely prepare abstracts of articles that they find of interest. If the transcriptionist is able to help with this task, the physician may also dictate an abstract and have you transcribe it. The abstract is typed on a card on which the periodical, author, title, volume, date of publication, and page numbers are indicated. If abstract cards are kept, it is not necessary to clip and file the actual article.

The following are some journals in which abstracts can be found.

American Journal of Medical Sciences
American Journal of Medicine
American Journal of Public Health
Annals of Internal Medicine
Medical Clinics of North America
Clinical Pharmacology and Therapeutics
Journal of the American Medical Association (or JAMA)
New England Journal of Medicine
American Journal of Clinical Nutrition
Lancet
Postgraduate Medicine

A physician may be asked to write an abstract of his or her original article when submitting the article to a journal for publication. The contents of an abstract consist of the following:

1. Surname of the author, with initials or first name
2. Affiliations of the author, if any
3. Title of the article
4. Title of the journal
5. The year, volume, and page numbers of the journal
6. Text (body of the abstract)

If the author writes the abstract, it is signed "author's abstract." If another person writes the abstract, it is signed by that person followed by the name of the institution with which he or she is associated. In some instances, an abstract may be published without a signature.

16

16–2: SELF-STUDY

Directions: Type the following material in abstract form on a plain sheet of 8 1/2 × 11 inch paper for submission to the *Journal of the American Medical Association.*

The title of the abstract is "Treatment of Pain in Hemophilia" by R. A. Binder et al., Georgetown University Hospital, Washington, D.C. 20007. The complete article appeared in the *American Journal of Diseases of Children,* volume 127, pages 371–373, March 199X issue.

Aspirin alters platelet function, causing impairment of ~~large~~ *small* vessel hemostasia and prolongation of bleeding time. Therefore, aspirin should be *avoided* in those who have a tendency to bleed. In this stady [u], a standardized time bleeding, using the template method, was used to screen a number of *stet* common analgesics and anti-inflammatory agents (propoxyphene hydrochloride, salicylate choline, pentazocine hydrochloride, prednisone, and codeine)

Sp in ③ patients with hemophilia A and ⑩ normal volunteers. A comparison of the bleeding time, before and after ingestion of these drugs, showed no major differences. These agnts [e] are suggested for ~~treatment~~ *therapy* in those

Sp ptients [a] with pain ⑧ inflammation who are known to have hemophilia.

16

16–3: PRACTICE TEST

Directions: A rough draft of a manuscript page appears on page 383. Retype this draft as it would appear in final manuscript form, using a plain sheet of 8 1/2 × 11 inch paper. You will notice formal proofreading corrections and errors in spelling and punctuation. Pay special attention to placement of side headings and paragraph headings. The title of the manuscript is "Categories of Tumors." The author is Joan T. Bennett, MD, XYZ Medical Center, Philadelphia, Pennsylvania. Dr. Bennett wants to submit this manuscript to the *Journal of the American Medical Association* in Chicago, Illinois, for publication. Prepare a title page on a plain sheet of 8 1/2 × 11 inch paper. See Appendix A for answers to this test after you have completed it.

Categories of Tumors

There are ~~several~~ many categories of tumors. Epithelial tumors is the topic of interest. 1. Epethelial tumors. These tumors arise from the coelomic mesothelium which is capable of differentiating into both benign and malignant tumors. The transition from benign to malignant is not abrupt there is an a (borderline or intermediate) category. Distinguishing benign borderline or malignant tumors is important in terms of (tx &) prognosis. Epithelial malignancies represent 82% of all ovarian malignancies. a. The predominant cell types are: (1) Serous (a) One out of (3) serous tumors ~~are~~ is malignant. (b) Serous cancers are more (then) (3X) as common as the mucinous variety (& 7X) as common as the endometrioid variety. (c) Serous cyst-adenoma carcinoma the most common type of ovarian cancer tends to be bilateral in 35%–50% of cases. (2) Mucinous (a) One out of (5) mucinous tumors are malignant. (b) Mucinous tumors are bilateral in 10%–20% of cases. (3) Endometrioid (a) The microscopic pattern is similar to primary carcinoma of the endometrium. (b) areas of endometriosis in the ovary may be present. (c) The prognosis is much better (then) that of the serous (&) mucinous carcinomas. b. The prognosis for each stage of epithelial ovarian tumors is linked to the grade of the tumor; poorly differentiated tumors have a poor prognosis. Long-term survival of patients with borderline or well-differentiated cancers after primary surgery is common.

SPEECHES

If the paper is prepared for a lecture, double space it and use large type so the speech can be read easily. At the bottom of each page, in the bottom right corner, type the first two or three words that appear at the beginning of the next page.

BOOK REVIEWS

A physician may be asked to do a book review that is an evaluation of a current publication, with the good and bad points highlighted. These reviews are published in magazines, journals, or newspapers.

16–4: PRACTICE TEST

Directions: Complete the following statements by filling in the blanks.

1. The page in a manuscript that contains the report title, for whom the manuscript is prepared, the name of the author, and the date of the manuscript is called the ______________.
2. A manuscript title is typed in ______________ letters on the title page.
3. When a manuscript is submitted to a journal for publication, a ______________ should accompany it stating the estimated length.
4. The table of contents page indicates the topics in the manuscript and the ______________ of each topic.
5. The body of the manuscript is generally typed with ______________ spacing or ______________ format.
6. Quoted material within a report is normally typed with ______________ spacing.
7. References used to cite the source of quoted material are called ______________.
8. Footnotes are typed with ______________ spacing within the footnote and ______________ spacing between footnotes.
9. Give the abbreviations for the following terms used in footnotes and in the manuscript.
   a. and elsewhere, or, and others ______________
   b. in the same place ______________
   c. in the work cited ______________
   d. that is ______________
   e. for example ______________
10. The ______________ identifies sources or references quoted within the manuscript.
11. When there are three or more authors of a single work, the bibliographic entry gives the name of the first author, followed by the phrase ______________.
12. Indicate the top, bottom, and side margins in inches for the manuscript and provide the correct location of the page number.

	Top	*Bottom*	*Left*	*Right*	*Page Number*
a. Unbound report: Page 1	______	______	______	______	______
Other pages	______	______	______	______	______

16

b. Left-bound report:

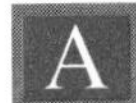

Page 1	______	______	______	______	______
Other pages	______	______	______	______	______

Answers to this test are in Appendix A.

A *Answers to* **16–2: SELF-STUDY**

TREATMENT OF PAIN IN HEMOPHILIA

R. A. Binder, et al. (Georgetown University Hospital, Washington, D.C. 20007), American Journal of Diseases of Children, 127: 371-373 (March) 1984.

Aspirin alters platelet function, causing impairment of small vessel hemostasia and prolongation of bleeding time. Therefore, aspirin should be avoided in those who have a tendency to bleed. In this study, a standardized bleeding time, using the template method, was used to screen a number of common analgesics and anti-inflammatory agents (propoxyphene hydrochloride, salicylate choline, pentazocine hydrochloride, prednisone, and codeine) in three patients with hemophilia A and ten normal volunteers. These agents are suggested for therapy in those patients with pain and inflammation who are known to have hemophilia. A comparison of the bleeding times, before and after ingestion of these drugs, showed no major differences.

Employment

CHAPTER

17

Applying for a Transcribing Position

OBJECTIVES

After reading this chapter and completing the assignments, you will be able to

1. List prospective employers.
2. Contact computerized job search data bases for on-line services.
3. Compose a cover letter to accompany your resume.
4. Prepare a resume.
5. Identify temporary jobs in your locale.
6. Prepare for an interview.
7. Explain professionalism.

INTRODUCTION

Now that you have learned the basic transcription skills, you are ready to hunt for a job and start your new career. There are many factors to consider in beginning your job search: typing your resume, locating prospective employers, and preparing for the interview. We discuss some traditional attitudes to guide those of you seeking a first job, and we give some pointers to those of you already working but planning to change jobs. Refresh your memory by reading through the job duties and responsibilities listed in the American Association for Medical Transcription model job description shown in Chapter 1, Figure 1–2.

PREPARE YOUR RESUME

A resume is a personal statement of "you." There is no exact format to be followed, but usually a resume is chronological or functional, or sometimes a combination of the two. A *chronological* resume is arranged historically (Fig. 17–1), stating recent experiences first, along with the dates and descriptive data for each job. A *functional* resume highlights the qualifications or various duties that an individual can perform (Fig. 17–2). This format is appropriate for you in that you will be applying for a specific job in a specific field, and when your resume is geared specifically to a certain job it is more likely that you will be successful in obtaining that position. A functional resume is also appropriate for those who have breaks in their work experience. The *combination* format emphasizes job skills as well as dates and places of employment (Fig. 17–3). The examples shown give you a few suggestions for organization as well as format.

A one-page resume is ample for a beginning transcriptionist, but someone in midcareer may require two or three pages. However, even if you have enough information for two or three pages, it is wise to try and condense it to one page. When not actively looking for a job, keep a few carefully prepared resumes on hand in case an opportunity arises unexpectedly.

Your resume should be professionally typed or printed on white bond paper. (Or, if you wish to catch the eye of a prospective employer, try using off-white paper.) Handwritten resumes are never acceptable. Carefully check your resume for spelling, punctuation, and typographical errors. If you have someone else proofread your resume, they may spot typographical errors and give you additional suggestions. Even one misspelled word or typographical error could discourage a prospective employer and negate your opportunity for an interview. Use wide, neat margins and balance the information well to produce an attractive page. If you need several copies of the resume, have it reproduced on a copy machine that produces excellent photocopies or have it printed profession-

CURRICULUM VITAE

NAME: Joan M. Seymour

ADDRESS: 4011 Jefferson Street
Belmont, XY 12345-0001

TELEPHONE: 013-487-2399

EDUCATION:

College:	Ventura Community College	Ventura, California	9-94 to 6-96
High School:	Oxnard High School	Oxnard, California	9-90 to 6-94

WORK EXPERIENCE:

John D. Avers, MD, 403 Sea Street, Oxnard, CA 93030 013-200-3921 7-96 to 6-97

<u>Position</u>
Medical Secretary. Made appointments; handled telephone, billing, and insurance form completion; purchased supplies, filed and typed correspondence.

PROFESSIONAL AFFILIATIONS:

Member of the American Association for Medical Transcription, Modesto, California.
Member of the American Association of Medical Assistants, Chicago, Illinois.

REFERENCES:

Available upon request.

Figure 17–1. Example of a chronological resume. The statements of birthdate, height, weight, marital status, and physical condition have been omitted to conform to the Civil Rights Act of 1964, enforced by the Equal Employment Opportunity Commission (EEOC).

17

BIOGRAPHICAL SKETCH

Personal Details

Name:	Harriet B. Stacy
Address:	5301 Upland Street Chatsworth, XY 12345-0002
Telephone:	013-430-2199

Education

Oxnard Community College	Oxnard, California	Attended 9-94 to 6-96
St. Mary's High School	Ventura, California	Attended 9-90 to 6-94

Work Experience

William A. Berry, MD June 1996 to August 1997.
Duties: Receptionist, transcriptionist, insurance clerk.

Skills

Typing: 65 wpm. Transcription: 100 lines/hr. WordPerfect 5.1. Excellent editing and composition skills. Pleasant telephone voice. Conversational Spanish.

(A functional resume does not list specific jobs or specific dates. It is organized to highlight the qualifications of the applicant. Stress selected skill areas, such as typing words per minute, transcription speed, editing skills, writing skills, operating types of equipment, and so forth. If you have had previous jobs, you can emphasize or play down past job duties.)

References

Mrs. Lynn D. Lamb, 431 J Street, Oxnard, California. Telephone: 913-320-1200 (teacher)
John Camp, MD, 320 Main St., Ventura, California. Tel: 013-430-4300 (former employer)

(List two or three. You may include former employers, teachers, former business associates, or other professional persons. Do not use relatives as a reference.)

Figure 17–2. Example of a functional resume.

ally. If using a computer, generate it via a laser printer for a professional appearance of highest quality.

The title for your resume can be Resume, Personal Data Sheet, Biographical Sketch, or Curriculum Vitae. The body of the resume should begin with your name, address, and telephone number. The Civil Rights Act of 1964 allows you to exclude your age, birthdate, marital status, height, weight, and physical condition, but sometimes listing these can enhance your chances of getting a job. However, if you do indicate your age, use your birthdate so that your resume will be current for longer than one year.

The second major subject of your resume should be your educational background. Include the high school, college, and any business school that you may have attended. If you received any awards or scholastic honors, these should also be included.

After your education, list your work experience. Begin with your latest place of employment and end with your first position. Include summer, full-time, part-time, and temporary jobs as well as volunteer work, and be sure to list past job accom-

PERSONAL DATA SHEET

Jose F. Espinoza
42 Colonia Drive
Oxnard, California 93030-4230
013-499-2399

RESUME SUMMARY: Medical transcriptionist with 240-hour externship experience. Major skills include excellent speller, knowledge of medical terminology, very good proofreader, keyboard 80 wpm, WordPerfect 5.1, and grammar and punctuation skills.

EDUCATION: Justin College, Oxnard, California. Graduated 1996 with an A.A. degree.

Emory High School, Oxnard, California. Graduated 1994. Diploma awarded.

WORK EXPERIENCE: James Henson, MD, 211 Mary Street, Oxnard, California. Telephone: 013-480-2311. Trainee transcriptionist (externship) 240 hours from 2-96 to 8-96.

SKILLS:
Type 80 words per minute.
Knowledge of medical terminology.
Excellent speller.
Able to transcribe.
Able to speak Spanish very well.
Excellent proofreader.
(List those skills that would be of value in the employment you are seeking.)

REFERENCES: Furnished upon request.

Figure 17–3. Example of the combination-format resume. Note beginning summary statement that emphasizes why the reader should be interested in this applicant. Personal data may be excluded, if you wish, as a result of the Civil Rights Act of 1964, enforced by the EEOC.

17

plishments. Describe briefly the duties that you had in each position. It is not necessary to state reasons why you left a job; this question may be asked during the interview or may appear on a job application form. Job hopping or gaps of several months between jobs will be scrutinized; if you wish, this can be dealt with during an interview. References may be listed, or you may state, "References furnished upon request." Choose references from former employers and teachers, a family physician, or a professional friend. Always ask permission to use the names of your references on your resume. Indicate what your relationship is/was with each reference, i.e., former (or current) instructor, employer, supervisor, friend for _______ years, and so on.

When applying for a position as a transcriptionist, list your typing skill in words per minute and your transcription speed in lines or characters per hour. Remember to list all business machines you know how to operate. State your membership in professional organizations, along with any offices or leadership positions held. It is optional for you to mention hobbies or special interests because this is irrelevant material. However, if you are fluent in another language, be sure to insert this information on your resume. You might insert a brief statement of career goals for the next five or ten years. A current photograph of yourself included with the resume is helpful to the interviewer when trying to recall an applicant. It, too, is optional, however. When telephoning a prospective employer, inquire whether they prefer the resume to be faxed or mailed. In a competitive employment atmosphere where time is important, it is wise to use every advantage possible.

Your present address
City, State, Zip code
Date of typing this letter

John Doe, MD or
Personnel Director
Street Address
City, State, Zip code

Dear Dr. Doe:

1st paragraph - Tell how you heard of the position. Tell why you are writing by naming the position, medical transcriptionist.

2nd paragraph - State one or two qualifications you consider to be of greatest interest to the doctor or hospital. Explain why you are interested in his or her practice, location, or type of work. If you have past experience or special training, be sure to mention this.

3rd paragraph - Refer the reader to the resume or application form enclosed.

4th paragraph - End the letter by asking for an interview and suggesting a date and time or that you will call for an appointment. If this letter is to request further information about the job opening, enclose a self-addressed, stamped envelope as a courtesy. The closing statement should not be vague but should give the reader a specific action to take.

Sincerely,

(your handwritten signature)

Type your name

Enclosure

Figure 17–4. Suggested content for a cover letter to accompany a resume.

17

Cover Letters

If you are sending your resume to a prospective employer, it is important to compose a letter of introduction or cover letter that is attractive and flawlessly typed. It should be composed for a specific job opening and should contain information not already in your resume or information that you may want to highlight and bring to the interviewer's attention (Fig. 17–4). The letter should be addressed to an individual, if possible, and mailed with the resume. Both letter and resume should contain your name, address, and telephone number. Ask for an interview before you close your letter. Carefully proofread the letter for typographical errors and errors in spelling, punctuation, and grammar.

PROSPECT SOURCES

First, tell everyone you know—friends, relatives, and professional contacts—that you are now available for work. Remember, most jobs are not advertised. When you visit a medical facility on business, let the staff members know that you are looking for a position and would appreciate any leads. Make frequent visits to hospitals and large medical clinics and check the personnel bulletin board. Openings are listed in this manner before they are publicized. Provide your instructor or school placement office with your resume so that they will have it handy and be truly knowledgeable about your background if they are contacted by a prospective employer. School counselors may give you a lead on where to look for a job. Go to the personnel offices of local hospitals, medical clinics, transcription businesses, and word processing centers and complete a job application to be filed in the event that an opening occurs in the future. Many large institutions have job lines, and you may telephone and hear information about any openings for employment. The title and salary range are usually given. Some large private medical buildings will permit you to leave resumes with the switchboard operator or pharmacist. Check with your local medical society to see if it has a provision for supplying you with leads. Consult the telephone directory or medical society roster for sources, and make a blind mailing of your resume to possible prospects. In the *Yellow Pages* of your telephone directory, physicians are listed under "Physicians and Surgeons," and typing services are generally listed under "Secretarial Services." The state employment department may have a list of available jobs, and there is no charge for their service. If you use a professional employment agency, you must be prepared to pay a fee if they place you. Join a chapter of the American Health Information Management Association, American Association of Medical Assistants, Inc., or American Association for Medical Transcription. By attending meetings and receiving their professional magazines and bulletins, you may hear of a job opportunity. Place a notice in your local chapter newsletter that you are looking for a job. Contact the national headquarters of each association for further information about local chapters.

American Association of Medical Assistants, Inc.
20 North Wacker Drive, Suite 1575
Chicago, IL 60606
Telephone: 800-228-2262

17

American Association for Medical Transcription
P.O. Box 576187
Modesto, CA 95357
Telephone: 800-982-2182
Fax: 209-551-9317

American Health Information Management Association
875 North Michigan Avenue, Suite 1850
Chicago, IL 60611
Telephone: 212-870-3136

If you plan to work in Canada, contact the following resources:

Canadian Association of Medical Transcriptionists
P.O. Box 396
Vancouver, BC, Canada V5Z 4C9

Ontario Medical Secretaries' Association
250 Bloor Street East, Suite 600
Toronto, Ontario, Canada M4W 1G6

Canadian Medical Association
P.O. Box 8650
Ottawa, Ontario, Canada K1G 0G8

Canadian Health Record Association
250 Ferrand Drive, Suite 909
Don Mills, Ontario, Canada M3C 3G8

Medical Office Assistants' Association of British Columbia
c/o British Columbia Medical Association
115-1665 West Broadway Street
Vancouver, BC, Canada V6J 1X1

ELECTRONIC JOB SEARCH

There are a few ways to approach the use of computer technology to find a job. One method is to subscribe monthly or annually to one or more on-line computer services, such as America Online, Prodigy, CompuServe, and so on. These services have bulletin boards for those interested in medical transcription, and you can post a notice or resume. Discard traditional resume-writing techniques (action verbs) and focus on action words (nouns), such as "transcriptionist" and "manager." Use labels or key words, such as "education," "experience," "skills," "knowledge," and "abilities." Avoid decorative or uncommon typefaces; do not underline. Minimize the use of abbreviations except for CMT (certified medical transcriptionist). Forget the one-page rule, and use three or four pages for an electronic resume.

Another method is to register with a computerized program that compiles your answers to a series of questions about a particular position and then sends your profile to prospective employers via the computer. American Computerized Employment Service has entered the job placement field with a trademarked system called TeleRecruiting. Job candidates register for no charge after completing an extensive profile questionnaire covering experience, skills, and job-related factors, such as maximum commuting distance and flextime requirements. This company acts as a liaison between employers and applicants. Employers use a touch-tone telephone to access the computer and search for candidates meeting their requirements through the use of annual subscription, pay-per-search, or package searches. Applicants may update their data from time to time when new skills and additional qualifications have been acquired and may register under more than one category. The data remain on-line after a job is obtained, so the service is helpful when advancing in a present career or making a change in career.

American Computerized Employment Service
17801 Main Street, Suite A
Irvine, CA 92714
Telephone: 714-250-0221

Hundreds of jobs may be found on the Internet's World Wide Web. Go to a Web index, such as Yahoo (www.yahoo.com/) which lists many different options for you to explore. To browse through some national job openings with postings by field, location, and career type, try the following:

America's Job Bank (http://www.ajb.dni.us)
Career Magazine (www.careermag.com/careermag/)
E-Span Employment Database Search (www.espan.com/)

A book on this topic is Kennedy, Joyce L.: *Hook Up, Get Hired! The Internet Job Search Revolution*, published by John Wiley & Sons, New York, 1995.

Other Web sites of particular interest to a medical transcriptionist that may or may not have job opportunities from time to time are:

American Association for Medical Transcription: http://www.aamt.org/aamt
Mary Morken, Web Monitor, a Networking Center,
MT Daily I: http://angelfire.com/mt
MT Daily II: http://angelfire.com/mt2/next.html
Medical Transcription Industry Alliance: http://www.wwma.com/a2/mtia/

TEMPORARY JOBS

There are reasons to work temporarily or as a permanent part-time employee. It may be difficult to decide exactly where you want to work, or perhaps you have small children at home and are unable to work full time. You may need an income to meet monthly bills while you are waiting for a full-time position. As a medical transcriptionist, you can work for various employers or for one particular office or hospital, doing overflow work. With the proper equipment, transcribing can be done in your home. Depending on the need for transcriptionists, many communities can use part-time transcriptionists.

Usually you can find this type of work from the sources mentioned, or you can be hired by a company that places you. Some of these national companies are Kelly Services, Manpower Incorporated, TOP Services, Western Temporary Services, Incorporated, and Olsten Temporary Services. Some have branch offices in foreign countries. Your community may have other local and regional temporary employment firms. Look in the *Yellow Pages* of your phone directory under the heading "Employment-Temporary." There are some advantages in applying to such a company because it will screen you, test your skills, place you into a job category or categories, and have incentive plans to encourage you to remain with it instead of taking a full-time job. Obtain a typing speed certificate while you are still in school to avoid taking a typing test under stress. Rather than being isolated in one office, you can have the experience of working in many offices and learn a variety of procedures. There is less chance that routine work will become boring or stale. Work schedules are flexible, and if you are called for a job and cannot report that day or week, you are not obliged to take the job. If a business has to cut costs, it tends to use "temporaries" rather than hire permanent employees to handle short-term increases in work load. Physicians whose offices are near resort areas may have to handle seasonal peak volumes of work and will need temporary help. Temporary firms do not encourage it, but if an employer wishes to hire you full time, there can be allowances in the contract for you to accept such a position.

Because medical transcription is a specialized and technical position, a "temporary" with medical transcribing skills can often command higher wages than other employees who receive close to minimum wage. Workers' compensation insurance is provided through temporary agencies, but group health insurance is not. Fringe benefits are likely to be cash bonuses for long or exceptional service or for recruiting other employees to the temporary employment firm. Some firms offer their employees profit-sharing plans and paid vacations. If travel is an objective, you can obtain work through national and international firms and work out of any of their branches. In some cases, retesting may not be required.

PREPARE FOR THE INTERVIEW

To prepare for an interview, find out as much as you can about the job and the organization to which you are going for the interview. If it has a personnel office, ask if you can be permitted to read the job description for the position for which you are applying. Brush up on any technical jargon or terminology associated with the medical specialty of the physician. If you visit an office for an application and are asked to remain for an interview, make an appointment so you can prepare for it.

One way to prepare yourself for an interview is by role playing. You may be interviewed by one individual or by a panel of individuals, so be prepared for either event. Ask yourself questions in front of a mirror so that you will be prepared and will not stumble on the answers (or give a friend a list of questions to ask you). Use a tape recorder and then replay the tape to see how you sounded when you asked yourself the questions. Here are some questions for role playing that may be of some help. See if you can answer them spontaneously and honestly.

EXAMPLE

Employer:
"If you get this job, how will you want me to assist you in your work?"

Job candidate:
"I would expect you to help me learn your policies and procedures, and then I'd ask for help if I didn't understand something."

This type of answer would indicate to the employer a job candidate's ability to work on his or her own and willingness to seek advice when he or she needs it.

1. Tell me something about yourself.
2. What is your major weakness?
3. Why do you want to work for me? Or for us?
4. Why do you think you would like this job?
5. What special qualifications do you have that make you feel you will be successful?
6. What have you done that shows initiative and willingness to work?
7. Will you be able to work overtime?
8. What salary do you expect?
9. How did you obtain your last job, and why did you leave it?
10. What does success mean to you?
11. What type of person do you like to work for?
12. How is your health? (Although it is illegal to ask, how would you respond to this type of question?)
13. Do you like routine work?
14. What do you plan to be doing five years from now?
15. Have you any plans to further your education?

17

When asked a question, reply in a manner that will bring out your strong points and assets. Do not reply immediately; *think* carefully and be alert to the reply you know the interviewer wishes to hear, but be aware of your handicaps and be ready to emphasize your best qualities. For example, if the interviewer notes that your typing speed is not high, you might emphasize that your accuracy is very high (if that is the case). If you are short on practical experience, point out your excellent school record. This is the one time when you may be completely frank about your qualifications without being a boaster or braggart. Do not sell yourself short or make negative statements about yourself. Do not discuss personal problems. Be enthusiastic and *ask* for the position if you want it. For questions that a prospective employer cannot ask, refer to the section on Application Blanks.

THE INTERVIEW

Arrive early to allow time for parking, finding the proper office, relaxing, and catching your breath. Take a pen, note pad, and your resume.

Dress carefully for the interview. Remember all the truisms about "first impressions." Because you do not know the attitude of the interviewer, you should always be appropriately attired. Women should wear a clean skirt, dress, or tailored suit and nylon stockings with low-heeled pumps. Men should wear a clean dark-gray or navy suit or plain slacks with shirt and tie, plain socks, and well-shined shoes. Men should avoid a lot of facial hair, long hair, earrings, and heavy aftershave lotion. Women should style their hair in a conservative and becoming manner and wear jewelry sparingly. They should avoid heavy makeup, low-cut necklines, sleeveless dresses, strong perfume, and dark or bright nail polish. Do not smoke or chew gum. Use a suitable deodorant. Try to eliminate nervous habits, such as thumping your fingers on the table, wringing your hands, or clicking the lid on a pen. Do not take anyone with you to the interview. Make up a checklist of questions on a note pad or 3×5 cards so you do not forget to ask the interviewer any questions you may have about the position. Once you are introduced to the interviewer, make a point to remember his or her name, and refer to the name in your conversation. Look the interviewer in the eye when answering questions, being careful not to avert your eyes. Maintaining eye contact implies sincerity.

Some jobs have fringe benefits about which you may have questions. Here are several pertinent ones. However, be careful not to appear too interested in benefits.

1. What is the salary? (If the interviewer does not bring up salary, you are entitled to ask what he or she can offer.)
2. What are the duties of this job?

3. Does the firm encourage or provide continuing education for its employees?
4. Will the employer pay tuition for courses to further skills?
5. What are the opportunities for advancement?
6. What types of insurance plans are available? Does this facility contribute to them? Is group health insurance, a pension, or profit sharing available?
7. What are the starting and quitting times?
8. Is there an incentive pay program?
9. Is overtime often required? What is the pay for it if any?
10. How long must one be employed before paid vacation time is available?
11. Are sick days given?
12. Do you have a company cafeteria? How much time are employees allowed for lunch or coffee breaks?
13. What kind of equipment is provided?
14. How and when can one qualify for a raise?
15. What is the ceiling salary in this job description?
16. Are there any dress restrictions that employees must observe?
17. Do you pay for membership fees in professional organizations?

There are many questions that may be considered discriminatory when applying for a job. A prospective employer cannot ask the following:

1. Your age
2. Date of birth
3. Birthplace
4. Ethnic background
5. Religious beliefs
6. Native language
7. Maiden name
8. Marital status
9. Date of marriage
10. Whether your spouse is employed
11. How much your spouse earns
12. If female, whether you are pregnant
13. If female, whether you have had an abortion
14. The number of dependent children living with you
15. To explain all the gaps in your employment record (i.e., to find out if you have taken time off to have children)
16. Whether you have any physical or emotional defects (but an interviewer can ask whether you have any job-related defects)
17. Provision for child care
18. Club memberships
19. Height or weight
20. Credit rating
21. Home and automobile ownership
22. Family planning

A question about whether you smoke is not considered discriminatory. Three suggestions for handling an illegal question are

1. Answer the question and ignore the fact that you know it is illegal.
2. Answer with "I think the question is not relevant to the requirements of this position."
3. Refuse to answer and contact the nearest Equal Employment Opportunity Commission office.

If a question is asked about why you left a previous employer and you had some difficulty in that position, you can state "for personal reasons." This can then be discussed in further detail if the interviewer wishes to know the particulars.

If the job is offered to you at the time of the interview and you are not sure you want it, you might ask, "May I have some time to think it over?" or "How soon do you need to know?" This will give you time to think about the job before you commit yourself.

Portfolio

When going for an interview, take along a document file or portfolio. A portfolio gives the interviewer the impression that the applicant is organized and serious about getting the job. It should contain extra copies of your resume, school diplomas or degrees, certificates, Social Security card, timed typing test certified by an instructor, a few select transcripts or work samples showing knowledge of format, alphabetical notebook of words, letters of recommendation (from former employers, teachers, family physician, professional friends, or community leaders), names and

4021 Madison Road
El Cajon, XY 12345-0002
January 10, 199x

Harris M. Peterson, MD
3200 Main Street
La Mesa, XY 12346-0003

Dear Dr. Peterson:

Thank you for giving me so much time yesterday to discuss the medical transcribing position in your office.

I hope that you will give me the opportunity to prove my ability as I feel that I can perform the work to your satisfaction; I am very eager to try.

Please let me hear from you in the near future (013-486-3200).

Sincerely yours,

(Mrs.) Jane Simon

Figure 17–5. Example of a thank-you letter after an interview.

addresses of references, and anything related to your prior education and work experience that is relevant to your current job campaign. This information can be placed in a manila envelope or report folder with a transparent cover.

After the Interview

Immediately after the interview, write a thank-you note to the interviewer, thanking him or her for the interview. Restate your interest in the position, and ask for consideration for employment (see Fig. 17–5, which will give you an idea of how the letter should appear and what it should contain).

APPLICATION FORMS

Read the application form entirely before you begin. Use a pen to complete the form, and follow the directions carefully, such as "Please print," "Complete in your own handwriting," or "Put last name first." This indicates your ability to follow instructions. Copy from your resume. This will help you to be accurate and consistent. Make the form look exceptionally neat. When you leave, this paper may be all that is left to represent you. Complete all the blanks accurately and honestly; if a question does not apply, put in "NA" (not applicable). Attach additional sheets of paper to answer a question completely rather than trying to squeeze your answer into a tiny space or answering it incompletely. Be sure to sign the form. After an interval, reread the form all the way through, word for word, to catch possible errors of omission or commission. You do not want to have to explain or apologize during the interview for a mistake. Remember that lies or misrepresentations may be automatic grounds for firing. If a question appears on an application form regarding salary, a proper answer might be "negotiable" or "flexible" so that this can be discussed during an interview. You want to avoid overpricing or underpricing yourself. Before the interview, do some research to see if the salary (when offered) is acceptable. In negotiating a salary, you may decide to accept a salary that is lower than what you want with an understanding that after a three- to six-month period your work will be evaluated for an increase of pay.

If you are an immigrant or alien, you will need to establish citizenship with a birth certificate or a Social Security card and your identity with a driver's license with a photograph. If you have a document that establishes both identity and authorization to work, take it with you when you apply for a job, i.e., a U.S. passport, a naturalization certificate, an alien registration card, a temporary resident receipt card, or an employment authorization card. Employers must conform to the Immigration Reform and Control Act of 1986 and will request documents from you, or they can be fined, imprisoned, or both, for repeated violations.

PROFESSIONALISM

The dictionary defines *professionalism* as the conduct, aims, or qualities that characterize or mark a profession. Because professionalism is intangible, it is difficult to put into words, but "you know it when you see it." Professional means more than being proficient at medical transcription. It is that extra effort you take in retyping a sloppy report (even when you are paid on production) or looking up a word when you are not sure of the spelling. Other qualities shared by true professionals are having enthusiasm for work, being courteous and dependable, having the right attitude, and being able to get along with others. As a professional, you want to reflect an image and convey a message that you are bright, alert, capable, and top-notch; so look the part. Professionals are self-confident, honest, and fair in their dealings with others.

An important aspect of professionalism is a willingness to continue learning even after long experience. To keep abreast of new medical terms, techniques, and procedures, consider joining a chapter, the national association, or both of the American Association for Medical Transcription (AAMT). Participate in their continuing medical education program by becoming certified. Refer to Chapter 1 for details regarding the requirements to become a certified medical transcriptionist (CMT). Categories of membership include active, associate, institutional, and student.

Aim for personal and professional success.

TIPS FOR HOLDING A JOB

Here are some suggestions on how to keep that good job now that you have landed it.

1. Be punctual in reporting for work.
2. Report fit and alert, being absent only when absolutely necessary.
3. Be well groomed at all times; dress attractively and appropriately.
4. Do not criticize your employer. If you do not like where you are working, find another employer.
5. If there are job assignments for which you do not particularly care, accept your share of the responsibility for these without complaints. Every job will have its good and bad points.
6. Stay within the time limit for coffee breaks and lunch period.
7. Limit personal telephone calls made or received to those that are absolutely necessary.
8. If you are not busy, offer to assist someone else who is.
9. Social visits with other employees should occur only after or before working hours.
10. Keep your personal problems to yourself.
11. Always do the job the boss's way. Later, when your experience and skills are established, your ideas and suggestions will be welcomed, but not in the beginning.
12. Keep a learning attitude. Stay flexible and adjust to new changes.

JOB EVALUATION

During our many years of teaching, a number of students have asked how a medical transcription supervisor evaluates their performance after they are hired. Usually employers have job descriptions that list job responsibilities for each employee. Job descriptions assist managers, supervisors, and others in recruiting, supervising, and evaluating individuals in their positions. Figure 1–2 in Chapter 1 is a model job description for a medical transcriptionist that was developed by the American Association for Medical Transcription. It is not a complete list of specific duties and responsibilities but is to be used as an aid in developing a job description by employers for their medical transcriptionist.

17

Evaluation of the relative and comparable worth of a beginning medical transcriptionist may affect your career growth within an organization and involves a number of factors. First, does the employer have a job evaluation plan? This is foremost because without job evaluation, there is no valid way to determine the relative worth of different positions within an organization. The relative worth of any position is determined by what the employee actually does. To compare position levels based only on job titles is misleading. The title "medical secretary" may cover different levels of responsibility ranging from "medical typist," "medical transcriptionist," or "insurance specialist" to "administrative or executive medical assis-

PROOFREADING STATEMENT

MT/CMT name: ______________________ Date proofed: ______________

Client: ______________________ Date transcribed: ______________

Total pages/document name: ______________________

Findings: ______________________

____

____

____

Proofreader: ______________________

MT/CMT signature: ______________________

SCORING SYSTEM FOR INTERNAL AUDIT

Major errors:	content only	1 point
Minor errors:	punctuation, paragraph assembly, grammar	½ point
	transposed letters, letters left out of words	¼ point

	score
0 points per 100 lines without blank lines	100
1 point per 100 lines without blank lines	90
2 points per 100 lines without blank lines	80
3 points per 100 lines without blank lines	70
4 points per 100 lines without blank lines	60
5 points per 100 lines without blank lines	Poor

Any audit with a score of 70 or below: MT needs to study more and must be audited again within 30 days to evaluate.

All audit sheets are submitted to the manager or department head on completion for review. Employees who are audited can then be interviewed and the results of the audit discussed. Audit sheets then become part of the medical transcriptionist's personnel records, and a schedule is developed by personnel for the next audit. A complete audit schedule is given to the audit supervisor for future reference.

AUDIT STATEMENT

MT's name: ______________________

Date of audit: ______________________

Account: ______________________

Document name: ______________________

Character count: ______________________

Line count w/o blanks: ______________________

Total pages: ______________________

Total number of errors: ______________________

Additional comments: ______________________

____

____

Employee's signature: ______________________

Date: ______________________

AUDIT LOG SHEET

Date	MT's Initials	Document Name	Auditor's Initials

Figure 17–6. Examples of proofreading statement and an audit (evaluation) statement and log, along with scores illustrating important points considered during internal audits. (Reprinted with permission from Journal of the American Association for Medical Transcription, May-June 1992, page 33.)

tant." You might be asked to write a job description listing some of the following:

1. What do you actually do when working; if you transcribe, how much do you accomplish per day?
2. What are the most complex duties that you perform?
3. What skills and experience are required? Since hired, have your skills improved?
4. To what extent, or in what areas, is independent judgment required?
5. What are the likelihood and impact of errors? Since hired, have your errors diminished in frequency?
6. With whom do you interact? Is the interaction positive or negative, compatible or incompatible?
7. What physical effort or manual dexterity is required?
8. What unusual working conditions exist?
9. What supervisory responsibilities are involved?

The employer must also have developed quantity (productivity) standards and quality standards. From the cost containment standpoint, this is important because a document with content, typographical, grammar, and punctuation errors may be returned for correction. Redoing the report increases production costs. Proofreading the document while it is on the computer screen instead of when it is printed is the most cost-effective way to ensure quality. Your transcripts will be carefully scrutinized during your 90-day probationary period to see whether you measure up to the employer's standards and whether you are meeting the turnaround time. In addition, your supervisor may take into account your independent action, whether your attendance at work was perfect or whether you missed work days due to illness, or whether you stayed overtime to transcribe STAT reports without complaints.

Figure 17–6 shows examples of a proofreading statement and an audit (evaluation) statement and log, along with scores for internal audit to give you an idea of how audits are accomplished.

SELF-EMPLOYMENT OR FREELANCING

Starting a Business

After sufficient transcription experience, you may want to be your own boss and have a flexible work schedule. This means full-time commitment, a lot of hard work, and long hours to develop a number of clients. Estimate how much money you will need in the start-up months, taking into consideration equipment, overhead, taxes, and final profit. Some transcriptionists work from their homes in the beginning, thereby reducing the overhead. However, working at home involves a certain amount of self-discipline. Time management is essential, so make out a schedule. When you are the boss, you are responsible for everything—advertising, billing, bookkeeping, obtaining clients, and so on. It is wise to have a cushion of money to run your business for six months to a year before you quit your regular job. One of the most common reasons that businesses fail is they are undercapitalized from the beginning. It usually takes at least a year before you make any real profit, so be patient. If you are weak in accounting, take a bookkeeping course. Attend seminars on starting a business offered by financial institutions, universities, community colleges, or private institutions. Set up detailed financial records from day one, even if you intend to hire an accountant. Get expert advice. Consult a lawyer or accountant or both about the best way of legally setting up your business and the tax pros and cons of each option.

Equipment

Equipment to consider would be a computer with modem, transcription equipment, telephone-answering machine, Fax machine, computer table, filing cabinet, and calculator. Investigate transcription equipment that has the capacity to handle standard cassettes and microcassettes. Thoroughly explore the equipment available, and talk to those already using the equipment about maintenance (service contracts), purchase, and lease options. To handle a large volume of transcription and expand your service, a word processor and a direct telephone-in line would be considered as well as faxing documents back to clients. A large percentage of clients like this method because of convenience and the rapid turnaround time in furnishing reports. Some companies have equipment that emits a beep for purposes of confidentiality if someone comes on the line. Because this equipment is more expensive as far as purchase and upkeep, investigate possible loan sources: commercial and savings banks, government-sponsored small business loans, finance companies, family, and friends. Obtaining loans from individual investors or venture capital can mean a percentage of the business or profits going to the investor, depending on the contractual agreement. Low-interest government Small Business Administration (SBA) loans and loans to physically challenged individuals are available to those who qualify.

Develop Clientele

Call local competitors and obtain information on range of fees regarding character count, line count, page count, stroke count, or hourly rates so you have an idea of what to charge as a fee for your work. Research your market area to see who will use your services in the community, such as physicians' offices (e.g., orthopedists, cardiologists), hospitals (medical record, pathology, or radiology departments), clinics, nurse practitioners, and so on. You can find work by substituting for transcriptionists who are ill, on vacation, or overloaded. Other professionals in search of transcriptionists are chief residents going into private practice, new

LETTERHEAD

DATE

Client's Name
Address
City, State, ZIP Code

Dear__________:

For___years, I have worked as a medical transcriptionist for _____________.
I am now establishing my own business. Perhaps your office or hospital has an overload or your medical transcriptionist is ill or planning a vacation. Maybe you have a manuscript you need typed for a medical journal or need a personnel manual, grant proposal or research paper typed.

You can be assured of the following:

1. Consultation rendered at no charge.
2. Accurate, complete, and speedy medical transcription. All work is proofread.
3. Courier service (pick up and delivery available). Your transcripts will be delivered to you on the day and at the hour you specify. Special RUSH pick up when required.
4. Low competitive rates.
5. Premium pay for overtime work eliminated on in-house transcription.
6. In-house office space and equipment requirements reduced, or eliminated.
7. Confidentiality of work guaranteed.
8. Personal, professional, dependable service provided on a temporary "fill-in" basis.
9. Service available 24 hours a day, 7 days a week, including holidays.
10. Call-in dictation from any location available.
11. Retyping of a report at no charge, if you are not satisfied with the transcript.

My business equipment includes_________typewriter or word processor and transcription equipment adaptable to standard, micro- and mini- cassettes.

Professional references will be supplied on request. I am a Certified Medical Transcriptionist (CMT) and a member of the American Association for Medical Transcription.

I welcome the opportunity to speak with you personally about this new service and will call you to set up an appointment in the near future. If you need my services immediately, please call________and leave a message. Please keep my telephone number on file in case you need my services in the future.

Sincerely,

Figure 17–7. Example of a letter to prospective clients.

17

LETTERHEAD

DATE

Client's Name
Address
City, State, ZIP code

Dear____________:

This is to confirm my conversation with you yesterday regarding transcription of your medical reports.

I agree to deliver completed transcripts to your office the day after pick up of the dictation. The rate is $________ per page with proration applied to those pages with less than half a page.

Please call me anytime you need my service. I look forward to transcribing for you.

Sincerely yours,

Note: You may wish to make the second paragraph specific by stating "I agree to pick up dictation on __Tuesday__ and deliver on __Thursday__."

Figure 17–8. Example of a letter outlining terms of an agreement.

physicians in town, a physician appointed to head an association, or physicians who are changing offices or adding colleagues, visiting nurse associations, marriage and family counselors, clinical psychologists, and medical researchers. Send prospective clients a letter (Fig. 17–7). Your major responsibility is to convince clients that your service is better than the competition, stressing dependability; efficient service; professional, prompt turnaround of quality work; direct telephone-in line, courier service (pick up and delivery); and so on. Misunderstandings about agreements can occur, so put everything in writing. If you change the terms of the agreement, write a letter outlining the new terms (Fig. 17–8).

Professional Fees

Some self-employed medical transcriptionists consider a standard page as 30 single-spaced lines. First pages are counted as a whole page, even when the letter or report is half a page. The final page of the work is prorated—anything under 15 lines is a half page, and anything over 15 lines is considered a full page. The monthly statement to the client should consist of a detailed record of patients' names, date of each report, and number of pages or hours depending on how you structure your fees (Fig. 17–9). You might want to establish a minimum charge. In trying to obtain a client, you might state the following:

> "My charge is computed on a per-page level, as this is quicker for you to check and for me to compute. I am currently charging ________ cents a line on full, single-spaced pages. This works out to $ ________ a full page for billing purposes."

17

Subcontracting

If someone who is self-employed gets too much work and asks you to pitch in, you are subcontracting. The self-employed individual will pay you so much per line, per page, or hourly and keep a percentage. Payment should be made at the time of delivery of the work to the self-employed individual, since you, the subcontractor, are not dealing directly with the client.

LETTERHEAD

Date

Client's Name
Address
City, State, ZIP code

BILLING STATEMENT

Tapes	Patient's Name	Report* Code No.	Pickup Date	Delivery Date	Pages or Hours	Balance Due
1	Mary Brown	3	11-22-9x	11-23-9x	13.5 pages	
2	Sue Morse	4	11-22-9x	11-23-9x	4.0 pages	
3						
4						
5						
6						
TOTALS		2			17.5	$

RATE: $_____per full singlespaced page (equals_____cents per line).

TERMS: *Terms should be stated on the billing statement, such as payable on delivery, net 30, net 15 days from invoice, end of month, payment due within 15 days of invoice, and so forth.*

*Report Code No. 1 = Chart note
2 = Consultation
3 = Discharge Summary
4 = History and Physical
5 = Letter
6 = Operative Report
7 = Other

17

Figure 17–9. Example of a monthly billing statement to a client.

Publications

As an independent (self-employed) contractor who establishes a business at home, you get a few dozen deductions for a home office. Obtain the Internal Revenue Service Publication No. 587 entitled "Business Use of Your Home." Each year you must pay a self-employment tax on net income. You also have to make estimated tax payments quarterly once your net income amounts to $500 or more. To avoid headaches at tax time, retain all receipts and keep careful, complete records of income and expenses.

A comprehensive guide on how to start and successfully run your own professional transcription business is available entitled *The Independent Medical Transcriptionist* by Donna Avila-Weil and Mary Glaccum (Rayve Productions, Inc., P.O. Box 726, Windsor, CA 95492; telephone toll-free 800-852-4890).

NEW BUSINESS CHECKLIST

1. Decide what address you will use; you may want to obtain a post office box number instead of using your home address.
2. Obtain a business license from the business license section of your city hall. Regulations vary in each city licensing office. You might have to obtain a home occupation permit from the planning department and have it signed by your landlord if you are renting. The city may have guidelines on hours of business, pedestrian and vehicular activity, noise, and so on in the residential area.
3. File a fictitious business name (*doing business as* [DBA]) at the county clerk's office by obtaining the proper form for completion. If you use your given name, you do not have to file a fictitious business name.
4. Publish the fictitious name in a local newspaper.
5. Contact the Internal Revenue Service (IRS) for an employer identification number and/or tax information. Obtain the booklet *Tax Guide for Small Business* No. 334 to determine business expenses that are deductible. Depending on how you set up your business, some possible tax breaks are depreciation of office equipment; declaring a room of your home as an office; subscriptions to professional publications; dues to professional associations; expenses associated with your automobile; telephone, photocopying, office supplies (stationery, books, photocopy and fax paper, and so on); promotion and advertising (postage, meals with business associates, and so on); and any expenses pertaining to meetings, conventions, workshops, or seminars (registration fees, lodging, meals, transportation, parking, and so on).
6. If you have no employees, contact the State Franchise Tax Board for the form used for estimating state withholding taxes for yourself. This must be filed quarterly. If you build up your business and have employees, obtain the proper forms and information for employees (state income tax, and state disability and unemployment insurance).
7. Obtain the insurance that you need: health insurance, disability insurance, life insurance, liability insurance, workers' compensation (if you have employees), and so on. Insurance is available to protect you against loss of material called "Release of Information Insurance" or "Errors and Omissions Insurance" with a "Hold Harmless" clause. You might want to consider a retirement plan, such as an Individual Retirement Account (IRA) or Keogh plan.
8. Contact the telephone company for telephone equipment. Do this early because there is often a delay in hook-up. You might consider using your existing telephone number and switching to a business listing. This allows you to be listed in the *Yellow Pages* of your telephone directory.
9. Open a bank account. If you want your telephone number on your checks, put the checks on hold until the telephone is confirmed.
10. Order business cards, stationery, billing forms, and reference books.
11. Begin to advertise your business by some of the following methods: newspaper, radio, flyers, announcements, signs, word of mouth, and letters to prospects (hospitals, clinics, and physician's offices).
12. Begin to assemble a library to include English and medical dictionaries; word books in surgery, general medicine, and medical specialties; laboratory terminology books; and pharmaceutical references.

There are some additional points to consider if you are ready to expand to a location outside of your home.

1. Check the zoning of the location at your city hall's planning department or, if you are in the county, the county's planning department. Sign a lease contingent on proper zoning and on meeting all federal, state, county, and city building safety and health requirements. Inquire about parking and sign restrictions at the planning department. Find out if you need any permits (building permit, certificate of occupancy, health permit, and so on). City and county offices may require a sign permit for new signs and changes on old ones.
2. If you have opened an office at a location, make a deposit for water, gas, and electricity. Rent, renovation, and janitorial or trash services must be considered.
3. Call the assessor's office and ask to be put on the mailing list for business property tax (inventory tax).
4. Contact the various inspectors: health, building and safety, and sign to have all completed work inspected and the necessary permits signed off.

HOW TO LEAVE A JOB

After working several years for one employer, some transcriptionists may wish to change jobs for a different environment. For example, working in a hospital setting is certainly different from working in a physician's office for one or two dictators. Factors beyond your control can arise, such as pregnancy, a spouse's transfer to another location, and so on. Before considering such a move, it is important to consider all aspects of your total compensation and working environment. It is also wise to obtain a new position before leaving your present one, giving at least two weeks' notice, depending on the hospital or office policy. You can complete the form below to discover your true earnings before contemplating a move.

If you know of a well-qualified person to take your place, suggest his or her name to your supervisor. This will communicate to your employer that you see the situation from his or her viewpoint. Make it easy for the replacement to step in. No one is indispensable, yet some employees want their presence to be missed so much that they destroy any helpful guides for the new employee. You will be thought of more kindly and will leave a good impression if you leave information that might be helpful to the new employee. Clean out your work station so that someone else does not have to finish the job before he or she moves in. If you do not like your employer, keep the negative thoughts to yourself and do not make derogatory remarks to your peers. Do not neglect any of your responsibilities or skip any last-minute commitments.

Remember to say "thank you" to your supervisor, employer, or both and to those who helped you in some way or made your job easier and more pleasant. Let your supervisor know what you are doing as your career progresses. Your paths may cross again directly or indirectly. Perhaps he or she will be in a position to recommend you for a job in the future. Keep your record unblemished because it may have taken you several years to build up your reputation. Be courteous. Be thoughtful. Be professional.

DIRECT COMPENSATION

Salary $ ____________

Bonuses ____________

Paid vacation ____________

17

Sick pay and/or compensation for unused days ____________

Incentive compensation ____________

Parental leave ____________

EMPLOYEE BENEFIT PLANS FULLY OR PARTIALLY PAID BY EMPLOYER—INSURED

Medical/dental insurance ____________

Group term life insurance ____________

Additional accidental death and dismemberment ____________

Long-term disability ____________

Workers' compensation insurance ____________

Federal unemployment taxes (FUTA) ____________

State unemployment taxes (SUI and ETT) ____________

EMPLOYEE BENEFIT PLANS—UNINSURED

Medical reimbursement ______________

Free medical care for employee ______________

Free medical care for family ______________

RETIREMENT CONTRIBUTIONS

Pension plan ______________

Profit-sharing plan ______________

FICA (Social Security)—employer paid ______________

MISCELLANEOUS

Mileage allowance ______________

Uniform allowance ______________

Continuing medical education ______________

(tuition, registration fees, dues)

TOTAL COMPENSATION $ ______________

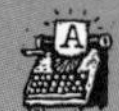

17–1: ASSIGNMENT

Directions: Prepare your resume by selecting one of the formats shown in Figures 17–1, 17–2, and 17–3. Rough draft it first and let your instructor read through it. Then do a final draft after the constructive criticism.

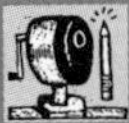

17–2: SELF-STUDY

Directions: The following advertisement appeared in your local newspaper. Compose a cover letter to go with your resume. Refer to Figure 17–4 for guidance in organizing your thoughts.

FULL TIME

Job No.	Description
1311	Medical transcriptionist. Working in medical records. A thorough knowledge of medical terminology with fast, accurate typing required and knowledge of WP5.1. CMT preferred. Excellent incentive pay program and fringe benefits. Send resume or call Personnel Dept., St. Anne's Hospital, 4021 Main Street, Oxnard, CA 94040 013/480-2349.

17

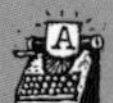

17–3: ASSIGNMENT

Directions: Type a list of where you could go for temporary jobs in your locale. Then meet at least three people who have a job that you would like. Obtain their name, place of employment, job title, and any special skills they needed to obtain the job. Type and hand this list in to your instructor.

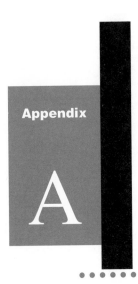

Answers to Practice Tests

A *Answers to* **3–3: PRACTICE TEST**

1. No commas; everything here is essential.
2. Place a comma after *prostate.* The phrase that follows is nonessential and simply adds further information.
3. Enclose *who is a senior this year* in commas. This is nonessential. *Pat,* as a one-word appositive, is not enclosed in commas. Also consider that there could be more than one daughter; we need to know which one.
4. No commas; everything here is essential. We must answer the question "*which* children?"
5. Enclose *Ralph Birch* in commas. It is a nonessential appositive.
6. The phrase *not to operate* is essential and so is not enclosed in commas. It answers the question "*which* decision?" However, there is a comma after *hasty* to set off *if you ask me,* a parenthetical expression.
7. Enclose *which is a carbon* in commas because it is nonessential.
8. No commas; everything here is essential. We need to know *when* to contact the anesthesiologist.
9. Enclose *my textbook* in commas as a nonessential appositive.
10. Enclose *Bright's disease* in commas; it is a nonessential appositive.

A

11. Place a comma after *Charles,* to set off the nonessential appositive *the new resident.*
12. No commas; everything here is essential. We need to know *which* patients.
13. No commas; everything here is essential.
14. Place a comma in front of *however* to show that it is nonessential. Be sure that you do not enclose *who fail to attend the meeting* because it is essential. We need to know *which* staff members.
15. Enclose the nonessential *not the receptionist* in commas.
16. Place a comma after *furthermore.* It is a parenthetical expression.
17. No commas; *Ethel Clifford* is an essential appositive. We need to know which patient because the person being addressed surely has more than one!
18. Place commas around *your patient* because it is a nonessential appositive.

A *Answers to* **3–5: PRACTICE TEST**

1. No commas. Everything is essential and there is no introductory phrase.
2. No commas. Everything is essential and there is no introductory phrase.
3. Enclose the nonessential appositive, *the pathologist,* in commas.
4. Enclose the nonessential appositive, *a girl,* in commas.
5. Place a comma after *furthermore,* a parenthetical expression.
6. Place a comma after *opportunity,* the final word of an introductory phrase.
7. Place a comma after *safe,* the final word of an introductory phrase.
8. Place an optional comma after *lunch,* the final word of a short introductory phrase.
9. Place a comma after *home,* the final word of an introductory phrase.
10. No commas. Everything is essential and there is no introductory phrase. Do not separate the subject from the verb with a comma after *word.*

A *Answers to* **3–7: PRACTICE TEST**

1. i—comma after *time.*
2. i—comma after *well.*

3. d—comma after *week.*
4. There are no commas in this sentence.
5. i—comma after *Hospital.*
6. There are no commas.
7. g and j—commas around *MD* and *Arizona.*
8. e—commas around *1994.*
9. f—optional comma after *Group.*
10. d and h—commas after *examination* and *well-developed.* Note: There is no comma between *well-nourished and white,* the last modifier in the set.
11. h—comma after *effort* and *breath.* (The second comma is optional.)
12. a and e—commas around *with your concurrence* and *July 1;* a comma after *199x.*

13. d—comma after *Jones* Note: No comma after *this* because it is the first part of the phrase.
14. c or d, g, b—commas after *know, Briggs, MD,* and *partner.*
15. e, a—Notice that the expression *which required intravenous antibiotics* simply adds information and does not qualify as being essential. Commas around *199x* and a comma after *bronchopneumonia.*

A *Answers to* 3–8: PRACTICE TEST

September 16, 199x	1. date
Tellememer Insurance Company 25 Main Street, Suite R Albuquerque, NM 87122	2. city, state
Gentlemen:	
RE: Ron Emerson	
I understand from Mr. Emerson that the insurance company feels that the charges for my services on June 30, 199x, are excessive.	4/3. date
Mr. Emerson was seen on an early Sunday morning with a stab wound in his chest, which had penetrated his lung producing an air leak into his chest wall. In addition, he had a laceration of his lung.	5. introductory
After consultation and review of his x-rays, his laceration was repaired. He was observed in the hospital for two days to be sure that he did not have continuing hemorrhage or collapse of his lung.	6. introductory
I feel that the bill given to Mr. Emerson is a fair one. We received, on July 31, 199X, a Tellememer Insurance Company check for $40, and I feel that your payment of $40 is unreasonable. It is doubtful that one could get a plumber to come out early Sunday morning to fix a leaky pipe for $40, and Mr. Emerson's situation, in my opinion, was much more serious than would be encountered by a plumber.	7. nonessential 8/9. date 10. compound 11. compound 12/13. parenthetical
We will bill Mr. Emerson for the remainder of the $200 balance on his account, but I want you to know that we feel that your payment is insufficient. If he feels that the bill is excessive, we would be glad to submit to arbitration through the County Medical Society Fee Committee. If this fails, I suggest we seek help through the New Mexico Insurance Commission.	14. compound 15. introductory 16. introductory
Sincerely yours,	17. close
William A. Berry, MD rl Enclosed: X-ray report; history and physical report Copy: Mr. Ron Emerson	18. degree

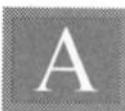

Answers to 3–11: PRACTICE TEST

1. Rule d. Semicolon after *yet.*
2. Rules a and c. Period after *Mr.* and semicolon after *disease.*
3. Rules g and b. Colon after *follows.* Decimal point after *$650.*
4. Rules g, a, f. Colon after *staff,* periods after *Dr., A., Dr., R., Jr., Mrs.* Semicolons after *resident, director, supervisor.*
5. Rule h. Colon after *man.*
6. Rules b and e. Decimal point after *101;* semicolon after *nausea.*
7. Rule b. Decimal point after the zero in *0.5%.*
8. Rule c. Semicolon after *normal.*
9. Rule e. Semicolon after *normal.*
10. Rule i. Colons after *diagnosis* and *discharge.*

A

Answers to 3–13: PRACTICE TEST

1. Mrs. Gail R. Smith-Edwards was hospitalized this morning. She is the 47-year-old woman Dr. Blake admitted with a self-inflicted knife wound. Her blood pressure was 60/40. *(sixty over forty)*
   Rule c, a, or b, a, j
2. Barbara Ness' happy-go-lucky personality was missed when she was transferred from Medical Records.
   Rule e, a, optional h (quotes around "happy-go-lucky")
3. Glen Mathews, the well-known trial lawyer, and the hospital's Chief-of-Staff, Dr. Carlton Edwards, will appear together (if you can believe that) on TV's latest talk show tonight. It's the only subject on the hospital's "gabfest." *Note:* Make sure your period is placed within the quotes.
   Rule a, e, c, i, e, f, e, h
4. I want a stamped, self-addressed envelope enclosed with this letter and sent out with today's mail.
   Rule a, e
5. Dr. Davis said his promotion was a good example of being "kicked upstairs." He obviously didn't want to leave his job in the X-ray Department. *Note:* Make sure your period is placed within the quotes.
   Rule h, f, b
6. Haven't you ever seen a Z-fixation? Bobbi-Jo will be happy to explain it to you. *Note*: Do not worry if you overlooked the hyphen in *Bobbi-Jo.* We could not be expected to know that unless we are familiar with her name.
   Rule f, b, c
7. We're all going to the CCU at 4 o'clock for instructions on mouth-to-mouth resuscitation.
   Rule f, f, a

A

8. Right eye vision: 20/20
   Left eye vision: 10/400
   Right retinal examination: Normal
   Left retinal examination: Inferior retinal detachment
   Rule j

9. You were seen on September 24 at which time you were having some stiffness at the shoulders which I felt was due to a periarthritis (a stiffness of the shoulder capsule); however, x-ray of the shoulder was negative. Notice that commas would not be a good substitute for the parentheses because of the semicolon needed before *however.*
   Rule i, b

10. After he completed the end-to-end anastomosis, he closed with #1 silk through-and-through, figure-of-eight sutures.
    Rule a, a, a

11. Dr. Chriswell's diagnosis bears out the assumption that the red-green blindness is the result of an X-chromosome defect.
    Rule e, a or d, b

12. After his myocardial infarction (MI), his blood test showed high level C-reactive protein.
    Rule i, b

A *Answers to* **3–15: PRACTICE TEST**

1. She inadvertently sterilized the Smith-Petersen nail instead of the V-medullary. (Needs 3 marks)
2. She has had no further spells, but she did have two episodes (prior to this one) several years ago. (Needs 4 marks)
3. The patient presents as a well-developed, asthenic, elderly, extremely bright, and oriented Caucasian female. She is fully alert and able to give an entirely reliable history; however, she is somewhat anxious and concerned over her present condition. (Needs 9 marks)
4. The patient has just moved to this community from Anchorage, Alaska, where he was engaged in the lumber industry. He had an emergency appendectomy performed at some remote outpost in January 1986. According to the patient, he has always felt like "something's hung up in there." Roentgenograms taken July 17, 199X, failed to reveal anything unusual. (Needs 12 marks)
5. He is a 35-year-old, well-developed, well-nourished black truck driver, oriented to time, place, and person. (Needs 10 marks)
6. The X-chromosome defect resulted in her ovarian aplasia, undeveloped mandible, webbed neck, and small stature: Morgagni-Turner syndrome. (Needs 7 marks)
7. Vital signs: Blood pressure: 194/97; pulse: 127; respirations: 32, regular, and gasping. General: Healthy-appearing male, looking his stated age, in moderately severe respiratory distress, with slightly dusky-colored lips. (Needs 17 marks)
   Also correct to use periods and capital letters as follows:
   Vital signs: Blood pressure: 194/97. Pulse: 127. Respiration: 32, regular, and gasping. (In some cases, it is also correct to abbreviate *blood pressure* as BP.)

A

A

Answers to **3–17: PRACTICE TEST**

You may use a semicolon or a comma after *station* in the final sentence of paragraph 3. You may use a comma or a semicolon after *times* in the final sentence of paragraph 4.

William A. Berry, MD
3933 Navajo Road
San Diego California 92119

463-0000

August 13, 199X

John D. Mench, MD
455 Main Street
Bethesda, MD 20034

Dear Dr. Mench:

Re: Debra Walters

This letter is to bring you up to date on Mrs. Walters who was first seen in my office on March 2, 199X, at which time she stated that her last menstrual period had started August 29, 199X. Examination revealed the uterus to be enlarged to a size consistent with an estimated date of confinement of June 5, 199X.

The pregnancy continued uneventfully until May 19, at which time the patient's blood pressure was 130/90. Hygroton was prescribed, and the patient was seen in one week. Her blood pressure at the next visit was 150/100, and additional therapy in the form of Ser-Ap-Es was prescribed in addition to other antitoxemic routines. Her blood pressure stabilized between 130 and 140/90.

The patient was admitted to the hospital on June 11, 199X, with ruptured membranes, mild preeclampsia, and a few contractions of poor quality. Intravenous oxytocics were started; and after two hours of stimulation, there was no change in the cervix, with that structure continuing to be long, closed, and posterior. The presenting part was at a -2 to a -3 station, and the amniotic fluid had become brownish-green in color, suggesting some degree of fetal distress.

Consultation was obtained, and it was recommended that a low cervical cesarean section be performed. A female infant was delivered by cesarean section. It was noted at the time of delivery that the cord was snugly wrapped around the neck of the baby three times, and this might have contributed to the evidence of fetal distress, as evidenced by the color of the amniotic fluid.

The patient's postoperative course was uneventful, and she and the baby were discharged home on the fifth postpartum day.

Sincerely yours,

William A. Berry, MD

mlo

A

A

Answers to LET'S HAVE A BIT OF FUN (CHAPTER 3)

1. b
2. b
3. a
4. a
5. a
6. b
7. b
8. both
9. a
10. b
11. b

A

Answers to 4–2: PRACTICE TEST

1. the right rev. michael t. squires led the invocation at the graduation ceremony for greenlee county's first paramedic class. (Right is an unusual title.)
2. nanci holloway, a 38-year-old caucasian female, is scheduled for a cesarean section tomorrow.
3. the internist wanted him to have meprobamate so he wrote a prescription for miltown. (Meprobamate is generic, and Miltown is a brand name.)
4. johnny temple had chickenpox, red measles, and german measles his first year in school.
5. unfortunately, the patient in icu whom dr. berry saw this morning has hodgkin's disease.
6. the pathology report showed a class IV malignancy on the pap sear. (Pap is an unusual abbreviation. It is not incorrect to use a lower case letter for class.)
7. some patients have been very sick with kaposi's sarcoma, the rare and usually mild skin cancer that seems to turn fierce with aids victims.
8. the mustard procedure is often used to reroute venous return in the atria. (Mustard is an eponym.)
9. the young man was an alert, asthenic, indochinese male who was well-oriented to time and place.
10. the gynecologist wrote a prescription for flagyl for the patient with trichomonas vaginalis. (Flagyl is the brand name for a drug.)
11. please note on mrs. stefandatter's chart that she is allergic to phenobarbital. (Phenobarbital is a generic drug name.)
12. dr. collier recommended a combination of gentamicin and a penicillin such as bicillin for our patient with endocarditis.
13. barbara, our lpn, is the new membership chairman for the local now chapter; she asked me to join.
14. the od victim was brought to the er by his roommate.
15. rhonda keller, mr. zimmer's executive secretary, spoke to the aama about good telephone manners.

A

A

Answers to **4–4: PRACTICE TEST**

William A. Berry, MD
3933 Navajo Road
San Diego, California 92119

463 - 0000

may 6, 199x

mrs. adrianne l. shannon
316 rowan road
clearwater, florida 33516 FL is the correct abbreviation

dear mrs. shannon:

dr. berry asked me to write to you and cancel your appointment for friday, may 15. we hope this will not inconvenience you, but dr. berry has made plans to attend the american college of chest physicians meeting in kansas city at that time. i have tentatively rescheduled your appointment for monday, may 18, at 10:15 a.m.

by the way, you might be interested to know that dr. berry has been asked to read the paper that he wrote entitled "the ins and outs of emphysema." i believe that you asked him for a copy of this article the last time you were in the office.

sincerely yours,

(ms.) laverne shay
secretary

A

William A. Berry, MD
3933 Navajo Road
San Diego California 92119

619-463-0000 Fax 619-463-0000

march 3, 199x

state compensation insurance fund
p. o. box 2970
winnetka, illinois 60140 IL is the correct abbreviation
attention ralph byron, inspector

gentlemen:

re: james r. gorman

the above-referenced patient was seen today for presurgical examination in the office. he has an acute upper respiratory infection with a red left ear and inflamed tonsils. therefore, his surgery was cancelled, and he was placed on keflex, 250 mg every six hours.

mr. gorman's surgery was rescheduled for march 15 at mercy hospital. he will be rechecked in the office on march 14.

very truly yours,

william a. berry, md

ref

A

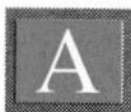

Answers to **5–2: PRACTICE TEST**

1. On September 26, 1990, she had a left lower lobectomy.
2. Two sutures of 000 (or 3–0) cotton were placed so as to obliterate the posterior cul-de-sac. (Notice hyphens in the expression "cul-de-sac.")
3. He smoked 1 1/2 packs of cigarettes a day. (leave out the word "and")
4. There was a tear in the iris at about 6 o'clock. (See Rule 5.12.)
5. The resting blood pressure is 76/40.
6. Please mail this to Dr. Ralph Lavton at 10 Dublin Street, Bowling Green, Ohio 43402. (Ten Dublin Street is also correct.)
7. We had 7 admissions Saturday, 24 Sunday, and 3 this morning. (See Rule 5.11.) (a.m. is used only with the time of day.)
8. In the accident, the spine was severed between C4-5. ($C_{4\text{-}5}$ also correct; C4 and C5 also correct.)
9. The child was first seen by me in the X-ray Department on the evening of May 11, 1990. (Military or European dating is not used in narrative copy except in military documents prepared in the military service.)
10. I recommend a course of cobalt-60 radiation therapy. (Notice the hyphen.)

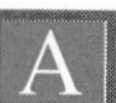

Answers to **5–4: PRACTICE TEST**

1. He has a grade I arteriosclerotic retinopathy and a grade IV hypertensive retinopathy. (*Grade I* and *Grade IV* are also correct.)
2. She was a Gravida V Para I Abortus IV and denied venereal disease but gave a history of vaginal discharge. (Note that there are no commas separating gravida, para, or abortus. These words may also be typed in lower case letters, although many dictators prefer the use of capital letters. It is also correct to use the figures 5, 1, and 4 instead of the roman numerals. Be consistent; do not mix.)
3. I can see only 15-20 patients a day. (15 to 20 also correct.) (See Rule 5.10.)
4. Please order 12 two-gauge needles. (twelve 2-gauge also correct.)
5. Use only one-eighth teaspoonful. (Notice the hyphen.) (See Rule 5.5.)
6. The dorsalis pedis pulses were 2+ and equal bilaterally.
7. The ear was injected with 2% Xylocaine and 1:6000 Adrenalin.
8. Please check the reading in V_4 again. (V4 also correct.)
9. This is her third C-section.
10. She quickly advanced from a Stage II to a Stage IV lymphosarcoma. (One may use *stage II* and *stage IV,* but the capitals look better with the capitalized roman numerals.)

A

A *Answers to* **5–7: PRACTICE TEST**

1. Hemoglobin (*Hb* would be incorrect) on July 27 (*7-27* or *7/27* would be incorrect) was 11.2 gm; hematocrit (*hct* would be incorrect) was 37.
2. Did you know that the postal rates were 25 cents (not *25¢*) for the first ounce (not *oz*) and 20 cents for each additional ounce to mail something first class in 1989? (*First Class* also correct.)
3. The protein was 65 mg%.
4. Electromyography shows a 3+ sparsity in the orbicularis oris.
5. An estimated 0.2 cc of viscid fluid was removed from the middle ear cavity. (Please notice the zero in front of the decimal point.)
6. He entered the ER at 4 a.m. (*AM* also correct) with a temperature of 99°F.
7. There was a reduction of the angle to within a two-degree difference. (*2-degree* also correct; 2° also correct.)
8. Take 50 mg/day. (*50 mg per day* also correct.)
9. I then placed two 4 x 4 sponges over the wound.
10. The TB skin test was diluted 1:100.
11. Drainage amounts to several cubic centimeters a day. (*cc's, ccs,* and *cc* all incorrect.)

A *Answers to* **6–6: TYPING PRACTICE TEST**

See the letter on page 418 properly prepared. The numbers in the margin refer to the comments below.

1. This is the correct placement of the reference line. However, it would also be correct to place it a double space under the salutation.
2. This is the appropriate paragraph break. To begin your second paragraph with "She brought the x-ray films . . . " is very weak.
3. Notice the insert of the "afterthought postscript." This would be the appropriate place to insert it when we have a rough draft. It is not incorrect to use it as a P.S. at the end of your document. It is just better at this place in the letter and the dictator appears better organized.
4. This is the appropriate paragraph break. However, it would be correct to attach it to either paragraph 2 or 4. It is attractive to have this one-sentence paragraph in the middle of the letter, however, and when we do have a choice like this, it is nice to take the option for appearance.
5. We hope this has now become an obvious paragraph break.
6. The parentheses at the end of this sentence are not the only way to handle this last comment. A comma at the end of "health" would also be appropriate. This is the correct paragraph break.
7. This final paragraph could have been joined to paragraph 6 since we are talking about "seeing" the patient in both. It does, however, make a nice balance with the one-line paragraph 3.
8. This enclosure line becomes necessary when the postscript has been eliminated and the data inserted into the body of the letter. If you left the postscript, it would appear here and the enclosure notice would be redundant.

JON L. MIKOSAN, MD
6244 APPLEGATGE ROAD
MILWAUKEE, WI 53209

May 1, 199X

Ian R. Wing, MD
2261 Arizona Avenue, Suite B
Milwaukee, WI 53207

RE: Mrs. Elvira Martinez (1)

Dear Dr. Wing:

I saw your patient Mrs. Elvira Martinez in consultation in my office today. She brought the x-rays from your office with her. She was afebrile today but, on questioning, admitted a low-grade fever over the past few days. (2)

I removed the fluid, as seen on your film of April 30, from the right lower lung field, and she felt considerably more comfortable. On thoracentesis, there was 50 cc of straw-colored fluid. I am enclosing a copy of the pathology report on the fluid; as you can see, it is negative. (3)

Her history is well known to you so I will not repeat it. (4)

On physical examination, I found a well-developed, well-nourished white female with minimal dyspnea. There was no lymphadenopathy. Breath sounds were diminished somewhat on the right; there was dullness at the right base; the left lung was clear to percussion and auscultation. The remainder of the examination was negative. (5)

Because of her history of chronic asthma, I suggested she might consider bronchoscopy if this fluid reaccumulates. Because she is a heavy smoker, I insisted she stop smoking completely. If she does not, she will not enjoy continuing good health (although I have no idea of the actual prognosis). (6)

Mrs. Martinez has been returned to you for her continuing care. I will be glad to see her again at any time you think it necessary.

Thank you for letting me see this pleasant lady with you. (7)

Sincerely yours,

Jon L. Mikosan, MD

your initials

Enclosure: Pathology report (8)

A

A *Answers to* 6–7: TYPING PRACTICE TEST

The markings are a facsimile for proper placement on the #10 envelope.

1.

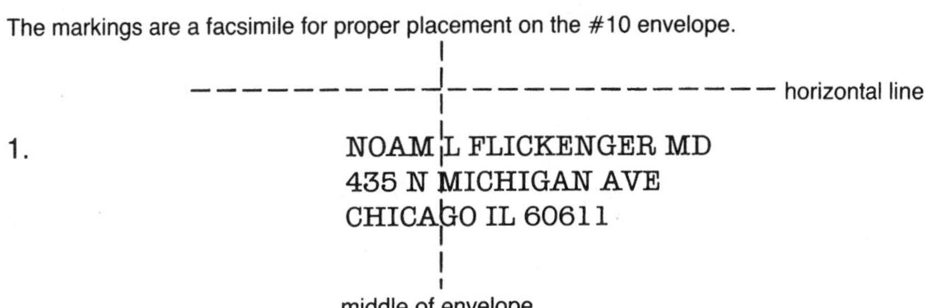

SPECIAL DELIVERY or Special Delivery is typed under the postage area leaving plenty of room for stamp or meter impression placement.

2.

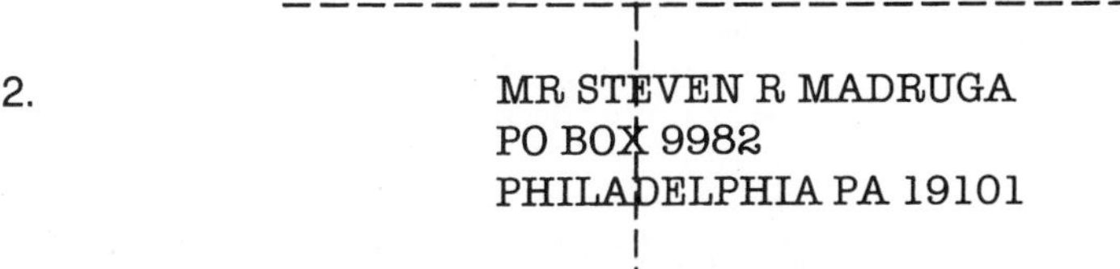

MR STEVEN R MADRUGA
PO BOX 9982
PHILADELPHIA PA 19101

3.

ATTN MRS SYLVIA FARQUAR
OCCIDENTAL LIFE INSURANCE CO
1150 S OLIVE SUITE 16
LOS ANGELES CA 90015

Be sure that the "attention line" is positioned properly either here or just below the name of the firm.

4.

MS MARIJANE N WOODS
MGR DESERT REALTY (also MANAGER DESERT REALTY)
2036 E CAMELBACK RD
PHOENIX AZ 85018

Be sure that the "confidential" notation is placed under the return address area in the upper left hand corner of the envelope.

A

A *Answers to* **7–4: PRACTICE TEST**

September 15, 199X

Carroll W. Noyes, MD
2113 Fourth Avenue, Suite 171
Houston, TX 77408

RE: Erma Hanlyn

Dear Dr. Noyes:

I first saw Erma Hanlyn, your patient, on July 18, 199X, with a history of a thyroid nodule since March of this year. This 35-year-old woman had it diagnosed at Alvarado Hospital where they urged her to have surgery, I guess.

She gave a history that the nodule was quite tender when she was seen there, and that she was on thyroid when they took her scan. However, when I saw her, the tenderness was gone. I could not feel any nodule.

We have had her stay off the thyroid so that we could get an accurate reading, and on September, 8, 199X, we had another scintigram done at Piikea General Hospital which revealed a symmetrical thyroid; it was free of any demonstrable nodules. All of the tenderness is gone and she feels well. She is elated over the fact that she has avoided surgery.

In my opinion, Mrs. Hanlyn probably had a thyroiditis when she was seen at Alvarado, and the radioactive iodine that she was given for the test is responsible for the cure.

Thank you very much for letting me see her with you, and I will be happy to see her again at any time you or she feel it is necessary.

Sincerely,

Kwei-Hay Wong, MD

student's initials

A

A *Answers to* **7–5: PRACTICE TEST**

1. he had one **slight** dyspnea	one-flight
2. she uses oxygen **binasal** prongs	by nasal
3. the neck is **subtle**	supple
4. he had a **mild cardial** infarction	myocardial
5. sutured along the **buckle** sulcus	buccal
6. Dx: Hypertension, **ideology** unknown	etiology
7. **palette** and tongue are normal	palate

8. **by manual** examination of the uterus	bimanual
9. no change in **gate** or stance	gait
10. unable to **breath**	breathe
11. pressure at the **sight** of the bleeding	site
12. one **sinkable** episode	syncopal
13. **bleeding** of the amniotic fluid	leaking
14. the right **plural** space	pleural
15. receptive **aphagia** for verbal commands	aphasia
16. **planter** reflex is negative	plantar
17. deep tendon **refluxes are in tact**	reflexes are intact
18. no rales or **bronchi**	rhonchi
19. retinal exam revealed **papal edema**	papilledema
20. a grey **whirling** tumor	whorling

A *Answers to* 8–2: PRACTICE TEST

1. maneuver	Pinard's	6. membrane	diphtheritic
2. acid	salicylic	7. disease	idiopathic
3. test	Wassermann	8. carcinoma	scirrhous or scirrhus
4. duct or gland	Bartholin's	9. tunica	adventitia
5. vas	spirale	10. disease	Alzheimer's

A *Answers to* 8–3: PRACTICE TEST

1. Colles'
   Book D Section orthopedic
   Book H Section C
   Book M Section Chapter 3
   Comments: Answers will vary. "Last entry because I don't know if I should use the apostrophe."

2. Albuquerque
   Book F Section A
   Comments: Answers will vary. "I would write it in my reference book."

3. Castroviejo
   Book K Section scissors
   Book I Section C
   Book D Section eye
   Comments: Answers will vary. "I knew this last one because I remembered they are used in eye surgery."

4. extirpative
   Book E Section e
   Book K Section miscellaneous
   Book N Section e
   Comments: Answers will vary. "I have this one already."

5. 15 mg or 50 mg
   Book A Section drug name
   Comments: Answers will vary.

A

6. mucous — Book M Section homonyms Appendix A
Book D Section skin
Comments: Answers will vary. Actually *mucus* is also a correct word here.

7. pylorus — Book D Section GI
Book E Section P
Comments: Answers will vary.

8. D&C — Book C Section D
Book M Section Chapter 5
Comments: Answers will vary. "I cannot remember if the spacing with the letters is correct."

9. aphasia — Book M Section homonyms Appendix B
Book D Section neurology
Comments: Answers will vary.

10. Darvocet-N — Book B Section D
Comments: Answers will vary. "I always use this one."

11. 120 over 80 — Book M Section Chapter 5
Comments: Answers will vary. "Not written correctly. It is 120/80."

12. pH — Book C Section P
Book D Section laboratory
Comments: Answers will vary. "We also have a laboratory reference in the classroom and I know this one anyway."

13. Mycobacterium — Book M Section Appendix B
Book D Section respiratory
Comments: Answers will vary.

14. Tms — Book C Section T
Book D Section ears
Comments: Answers will vary.

15. PERRLA — Book C Section P
Book D Section eyes
Comments: Answers will vary.

A *Answers to* 8–5: PRACTICE TEST

1. eject	do not divide	8.11, 8.14
2. couldn't	do not divide or spell out could not	8.16
3. page 590	do not divide	8.18
4. impossible	im/possible or impos/sible	8.9
5. scheme	do not divide	8.13
6. 7 o'clock	do not divide or spell out seven/o'clock	8.18
7. today	do not divide	8.11
8. doesn't	do not divide or spell out does not	8.16
9. 2480 Ames Drive	2480 Ames/Drive	8.17
10. CHAMPUS	do not divide	8.16
11. t.i.d.	do not divide	8.16
12. shipped	do not divide	8.13
13. around	do not divide	8.14
14. 7,201,082,976	do not divide	8.16
15. John Jeffers, M.D.	do not divide or John/Jeffers, M.D.	8.6
16. 35-year-old	35-/year-old or 35-year-/old	8.7

Answers to 8–6: PRACTICE TEST

1. claustrophobia claustro/phobia
2. infraorbital infra/orbital
3. leukopenia leuko/penia
4. postoperative post/operative
5. posterolateral postero/lateral
6. tuberosity tuber/osity
7. acromion acro/mion
8. metatarsus meta/tarsus
9. myoplasty myo/plasty
10. bursitis burs/itis or bur/sitis
11. edema do not divide
12. viruses vi/ruses

Answers to 8–7: PRACTICE TEST

1. b (preferred) (all right)
2. a (supersede)
3. b (embarrassed)
4. b (drunkenness)
5. a (irresistible)
6. b (occurrence)
7. a (ecstasy)
8. a (anoint)
9. b (occasion)
10. a (disappoint)
11. b (analyze)
12. a (tyranny)
13. a (inoculate)
14. b (coolly)
15. a (indispensable)
16. a (superintendent)
17. a (battalion)
18. a (perseverance)
19. a (iridescent)
20. b (recommend)

Answers to 8–8: PRACTICE TEST

	Remember the Silent	*Spelling*
1.	g	gnathodynia
2.	p	pterygium
3.	p	pneumatic
4.	c	cnemial
5.	k	knock-knee
6.	rh	dysmenorrhea
7.	rh	hemorrhage
8.	e	cacogeusia
9.	rh	metrorrhexis
10.	rh	menometrorrhagia

Answers to 8–10: PRACTICE TEST

1. altogether
2. all together
3. anyone
4. anyway
5. any way
6. Although
7. all right
8. some day
9. someday
10. all ready
11. already
12. any time
13. anytime
14. everyday
15. some time
16. sometime
17. any more
18. anything
19. awhile
20. anywhere
21. everything
22. anybody

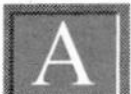

Answers to 8–13: PRACTICE TEST

Note: Answers to this test may vary depending on the edition of the *Physicians' Desk Reference* (PDR) that is used to look for answers. Remember that some generic names have been adopted by drug manufacturers as brand names, but the generic form is to be used when transcribing reports unless the employer specifies otherwise. Some generic names may sound like a brand name but may be spelled differently (e.g., *adrenaline* with an "e" on the end is the generic and *Adrenalin* without an "e" is the brand name).

1. Depending on the PDR edition, the answer may be one of the following: Brand and Generic Name Index (1996), Product Name Index, or Alphabetical Index (pink) Brand Names.
2. a. Valium (tablets or injectable), Valrelease (capsules)
   b. atenolol
   c. simvastatin
   d. Mevacor (tablets)
   e. Tenormin (tablets or injectable), Tenoretic (tablets)
   f. warfarin sodium
3. Lanoxin; flag the location in the document and check with the physician/dictator of the report.

A *Answers to* 8–14: PRACTICE TEST

1. Thorazine	chlorpromazine
2. Benadryl	diphenhydramine HCl
3. Hygroton	chlorthalidone
4. Dilantin	phenytoin sodium
5. Provera	medroxyprogesterone acetate
6. Gantrisin	sulfisoxazole diolamine
7. Tofranil	imipramine HCl
8. Lomotil	diphenoxylate HCl
9. Pyridium	phenazopyridine HCl
10. Mellaril	thioridazine

A *Answers to* 10–2: PRACTICE TEST

1. advise
2. lay
3. compliment
4. Whose
5. Your, too
6. razed
7. surge, forth
8. cite
9. course
10. here, hear
11. stationery
12. effect
13. effect
14. then
15. than
16. correspondence
17. break
18. principal, site
19. accept
20. effected
21. there
22. They're, They are
23. their

A *Answers to* 10–4: PRACTICE TEST

1. opposition
2. apposition
3. position
4. abrasion
5. aberration
6. dysphagia
7. dysphasia
8. absorption
9. adsorption
10. adherents
11. adherence

A

A *Answer to* 11–2: PRACTICE TEST

Maryellen Mawson — Age: 6

(Today's date) This is a 6-year-old who has had a 3-week history of polydipsia, polyuria, polyphagia, and weight loss. The child has become progressively more lethargic over the past 24 hours and 12 hours ago, the parents noticed she was breathing rapidly.

PX: Height: 127 cm. Weight: 33 kg. Temp: 99°F. Pulse: 112. BP: 95/70. The child was semicomatose. She has dry mucous membranes but good skin turgor and full peripheral pulses.

STAT Lab: Sodium: 138 mEq/L. Potassium 3.3 mEq/L. Chloride: 97 mEq/L. Total CO_2: 5 mEq/L. Blood glucose: 700 mg%.

PLAN: Admit STAT to Childrens Hospital.

(student's initials)

Eugene W. Gomez, MD

A *Answers to* **12–2: PRACTICE TEST**

Joseph R. Balentine
423-12-22
Copy: Stuart L. Paulson, MD

HISTORY

CHIEF COMPLAINT: This patient is a 25-year old male complaining of recurring epistaxis.

PRESENT ILLNESS: This patient reports that yesterday he had onset of epistasis in the left side of his nose. This was intermittent throughout the day, and at 4:30 this morning, he came in to the ER.

PAST HISTORY;
ALLERGIES None.
ILLNESSES: The patient had a collapsed lung about five years ago and subsequently had surgery but does not know the exact etiology of the problem or the exact name of the surgery. There is no bleeding history except for PI.
MEDICATIONS: None.

FAMILY HISTORY: Essentially unremarkable. Father, mother, siblings are all well and healthy.

REVIEW OF SYSTEMS:
SKIN; No rashes or jaundice.
HEENT: See PI
CR: See Past History. No history of pneumonia, tuberculosis, chronic cough, or hemoptysis. No history of pedal edema.
GI: Weight is stable, He denies any nausea, vomiting, diarrhea, or food intolerance.
GU: No history of GU tract infections, dysuria, hematuria, pyuria.
ENDOCRINE: No polyuria or polydipsia.
NEUROLOGIC: No history of psychiatric disorder

mlo
D: 11-16-XX
T: 11-16-XX

Benjamin B. Abboud, MD

(You should check to ensure that the format is that indicated: block. Check to be sure that all lines are blocked, main topics are typed in full caps and underlined, and subtopics are indented and typed in full caps. You may double space between main topics and subtopics, single space between subtopics. Be sure that the copy notation is made at either the top or the bottom. Patient and ID number of patient at top of page. Assignment should be neat, attractive, with narrow margins.)

Student: If you are preparing an outline of this sort and the main topic or subtopic dictated is too long, consider using two lines for it. It would appear like this, for example:

MEDICATIONS AND DRUGS: The patient is a social drinker except on the weekends when he may "binge" on "a couple of six-packs." He denies use of recreational drugs and is taking Paxil for depression. He takes Motrin p.r.n. for headaches.

It is also acceptable to make two topics as illustrated:

DRUGS: The patient is a social drinker except on the weekends when he may "binge" on "a couple of six-packs." He denies use of recreational drugs.

MEDICATIONS: Paxil for depression. He takes Motrin p.r.n. for headaches.

A *Answers to* **12–5: PRACTICE TEST**

Copies: Be sure that the copies are designated properly to Willow Moran, MD and Gordon Bender, MD. (These are given as Dr. Willow Moran and Dr. Gordon Bender in the directions. By now, you should be able to make the proper title change.)

Topics and Subtopics: Check these carefully as all were not "dictated." The Review of Systems is called the "Functional Inquiry" in this exercise.

Continuation: Be sure that the first page is marked "continued" and the second page carries all the vital patient data. (See Figure 12–6.)

Impression: These should be numbered 1 through 4 although the "dictator" failed to designate them in other than individual sentences.

Lily Mae Jenkins
5980-A
Copies: Willow Moran, MD
Gordon Bender, MD

HISTORY

CHIEF COMPLAINT: Rectal bleeding, one day.

PRESENT ILLNESS: This 90-year-old lady has been looking after her own personal affairs and living with her daughter for the last three years. Last night, she had a bowel movement that had some bright rectal blood mixed in with it. This morning, she had another bowel movement, and it consisted mostly of bright-red blood. She has a history of gallbladder disease, dating back over 50 years. She refused to have her gallbladder taken out but has been on a low-fat diet ever since that time. Her daughter describes numerous gallbladder attacks, lasting for several days, consisting of severe, right upper quadrant pain. She has had occasional, intermittent right lower quadrant pain that does not seem similar to the gallbladder attacks.

PAST HISTORY: Operations: In 1927, she had enucleation of the left eye. She had surgery in 1986 for glaucoma in the right eye. Medical: 1976, Colles' fracture, right wrist. 1980's, severe arthritis of her spine.

MEDICATIONS: Patient is presently taking Peritrate, 1 capsule, b.i.d. Reserpine-A, 1 tablet q a.m. Indocin, 1 tablet, t.i.d. She takes Bufferin p.r.n. for pain. She takes nitroglycerin, 2–3 tablets per week for chest pain and has done so for 5 years.

FAMILY: Both of her parents lived until their nineties. She had 6 children: 1 died at age 3, the result of injuries sustained in an automobile accident, 1 died at age 56 of carcinoma of the breast. Otherwise, the family history is unremarkable. There are 4 children who are alive and well.

(continued)

Lily Mae Jenkins
5980-A
Physical Examination, page 2

FUNCTIONAL INQUIRY: HEENT: Hearing in her right ear is absent. Hearing in her left ear is decreased. There is an artificial eye in the left and there is only slight vision in her right eye if one comes exactly in the middle of her visual field. Patient has been edentulous for several years.
CHEST: Nonsmoker.
CV: Patient has had angina for over five years and abnormal cardiograms for the last three. She is cold all of the time and is constantly bundling herself up in an effort to keep warm.
GI: Her bowel movements have been normal. See History of Present Illness.
GU: She has no history of any bladder or kidney infections, despite the fact that she had a history of kidney failure last year.
NM: Patient has shooting, severe pains up her spine, which are relatively incapacitating, but she manages to keep going by just taking Bufferin.

PHYSICAL EXAMINATION

GENERAL: This is a 90-year-old black woman in no obvious distress, who is hard of hearing but can answer questions.

HEENT: Ears: There is wax in both ears. The drums, beyond the wax, appear within normal limits. There is no hearing in the right ear and only slight hearing in the left. Eyes: The left eye is artificial. The right eye is pinpoint. There is no scarring in the right eye, consistent with an iridectomy. She has a cataract in the right eye, as well. Nose: Unremarkable. Mouth: Edentulous. Neck: There are no carotid bruits. No jugular venous distention. Thyroid is palpable and unremarkable. Range of motion of the neck is generally slightly restricted.

CHEST: Clear to percussion and auscultation. Heart: The apex beat is not palpable. There is some tenderness over the costochondral cartilages on the left side. Heart size is not enlarged to percussion. There is muffled heart sound. There is no third or fourth heart sound. There are no murmurs heard in the supine position. Breasts: Palpable and there are no masses noted.

ABDOMEN: Soft. There are marked senile keratoses over the abdominal wall. There is some diffuse tenderness on deep palpation over the cecum in the right lower quadrant. There is no other tenderness noted or abnormal bowel sounds noted in the abdomen. Bowel sounds are within normal limits.

PELVIC: Not done.

RECTAL: Full sigmoidoscopic examination to 25 cm revealed fresh blood in the sigmoid area with no obvious bleeding source noted.

EXTREMITIES: There is essentially no motion in the back. Range of motion of the hips is within normal limits and painless. There is only a +1 dorsalis pedis on the right; otherwise, there are no peripheral pulses present. There is marked coldness of both feet.

CNS: The patient's strength is within normal limits. The reflexes are within normal limits. Coordination is not tested. There is an involuntary shaking, consistent with the diagnosis of old Parkinson's disease.

IMPRESSION:
1. Acute gastrointestinal hemorrhage, etiology not yet diagnosed.
2. Chronic cholecystitis.
3. Severe osteoarthritis of spine.
4. Arteriosclerotic heart disease with angina pectoris.

(student's initials)
D: *(today's date)*
T: *(today's date)*

Philip D. Quince, MD

A

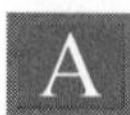

Answer to **13–2: PRACTICE TEST**

This assignment is to be set up using indented format with no variations.

Date: January 4, 19––

Dwight, John P.
86-30-21
Room No. 582-B

OPERATIVE REPORT

PREOPERATIVE DIAGNOSIS: Otosclerosis, left ear.

POSTOPERATIVE DIAGNOSIS: Otosclerosis, left ear.

OPERATION: Left stapedectomy.

FINDINGS: Otosclerosis footplate.

PROCEDURE: Under local anesthesia, the ear was prepared and draped in the usual manner. The ear was injected with 2% Xylocaine and 1:6,000 Adrenalin. A stapes-type flap was elevated from the posterosuperior canal wall, and the bony overhang was removed with the stapes curet. The chorda tympani nerve was removed from the field. The incudostapedial joint was separated. The stapes tendon was cut. The superstructure was removed. The mucous membrane was reflected from the ear, stapes, and the facial nerve promontory. The footplate was then reamed with small picks and hooks. A flattened piece of Gelfoam was placed over the oval window and a 5 mm wire loop prosthesis was inserted and crimped in the incus. The drum was reflected and a small umbilical tape was placed in the ear canal. The patient tolerated the procedure well.

Surgeon ______________________
Felix A. Konig, MD

(student's initials)
D: *1–4-year*
T: *(current date)*

Line 11: Some physicians dictate "same" for the postoperative diagnosis. Although it is not incorrect to type it, the preferred style is to spell out the diagnosis again.

Line 18: Adrenalin is the brand and epinephrine is the generic name; Xylocaine is the brand name for lidocaine.

A

Answer to **13-3: PRACTICE TEST**

This assignment is to be set up using modified block format and no variations.

PATHOLOGY REPORT

DATE:	June 6, 199–	PATHOLOGY NO. 532009	
PATIENT:	Joan Alice Jayne	ROOM NO.	453-A
PHYSICIAN:	John A. Myhre, MD	HOSPITAL NO.	72-11-03

SPECIMEN(S): The specimen consists of a 4.5 cm in diameter nodule of fibro-fatty tissue removed from the right breast at biopsy, and enclosing a central, firm, sharply demarcated nodule 1 cm in diameter. Surrounding breast parenchyma reveals dilated ductiles (microcystic disease).

FROZEN SECTION IMPRESSION: Myxoid fibroadenoma of breast.

MICROSCOPIC AND DIAGNOSIS: Myxoid fibroadenoma occurring in right parenchyma, the site of microcystic disease of right breast.

Pathologist ______________________________
James T. Rodgers, MD

(student's initials)
D: *6-6-year*
T: *(current date)*

A

A *Answer to* **13–5: PRACTICE TEST**

This assignment is to be set up using modified block format with indented paragraphs and mixed punctuation.

Letterhead

Current Date

Glen M. Hiranuma, MD
2501 Main Street
Ventura, CA 93003

RE: Mrs. Hazel R. Plunkett

Dear Dr. Hiranuma:

Thank you for referring your patient Mrs. Hazel R. Plunkett for neurological consultation, evaluation, and treatment of chronic and recurrent headaches.

In the past, the patient has had episodes of probably typical migraine occurring perhaps six or eight times in her life. She remembers that her mother had a similar complaint. This would begin with loss in the field of vision; and then, approximately fifteen minutes thereafter, she would have a relatively typical, unilateral throbbing pain of a significant degree which would often incapacitate her. These headaches disappeared many years ago and have never returned.

However, for the last eight years approximately, the patient has had recurrent daily headaches, always right-sided, with associated pain beginning in the back of the neck with stiffness of the right side of the neck, radiating forwards over the vertex to the right orbit, the nose, and the jaw. She also notes some pain in the right trapezius area. The pain tends to appear from 10 a.m. to noon, when she will take a Fiorinal, and often after she goes to sleep at night (at about 12:30 a.m.). She controls this pain by taking Fiorinal, one to four a day, and Elavil, 75 mg at bedtime. She estimates that the headaches occur approximately twice daily, are relatively short-lived, but occasionally last a full day. The pain is dull and heavy, not throbbing, and worse at some times than at others.

On examination she was a quiet woman, not in acute distress, and somewhat dour; but she gave a careful and concise history. Her gait and station were normal. The head functions were basically intact. The fundi showed only modest arteriosclerotic changes. The temporal arteries were normal. Facial motility and sensation were normal. There was a significant right carotid bruit present, which was persistent and could be heard all along the course of the right carotid artery. It was not transmitted from the neck. There were moderate pain and tenderness at the insertion of the great muscles of the neck and the occiput, and palpation over this area consistently reproduced the patient's symptoms. She also had a persistent area of tenderness in the right trapezius muscle. Otherwise, power, size, and symmetry of the arms and legs were essentially normal. The deep tendon reflexes were brisk. There were no long tract or focal signs, and sensation was intact.

Impression:
1. Muscle contraction headaches, chronic.
2. Localized myositis, right side of the neck, right shoulder girdle.
3. Right carotid bruit, silent, asymptomatic.

A

RE: Mrs. Hazel R. Plunkett
Page 2
(Current Date)

Comment: The findings were discussed in detail with the patient, but no neurological studies were done. I suggested simple measures of physical therapy to the neck including the use of heat, hot packs, and massage and advised also that she purchase a cervical pillow on which to rest during the day. Motrin, 400 mg twice daily and Maolate, 400 mg at night were suggested in an attempt to provide anti-inflammatory and muscle relaxant properties. It may also be necessary to inject these tender areas which are quite well localized. This can be determined after 30 to 60 days on the treatment regimen outlined above.

The patient also has what seems to be a silent right carotid bruit. Certainly she is without symptoms. This should be brought to the attention of those who are caring for her, so that if transient ischemic attacks appear in the future, appropriate steps can be taken. I do not think that the right carotid bruit has anything to do with the patient's headaches, which are not vascular, and certainly there is no sign of cranial arteritis.

She was referred back to you for continuing medical service. Thank you for the opportunity of seeing this patient.

Sincerely,

Margo A. Wilkins, MD

(student's initials)

A *Answer to* **14–2: PRACTICE TEST**

WHY:	Dr. Berry has received her request and has agreed to make an abstract of her record. He wishes to meet with her and discuss the abstract. He wishes to answer any questions she may have.
WHO:	Obtain complete name and address of patient.
WHAT:	Find out how much time Dr. Berry wishes to save for the conference. $40 fee for the conference and abstract. Choose a date and time for the conference.
REACTION:	Patient is to call if the plans are suitable or make new arrangements.
	(and a special note for myself:
FOLLOW-UP:	Be sure abstract is dictated and transcribed in time for the conference.)

A

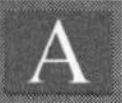

Answer to **15–1: PRACTICE TEST**

MEMO

DATE: May 7, 199X

TO: Your name, Office Manager
Mary Connors, CMT
Sue Marcos, RN
Joan Taylor, CMA-A

FROM: Dr. Berry

SUBJECT: Use of photocopy equipment

Attached is a brochure outlining in detail our new photocopy equipment. Please become familiar with its operation and upkeep.

The machine is to be used only for the following:

1. To reproduce billing statements.
2. To make copies of completed insurance claims.
3. To make copies of chart documents when required.
4. To make copies of correspondence.

Please ask me for permission for any personal use of the machine.

(your initials)

A *Answers to* **15–3: PRACTICE TEST**

HOLTER MONITOR CV-15

OBJECTIVE:

To obtain a magnetic tape record of a patient's electrocardiographic activity over a 24-hour period.

EQUIPMENT:

1. Holter monitor.
2. Battery.
3. Tape.
4. Patient cable.
5. Universal cable.
6. ECG machine.
7. ECG electrodes.
8. 2 × 2 pads, alcohol, and Redux paste.
9. Transpore tape.
10. Patient diary.
11. Shaving prep kit.

PROCEDURE:

1. Verify the physician's order by checking the medical chart.
2. Assemble all equipment and bring to the patient's bedside.
3. Introduce yourself to the patient and thoroughly explain what you are about to do.
4. Verify the patient's identity by checking the patient's I.D. bracelet.
5. Have the patient remove all clothing covering his or her chest.
6. Locate the necessary anatomical landmarks and prepare the five areas as follows:
   a. Shave all hair.
   b. Cleanse the area with alcohol.
   c. Scrub the cleansed area with Redux paste.
   d. Remove the Redux paste with alcohol.
7. Attach the electrodes to the patient's chest.
   a. 2nd rib space on the right side of the sternum.
   b. 2nd rib space on the left side of the sternum.
   c. Over the xiphoid process.
   d. Right V4—Right mid-clavicular at the 5th intercostal space.
   e. Left V4—Left mid-clavicular at the 5th intercostal space.
8. Attach the electrode cables to the patient:
   a. White—right arm.
   b. Brown—left arm.
   c. Black—V1.
   d. Green—right leg.
   e. Red—left leg.
9. Tape the electrode cables in a loop on the patient's abdomen allowing the cable to hang free.
10. Place a tape in the Holter monitor unit.
11. Place a battery in the Holter monitor unit.
12. Attach the recorder to the belt or shoulder strap (patient's preference).
13. Plug Universal cable into recorder.
14. Connect RA, LA, RL, LL, and V1 from ECG machine to Universal cable.
15. Connect patient cable to recorder.
16. Run a short strip on the ECG machine to verify the quality of the tracing (L1, L2, L3, AVR, AVL, AVF, and V1).
17. Disconnect Universal cable from recorder unit.
18. Set time on recorder and start Holter monitor.
19. Record starting time in the patient diary and explain the importance of the diary to the patient.
20. If an outpatient, remind the patient of the importance of returning in 24 hours.
21. After 24 hours, record ending time in the patient's diary.
22. Remove the cable from the recorder.
23. Remove the cable and electrodes from the patient.
24. Prepare the tape for scanning.

A

<u>CARE OF EQUIPMENT:</u>

1. Exercise caution when handling unit to avoid dropping.
2. Instruct patient not to bathe, shower, or go swimming while attached to the unit.
3. Clean recording heads and capstan with alcohol after each patient use.

<u>IMPORTANT POINTS:</u>

1. Proper preparation of the patient's chest is important to a good recording.
2. Run a short strip with the ECG machine to insure that the electrodes are placed correctly.
3. Make sure the patient thoroughly understands the importance of the diary.

Approved: ____________________ Policy Number 90-202

Effective date: (current date) Revised:
Reviewed: Revised:

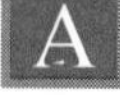

Answers to **16–1: PRACTICE TEST**

COCKTAILS CAN CAUSE CARDIAC COMPLICATIONS

A Manuscript Prepared

for

Modern Medicine

Chicago, Illinois

by

Roger Balor, MD

Mount Sinai Hospital and Mount Sinai School of Medicine

of the City University of New York

New York City, New York

Current Date

COCKTAILS CAN CAUSE CARDIAC COMPLICATIONS[1]

Prolonged, heavy ingestion of alcohol by certain individuals, even though they are well nourished, may result in cardiac abnormalities that are evident clinically or electrocardiographically, or both. Electrocardiographic abnormalities in these patients may indicate the early developmental stages of cardiomyopathy, a process that may be reversed if the patient abstains from ingestion of alcohol.

Cardiac abnormalities in well-nourished alcoholics may include resting tachycardia, sinus tachycardia or bradycardia, premature ventricular contractions, premature atrial contractions, paroxysmal atrial fibrillation, or a rhythm varying between sinus rhythm with frequent premature beats and atrioventricular dissociation. First-degree atrioventricular block also may be found.

Notched or tall P waves may be present on the electrocardiogram. In addition, the QRS complex may show some abnormality, as may the S-T segment and T wave. T-wave abnormalities may consist of diminished wave amplitudes, diphasic waves, or frank wave inversion. Some patients may have enlarged hearts.

The electrocardiograms of 50 randomly chosen, well-nourished alcoholics were studied and compared with those from 50 nonalcoholic controls. No subject in either group had any known heart disease.

The electrocardiogram was considered to be within normal limits in 36 alcoholic patients but was clearly abnormal in four others. Only one control patient had an abnormal electrocardiogram.

---

1. George J. Sanna, MD, Quarterly Journal for the Study of Alcoholism, 34: 774-785, 1984.

A

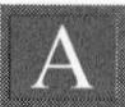

Answers to **16–3: PRACTICE TEST**

CATEGORIES OF TUMORS

A Manuscript Prepared

for

Journal of the American Medical Association

Chicago, Illinois

by

Joan T. Bennett, MD

XYZ Medical Center

Philadelphia, Pennsylvania

Current Date

A

CATEGORIES OF TUMORS

There are many categories of tumors. Epithelial tumors is the topic of interest.

1. Epithelial tumors. These tumors arise from the coelomic mesothelium, which is capable of differentiating into both benign and malignant tumors. The transition from benign to malignant is not abrupt; there is an intermediate or borderline category. Distinguishing benign, borderline, or malignant tumors is important in terms of treatment and prognosis. Epithelial malignancies represent 82% of all ovarian malignancies.
   a. The predominant cell types are:
      (1) Serous
         (a) One out of three serous tumors is malignant.
         (b) Serous cancers are more than three times as common as the mucinous variety and seven times as common as the endometrioid variety.
         (c) Serous cystadenoma carcinoma, the most common type of ovarian cancer, tends to be bilateral in 35%–50% of cases.
      (2) Mucinous
         (a) One out of five mucinous tumors is malignant.
         (b) Mucinous tumors are bilateral in 10%–20% of cases.
      (3) Endometrioid
         (a) The microscopic pattern is similar to primary carcinoma of the endometrium.
         (b) Areas of endometriosis on the ovary may be present.
         (c) The prognosis is much better than that of the serous and mucinous carcinomas.
   b. The prognosis for each stage of epithelial ovarian tumors is linked to the grade of the tumor; poorly differentiated tumors have a poor prognosis. Long-term survival of patients with borderline or well-differentiated cancers after primary surgery is common.

A

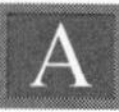

Answers to **16–4: PRACTICE TEST**

1. title page
2. capital
3. letter of transmittal
4. page number
5. double spacing or manuscript format
6. single
7. footnotes
8. single spacing within the footnote and double spacing between footnotes
9. a. et al.
   b. ibid.
   c. i.e.
   d. e.g.
10. bibliography
11. et al.
12.

	Top	Bottom	Left	Right	Page Number
a. Unbound report:					
Page 1	2″	1″	1″	1″	none
Other pages	1″	1″	1″	1″	upper right or centered at top of page
b. Left-bound report:					
Page 1	2″	1″	1½″	1″	none
Other pages	1½″	1″	1½″	1″	upper right or centered at top of page

A

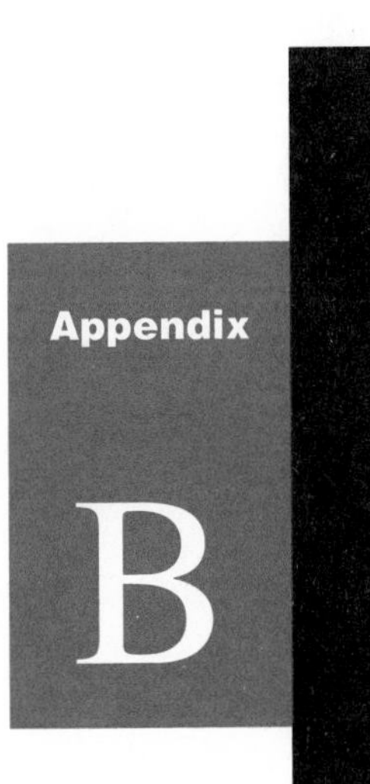

Reference Materials

CONTENTS

INTRODUCTION

The information in this section has been given on perforated pages so they can be torn out and placed into your personal standard-sized binder/transcriptionist notebook for easy and quick reference. These pages are merely the beginning of your collection, and you are encouraged to add to it on a daily basis as you encounter new information. The notebook will become an important and valuable tool that you will use as you develop the skill of transcription.

ABBREVIATIONS COMMONLY USED

This brief list contains some abbreviations that are commonly used in office chart notes and hospital records. You may want to remove it from the book or photocopy it and place it into your reference book so you can refer to it at any time. Later, you may want to add new abbreviations and institution-approved lists to your collection. Some abbreviations are said as a word (*cabbage* for *CABG* and *hope* for *HOPE*); others are said as an entire word that is turned into an abbreviation (*milligram* for *mg* and *see section* for *C-section*); and for some, each letter of the abbreviation is spoken (*b.i.d.* and *L&W*).

@	at
A, B, AB, O	these are blood types and can also be dictated with subscript numbers
A_1 or A1	first aortic sound
A_2 or A2	aortic second sound
AB/ab	abortion
ABGs	arterial blood gases
a.c.	before meals
ACh	acetylcholine
ACTH	adrenocorticotrophic hormone
a.d. or AD	right ear
a.d.	alternating days
A&D	ascending and descending (each letter is said: *ay-en-dee*)
ad lib.	freely (usually refers to drug or modality)
ADH	antidiuretic hormone; vasopressin
ADL	activities of daily living
ADT	admission, discharge, transfer
AFB	acid-fast bacillus (TB organism)
Ag	silver
AIDS	acquired immune deficiency syndrome (whole word is said: *aids*)
a.m. or AM	in the morning or before noon
AMA	against medical advice; American Medical Association
AP	anteroposterior (each letter is said: *ay-pee*)
A&P	auscultation and percussion
APC	acetylsalicylic acid (aspirin), phenacetin, and caffeine
Aq	water
ARC	AIDS-related complex (whole word is said: *ark*)
ARD	acute respiratory disease
ARDS	adult respiratory disease syndrome
a.s. or AS	left ear
ASAP	as soon as possible (see STAT)
ASCVD	atherosclerotic cardiovascular disease
ASD	atrial septal defect
Au	gold
AV	atrioventricular
A&W	alive and well
Ba	barium
baso	basophils
BBB	bundle-branch block
BCC	basal cell carcinoma
BE	barium enema
bib	drink
b.i.d.	twice a day (each letter is said)
BLE	both lower extremities
BLT	bilateral tubal ligation

B

BM	bowel movement
BP or B/P	blood pressure
BPH	benign prostatic hypertrophy
BS	blood sugar; bowel sounds
BUN	blood urea nitrogen (each letter is said)
BUS	Bartholin urethral and Skene (glands) (this is not said as a word)
BVE	bachelor of vocational education
Bx	biopsy
c̄	with
C or °C	Celsius
C_1 or C1	first cervical vertebra (continues through C7)
Ca	calcium
Ca or CA	carcinoma (each letter is said)
Ca^{++} or Ca^{2+}	calcium ion
CABG	coronary artery bypass graft surgery (said as *cabbage*)
CAD	coronary artery disease
CAT	computerized axial tomography
CBC	complete blood count
CC	chief complaint
cc	cubic centimeter (same as mL; said as *see-see* or *cubic centimeter*)
CCU	coronary care unit; critical care unit
CDC	Centers for Disease Control and Prevention
CF	complement fixation
CHD	coronary heart disease; chronic heart disease; congestive heart disease
CHF	congestive heart failure
cm	centimeter
CMA-A	certified medical assistant, administrative
CMA-C	certified medical assistant, clinical
CMT	certified medical transcriptionist
CNS	central nervous system
CO	carbon monoxide
Co	cobalt
CO2 or CO_2	carbon dioxide
COD	condition on discharge
COPD	chronic obstructive pulmonary disease
CPR	cardiopulmonary resuscitation
CPX	complete physical examination
CR	cardiorespiratory
C-section	cesarean section
CSF	cerebrospinal fluid
CT	computed tomography
Cu	copper
CVA	costovertebral angle; cerebrovascular accident
CXR	chest x-ray
D/C	discontinue
D&C	dilation and curettage (each letter is said: *dee-en-see*)
DD	differential diagnosis
D_5W or D5W	dextrose and water (each character is said)
DOA	dead on arrival
DOB	date of birth
DOE	dyspnea on exertion
DPM	doctor of podiatric medicine
DPT	diphtheria-pertussis-tetanus

B

DRG	diagnosis related group
DSM	*Diagnostic and Statistical Manual of Mental Disorders*
DTR	deep tendon reflexes
D/W	dextrose and water
Dx	diagnosis
EAC	external auditory canal
ECG	electrocardiogram
ECMO	extracorporal membrane oxygenation (said as *ek-moe*)
ED	emergency department
EDC	estimated date of confinement; due date for baby
EEG	electroencephalogram
EENT	eyes, ears, nose, throat
e.g.	example given (each letter is said: *e-gee*)
EKG	electrocardiogram
ELISA	enzyme-linked immunosorbent assay (said as a word)
EMG	electromyogram
EMI	see CAT
EMS	emergency medical services
EMT	emergency medical technician or emergency medical treatment
ENT	ear, nose, throat
EOM	extraocular movements
eos	eosinophils
eq.	equivalent
ER	emergency room
Esq.	esquire
ESR	erythrocyte sedimentation rate
et al.	and others (both words are said)
F or °F	Fahrenheit
FB	foreign body
FBS	fasting blood sugar
Fe	iron
FH	family history
FHT	fetal heart tone
fl oz	fluid ounce
FSH	follicle-stimulating hormone
ft	foot
5-FU	5-Fluorouracil (chemotherapy drug)
FUO	fever of unknown origin
Fx	fracture
G	gravida (pregnant)
gm or g	gram (authors prefer gm to avoid misunderstanding value)
G neg.	gram-negative
G pos.	gram-positive
GB	gallbladder
GC	gonorrhea
GH	growth hormone
GI	gastrointestinal
GP	general practitioner
gtt	drop(s)
GU	genitourinary
GYN or Gyn	gynecology/gynecologist
h	hour
H	hour or hydrogen

B

H^+	hydrogen ion
H_2O or H2O	water
Hb	hemoglobin (also hgb)
HCG	human chorionic gonadotropin
HCl	hydrochloric acid
Hct or hct	hematocrit
HDL	high-density lipoprotein
HEENT	head, eyes, ears, nose, and throat
Hg	mercury
hgb	hemoglobin
H&H	hemoglobin and hematocrit (test on rbcs)
HIV	human immunodeficiency virus
HOPE	Health Opportunities for People Everywhere (said as *hope*)
H&P	history and physical (words are said or each letter is said: *h-en-pee*)
HPF or hpf	high-power field
HPI	history of present illness
h.s.	bedtime (hour of sleep)
Hx	history
I	iodine
ibid.	in the same place
ICD–9–CM	International Classification of Diseases, Ninth Revision, Clinical Modification
ICU	intensive care unit
I&D	incision and drainage (each letter is said: *eye-en-dee*)
i.e.	that is (each letter is said: *eye-e*)
IgA	alpha immunoglobulin (also IgG, IgB, and IgE)
IM	intramuscular
IMP	impression
in.	inch
I&O	intake and output
IOP	intraocular pressure
IPPB	intermittent positive pressure breathing
IV or I.V.	intravenous
IVP	intravenous pyelogram
K	potassium
K^+	potassium ion
kg	kilogram
km	kilometer
KUB	kidneys, ureters, bladder
L	liter
L&A	light and accommodation
L1 or L_1	first lumbar vertebra (continues through L5)
lb	pound
LBBB	left bundle-branch block
LDL	low-density lipoprotein
LH	luteinizing hormone
LLQ	left lower quadrant
LMP	last menstrual period
LP	lumbar puncture
LPN	licensed professional nurse
LSH	lutein-stimulating hormone

B

LTH	lactogenic hormone, prolactin
LUQ	left upper quadrant
LVN	licensed vocational nurse
L&W	living and well
MDR	minimum daily requirement
mEq	milliequivalent
mg	milligram
Mg	magnesium
Mg^{++} or Mg^{2+}	magnesium ion
mg%	milligrams percent
MI	myocardial infarction
mL or ml	milliliter
MM	mucous membrane
mm	millimeter
mmHg or mm Hg	millimeters of mercury
monos	monocytes
MOPP	nitrogen mustard, Oncovin, prednisone, procarbazine (chemotherapy)
mOsm	milliosmol
MR	mitral regurgitation
MRI	magnetic resonance imaging
MS	masters degree in science
MS	multiple sclerosis
N	nitrogen
N^{+}	nitrogen ion
NA	not applicable
Na	sodium
Na^{+}	sodium ion
NG	nasogastric
NMI	no middle initial
NOS	not otherwise specified
NPC	near point of convergence (eyes); no previous complaint
NPH	no previous history
n.p.o.	nothing by mouth
NS	not significant
NSAID	nonsteroidal anti-inflammatory drug
NSR	normal sinus rhythm
NTP	normal temperature and pressure
NYD	not yet diagnosed
O_2 or O2	oxygen
OB	obstetrics
OB-GYN	obstetrics and gynecology
o.d.	right eye; every day
OD	right eye
OR	operating room
o.s. or OS	left eye
oz	ounce
P	phosphorus or pulse
P_1 or P1	pulmonic first sound (P1, P2, and so on)

B

P1	para 1 (and so on)
PA	posteroanterior
P&A	percussion and auscultation
Pap	Papanicolaou test/smear
PBI	protein-bound iodine
p.c.	after meals
pCO_2 or pCO2	pressure of carbon dioxide
PDR	*Physicians' Desk Reference* (drug reference)
PE	physical examination (also PX)
PERLA	pupils equal and reactive to light and accommodation
PET	positron emission tomography
PH	past history
pH	hydrogen ion concentration; degree of acidity or alkalinity
PI	present illness
PID	pelvic inflammatory disease
PIP	proximal interphalangeal (joint)
PKU	phenylketonuria (test given to newborns)
PM or p.m.	afternoon
PMH	past medical history
PMI	point of maximal impulse
PMS	premenstrual syndrome
PO	postoperative
p.o.	by mouth
pO_2 or pO2	pressure of oxygen
POC	products of conception
p.r.n.	as required or needed; as the occasion arises (each letter is said)
pt	patient
PTA	prior to admission
PVC	premature ventricular contraction
PX	physical examination (also PE)
Px	prognosis

q.	every
q.h.	every hour
q.2h.	every two hours
q.3h.	every three hours
q.4h.	every four hours
q.i.d.	four times a day (each letter is said)
QRS	complex in electrocardiographic study
qt	quart

R	respiration
r	roentgen
Ra	radium
RBBB	right bundle-branch block
RBC	red blood count
rbc	red blood cell
Rh (factor)	blood type (negative or positive factor antigen on the rbc)
RhoGAM	drug given to Rh negative women to avoid risk of blood titer (said as *row-gam*)
RLQ	right lower quadrant
RN	registered nurse
R/O	rule out

ROS	review of systems
RUQ	right upper quadrant
Rx	prescription or treatment
$\bar{s}$	without
SG	specific gravity
SGOT	serum glutamic pyruvic transaminase
SI	seriously ill
SIDS	sudden infant death syndrome (crib death)
sig.	directions
SMAC	automated analytic device for testing blood (said as *smack*)
SOAP	Subjective, Objective, Assessment, Plan used for patient notes
SOB	shortness of breath
sp. gr.	specific gravity
stat/STAT	immediately
S/S	signs and symptoms
STD	sexually transmitted disease
T1 or T_1	first thoracic vertebra (continues through T12)
T&A	tonsillectomy and adenoidectomy (said as *tee-en-ay*)
TAB	therapeutic abortion
TB	tuberculosis
TIA	transient ischemic attack
t.i.d.	three times a day
TM	tympanic membrane
TNTC	too numerous to count
TPR	temperature, pulse, respiration
TSH	thyroid stimulating hormone
TURP	transurethral resection of the prostate gland
Tx	treatment
U	unit (used in referring to measurement of blood)
U	uranium
UA	urinalysis
URI	upper respiratory infection
UTI	urinary tract infection
VA	visual acuity
VDRL	Venereal Disease Research Laboratory (test for syphilis)
VF	visual fields
viz	that is; namely
vs	versus
VS	vital signs
VSD	ventricular septal defect
V&T	volume and tension (pulse)
WBC	white blood count
wbc	white blood cell
w-d	well-developed
WF	white female
WM	white male
w-n	well-nourished
WNL	within normal limits
x	times
X match	cross-match

B

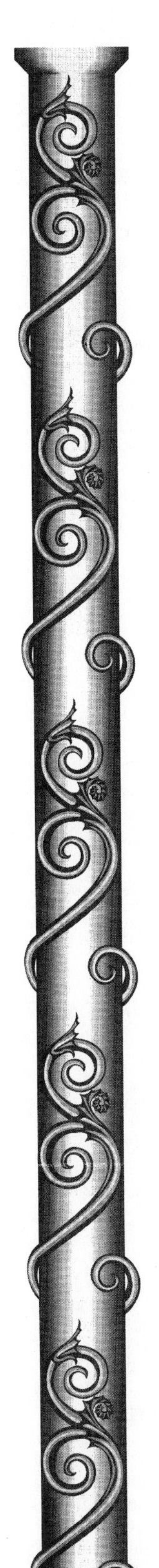

AAMT CODE OF ETHICS

Adopted July 10, 1995

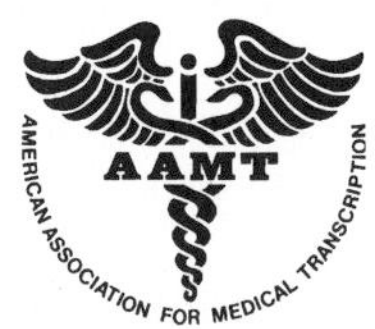

PART I
ASSOCIATION MEMBERSHIP

Preamble

Be aware that it is by our standards of conduct and professionalism that the American Association for Medical Transcription (AAMT) is evaluated. As members of AAMT we should recognize and observe the goals and objectives of the organization and the limitations and confinements imposed by its bylaws, policies, and procedures.

Scope of Member Conduct

AAMT members (in individual categories of membership) will:

1. Place the goals and purposes of the Association above personal gain and work for the good of the profession.

2. Discharge honorably and to the best of their ability the responsibility of any elected or appointed Association position.

3. Preserve the confidential nature of professional judgments and determinations made confidentially by the official bodies of the Association.

4. Represent truthfully and accurately (a) one's membership in the Association, (b) one's roles and functions in the association, and (c) any positions and decisions of the association.

B

PART II
PROFESSIONAL STANDARDS

Preamble

AAMT members are aware that it is by our standards of conduct and professionalism that the entire profession of medical transcription is evaluated. We should conduct ourselves in the practice of our profession so as to bring dignity and honor to ourselves and to the profession of medical transcription as medical language specialists. Therefore, the following standards are considered essential in the workplace:

1. A medical transcriptionist undertakes work only if s/he is competent to perform it.

2. A medical transcriptionist exhibits honesty and integrity in his/her professional work and activities.

3. A medical transcriptionist is reasonably familiar with and complies with principles of accuracy, authenticity, privacy, confidentiality, and security concerning patient care information.

4. A medical transcriptionist engages in professional reading and continuing education sufficient to stay abreast of important professional information.

5. A medical transcriptionist does not misrepresent or falsify information concerning medical records, his/her fees, work or professional experience, credentials, or affiliations.

6. A medical transcriptionist complies with applicable law and professional standards governing his/her work.

7. A medical transcriptionist does not assist others to violate ethical principles or professional standards of the medical transcription field.

8. If a medical transcriptionist learns of a significant unethical practice by another medical transcriptionist, s/he takes reasonable steps to resolve the matter.

9. A medical transcriptionist who agrees to serve in an official capacity in a professional association exhibits honesty and integrity in discharging his/her responsibilities.

10. AAMT members who are not medical transcriptionists should abide by the above principles where applicable.

AAMT CODE OF ETHICS POLICIES AND PROCEDURES

POLICY

The Code of Ethics is enforceable by the Ethics Committee as it applies to the members of the American Association for Medical Transcription. Professional standards are the basis of professional growth and development as they apply to the industry of medical transcription and to the medical transcriptionist as a medical language specialist. Issues involving actual or alleged ethical misconduct by an AAMT member will be resolved by the Ethics Committee by reference to interests of persons receiving healthcare services, those for whom transcriptionists provide services, the Association, and its members. Association and membership confidence must be safeguarded within the constraints of the law. The actions of the Association's members must be within the confines of the Code of Ethics. It is the duty of the Ethics Committee to place the welfare of those who receive healthcare services above all considerations. To this end, when and if an alleged ethical violation or act of misconduct is identified, the following process will apply.

B

COMPOSITION OF COMMITTEE

In accordance with the AAMT bylaws, the Ethics Committee Chair will be appointed by the President with the approval of the Board of Directors. The Committee will consist of 6 active AAMT members in good standing (who are not members of the Board of Directors) initially appointed by the Chair and the President; 3 members shall have 2-year terms and 3 members shall have 3-year terms. Appointments to fill vacancies will be made by the Chair and the President to complete the term vacated. Refer to criteria for selection of Committee members. The Ethics Committee is authorized to receive complaints, initiate a proceeding, conduct investigations, hold hearings, and make recommendations to the AAMT Board concerning instances of possible misconduct or violation of AAMT's Code of Ethics.

CONSIDERATIONS BROUGHT BEFORE THE COMMITTEE

The Ethics Committee may consider complaints in the following categories:

Member complaint: A complaint by a member of AAMT against another member must be in writing and signed by the complainant, and must describe the facts and ethical issues concerning the alleged misconduct.

Committee complaint: Of its own accord, the Ethics Committee may begin a proceeding if it becomes aware, through publicly available or governmental sources, of possible misconduct of a member.

COMMITTEE ACTIVITY

All complaints of violation of the Code of Ethics and/or an act of misconduct shall be addressed to the Chair of the Ethics Committee. Upon receipt of a member complaint or information that a complaint may be warranted, the Chair of the Committee shall consider the information and, after discussion with the President, Executive Director, and counsel, make a preliminary determination of whether a proceeding should be initiated, and if so, shall provide the respondent with a copy of the complaint, and request the complainant and the respondent to submit the names, addresses, and telephone numbers of each person who may have information on the matter.

AAMT, the AAMT Board of Directors, and the AAMT Ethics Committee shall take reasonable steps to maintain the confidentiality of all proceedings under the Code of Ethics so long as the affected member maintains the confidentiality of such proceedings.

If a proceeding is begun, the respondent shall receive a copy of the complaint and be advised by the Committee as to the apparent ethical questions of issue (additional questions may, however, be raised in the course of the process). The respondent shall be given 60 days (according to AAMT bylaws, Article IV, Section 3) in which to request the right to a hearing and to submit any information from all appropriate sources to the full extent available, consistent with the law and organizational rules. By availing himself/herself of the AAMT administrative process, the respondent agrees not to challenge it in any judicial proceeding until it is completed. Whether the respondent responds within 60 days or not, the Committee shall proceed with its investigation and make recommendations to the AAMT Board on the matter. The Committee shall be authorized to obtain the necessary information from all appropriate sources to the full extent consistent with the law and organizational rules.

If the member registering the complaint is a member of the Ethics Committee, or if the member against whom the complaint is registered is a member of the Ethics Committee, that Ethics Committee member shall be recused.

The Chair shall designate 1 member of the Committee to supervise and/or conduct the investigation in each case. The Committee member who supervises the investigation may not participate in the decision on the matter but may participate in the hearing. After preliminary investigation, if the Committee concludes that the information does not indicate any basis for a finding of misconduct, it shall promptly advise the respondent and the complainant and close the matter. If the Committee concludes that misconduct may or may not have occurred but any possible misconduct is not serious, or that the matter is unlikely to be susceptible to a clear resolution, it may send the member a letter expressing concern about the issue and suggest some form of disposition or resolution of the matter. If the member accepts the proposed disposition, the Ethics Committee shall recommend to the Board that the matter be resolved in this fashion. The Board can accept or reject the Committee's recommendation. If the matter is neither dismissed nor resolved, the Committee shall proceed to decide the matter or, if a hearing has been requested, proceed with the hearing process.

If the respondent resigns from AAMT during the pendency of a proceeding, the Committee may, in its discretion, continue or terminate the proceeding.

COMMITTEE HEARING

At least 30 days prior to the hearing on the matter of misconduct or violation of the Code of Ethics, the Ethics Committee shall prepare a record of all information gathered at that point and submit it to the respondent. The respondent shall then have 20 days in which to submit additional information, including statements of witnesses. All information submitted by all sources shall then be bound in a hearing record and maintained by AAMT. (See Glossary of Terms regarding hearing record.)

The following individuals may be allowed to attend the hearing at the AAMT office: Ethics Committee members, Association executive director and Association counsel, the respondent and respondent's counsel and witnesses, the complainant, and any other persons the Committee concludes have a legitimate purpose in attending. The respondent and the complainant, as well as the Committee, may be represented by counsel, make statements, present documentary evidence, and present and cross-examine witnesses, provided that the members of the Committee may not be examined. The respondent shall bear all costs of presenting his/her defense. The Committee may bear costs of other witnesses at its discretion. If the presence of a witness cannot be obtained for the hearing, his/her testimony may be presented in a notarized affidavit or other form of evidentiary documentation acceptable to the committee.

Formal judicial rules need not be applied by the Committee, and the Chair may conduct the hearing in a manner which efficiently elicits evidence consistent with fundamental fairness. The Chair may limit the length or manner of presenting evidence, or the scope of subjects addressed, or make any other rules necessary to conduct the hearing in a reasonable manner. A majority of the members of the Committee, excluding the one designated to supervise the investigation, shall constitute a quorum for hearing and deciding the matter.

DECISION AND RECOMMENDATIONS FROM THE COMMITTEE

The Committee shall make a recommendation to the board no later than 30 days after the close of the hearing. The decision shall be based only upon information within the hearing record. The decision for recommending a specific outcome shall be by majority of the voting members of the Committee. If the Committee decides that charges of misconduct against a member have not been proven by a preponderance of the evidence, it shall dismiss the matter and so inform the respondent, complainant, and any other parties deemed appropriate by the Chair. If the Committee decides that charges of misconduct against a member have been proven by a preponderance of the evidence, it shall issue its conclusions and recommendations to the AAMT Board with a copy to the respondent and complainant.

At the conclusion of the hearing, the hearing record shall be closed. This closed record shall be maintained at the AAMT administrative office and may be re-opened if there is another complaint related to the respondent within 7 years after the Board of Directors' final decision in the matter. (See below for Board of Directors decision-making process.) The hearing record shall be destroyed after 7 years. The Committee may recommend one or more of the following to the Board of Directors, with notification to member of recommended outcome:

a. The member be asked to not accept or hold any leadership position in AAMT or its component associations for a defined period.

b. The member be suspended from AAMT for a specified period of time, following which s/he may reapply.

c. The member be expelled from AAMT or agree to resign, in which case he/she may not reapply for a defined period.

d. Other appropriate sanctions.

e. No action to be taken.

➤

REPORTING MECHANISM FROM ETHICS COMMITTEE TO BOARD REGARDING COMMITTEE RECOMMENDATION

The Ethics Committee shall provide written recommendation to the AAMT Board of Directors as follows:

- Describe the issues concerning the alleged misconduct.
- Describe the investigative process concerning the alleged misconduct.
- Summarize the materials enclosed in the hearing record and confirm that the record has been closed and placed in the AAMT administrative office.
- Provide the recommended outcome and/or action to be taken.

BOARD OF DIRECTORS DECISION-MAKING PROCESS

The Association Board of Directors, in accordance with AAMT bylaws, shall receive from the Ethics Committee, in each case that results in an investigation, the following: (a) the entire written record of the case (including any hearing transcripts, any written statements submitted by the affected individual, and all relevant documents); (b) a report summarizing the Committee's investigation and findings; and (c) a formal recommendation regarding sanctions. If the Ethics Committee recommends against sanctions in a particular case, the Board must adopt the Committee's recommendation and the matter will be dismissed.

If the Ethics Committee recommends any type of sanction, the Board shall review the Committee's recommendations and report, and all other documents relevant to the case. The Board may, at its option, choose to obtain further information and/or clarification from the Ethics Committee or the individual who is the subject of the investigation. Based on its review of the case, the Board may adopt fully, adopt in part, modify, or reject the recommendation of the Ethics Committee. The Board may not, however, impose sanctions that are more severe than those recommended by the Ethics Committee. Sanctions shall take effect upon notice to the affected individual, but no earlier than 5 days after the Board's decision.

DENIAL OF MEMBERSHIP

An application for Association membership may be rejected upon a finding by a majority of the Association's Board of Directors that an applicant is not in compliance with the Association's Code of Ethics. If an application for membership is denied on that basis, the applicant may file a request for reconsideration with the Board. The Board, at its sole discretion, may choose to reconsider the application and may review as part of the reconsideration process any additional information presented by the applicant or other individuals having knowledge of the matter. The applicant shall not be entitled to a hearing. The Board may decide to either (a) not reconsider the initial determination; (b) reject the application following the reconsideration process; or (c) accept the application following the reconsideration process. The decision of the Board shall be final.

ETHICS COMMITTEE MEMBERS

SELECTION CRITERIA

- Must be a current Active member in good standing (and not a member of the Board of Directors) for a minimum of 3 consecutive years.

TERM OF OFFICE

- Of the 6 members of the Ethics Committee, 3 shall have 2-year terms, and 3 shall have 3-year terms.
- The Chair shall be selected by the President from among the members of the Committee and shall serve a 1-year term as Chair.
- Appointments to fill a vacancy shall be for the remaining term of the vacancy.

GLOSSARY OF TERMS

ACTIVE MEMBER IN GOOD STANDING: Any member who qualifies for the Active category of membership and whose dues have been currently paid, and who is not under any current probation or sanction.

APPROPRIATE SANCTIONS: Any one of a number of disciplinary measures that may be warranted in a particular case brought under this Code of Ethics. Examples of appropriate sanctions include (among others) expulsion or suspension from AAMT, restrictions on holding leadership positions, imposition of a probationary period, fines, and public apologies.

COMPLAINANT: Member registering written complaint against another member. May be a member of the Ethics Committee.

FUNDAMENTAL FAIRNESS: The standard governing all AAMT activities under this Code of Ethics, including hearings of the Ethics Committee. Among other things, fundamental fairness means that any AAMT member who is accused of violating this Code of Ethics will be given an opportunity to respond fully to the charges and will have his or her case adjudicated in an impartial and unbiased manner.

HEARING RECORD: Documentation of the opportunity to be heard with examination of charges and evidence with testimony and arguments presented so as to determine whether action is justified.

INDIVIDUAL CATEGORIES OF MEMBERSHIP: Those categories held by individual persons rather than by an entity other than a person. Includes Active, Associate, Student, Sustaining.

ORGANIZATIONAL RULES: The rules, policies and procedures that govern AAMT activities. Examples of organizational rules include AAMT's bylaws, this Code of Ethics, and resolutions of AAMT's Board and AAMT's House of Delegates.

INVESTIGATION: The act or process of the research. A searching inquiry for ascertaining facts by careful examination.

JUDICIAL PROCEEDING: Any dispute resolution proceeding that is adjudicated by individuals who are not members of, or otherwise affiliated with, AAMT. Lawsuits, arbitrations, and mediations are examples of judicial proceedings.

OFFICIAL BODIES OF THE ASSOCIATION: Board of Directors, House of Delegates, and councils and committees (including task forces) duly organized by the Board of Directors or House of Delegates.

PROCEEDINGS: Action or series of activities involved in the investigative and/or decision-making process.

RECUSED: Disqualified to participate as a member of Ethics Committee in a particular proceeding due to possible conflict of interest.

RESPONDENT: Member whose conduct is questioned by complainant. May be a member of the Ethics Committee.

B

BRAND AND GENERIC DRUGS MOST OFTEN PRESCRIBED

Accupril (quinapril HCl)
acetaminophen with codeine
Advil
albuterol
alprazolam
Ambien (zolpidem tartrate)
amitriptyline HCl
amoxicillin trihydrate
Amoxil (amoxicillin trihydrate)
Anaprox DS (naproxen sodium)
Ansaid (flurbiprofen)
atenolol
Ativan (lorazepam)
Atrovent (ipratropium bromide)
Augmentin (amoxicillin trihydrate, clavulanate potassium)
Axid (nizatidine)
Azmacort (triamcinolone acetonide)

Bactroban (mupirocin)
Beconase AQ (beclomethasone dipropionate)
Beepen-VK (penicillin V potassium)
Biaxin (clarithromycin)
Bumex (bumetanide)
BuSpar (buspirone HCl)

Calan (verapamil HCl)
Calan SR
Capoten (captopril)
Carafate (sucralfate)
Cardec-DM (dextromethorphan hydrobromide, pseudoephedrine HCl, carbinoxamine maleate)
Cardizem (diltiazem HCl)
Cardizem CD
Cardura (doxazosin mesylate)
carisoprodol
Ceclor (cefaclor)
Ceftin (cefuroxime axetil)
Cefzil (cefprozil)
cephalexin
Cipro (ciprofloxacin)
Claritin (loratadine)
Cleocin T (clindamycin phosphate)
Compazine (prochlorperazine maleate)
Contuss-XT (phenylpropanolamine HCl, phenylephrine HCl, guaifenesin, alcohol)
Corgard (nadolol)
Cotrim (sulfamethoxazole, trimethoprim)
Cotrim DS
Coumadin (warfarin sodium)
cyclobenzaprine HCl

Darvocet-N (propoxyphene napsylate, acetaminophen)
Daypro (oxaprozin)
Deltasone (prednisone)
Demulen (ethynodiol diacetate, ethinyl estradiol)
Depakote (divalproex sodium)
DiaBeta (glyburide)
diazepam
dicyclomine HCl
Diflucan (fluconazole)
Dilantin (phenytoin sodium)
doxycycline hyclate
Duricef (cefadroxil monohydrate)
Dyazide (hydrochlorothiazide, triamterene)
DynaCirc (isradipine)

E-Mycin (erythromycin)
E-Mycin 333 (erythromycin)
EES (erythromycin ethylsuccinate)
Elocon (mometasone furoate)
Entex LA (phenylpropanolamine HCl, guaifenesin)
Ery-Tab (erythromycin)
Erythrocin Stearate (erythromycin stearate)
erythromycin
Estrace (estradiol)
Estraderm (estradiol)

Fiorinal with Codeine (codeine phosphate, acetaminophen, caffeine, butalbital)
Floxin (ofloxacin)
furosemide

gemfibrozil
Glucotrol (glipizide)
Glynase PresTabs (glyburide)
guaifenesin/PPA

Halcion (triazolam)
Hismanal (astemizole)
Humulin N (isophane insulin)
hydrochlorothiazide (HCT, HCTZ)
Hydrocodone-APAP (hydrocodone bitartrate, acetaminophen)
hydroxyzine HCl
Hytrin (terazosin HCl)

IBU (ibuprofen)
Iletin NPH (insulin)
Inderal (propranolol HCl)

B

Intal (cromolyn sodium)
Iophen-DM (iodinated glycerol, dextromethorphan hydrobromide)
Isoptin (verapamil HCl)
isosorbide dinitrate

K-Dur (potassium chloride)
Klonopin (clonazepam)
Klor-Con (potassium chloride)

Lanoxin (digoxin)
Lasix (furosemide)
Levoxine (levothyroxine sodium)
Levoxyl (levothyroxine sodium)
Lo/Ovral (ethinyl estradiol, norgestrel)
Lodine (etodolac)
Loestrin Fe (norethindrone acetate, ethinyl estradiol, ferrous fumarate)
Lopid (gemfibrozil)
Lopressor (metoprolol tartrate, hydrochlorothiazide)
Lorabid
lorazepam
Lorcet 10/650 (hydrocodone bitartrate, acetaminophen)
Lorcet Plus (hydrocodone bitartrate, acetaminophen)
Lortab (hydrocodone bitartrate, acetaminophen)
Lotensin (benazepril HCl, hydrochlorothiazide)
Lotrisone (betamethasone diproprionate, clotrimazole)
Lozol (indapamide)

Macrobid (nitrofurantoin macrocrystals, nitrofurantoin monohydrate)
Maxzide (triamterene, hydrochlorothiazide)
methylphenidate HCl
methylprednisolone
metoprolol tartrate
Mevacor (lovastatin)
Micro-K (potassium chloride)
Micronase (glyburide)
Motrin (ibuprofen)

Naprosyn (naproxen)
naproxen
Nasacort (triamcinolone acetonide)
neomycin
Nicoderm (nicotine)
Nitro-Dur II (nitroglycerin)
Nizoral (ketoconazole)
Nizoral Cream
Nolvadex (tamoxifen citrate)
Nordette (ethinyl estradiol, levonorgestrel)
nortriptyline HCl
Norvasc (amlodipine)

Ogen (estropipate sulfate)
Orasone (prednisone)
Ortho-Cept 28 (desogestrel, ethinyl estradiol)
Ortho-Novum 7/7/7 (norethindrone, ethinyl estradiol)
Ortho-Novum 7/7/7-28
Oruvail (ketoprofen)
Ovcon (ethinyl estradiol, norethindrone)

Pamelor (nortriptyline HCl)
Paxil (paroxetine HCl)
PCE (polymer-coated erythromycin)
Pen-Vee K (penicillin V potassium)
penicillin V
Penicillin VK (penicillin V potassium)
Pepcid (famotidine)
Percocet-5 (oxycodone HCl, acetaminophen)
Peridex (chlorhexidine gluconate)
Phenergan (promethazine HCl)
Poly-Histine DM
Polymox (amoxicillin trihydrate)
potassium chloride
Pravachol (pravastatin sodium)
prednisone
Premarin (conjugated estrogens)
Prilosec (omeprazole)
Principen (ampicillin trihydrate)
Prinivil (lisinopril)
Procardia (nifedipine)
Procardia XL (nifedipine)
Promethazine VC with Codeine (codeine phosphate, phenylephrine HCl, promethazine HCl, alcohol)
Propacet (propoxyphene napsylate, acetaminophen)
propoxyphene NAP with APAP
Propulsid (cisapride)
Proventil (albuterol)
Proventil Aerosol (albuterol sulfate)
Proventil Repetabs (albuterol sulfate)
Provera (medroxyprogesterone acetate)
Prozac (fluoxetine HCl)

Relafen (namubetone)
Retin-A (tretinoin)
Ritalin (methylphenidate HCl)
Roxicet (oxycodone HCl, acetaminophen)

B

Seldane-D (terfenadine, pseudoephedrine HCl)
Sinemet (carbidopa, levodopa)
Slo-bid (theophylline)
Slow-K (potassium chloride)
SMZ-TMP (sulfamethoxazole, trimethoprim)
Sumycin (tetracycline HCl)
Suprax (cefixime)
Synthroid (levothyroxine sodium)

Tagamet (cimetidine)
Tegretol (carbamazepine)
temazepam
Tenex (guanfacine HCl)
Tenormin (atenolol)
Terazol (terconazole)
Terazol 3 (terconazole)
Terazol 7 (terconazole)
Theo-Dur (theophylline)
thyroid
Timoptic (trimolol maleate)
TobraDex (dexamethasone, tobramycin)
Tobrex (tobramycin)
Toradol (ketorolac tromethamine)
Transderm-Nitro (nitroglycerin)
Trental (pentoxifylline)
Tri-Levlen (levonorgestrel, ethinyl estradiol)
triamterene with HCTZ
trimethoprim sulfate
Trimox (amoxicillin trihydrate)
Triphasil (levonorgestrel, ethinyl estradiol)
Triphasil-28 (levonorgestrel, ethinyl estradiol)
Tussionex Pennkinetic (hydrocodone polistirex, chlorpheniramine polistirex)
Tylenol with Codeine (acetaminophen, codeine phosphate)

Valium (diazepam)
Vancenase AQ (beclomethasone dipropionate)
Vanceril (beclomethasone dipropionate)
Vantin (cefpodoxime proxetil)
Vasotec (enalapril maleate)
Veetids (penicillin V potassium)
Ventolin (albuterol)
verapamil HCl
verapamil SR
Verelan (verapamil HCl)
Vicodin (hydrocodone bitartrate, acetaminophen)
Vicodin ES (hydrocodone bitartrate, acetaminophen)
Voltaren (diclofenac sodium)

Wymox (amoxicillin trihydrate)

Xanax (alprazolam)

Zantac (ranitidine HCl)
Zestril (lisinopril)
Zithromax Z-Pak (azithromycin dihydrate)
Zocor (simvastatin)
Zoloft (sertraline HCl)
Zovirax (acyclovir)

B

CAPITALIZATION RULE SYNOPSIS

Capitalize	*Rule*	*Page*
Abbreviations	4.18	100
Abbreviations for state names	4.5	96
Academic courses	4.21	101
Academic degrees	4.19	100
Acronyms	4.18	100
Allergies	4.22	101
Article titles	4.15	100
"Attention" lines	4.4	96
Avenue in addresses	4.2	96
Book titles	4.15	100
Boulevard in addresses	4.2	96
Brand names for drugs	4.10	98
Brand names for products	4.10	98
Capitals with colons	4.14	99
Cardiologic abbreviations	4.24	101
Cardiologic symbols	4.24	101
Colons with capital letters	4.14	99
Complimentary closes	4.1	96
Days of the week	4.16	108
Degrees	4.19	100
Departments in hospital	4.11	98
Direct quotes	4.14	99
Diseases	4.23	101
Drugs	4.10 and 4.22	98 and 101
Eponyms	4.7 and 4.23	97 and 101
Family titles	4.6	97
Genuses	4.9 and 4.23	98 and 101
Geographic locations	4.17	100
Headings	4.13	99
Historic events	4.16	100
Holidays	4.16	100
Languages	4.8	98
Military ranks	4.6	97
Months of the year	4.16	100
Names	4.7 and 4.23	97 and 101
Names for courses	4.21	101
Nicknames	4.7	97
Nouns	4.7	97
Nouns used as adjectives	4.9	98
Nouns with letters	4.12	99
Nouns with numbers	4.12	99
Numbers with words	4.12	99
Officers' titles	4.20	100
Organizations' names	4.20	100
Outlines	4.13	99
People's titles	4.3	96
People	4.8	98
Periodical titles	4.15	100
Place names	4.17	100
Political titles	4.6	97
Professional titles	4.6	97
Proper nouns	4.7 and 4.23	97 and 101

B

B

GENUS AND SPECIES NAMES COMMONLY USED

Genus and Species	*Common Term (If Any)*
Actinomyces muris	
Amoeba proteus	
Amoeba urinae granulata	
Ancylostoma duodenale	hookworm
Ascaris lumbricoides	ascariasis
Aspergillus auricularis	aspergillosis
Aspergillus fumigatus	
Bacillus cereus	bacillosis
Bacillus proteus	
Bacteroides fragilis	bacteroidosis
Bacteroides funduliformis	
Bacteroides melaninogenicus	
Bordetella pertussis	
Borrelia buccalis	
Borrelia recurrentis	
Borrelia vincentii	
Brucella melitensis	brucellosis
Brugia malayi	
Campylobacter fetus	
Candida albicans	candidiasis
Cellvibrio fulvus	
Cellvibrio vulgaris	
Chromobacterium amythistinum	
Cladosporium carrionii	chromomycosis
Cladosporium trichoides	cladosporiosis
Clostridium botulinum	botulism
Clostridium perfringens	
Clostridium tetani	tetanus
Coccidioides immitis	coccidioidomycosis
Corynebacterium acnes	
Corynebacterium diphtheriae	diphtheria
Corynebacterium xerosis	
Coxiella burnetii	
Cryptococcus neoformans	
Cysticercus cellulosae	cysticercosis
Cysticercus ovis	

B

Genus and Species	*Common Term (If Any)*
Cysticercus tenuicollis	
Diplococcus mucosus	
Diplococcus paleopneumoniae	
Diplococcus pneumoniae	pneumonia
Echinococcus granulosis	echinococcosis/tapeworm
Endomyces capsulatus	
Entamoeba coli	entamebiasis
Entamoeba gingivalis	
Entamoeba histolytica	amebic dysentery
Enterobius vermicularis	enterobiasis/pinworm
Escherichia coli	
Fasciolopsis buski	fasciolopsiasis/flukes
Filaria labialis	
Giardia lamblia	giardiasis
Haemophilus aegyptius	
Haemophilus influenzae	
Haemophilus pertussis	
Haemophilus vaginalis	
Histoplasma capsulatum	histoplasmosis
Klebsiella friedländeri	
Klebsiella pneumoniae	
Lactobacillus acidophilus	
Lactobacillus bifidus	
Legionella pneumophila	
Leishmania caninum	leishmaniasis
Leptospira pomona	leptospirosis
Microsporum audouinii	ringworm/microsporosis
Microsporum canis	ringworm/microsporosis
Mycobacterium leprae	leprosy
Mycobacterium tuberculosis	
Mycoplasma pneumoniae	pneumonia
Necator americanus	hookworm
Neisseria gonorrhoeae	gonorrhea
Neisseria meningitidis	cerebrospinal meningitis
Neisseria mucosa	
Nocardia asteroides	nocardiosis

B

Genus and Species	*Common Term (If Any)*
Onchocerca volvulus	onchocerciasis/roundworm
Pasteurella tularensis	
Peptococcus magnus	
Plasmodium falciparum	
Plasmodium malariae	malaria
Plasmodium vivax	
Pneumocystis carinii	
Proteus morganii	
Proteus vulgaris	
Pseudomonas aeruginosa	
Rickettsia akari	
Rickettsia burnetii	
Rickettsia prowazekii	
Rickettsia quintana	
Rickettsia rickettsii	Rocky Mountain spotted fever
Saccharomyces capillitii	saccharomycosis
Salmonella choleraesuis	
Salmonella enteritidis	salmonellosis
Salmonella typhi	typhoid fever
Schistosoma haematobium	
Schistosoma japonicum	
Schistosoma mansoni	
Serratia marcescens	
Shigella boydii	
Shigella dysenteriae	shigellosis
Shigella flexneri	
Staphylococcus aureus	
Streptococcus faecalis	
Streptococcus pneumoniae	
Streptococcus pyogenes	
Strongyloides stercoralis	strongyloidiasis/threadworm
Taenia lata	tapeworm
Taenia saginata	
Taenia solium	
Toxoplasma gondii	toxoplasmosis
Treponema pallidum	syphilis

B

Genus and Species	*Common Term (If Any)*
Trichinella spiralis	trichiniasis/trichinosis
Trichomonas hominis	trichomoniasis
Trichomonas vaginalis	
Trichophyton tonsurans	ringworm
Trichophyton violaceum	
Trichuris trichiura	trichuriasis/whipworm
Trombicula akamushi	
Trypanosoma cruzi	
Wuchereria bancrofti	

B

HOMONYMS

The following words are commonly encountered in medical transcription. You will notice that they are in alphabetical sequence with the homonyms listed indented below each word. Phonetics are shown and the stress point of the word is capitalized. Abbreviated definitions are listed so that you do not have to refer to your medical dictionary unless you wish a more detailed meaning.

Word	Phonetics	Definition
abduction *addiction* *adduction* *subduction*	ab-DUK-shun	A drawing away from the midline.
aberrant *afferent* *apparent* *efferent* *inferent*	ab-ER-ant	Wandering or deviating from the normal course.
aberration *abrasion* *erasion* *erosion* *operation*	ab″er-A-shun	Deviation from the usual course.
abrasion *aberration* *erasion* *erosion* *operation*	ah-BRA-zhun	Denudation of skin.
abscess *aphthous*	AB-sess	A localized collection of pus, caused by infection.
absorption *adsorption* *sorption*	ab-SORP-shun	The uptake of substances into tissues.
addiction *abduction* *adduction*	ah-DIK-shun	Dependence on a drug or some habit.
adduction *abduction* *addiction*	ah-DUK-shun	A drawing toward the midline.
adherence *adhered to* *adherent* *adherents*	ad-HĒR-ens	The act or quality of sticking to something.
adsorption *absorption* *sorption*	ad-SORP-shun	To collect in condensed form on a surface.
affect *effect*	af-FEKT	To have an influence on; the feeling experienced in connection with an emotion.
afferent *aberrant* *efferent*	AF-er-ent	Conveying toward a center.

B

alveolar *alveolate* *alveoli* *alveolus* *alveus* *alvus* *areolar*	al-VE-o-lar	Pertaining to an alveolus.
alveoli *alveolar* *alveolate* *alveolus* *alveus* *alvus* *areolar*	al-VE-o-li	Plural of alveolus.
alveolus *alveolar* *alveolate* *alveoli* *alveus* *alvus* *areolar*	al-VE-o-lus	A small saclike dilatation.
alveus *alveolar* *alveolate* *alveoli* *alveolus* *alvus* *areolar*	AL-ve-us	A trough or canal.
alvus *alveolar* *alveolate* *alveoli* *alveolus* *alveus* *areolar*	AL-vus	The abdomen with its contained viscera.
amenorrhea *dysmenorrhea* *menorrhagia* *menorrhea* *metrorrhagia*	ah-men″o-RE-ah	Stoppage of the menses.
antiseptic *asepsis* *aseptic* *sepsis* *septic*	an″tĭ-SEP-tik	Preventing decay or putrefaction.
aphagia *abasia* *aphakia* *aphasia*	ah-FA-je-ah	Abstention from eating.
aphakia *aphagia* *aphasia*	ah-FA-ke-ah	Absence of the lens of the eye.

B

aphasia *abasia* *aphagia* *aphakia*	ah-FA-ze-ah	Loss of the power of expression by speech, writing, or signs.
aphthous *abscess*	AF-thess	Adjective form of aphthae referring to small ulcers of oral mucosa.
apophysis *epiphysis* *hypophysis* *hypothesis*	ah-POF-e-sis	Bony outgrowth or process of a bone.
apposition *opposition*	ap″o-ZISH-un	The placing of things in juxtaposition or proximity.
arrhythmia *erythema* *eurhythmia*	ah-RITH-me-ah	Variation from the normal rhythm of the heartbeat.
arteriosclerosis *arteriostenosis* *atherosclerosis*	ar-te″re-o-skle-RO-sis	A disease characterized by thickening and loss of elasticity of arterial walls.
arteriostenosis *arteriosclerosis* *atherosclerosis*	ar-te″re-o-ste-NO-sis	The narrowing or diminution of the caliber of an artery.
atherosclerosis *arteriosclerosis* *arteriostenosis*	ath″er-o″skle-RO-sis	Deposits of yellowish plaques containing cholesterol and lipoid material formed on the inside of the arteries.
aural *aura* *ora* *oral*	AW-ral	Pertaining to or perceived by the ear.
auscultation *oscillation* *oscitation* *osculation*	aws″kul-TA-shun	The act of listening for sounds within the body.
bare *bear*	baer	Naked.
border *boarder* *quarter*	BOR-der	A rim, margin, or edge.
bowel *bile* *vowel*	BOW-el	The intestine.
breath *breadth*	breth	The air taken in and expelled by the expansion and contraction of the thorax.
breathe *breed*	brēth	To take air into the lungs and let it out again.
bronchoscopic *proctoscopic*	brong″ko-SKOP-ik	Pertaining to bronchoscopy or to the bronchoscope.

B

bruit *brute*	brwe, broot	A sound or murmur heard in auscultation.
calculous *calculus* *caliculus* *callous* *callus*	KAL-ku-lus	Pertaining to, of the nature of, or affected with calculus.
calculus *calculous* *caliculus* *callous* *callus*	KAL-ku-lus	Any abnormal stony mass or deposit formed in the body.
callous *calculous* *calculus* *callus* *talus*	KAL-us	Pertaining to a hardened, thickened place on the skin.
callus *calculous* *calculus* *callous* *talus*	KAL-us	A hardened, thickened place on the skin; formation of new bone between broken ends of a bone.
cancellous *cancellus* *cancerous*	KAN-sĕ-lus	Of a reticular, spongy, or lattice-like structure.
cancellus *cancellous* *cancerous*	kan-SEL-us	Any structure arranged like a lattice.
cancer *canker* *chancre*	KAN-ser	Malignant tumor.
cancerous *cancellous* *cancellus*	KAN-ser-us	Pertaining to cancer.
canker *cancer* *chancre*	KANG-ker	Ulceration, chiefly of the mouth and lips.
carbuncle *caruncle* *furuncle*	KAR-bung-kl	A cluster of boils; furuncles.
carpus *carpal* *corpus*	KAR-pus	The wrist.
caruncle *carbuncle* *furuncle*	KAR-ung-kl	A small fleshy eminence, whether normal or abnormal.
chancre *cancer* *canker*	SHANG-ker	The primary sore of syphilis.

B

cirrhosis *cillosis* *psilosis* *sclerosis* *serosa* *xerosis*	sir-RO-sis	A degenerative disease of the liver.
coarse *course* *force*	kors	Not fine or microscopic; rough or crude.
contusion *concussion* *confusion* *convulsion*	kon-TU-zhun	A bruise.
cord *chord* *cor*	kord	Any long, rounded, flexible structure. Also spelled chord and chorda.
corneal *cranial*	KOR-ne-al	Pertaining to the cornea of the eye.
corpus *carpus* *copious* *core* *corps* *corpse*	KOR-pus	A human body; the body (main part) of an organ.
cranial *corneal*	KRA-ne-al	Pertaining to the cranium (skull).
cytology *psychology* *sitology*	si-TOL-o-je	The study of cells.
diaphysis *apophysis* *diastasis* *diathesis* *epiphysis*	di-AF-ĭ-sis	Shaft of a long bone.
diastasis *diaphysis* *diathesis*	dye-AS-te-sis	Dislocation or separation of two bones that are normally attached.
diathesis *diaphysis* *diastasis*	di-ATH-ĕ-sis	A predisposition to certain diseases.
dilatation *dilation*	dil-ah-TA-shun	A dilated condition or structure.
dilation *dilatation*	di-LA-shun	The process of dilating or becoming dilated.
dysphagia *dysbasia* *dyscrasia* *dysphasia* *displasia* *dyspragia*	dis-FA-je-ah	Difficulty in swallowing

Term	Pronunciation	Definition
dysphasia *dysbasia* *dyscrasia* *dysphagia* *dysplasia* *dyspragia*	dis-FA-ze-ah	Impairment of the faculty of speech.
dysplasia *dysbasia* *dyscrasia* *dysphagia* *dysphasia* *dyspragia*	dis-PLA-se-ah	Abnormality in development of tissues or body parts.
dyspragia *dysphagia* *dysphasia* *dysplasia*	dis-PRA-je-ah	Painful performance of any function.
dyspraxia *dystaxia*	dis-PRAK-se-ah	Partial loss of ability to perform coordinated acts.
ecchymosis *achymosis* *echinosis* *echomosis*	ek″ĭ-MO-sis	A bruise.
effect *affect* *defect*	e-FEKT	The result; to bring about.
efferent *aberrant* *afferent*	EF-er-ent	Conveying away from a center.
elicit *illicit*	e-LIS-it	To cause to be revealed; to draw out.
embolus *bolus* *embolism* *thrombus*	EM-bo-lus	A blood clot carried in the bloodstream.
endemic *ecdemic* *epidemic* *pandemic*	en-DEM-ik	A disease native to a particular region.
enervation *denervation* *innervation*	en″er-VA-shun	Lack of nervous energy; removal or section of a nerve.
enteric *icteric*	en-TER-ik	Pertaining to the small intestine.
epidemic *ecdemic* *endemic*	ep″ĭ-DEM-ik	The rapid spreading of a contagious disease.
epiphysis *apophysis* *hypophysis* *hypothesis*	e-PIF-e-sis	Growth center at the end of a long bone.

B

erythema *arrhythmia* *erythremia* *eurhythmia*	er″i-THE-mah	Redness of the skin due to a variety of causes.
eschar *a scar* *escharotic* *scar*	ES-kar	A slough produced by a thermal burn or by gangrene.
everted *inverted*	e-VER-ted	Turned outward.
facial *basal* *fascial* *faucial* *racial*	FA-shal	Pertaining to the face.
fascial *facial* *falcial* *fascia* *fashion* *faucial*	FASH-e-al	Pertaining to fascia.
fauces *facies* *feces* *foci* *fossa* *fossae*	FAW-sēz	The throat.
fecal *cecal* *fetal* *focal* *thecal*	FE-cal	Pertaining to or of the nature of feces.
fetal *fatal* *fecal*	FE-tal	Pertaining to a fetus.
flexor *flexure*	FLEK-sor	Any muscle that flexes a joint.
flexure *flexor*	FLEK-sher	A bent position of a structure or organ.
fundi *fungi*	FUN-di	Plural of fundus, a bottom or base.
furuncle *carbuncle* *caruncle*	FU-rung-k'l	A boil.
gastroscopy *gastrostomy* *gastrotomy*	gas-TROS-ko-pe	Inspection of the stomach with a gastroscope.
gastrostomy *gastroscopy* *gastrotomy*	gas-TROS-to-me	Artificial opening into the stomach.

B

gavage *lavage*	gah-VAHZH	Feeding by stomach tube.
glands *glans*	glands	Groups of cells that secrete or excrete material not used in their metabolic activities.
glans *glands*	glanz	Latin for gland.
hypercalcemia *hyperkalemia* *hypocalcemia*	hi″per-kal-SE-me-ah	An excess of calcium in the blood.
hyperinsulinism *hypoinsulinism*	hi″per-IN-su-lin-izm″	Excessive secretion of insulin by the pancreas; insulin shock.
hyperkalemia *hypercalcemia* *hyperkinemia* *hypokalemia*	hi″per-kah-LE-me-ah	Abnormally high potassium concentration in the blood.
hypertension *Hypertensin* *hypotension*	hi″per-TEN-shun	High blood pressure.
hypocalcemia *hypercalcemia* *hyperkalemia*	hi″po-kal-SE-me-ah	Reduction of the blood calcium below normal.
hypoinsulinism *hyperinsulinism*	hi″po-IN-su-lin-izm	Deficient secretion of insulin by the pancreas.
hypokalemia *hypercalcemia* *hyperkalemia* *hyperkinemia*	hi″po-ka-LE-me-ah	Abnormally low potassium concentration in the blood.
hypophysis *apophysis* *epiphysis* *hypothesis*	hi-POF-e-sis	Pituitary gland.
hypotension *hypertension*	hi″po-TEN-shun	Low blood pressure.
hypothesis *apophysis* *epiphysis* *hypophysis*	hi-POTH-e-sis	An unproved theory tentatively accepted to explain certain facts or to provide a basis for further investigation.
icteric *enteric* *mycteric*	ik-TER-ik	Pertaining to or affected with jaundice.
ileum *ilium*	IL-e-um	Part of the small intestine.
ilium *ileum*	IL-e-um	The flank bone or hip bone.
illicit *elicit*	i-LIS-it	Illegal.

B

infarction *infection* *infestation* *infraction* *injection*	in-FARK-shun	The formation of an infarct.
infection *infarction* *infestation* *inflection* *inflexion* *in flexion* *injection*	in-FEK-shun	Invasion of the body by pathogenic microorganisms.
infestation *infarction* *infection* *injection*	in-fes-TA-shun	Invasion of the body by small invertebrate animals, such as insects, mites, or ticks.
injection *infarction* *infection* *infestation* *ingestion*	in-JEK-shun	Act of forcing a liquid into a part or an organ.
innervation *enervation*	in″er-VA-shun	The distribution of nerves to a part.
insulin *inulin*	IN-su-lin	Protein formed by the islet cells of Langerhans in the pancreas.
inulin *insulin*	IN-u-lin	A vegetable starch.
inverted *everted*	in-VERT-ed	Turned inside out or upside down.
keratitis *keratiasis* *keratosis* *ketosis*	ker″ah-TI-tis	Inflammation of the cornea.
keratosis *keratitis* *keratose* *ketosis*	ker″ah-TO-sis	Any horny growth, such as a wart or a callosity.
ketosis *keratitis* *keratosis*	ke-TO-sis	Abnormally high concentration of ketone bodies in the body tissues and fluids.
laceration *maceration* *masturbation*	las″er-A-shun	Act of tearing; wound made by tearing.
lavage *gavage*	lah-VAHZH	The irrigation or washing out of an organ.
lipoma *fibroma* *lipomyoma* *lymphoma*	li-PO-mah	A benign tumor composed of mature fat cells.

B

lithotomy *lithotony*	lith-OT-o-me	Incision of an organ for removal of a stone.
lithotony *lithotomy*	lith-OT-o-ne	Creation of an artificial vesical fistula that is dilated to extract a stone.
liver *livor* *sliver*	LIV-er	A large gland of dark-red color in the upper part of the abdomen on the right side.
livor *liver*	LIV-or	Discoloration.
lymphoma *lipoma*	lim-FO-mah	Any neoplastic disorder of the lymphoid tissue.
maceration *laceration* *masturbation*	mas″er-A-shun	The softening of a solid by soaking.
mastitis *mastoiditis*	mas-TI-tis	Inflammation of the mammary gland, or breast.
mastoiditis *mastitis*	mas″toi-DI-tis	Inflammation of the mastoid antrum and cells.
masturbation *laceration* *maceration*	mas″tur-BA-shun	Production of orgasm by self-manipulation of the genitals.
menorrhagia *menorrhea* *metrorrhagia*	men″o-RA-je-ah	Excessive uterine bleeding at menstruation time.
menorrhea *amenorrhea* *dysmenorrhea* *menorrhagia* *metrorrhagia*	men″o-RE-ah	The normal discharge of the menses.
metacarpal *metatarsal*	met″ah-KAR-pal	Pertaining to the metacarpus.
metastasis *metaphysis* *metastases (plural)* *metastasize* *metastatic*	mĕ-TAS-tah-sis	The transfer of disease from one site to another not directly connected with it.
metastasize *metastases* *metastasis* *metastatic*	me-TAS-tah-size	To form new foci of disease in a distant part by metastasis.
metastatic *metastases* *metastasis* *metastasize*	met″ah-STAT-ik	Pertaining to metastasis.
metatarsal *metacarpal*	met″ah-TAR-sal	Pertaining to the metatarsus.

B

Term	Pronunciation	Definition
metrorrhagia *menorrhagia* *menorrhea*	me″tro-RA-je-ah	Uterine bleeding at irregular intervals sometimes being prolonged.
mucoid *Mucor* *mucosa* *mucosal*	MU-koid	Resembling mucin.
mucosa *mucosal* *mucosin* *mucous* *mucus*	mu-KO-sah	A mucous membrane.
mucosal *mucosa* *mucous* *mucus*	mu-KO-sal	Pertaining to the mucous membrane.
mucous *mucosa* *mucosal* *mucus*	MU-kus	The adjective that means pertaining to mucus.
mucus *mucosa* *mucosal* *mucous*	MU-kus	The noun that means a viscid watery secretion of mucous glands.
myogram *myelogram*	MI-o-gram	A recording or tracing mode with a myograph.
necrosis *narcosis* *nephrosis* *neurosis*	ne-KRO-sis	Death of tissue.
nephrosis *necrosis* *neurosis* *tephrosis*	ne-FRO-sis	Any disease of the kidney.
neurosis *necrosis* *nephrosis* *urosis*	nu-RO-sis	Disorder of psychic or mental constitution.
obstipation *constipation* *obfuscation*	ob″sti-PA-shun	Intractable constipation.
oral *aura* *aural*	O-ral	Pertaining to the mouth.
oscillation *auscultation* *oscitation* *osculation*	os″i-LA-shun	A backward and forward motion; vibration.

B

oscitation *auscultation* *excitation* *oscillation* *osculation*	os″i-TA-shun	The act of yawning.
osculation *auscultation* *escalation* *oscillation* *oscitation*	os″ku-LA-shun	To kiss; to touch closely.
palpation *palliation* *palpitation* *papillation*	pal-PA-shun	The act of feeling with the hand.
palpitation *palliation* *palpation* *papillation*	pal″pi-TA-shun	Regular or irregular rapid action of the heart.
parasthenia *paresthesia*	par″as-THE-ne-ah	A condition of organic tissue causing it to function at abnormal intervals.
paresthesia *pallesthesia* *parasthenia* *paresthenia*	par″es-THE-ze-ah	An abnormal sensation, such as burning or prickling.
parietitis *parotiditis* *parotitis*	pah-ri-ĕ-TI-tis	Inflammation of the wall of an organ.
parotiditis *parietitis* *parotitis*	pah-rot″ĭ-DI-tis	Inflammation of the parotid gland.
parotitis *parietitis* *parostitis* *parotiditis*	par″o-TI-tis	Inflammation of the parotid gland.
parous *Paris* *pars* *porous*	PA-rus	Having brought forth one or more living offspring.
pedicle *medical* *particle* *peduncle* *pellicle*	PED-ĭ-k′l	A footlike or stemlike structure.
perineal *pectineal* *peritoneal* *peroneal*	per″i-NE-al	Pertaining to the perineum.
perineum *peritoneum*	per″i-NE-um	The region at the lower end of the trunk between the thighs.

Term	Pronunciation	Definition
peritoneum *perineum*	per″i-to-NE-um	The serous membrane lining the abdominal walls.
peroneal *pectineal* *perineal* *peritoneal* *peronia*	per″o-NE-al	Pertaining to the fibula or outer side of the leg.
pleural *plural*	PLOOR-al	Pertaining to the pleura.
prostate *prostrate*	PROS-tāt	A gland in the male that surrounds the neck of the bladder and the urethra.
prostrate *prostate*	PROS-trāt	Lying flat, prone, or supine.
psychology *cytology* *sitology*	si-KOL-o-je	The science dealing with the mind and with mental and emotional processes.
pyelonephrosis *pyonephrosis*	pi″e-lo-nĕ-FRO-sis	Any disease of the kidney and its pelvis.
pyonephrosis *pyelonephrosis*	pi″o-nĕ-FRO-sis	Suppurative destruction of the parenchyma of the kidney.
pyrenemia *pyoturia* *pyuria*	pi″rĕ-NE-me-ah	The presence of nucleated red cells in the blood.
pyuria *paruria* *pyorrhea* *pyoturia* *pyrenemia*	pi-U-re-ah	The presence of pus in the urine.
radical *radicle*	RAD-ĭ-kal	Directed to the source of a morbid process, as radical surgery.
radicle *radical*	RAD-ĭ-k′l	Any one of the smallest branches of a vessel or nerve.
recession *resection*	re-SESH-un	The act of drawing away or back.
reflex *efflux* *reflux*	RE-fleks	A reflected action; an involuntary muscular movement.
reflux *efflux* *reflex*	RE-fluks	A backward or return flow.
resection *recession*	re-SEK-shun	Excision of a portion of an organ or other structure.
rhonchi *bronchi* *ronchi*	RONG-kī	Plural of rhonchus, a rattling in the throat; a dry, coarse rale.

B

scar *a scar* *eschar* *scarf*	skahr	A mark remaining after the healing of a wound.
scirrhous *cirrhosis* *cirrus* *scirrhus* *sclerous* *serious* *serous*	SKIR-us	Pertaining to a hard cancer.
scirrhus *cirrhosis* *cirrus* *scirrhous* *sclerous* *serious* *serous*	SKIR-us	Scirrhous carcinoma.
sedentary *sedimentary*	SED-en-ter″e	Sitting habitually.
sedimentary *sedentary*	sed-ĭ-MEN-ter-e	Of, having the nature of, or containing sediment.
separation *suppression* *suppuration*	sep-ah-RA-shun	Break; division; gap.
sepsis *antiseptic* *asepsis* *aseptic* *septic* *threpsis*	SEP-sis	The presence in the blood of pathogenic microorganisms or their toxins.
septic *antiseptic* *asepsis* *a septic* *aseptic* *sepsis* *septal* *septile* *skeptic*	SEP-tik	Owing to decomposition by microorganisms.
serosa *cirrhosis* *xerosis*	se-RO-sah; se-RO-zah	Any serous membrane (tunica mucosa); tunica serosa; the chorion.
serous *cirrus* *scirrhous* *scirrhus* *sclerous* *sera* *serious* *serose*	SE-rus	Pertaining to serum.

B

sight *cite* *cyte* *side* *site* *slight*	sīt	The act of seeing; a thing seen.
stasis *bases* *basis* *station* *status* *staxis*	STA-sis	A stoppage of the flow of blood.
staxis *stasis*	STAK-sis	Hemorrhage.
stroma *soma* *stoma* *struma* *trauma*	STRO-mah	The supporting tissue of an organ.
struma *stoma* *stroma*	STROO-mah	Goiter.
suppression *separation* *suppuration*	sŭ-PRESH-un	The sudden stoppage of a secretion, excretion, or normal discharge.
suppuration *separation* *suppression* *susurration*	sup″u-RA-shun	The formation of pus.
sycosis *psychosis*	si-KO-sis	A disease marked by inflammation of the hair follicles; a kind of ulcer on the eyelid.
tenia *taenia* *Taenia* *tinea*	TE-ne-ah	A flat band or strip of soft tissue.
thenar *femur* *thinner*	THE-nar	The mound on the palm at the base of the thumb.
thrombus *embolus*	THROM-bus	A blood clot that remains at the site of formation.
tinea *linea* *linear* *taenia* *Taenia* *tenia*	TIN-e-ah	Ringworm.
trachelotomy *tracheophony* *tracheotomy*	tra″ke-LOT-o-me	The surgical cutting of the uterine neck.

B

tracheophony *trachelotomy* *tracheotomy*	tra″kĕ-OF-o-ne	A sound heard in auscultation over the trachea.
tracheotomy *trachelotomy* *tracheophony*	tra″ke-OT-o-me	Incision of the trachea through the skin and muscles of the neck.
track *tract*	trak	Series of marks or pathway, e.g., needle track found on drug addicts or patients on dialysis.
tract *track*	trakt	A system of organs having some special function, e.g., gastrointestinal tract; abnormal passage through tissue.
tympanites *tympanitis*	tim″pah-NI-tēz	Distention of the abdomen due to gas or air in the intestine or in the peritoneal cavity.
tympanitis *tenonitis* *tinnitus* *tympanites*	tim″pah-NI-tis	Inflammation of the middle ear.
ureter *ureteral* *urethra* *urethral*	u-RE-ter	The tube that conveys the urine from the kidney to the bladder.
ureteral *ureter* *urethra* *urethral*	u-RE-ter-al	Pertaining to the ureter.
urethra *ureter* *ureteral*	u-RE-thrah	The canal conveying urine from the bladder to the outside of the body.
urethral *ureter* *ureteral* *urethra*	u-RE-thral	Pertaining to the urethra.
urethrorrhagia *ureterorrhagia*	u-re″thro-RA-je-ah	A flow of blood from the urethra.
uterus *ureter* *urethra* *urethral*	U-ter-us	The womb.
vagitis *vagitus*	va-JI-tis	Inflammation of the vagal nerve.
vagitus *vagitis*	vah-JI-tus	The cry of an infant.
vagus *valgus*	VA-gus	The tenth cranial nerve.

B

valgus *vagus* *varus* *vastus*	VAL-gus	Bent outward, twisted, as in knock-knee (genu valgum).
variceal *varicella*	var″ĭ-SE-al	Pertaining to a varix, an enlarged artery or vein.
varicella *variceal*	var″ĭ-SEL-ah	Chickenpox.
varicose *verrucose* *very close* *very coarse*	VAR-ĭ-kos	Pertaining to a varix, an enlarged artery or vein.
variolar *variola*	vah-RI-o-lar	Pertaining to smallpox.
venous *Venus*	VE-nus	Pertaining to the veins.
Venus *venous*	VE-nus	The goddess of love and beauty in Roman mythology; the planet second from the sun.
verrucose *varicose* *verrucous* *vorticose*	VER-oo-kōs	Rough; warty.
verrucous *varicose* *verrucose* *vorticose*	VER-oo-kus	Rough; warty.
vesical *fascicle* *vesica* *vesicle* *vessel*	VES-ĭ-kal	Pertaining to the bladder.
vesicle *fascicle* *vesica* *vesical* *vessel*	VES-ĭ-k′l	A small bladder or sac containing liquid.
vessel *vesical* *vesicle*	VES-′l	A tube or duct containing or circulating a body fluid.
villous *villose* *villus*	VIL-us	Shaggy with soft hairs.
villus *villose* *villous*	VIL-lus	A small vascular process or protrusion.
viscera *visceral* *viscus*	VIS-er-ah	Plural of viscus.

B

viscus *discus* *vicious* *viscera* *viscose* *viscous*	VIS-kus	Any large interior organ in any one of the three great cavities of the body.
womb *wound*	wōōm	The uterus.
wound *womb*	wōōnd	An injury to the body caused by physical means.
xerosis *cirrhosis* *serosa*	ze-RO-sis	Abnormal dryness.

B

LABORATORY TERMINOLOGY AND NORMAL VALUES

Remember the following rules when transcribing laboratory data and values. Some physicians dictate the word *lab* as a short form for *laboratory,* which is acceptable except in headings and subheadings. When laboratory tests are ordered, it is common to hear, for example, "Dr. Mendez ordered a SMAC test on Mrs. Garcia." The equipment that is used, the Sequential Multiple Analyzer Computer, may be abbreviated and typed as SMAC, SMA, or Chem (for chemistry). This study is a panel of chemistry tests; from four to as many as 22 tests may be performed on the blood specimen (e.g., SMAC-8, SMA-5, Chem-9, and so on). Use numbers to express laboratory values, but never begin a sentence with a number. As discussed in Chapter 4, always place a zero (0) before a decimal (e.g., 0.6, not .6). Do not use commas to separate a laboratory value from the name of the test (e.g., hemoglobin 14.0). When typing several laboratory tests, separate related tests by commas and separate unrelated tests by periods. If you are uncertain whether the tests are related, use periods. Use semicolons when a series of internal commas are present.

EXAMPLES

Red blood count 4.2, hemoglobin 12.0, hematocrit 37, urine specific gravity 1.003, pH 5, negative glucose.

Differential showed 60 segs, 3 bands, 30 lymphs, 5 monos, and 2 basos; hemoglobin 16.0; and hematocrit 46.1.

Because normal values vary slightly from one laboratory to another depending on the type of equipment that is used, the figures given throughout this section are approximate. Many values increase from three- to ten-fold during pregnancy. The brief forms and abbreviations given in parentheses are acceptable for use in laboratory data sections of medical documents. The normal values shown here are expressed in conventional units.

Hematology

Blood consists of the following components.

- Formed elements: red blood cells (erythrocytes that carry oxygen), white blood cells (leukocytes that fight infection), and platelets, or thrombocytes (aid in blood coagulation)
- Fluid portion: plasma contains 90% to 92% water and 8% to 10% solids (e.g., carbohydrates, vitamins, hormones, enzymes, lipids, salts)

Hematology Vocabulary

The following information will introduce you to laboratory terms used in medical reports that contain patient blood data.

Test	*Normal Values*	*Clinical Significance*
Haptoglobin	40 to 336 mg/100 mL	Decreases in hemolytic anemia; increases with certain infections
Hemoglobin (H, Hg, HGB)	Male, 14.0 to 18.0 gm/dL Female, 12.0 to 16.0 gm/dL 10 Year old, 12 to 14.5 gm/dL	Increases with polycythemia, high altitude, chronic pulmonary disease; decreases with anemia, hemorrhage

B

Test	*Normal Values*	*Clinical Significance*
Methemoglobin (m-Hg)	1 to 130 mg/100 mL	To evaluate cyanosis
Hematocrit (Crit, H, HCT)	Male, 40% to 54% Female, 37% to 47% Newborn, 50% to 62% 1 Year old, 31% to 39%	Increases with dehydration and polycythemia; decreases with anemia and hemorrhage
White blood cell count	4,200 to 12,000/mm^3 (also typed *4.2 thousand*)	Increases with acute infection, polycythemia, and other diseases; extremely high counts in leukemia; decreases in some viral infections and other conditions
Red blood cell count	Male, 4.6 to 6.2 million/mm^3 Female, 4.2 to 5.4 million/mm^3	Increases with polycythemia and dehydration; decreases with anemia, hemorrhage, and leukemia

Corpuscular Values of Erythrocytes (Indices):

Note: Normal values are different at different ages.

Mean corpuscular volume (MCV)	80 to 105 μm	Increases or decreases in certain anemias
Mean corpuscular hemo-globin (MCH)	27 to 31 pm/RBC	Increases or decreases in certain anemias
Mean corpuscular hemoglobin concentration (MCHC)	32% to 36%	Increases or decreases in certain anemias

Blood Gases

Blood gas values are used to measure the exchange and transport of the gases in the blood and tissues. Many disorders will cause imbalances, such as diabetic ketoacidosis.

	Arterial	*Venous*
pH	735 to 745	733 to 743
Oxygen (O_2) saturation	94% to 100%	60% to 85%
Carbon dioxide (CO_2)	23 to 27 mmol/L	24 to 28 mmol/L
Oxygen partial pressure (PO_2 or pO_2)	80 to 100 mmHg	30 to 50 mmHg
Carbon dioxide partial pressure (PCO_2 or pCO_2)	35 to 45 mmHg	38 to 55 mmHg
Bicarbonate (HCO_3)	22 to 26 mmol/L	23 to 27 mmol/L
Base excess	−2 to +2 mEq/L	

Coagulation Tests

Sedimentation rate (ESR or Sed Rate)	*Wintrobe method:* Male, 0 to 5 mm/hr	Increases with infections, inflammatory diseases,

B

Test	*Normal Values*	*Clinical Significance*
	Female, 0 to 15 mm/hr *Westergren method:* Male, 0 to 15 mm/hr Female, 0 to 20 mm/hr	and tissue destruction; decreases with polycythemia and sickle cell anemia
Prothrombin time (PT)	12.0 to 14.0 sec	Tests ability of blood to clot for patients receiving blood-thinning drugs (e.g., coumadin or heparin)
Partial thromboplastin time (PTT)	35 to 45 sec	Monitors heparin therapy
Fibrin split products (fibrin)	negative at 1:4 dilution	Increases with disseminated intravascular coagulopathy (DIC)
Fibrinogen	200 to 400 mg/100 mL	Increases with disseminated intravascular coagulopathy (DIC)
Fibrinolysis	0	Increases with disseminated intravascular coagulopathy (DIC)
Coombs test	Negative	Test for infants born to Rh negative mothers
Bleeding time		
Duke	1 to 5 min	Tests platelet function
Ivy	<5 min	Tests platelet function
Simplate	3 to 9.5 min	Tests platelet function
Clot lysis time	None in 24 hr	Tests for excessive fibrinolysis
Clot retraction time	30 to 60 min	Tests platelet function
Coagulation time (Lee-White)	5 to 15 min	Tests for abnormalities in clotting
Factor VIII	50% to 150% of normal	Deficient in classic hemophilia
Tourniquet test	Up to 10 petechiae	Vascular abnormalities

Differential

This blood smear study determines the relative number of different types of white blood cells present in the blood; the total should equal 100%. A blood smear contains red blood cells, platelets, and white blood cells. The size and shape (morphology) of these cells are also reported.

Polymorphonuclear neutrophils (polys, segs, stabs, bands)	54% to 62%	Increases with appendicitis, myelogenous leukemia, and bacterial infections
Lymphocytes (lymphs)	25% to 33%	Increases with viral infections, whooping cough, infectious mononucleosis, and lymphocytic leukemia

B

Test	Normal Values	Clinical Significance
Eosinophils (eos or eosin)	1% to 3%	Increases with allergenic reactions, allergies, scarlet fever, parasitic infections, and eosinophilic leukemia
Monocytes (monos)	3% to 7%	Increases with brucellosis, tuberculosis, and monocytic leukemia
Basophils (basos)	0% to 0.75%	
Myelocytes (myelos)	0%	
Platelets	150,000 to 350,000/mm^3	Increases with hemorrhage
Reticulocytes	25,000 to 75,000/mm^3	Decreases with leukemias

Morphology

The shape of the cells can be described with the following terms: aniso (anisocytosis), poik (poikilocytosis), macro (macrocytic), micro (microcytic), and hypochromia.

Chemistry

Test	Normal Values	Clinical Significance
Albumin/globulin (A/G) ratio	1.1 to 2.3	
Albumin	3.0 to 5.0 gm/dL	Decreases with kidney disease and severe burns
Blood urea nitrogen (BUN)	10.0 to 26.0 mg/dL	Diagnosis of kidney disease, liver failure, and other diseases
Calcium (Ca)	8.5 to 10.5 mg/100 mL	Assessment of parathyroid functioning and calcium metabolism and to evaluate malignancies
Cholesterol, serum	150 to 250 mg/100 mL	Increases with diabetes mellitus and hypothyroidism; decreases with hyperthyroidism, acute infections, and pernicious anemia
Creatinine, serum	0.7 to 1.5 mg/100 mL	Screening test of renal function
Electrolyte panel		
Bicarbonate, serum (bicarb or HCO_3)	23 to 29 mEq/L	
Chloride (Cl)	96 to 106 mEq/L	Diagnosis of disorders of acid/base balance

B

Test	*Normal Values*	*Clinical Significance*
Potassium (K)	1.5 to 2.5 mEq/L	Diagnosis of disorders of water balance and acid/base imbalance
Sodium (Na)	136 to 145 mEq/L	Diagnosis of acid/base imbalance occurring in many conditions
Fasting blood sugar	70 to 110 mg/100 mL	Screening test for carbohydrate metabolism
Gamma-glutamyl transpeptidase (GGTP)	8.0 to 35.0 milliunits/mL	
Globulin	1.5 to 3.7 gm/dL	
Glucose-tolerance test (GTT) fasting blood sugar	70 to 100 mg/dL 30 min, 120 to 170 mg/dL 1 hr, 120 to 170 mg/dL 2 hr, 100 to 140 mg/dL 3 hr, <125 mg/dL	Detection of disorders of glucose metabolism
Magnesium, serum	1.5 to 2.5 mEq/L	
Phosphate	3.0 to 4.5 mg/dL	
Immunoglobulins (Ig), Serum		
IgA	60 to 333 mg/dL	Involved in antibody responses
IgD	0.5 to 3.0 mg/dL	Involved in antibody responses
IgE	>300 ng/mL	Involved in antibody responses
IgG	550 to 1,900 mg/dL	Involved in antibody responses
IgM	45 to 145 mg/dL	Involved in antibody responses
Iron, serum	75 to 175 μg/dL	
Lipids, serum, total	450 to 850 mg/dL	
Liver functions		
Acid phosphatase (ACP)	0 to 7.0 milliunits/mL	
Alkaline phosphatase, serum (ALP or alk. phos.)	10 to 32 milliunits/mL	Diagnosis of liver and bone diseases
Bilirubin	0.3 to 1.1 mg/dL	Increases with conditions causing red blood cell destruction or biliary obstruction

B

Test	*Normal Values*	*Clinical Significance*
Lactate dehydrogenase (LDH)	80 to 120 units/mL	Diagnosis of myocardial infarction and differential diagnosis of muscular dystrophy and pernicious anemia
Alanine-aminotransferase (ALT [SGPT[1]])	0 to 17 milliunits/mL	Detection of liver disease; increases with acute pancreatitis, mumps, intestinal obstructions
Aspartate aminotransferase (AST[SGOT[2]])	<35 IU/dL	Detection of tissue damage; increases with myocardial infarction; decreases in some diseases; elevated in liver disease, pancreatitis, excessive trauma of skeletal muscle
Total protein	6.0 to 8.0 gm/dL	Increases with liver diseases
Triglycerides, serum (TG)	40 to 150 mg/100 mL	Elevation occurs in suspected atherosclerosis, liver disease, hypothyroidism, and diabetes mellitus
Uric acid	2.2 to 7.7 mg/dL	Evaluation of renal failure, gout, and leukemia
Radioassay Thyroid Functions		
Tri-iodothyronine (T_3)	25% to 38%	
Thyroxine (T_4)	4.4 to 9.9 μg/100 mL	
Thyroid-stimulating hormone (TSH)	0 to 7 μunits/mL	
Serology		
Antinuclear antibody (ANA) negative	Negative	Diagnosis of certain autoimmune diseases
C-reactive protein (CRP)	Negative	Inflammatory diseases
Rheumatoid arthritis (RA) latex	Negative	Arthritis
Rapid plasma reagin (RPR)	Negative	Diagnosis of venereal disease

[1]SGPT (serum glutamic-pyruvic transaminase) is no longer in use and has been replaced by ALT (alanine aminotransferase).
[2]SGOT (serum glutamic-oxaloacetic transaminase) is no longer in use and has been replaced by AST (aspartate aminotransferase).

B

Test	*Normal Values*	*Clinical Significance*
Venereal Disease Research Laboratory (VDRL)	Nonreactive	Diagnosis of venereal disease (syphilis)

Urinalysis

In a routine urinalysis, four types of examination are performed:

1. Physical examination consisting of volume, color, character, and specific gravity.
2. Chemical examination for determining alkaline or acidity (pH) reaction, glucose, and albumin (protein) content.
3. Chemical tests that include acetone, diacetic acid, urobilinogen, and bilirubin.
4. Microscopic examination for counting the white and red blood cells and identifying casts, cylindroids, epithelial (skin) cells, crystals, amorphous urates and phosphates, bacteria, and parasites.

Urinalysis Vocabulary

The following are laboratory terms used in medical reports that contain patient urine data.

Test	*Normal Values*	*Clinical Significance*
Physical Examination and Chemical Tests		
Color	Yellow, straw, or colorless	Red may mean blood
Turbidity (clarity)	Clear	Cloudy may mean bacteria or pus
Specific gravity (spec. grav.)	1.002 to 1.030	
pH	4.5 to 8.0	Acid or alkaline
Nitrite	Negative	Bacterial infection if present
Protein or albumin	Negative	Kidney function
Glucose (sugar)	Negative	Carbohydrate metabolism
Hemoglobin	Negative	Kidney function
Acetone or ketones	0 or negative	Fat metabolism disorder
Blood, occult	Negative	Kidney function
Bilirubin (bili)	0.02 mg/dL/negative	Liver function
Urobilinogen	0.1 to 1.0 Ehrlich Units/dL	Liver function

B

Test	Normal Values	Clinical Significance
Microscopy		
Cells		
Red blood cells per high-power field (RBC/hpf)	0 to 2/hpf	Increases with infections
White blood cells per high-power field (WBC/hpf)	5/hpf	Increases with infections
Epithelial cells/hpf (renal, caudate cells of renal pelvis, urethral, bladder, vaginal)	Few or moderate	Increases with infections
Bacteria/lpf (low-power field) (yeast and bacteria)	Few or moderate	Increases with infections
Casts (and Artifacts)		
Casts/lpf (granular, fine, coarse, hyaline, leukocyte, epithelial, waxy, blood)	Negative	
Cylindroids		
Mucous threads	Few or moderate	
Spermatozoa	None	Recent intercourse
Trichomonas vaginalis	None	Infection
Cloth fibers and bubbles	None	Poor collection

Crystals Found in Acid Urine

Note: Most crystals are normal; a few are considered abnormal and may be associated with diseases (e.g., cystine, tyrosine, leucine, and some drug crystals).

Test	Normal Values	Clinical Significance
Crystals/lpf (uric acid, amorphous urates, hippuric acid, calcium oxalate, tyrosine needles, leucine spheroids, cholesterin plates, cystine)	Few	
Crystals Found in Alkaline Urine		
Crystals/lpf (triple phosphate, ammonium and magnesium, triple phosphate going in solution, amorphous phosphate, calcium phosphate, calcium carbonate, ammonium urate)	Few	

B

PLURAL FORM SYNOPSIS

If The Singular Ending Is	Example	The Plural Ending Is	Example
a	bursa	ae (pronounce ae as i)	bursae
us	alveolus	i	alveoli
um	labium	a	labia
ma	carcinoma	mata	carcinomata*
on	criterion	a	criteria
is	anastomosis	es	anastomoses
ix	appendix	ices	appendices
ex	apex	ices	apices
ax	thorax	aces	thoraces
en	foramen	ina	foramina
nx	phalanx	ges	phalanges

*A simple "s" ending is also correct: *myomas.*

Exceptions to the Rules

arthritis	arthritides
calyx (calix)	calyces (calices)
comedo	comedones
cornu	cornua
corpus	corpora
embryo	embryos
epididymis	epididymides
femur	femora
genius	geniuses
index	indexes (indices for numeric expressions)
os	ora (when the meaning is *mouths*)
os	ossa (when the meaning is *bones*)
plexus	plexuses
pons	pontes
sinus	sinuses
virus	viruses
viscus	viscera

B

PUNCTUATION RULE SYNOPSIS

Use a Comma or Pair of Commas	*Rule*	*Page*
To set off a nonessential word or words from the rest of the sentence	3.1	60
To set off nonessential appositives	3.1a	61
To set off a parenthetical expression	3.1b	61
To set off an introductory phrase or clause	3.2a	64
	(See also Rule 3.2b)	
To set off the year in a complete date	3.3	65
To set off the name of the state when the city precedes it	3.4	66
To set off "Inc." or "Ltd." in a company name	3.5	66
To set off titles and degrees following a person's name	3.6	66
To separate words in a series	3.7	66
To separate two independent clauses	3.8	67
To set off the name of a person in a direct address	3.9	69
To separate certain modifiers	3.10	69
To avoid confusion	3.11	70
After the complimentary close	3.12	70
In certain long numbers	3.13	70
To separate the parts of a date in the date line of a letter	3.14	70

Use a Period		
At the end of a sentence	3.15	73
With single capitalized word abbreviations	3.16	73
When the genus is abbreviated	3.16	73
In certain lower case abbreviations	3.16	73
To separate a decimal fraction from whole numbers	3.17	73

Use a Semicolon		
Between two independent clauses when there is no conjunction	3.18	73
Between independent clauses if either or both are already punctuated	3.19	73
Before a parenthetical expression when it is used as a conjunction	3.20	74
Between a series of phrases or clauses when any item in the series has internal commas	3.21	74

Use a Colon		
To introduce a list or series of items	3.22	74
After the salutation in a business letter when using "mixed" punctuation	3.23	74
Between the hours and minutes indicating the time in figures	3.24	74
In ratios and dilutions	3.24	74
After the introductory word or words in a history and physical report	3.25	74
With the introductory words in an outline	3.25	74
To introduce an example or clarify an idea	3.26	75

Use a Hyphen		
When two or more words have the force of a single modifier	3.27	77
Between coordinate expressions	3.28	77
In a series of modifiers	3.29	77
When numbers are compounded with words	3.30	77
Within compound numbers 21 to 99 when they are written out	3.31	78
Between a prefix and a proper noun	3.32	78

B

B

SHORT FORMS, BRIEF FORMS, AND MEDICAL SLANG

An asterisk indicates that the short form should be written out. The remainder can be used as is, with site approval.

Short Form	*Means*
abd*	abdomen
abs*	abdominal muscles
adm*	admission
afib*	atrial fibrillation
alk*	alkaline
amt*	amount
anes*	anesthesia
ant*	anterior
approx*	approximately
appy*	appendectomy (also *hot appy,* meaning an acute appendicitis)
bact*	bacteria (pronounced *back-tee*)
bands	band neutrophils
basos	basophils (one of the family of white blood cells)
bili*	bilirubin
bio*	biology
caps	capsules
cath*	catheter
cauc*	Caucasian
consult	consultation
cric*	cricothyrotomy
crit*	hematocrit
cysto*	cystoscopy
defib*	defibrillated
diff*	differential
dig*	digitalis
doc*	doctor
echo*	echocardiogram and so on
echs*	ecchymoses (bruises)
emerg*	emergency
eos	eosinophils (one of the family of white blood cells)
epi*	epidural anesthesia
equiv*	equivalent
esp*	especially
eval*	evaluation
exam	examination
flu	influenza
fluoro*	fluoroscopy
frac*	fracture
frag*	fragment
freq*	frequency or frequent
glob*	globulin
hosp*	hospital
hot appy*	acute appendicitis
hypo*	hypodermic or injection
imp*	impression
infarct	infarction
inoc*	inoculate (pronounced *in-ock*)
inop*	inoperable (pronounced *in-op*)
kilo*	kilogram (kg; e.g., 6 kg, not 6 kilos)
lab	laboratory
lap*	laparotomy

B

Short Form	*Means*
lymphs	lymphocytes (one of the family of white blood cells)
lytes*	electrolytes
max*	maximum
meds*	medications
monos	monocytes (one of the family of white blood cells)
multip*	multipara (a woman who has borne more than one child)
narcs*	narcotics
neg*	negative
nitro*	nitroglycerin
norm	normal
nullip*	nullipara (a woman who has never borne a child)
Pap smear/test	Papanicolaou smear or test
path*	pathology
path lab*	pathology laboratory or department
pecs*	pectoral muscles
peds*	pediatrics
polys	polymorphonuclear leukocytes/granulocytes
pos*	positive
postop*	postoperative
preemie	premature infant
prep	to prepare
prepped	prepared
primip*	primipara (a woman who is bearing her first child)
pro time	prothrombin time (blood clotting time)
procto*	proctoscopy
psych*	psychology or psychiatry or mental health unit
psych eval*	psychiatric evaluation
quads*	quadriceps muscle
reg*	regular
Rx	prescription
script*	prescription
sec*	second or secondary
sed rate	sedimentation rate
segs	segmented neutrophils
spec*	specimen
stabs	stab cells (band cells)
staph	Staphylococcus (a bacterium)
strep	Streptococcus (a bacterium)
subcu*	subcutaneous (usually referring to an injection)
surg*	surgery or to perform surgery
tabby*	therapeutic abortion
temp*	temperature
tibs, fibs, pops*	tibial, fibular, and popliteal
trach*	tracheostomy
V fib*	ventricular fibrillation
V tach*	ventricular tachycardia

Add to the List

B

SOUND AND WORD FINDER TABLE

The following are some common examples of how English and medical terms sound phonetically together with clues as to how they would be spelled to help you locate them in the medical dictionary. If you cannot find a word when you look it up, refer to this table and use another combination of letters that has the same sound.

If the Phonetic Sound Is Like . . .	*Try the Spelling as in . . .*	*Examples*
a in fat	ai	plaid
	al	half
	au	draught
a in sane	ai	pain
	ao	gaol
	au	gauge
	ay	pay, x-ray, Tay-Sachs
	ue	suede
	ie	piedra
	ea	break
	ei	vein
	eigh	weigh
	et	sachet
	ey	they, peyote
a in care	ai	air, clairvoyant
	ay	prayer
	e	there
	ea	wear
	ei	their
a in father	au	aural, auricle, auscultation
	e	sergeant
	ea	heart
a in ago	e	agent
	i	sanity
	o	comply
	u	focus
	iou	vicious
aci in acid	acy	acystia
ak	ac	accident
	ach	achromatic
	acr	acromegaly
ark	arch	archicyte
b in big	bb	rubber
	pb	cupboard
bak sound in back	bac	bacteremia
bee	by	presbyopia
ch in chin	c	cello
	Cz	Czech
	tch	stitch
	ti	question
	tu	denture, fistula

B

If the Phonetic Sound Is Like . . .	*Try the Spelling as in . . .*	*Examples*
d in do	dd	puddle
	ed	called
die	di	diagnosis, diarrhea
dis	dis	discharge
	dys	dyspnea
dew	deu	deuteropathy
	dew	dewlap
	du	dura
e in get	a	any
	ae	aesthetic
	ai	said
	ay	says
	e	edema
	ea	head
	ei	heifer
	eo	leopard
	ie	friend
	oe	roentgen
	u	burial
e in equal	ae	haemoglobin
	ay	quay
	ea	lean
	ee	free
	ei	deceit
	eo	people
	ey	key
	i	hemicardia
	ie	siege
	oe	amoeba
	y	tracheotomy
e in here	ea	ear
	ee	cheer
	ei	weird
	ie	bier
ek	ec	lectotype, eczema
	ek	ekphorize
er in over	ar	liar
	ir	elixir
	or	author, labor
	our	glamour
	re	acre
	ur	augur
	ure	measure
	yr	zephyr
eri, ere, aire	ery	erythrocyte, erythema
you	eu	euphoria, eugenic
ex	ex	extravasation
	x	x-ray

B

If the Phonetic Sound Is Like . . .	*Try the Spelling as in . . .*	*Examples*
f in fine	ff	cliff
	gh	laugh, slough
	lf	half
	ph	physiology, prophylactic
fizz	phys	physical
floo, flu	flu	fluoride, fluoroscopy
g in go	gg	egg
	gh	ghost
	gu	guard
	gue	prologue
gli in glide	gly	glycemia
grew	grou	group
guy (also see jin)	gy	gynecomastia
h in hat	g	Gila monster
	wh	who, whooping cough
he	he	hematoma
	hae (British spelling)	haematology
hi in high	hy	hydrocele
i in it	a	usage
	e	English
	ee	been
	ia	carriage
	ie	sieve
	o	women
	u	busy
	ui	built
	y	laryngeal, nystagmus
i in kite	ai	guaiac
	ay	aye
	ei	height, meiosis
	ey	eye
	ie	tie
	igh	nigh
	is	island of Langerhans
	uy	buy
	y	myograph
	ye	rye
ik or ick	ich	ichthyosis
ink	inc	incubator
j in jam	d	gradual
	dg	judge
	di	soldier
	dj	adjective
	g	register, fungi
	ge	vengeance
	gg	exaggerate

B

If the Phonetic Sound Is Like . . .	*Try the Spelling as in . . .*	*Examples*
gin	gyn	gynecology
k sound in keep	c	eczema
	cc	account
	ch	chronic, tachycardia
	ck	tack
	cq	acquire
	cu	biscuit
	lk	walk
	qu	liquor
	que	plaque
key	che	chemotherapy
	chy	ecchymosis
ko	cho, co	cholecyst, colon
kon	chon	chondroma
	con	condyloma
kw sound in quick	ch	choir
	qu	quintuplet
l in let	ll	call
	sl	isle
la in lay	lay	layette
	le	lei
lack	lac	lacrimal
loo	leu	leukocyte
	lew	lewisite
m in me	chm	drachm
	gm	phlegm
	lm	balm
	mb	limb
	mm	hammer toe
	mn	hymn
mass	mac	macerate
mix	myx	myxedema
n in no	cn	cnemial
	gn	gnathic
	kn	knife
	mn	mnemonic
	nn	tinnitus
	pn	pneumonia
ng in ring	ngue	tongue
new	neu	neurology
	pneu	pneumococcus
o in go	au	mauve
	eau	beau
	eo	yeoman
	ew	sew

B

If the Phonetic Sound Is Like . . .	*Try the Spelling as in . . .*	*Examples*
o in go	oa	foam
	oe	toe
	oh	ohm
	oo	brooch
	ou	shoulder
	ough	dough
	ow	row
o in long	a	all
	ah	Utah
	au	fraud
	aw	thaw
	oa	broad
	ou	ought
off	oph	exophthalmos, ophthalmology
oi in oil	oy	boy
oks	occ	occiput
	ox	oxygen
oo in tool	eu	leukemia
	ew	drew
	o	move
	oe	shoe
	ou	group
	ough	through
	u	rule, tularemia
	ue	blue
	ui	bruise
oo in look	o	wolffian
	ou	would
	u	pull, tuberculosis
ow in out	ou	mouth
	ough	bough
	ow	crowd
p in put	pp	happy
pack	pach	myopachynsis, pachyderma
pi in pie	py	nephropyosis
r in red	rh	rhabdocyte
	rr	berry
	rrh	cirrhosis, hemorrhoid
	wr	wrong, wrist
re in repeat	rhe	rheostosis
	ri	malaria
	rrhe	otorrhea
rew	rheu	rheumatism
	rhu	rhubarb
rom	rhom	rhomboid
rye	rhi	rhinoplasty

B

If the Phonetic Sound Is Like . . .	*Try the Spelling as in . . .*	*Examples*
s in sew	c	cyst, foci
	ce	rice
	ps	psychology
	sc	sciatic, viscera
	sch	schism
	ss	miss
	sth	isthmus
sh in ship	ce	ocean
	ch	chancre
	ci	facial
	s	sugar
	sch	Schwann's cell
	sci	fascia
	se	nauseous
t in tea	pt	pterygium, ptosis
zh sound in azure	ge	garage, massage, curettage
	s	vision
	si	fusion
	zi	glazier
zi (rhymes with sigh)	zy	zygoma, zygote, enzyme
	x	xiphoid
zz	ss	scissors
	zz	buzz

As an additional spelling aid, here is a group of letter combinations that can cause problems when you are trying to locate a word.

If You Have Tried . . .	*Then Try . . .*
pre	per, pra, pri, pro, pru
per	par, pir, por, pur, pre, pro
is	us, ace, ice
ere	ear, eir, ier
wi	whi
we	whe
zi	xy
cks, gz	x
tion	sion, cion, cean, cian
le	tle, el, al
cer	cre
si	psi, ci
ei	ie
x	eks
z	xe

B

If You Have Tried . . .	*Then Try . . .*
dis	dys
ture	teur
tious	seous, scious
air	are, aer
ny	gn, n
ance	ence
ant	ent
able	ible
fizz	phys

B

STATE NAMES AND OTHER U.S. POSTAL SERVICE ABBREVIATIONS

Two-Letter State Abbreviations for the United States and Its Dependencies

Alabama	AL	Kentucky	KY	Oklahoma	OK
Alaska	AK	Louisiana	LA	Oregon	OR
Arizona	AZ	Maine	ME	Pennsylvania	PA
Arkansas	AR	Maryland	MD	Puerto Rico	PR
California	CA	Massachusetts	MA	Rhode Island	RI
Canal Zone	CZ	Michigan	MI	South Carolina	SC
Colorado	CO	Minnesota	MN	South Dakota	SD
Connecticut	CT	Mississippi	MS	Tennessee	TN
Delaware	DE	Missouri	MO	Texas	TX
District of Columbia	DC	Montana	MT	Utah	UT
Florida	FL	Nebraska	NE	Vermont	VT
Georgia	GA	Nevada	NV	Virginia	VA
Guam	GU	New Hampshire	NH	Virgin Islands	VI
Hawaii	HI	New Jersey	NJ	Washington	WA
Idaho	ID	New Mexico	NM	West Virginia	WV
Illinois	IL	New York	NY	Wisconsin	WI
Indiana	IN	North Carolina	NC	Wyoming	WY
Iowa	IA	North Dakota	ND		
Kansas	KS	Ohio	OH		

Common Address Abbreviations Approved by the U.S. Postal Service

Apartment, APT
Association, ASSN
Attention, ATTN
Avenue, AVE
Boulevard, BLVD
Building, BLDG
Center, CTR
Circle, CIR
Department, DEPT
Drive, DRV
East, E
Estate, EST
Expressway, EXPY
Floor, FL
Freeway, FWY
Garden, GDN
Glen, GLN
Harbor, HBR
Haven, HVN
Heights, HTS
Highway, HWY
Hospital, HOSP
Institute, INST
Island, IS
Junction, JCT
Lake, LK
Lakes, LKS
Lane, LN
Manager, MGR
Meadows, MDWS
Mountain, MTN
North, N
Northeast, NE
Northwest, NW
Orchard, ORCH
Palms, PLMS
Park, PK
Parkway, PKY
Place, PL
Plaza, PLZ
Point, PT
Port, PRT
Post Office, PO
President, PRES
Ridge, RDG
River, RIV
Road, RD
Room, RM
Route, RT
Rural, R
Rural Route, RR
Secretary, SECY
Shore, SH
South, S
Southeast, SE
Southwest, SW
Square, SQ
Station, STA
Street, ST
Suite, STE
Terrace, TER
Treasurer, TREAS
Turnpike, TPKE
Union, UN
Valley, VLY
Vice President, VP
View, VW
Village, VLG
West, W

Two-Letter Abbreviations for Canadian Provinces and Territories

Alberta	AB	Newfoundland	NF	Quebec	QC
British Columbia	BC	Northwest Territories	NT	Saskatchewan	SK
Labrador	LB	Nova Scotia	NS	Yukon Territory	YT
Manitoba	MB	Ontario	ON		
New Brunswick	NB	Prince Edward Island	PE		

B

SYMBOLS AND NUMBERS RULE SYNOPSIS

	Rule	*Page*
General		
Abbreviations and numbers	5.15	115
Date	5.1, 5.16	112, 116
Decimals	5.24, 5.25	118, 119
Dimensions	5.19	116
Fractions	5.5, 5.24	113, 118
Indefinite expressions	5.4	113
Large numbers	5.8, 5.10, 5.27	114, 114, 119
Money	5.13	115
Multiple use of numbers	5.2, 5.6, 5.11, 5.24, 5.26	113, 113, 114, 118, 119
Numbers in the address	5.1	112
Ordinal numbers (first, second)	5.1	112
Spelling out numbers	5.2 to 5.8	113, 114
Time of day	5.7, 5.9, 5.17	114, 114, 116
Unrelated numbers	5.26	119
Written-out numbers	5.2 to 5.8	113 to 114
Technical		
Abbreviations	5.30 to 5.40	123 to 125
Capitalization of abbreviations	5.37	124
Chemical abbreviations	5.38	125
Dilute solutions	5.22	118
Electrocardiographic leads	5.21, 5.28	117, 120
Figures with plus or minus	5.23	118
Foreign abbreviations	5.39	125
Greek letters	5.28	120
Metric abbreviations	5.36	124
Military time	5.17	116
Miscellaneous abbreviations		123
O'clock area	5.12	114
Punctuation with abbreviations	5.37	124
Ranges	5.22	118
Ratios	5.22	118
Roman numerals	5.28	120
Spacing with symbols		119
Spinal column and nerves	5.20	117
Subscript and superscript		117
Suture materials	5.18	116
Symbols	5.15, 5.29	115, 122
Units of measurement	5.14, 5.19, 5.22	115, 116, 118
Vital statistics	5.14	115
When not to abbreviate	5.30 to 5.32, 5.40	123, 125

TRADEMARKED FORMS (PACKAGING, DOSAGE FORMS, AND DELIVERY SYSTEMS)

Abbo-Pac
Accu-Pak
Act-O-Vial
ADD-Vantage
Adria-Oncoline
Chemo-Pin
ADT
AeroChamber
Aerotrol
Appli-Kit
Arm-A-Med
Arm-A-Vial
Aspirol
Atrigel
Autohaler
Back-Pack
bidCAP
Brik-Paks
Bristoject
caplet
Capsulets
Captabs
Carpuject
Carpuject Smartpak
Cartrix
Chemo-Pin
Chronosule
Chronotab
Clinipak
ControlPak
D-Lay
Delcap
Dermprotective Factor
DPF
Detecto-Seal
Dey-Dose
Dey-Lute
Dialpak
Dis-Co Pack
Disket
Dispenserpak
Dispertab
Dispette
Divide-Tab
Dividose
Dosa-Trol Pack
Dosepak
Dosette
Dospan
Drop-Dose
Drop-Tainers
Dropperettes
Dulcet
Dura-Tab
Duracaps
DuraSite
EN-tab
Enduret
Enseal
Entri-Pak
Expidet
Extencap
Extentab
Faspak
Fast-Trak
Filmlok
Filmseal
Filmtab
Flo-Pack
gelcap
Gelseal
Glossets
Gradumet
Gy-Pak
Gyrocap
Hyporet
Identi-Dose
Infatab
Inhal-Aid
Inject-all
Inlay-Tab
InspirEase
Intensol
Iofoam
Isoject
Kapseal
Kronocap
Lanacaps
Lanatabs
Lederject
Linguets
Liquid Caps
Liquid Tabs
Liquitab
Lozi-Tabs
Memorette
Min-I-Mix
Mistometer
Mix-O-Vial
Mono-Drop
NewPaks
Nursette
Ocudose
Ocumeter
Oralet
Ovoid
Pastilles
PenFill
Perle
Pilpak
Plateau Cap
Pockethaler
Prefill
Pulvule
Redi Vial
Rediject
Redipak
Release-Tabs
Repetab
Rescue Pak
Respihaler
Respirgard II
Robicap
Robitab
Rotacaps
℞ Pak
SandoPak
Sani-Pak
Secule
Select-A-Jet
Sequels
SigPak
Slocaps
SnapTab
Softab
softgels
Soluspan
Solvet
Spancaps
Spansule
Sprinkle Caps
Stat-Pak
Steri-Dose
Steri-Vial
StrapKap
Supprette
Supule
T-Tabs
Tabloid
Tabules
Tamp-R-Tel
Tel-E-Amp
Tel-E-Dose
Tel-E-Ject
Tel-E-Pack
Tel-E-Vial
Tembid
Tempule
Ten-Tab
TetraBriks
TetraPaks
Thera-Ject
Tiltab
Timecap
Timecelle
Timespan
Timesules
Titradose
Traypak
Tubex
Turbinaire
U-Ject
UDIP
Ultra Vent
Uni-Amp
Uni-nest
Uni-Rx
Unimatic
Unipak
Unisert
Unisom SleepGels
Univial
Vaporole
VCF
Viaflex
Visipak
Wyseal

Compiled from Drake E, Drake R: Saunders Pharmaceutical Word Book. 1995. Reprinted with permission of W.B. Saunders, Philadelphia.

UNUSUAL MEDICAL TERMS COMMONLY DICTATED IN MEDICAL REPORTS

After mastering a beginning terminology course and embarking on a transcription career, you will probably be taken aback when you hear the physician or dictator giving you an unusual expression, such as "coffee-ground stools." The dictation may be quite clear, and you will probably type the expression without difficulty but with a question in your mind concerning what you "really" heard. Or it could be that the dictation is not clear, and you forge ahead, looking for the words in a medical or English reference. Chances are that you will not find the expression. More than 100 unusual terms commonly dictated in medical reports are given here to help you with puzzling dictation.

Term	*Specialist/Definition*
acorn tipped catheter	urologist
Adam's apple	—
aerobic deafness	otolaryngologist
Ambu bag	a low-tech resuscitation tool in the emergency room
angle of Louis	surgeon
argyle tube	surgeon
ash leaf spots (eye)	ophthalmologist
BABYbird respirator	respiratory system
banana blade knife	orthopedist
banjo-string adhesions	surgeon
basement membrane	nephrologist, ophthalmologist
Best clamps	surgeon
bikini bottom	orthopedist
Billroth II (procedure)	gastroenterologist/surgeon
Bird machine (on the Bird)	respiratory system
black doggie clamps	clamps
black heel	orthopedist
blowout fracture	orthopedist
blue bloaters	radiologist
blueberry muffin baby	gynecologist, pediatrician
bony thorax	orthopedist
brawny edema or brawny induration	skin (a general term)
bread-and-butter heart	cardiologist
bubble hair	—
bucket-handle tear	orthopedist
buffy coat	pathologist
CABG (pronounced "cabbage") refers to coronary artery bypass graft	cardiologist
CAT scan	radiologist
café au lait spots	—
chain cystogram	urologist
charley horse	orthopedist
cherry angioma	dermatologist, plastic surgeon
chocolate agar	pathologist
chocolate cyst	—
choked disc (or disk)	ophthalmologist
cigarette (or cigaret) drain	surgeon
clap (gonorrhea)	gynecologist/urologist
clergyman's knee	orthopedist
clog (clot of blood)	cardiovascular surgeon
Coca-Cola-colored urine	—

B

Term	*Specialist/Definition*
coffee-ground stools or emesis	gastroenterologist
cogwheel rigidity or motion	hemologist
cottonoid patty	surgeon
COWS	refers to cold to the opposite, warm to the same—a mnemonic device used in otolaryngology for the Hallpike caloric stimulation response
crick (painful spasm in a muscle, usually in the neck)	orthopedist
currant jelly stools	gastroenterologist
Dandy scissors	surgeon
doll's eye movements	neurologist
fat pad	orthopedist
fat towels (wound towels)	surgeon
fern test (an estrogen test)	gynecologist
finger clubbing	pediatrician, orthopedist
fish fancier's finger	dermatologist
fish-mouthed cervix	obstetrician/gynecologist
flashers and floaters (eye exam)	ophthalmologist
49er brace	orthopedist (a knee brace)
frank breech position	obstetrician
gallops, thrills, and rubs	respiratory system
gimpy (lame)	orthopedist
glitter cells	pathologist
goose egg (swelling due to blunt trauma)	orthopedist
gull-wing sign	neurologist
gulper's gullet	otolaryngologist
gum ball headache	—
guy suture	surgeon
haircut (syphilitic chancre)	—
hammock configuration	—
hanging drop test	pathologist
hickey	dermatologist
His (bundle)	cardiologist
hot potato voice	otolaryngologist
jogger's nipples	orthopedist
joint mice	orthopedist
Kerley's B (costophrenic septal lines)	radiologist
Kerley's C lines	radiologist
kick counts	obstetrician
lacer cock-up (splint)	orthopedist
lemon squeezer (instrument)	vascular surgeon
Little lens	ophthalmologist
loofah folliculitis	dermatologist
loose body	orthopedist
maple syrup urine disease (MSUD)	gynecologist, pediatrician
Mill-house murmur	cardiologist
mouse (periorbital ecchymosis)	ophthalmologist
mouse units	laboratory
MUGA	cardiologist
mulberry molars	—
Mule vitreous sphere	ophthalmologist
musical bruit	cardiologist
Mustard procedure	vascular surgeon

B

Term	*Specialist/Definition*
napkin-ring obstruction	gastroenterologist
nutcracker esophagus	—
nutmeg liver	pathologist
octopus test	ophthalmologist
outrigger (orthopedic)	orthopedist
ox cell hemolysin test	pathologist
oyster (mass of mucus coughed up)	respiratory system
pants-over-vest (technique)	surgeon
parrot beak tear	orthopedist
patient flat lined ("expired" is preferred)	a general term
peanut (a small surgical gauze sponge)	surgeon
PERLA or PERRLA	(pupils equal, regular, react to light and to accommodation)
piggyback probe	—
pigtail catheter	cardiovascular surgeon
piles (hemorrhoids)	proctologist
pill esophagitis	otolaryngologist
pill-rolling (tremor)	neurologist
pink puffer (patient showing dyspnea but no cyanosis)	cardiologist
pins and needles (paresthesias)	neurologist
pollywogs (cotton pledgets or sponges with pointed ends)	surgeon
port-wine stain	gynecologist, pediatrician, plastic surgeon
prep or prepped (from the word "prepared")	surgeon
prostate boggy	urologist
proudflesh (granulation tissue)	surgeon
prune belly syndrome	endocrinologist
pulmonary toilet	pulmonologist
purse-string suture	surgeon
pycnic habit (short, stocky body build)	—
rice-water stools	—
rocker-bottom foot	orthopedist
romied, from an acronym: R = rule, O = out, M = myocardial, I = infarction	cardiologist
rooting reflex	pediatrician
rubber booties	surgeon
rugger jersey sign	—
runner's rump	orthopedist
running off (diarrhea)	gastroenterologist
sago spleen	—
salmon flesh excrescences	—
sand (encrusted secretions about the eyes)	ophthalmologist
saucerize (refers to suturing a cyst inside out so it will heal)	—
sausage fingers	—
scotty dog's ear	surgeon
sea bather's eruption	dermatologist
seagull bruit	respiratory system, cardiologist

B

Term	*Specialist/Definition*
shiner	black eye or hematoma of eye
shoelace suturing	surgeon
shotty nodes	a general term
silver fork deformity	orthopedist
simian crease (seen in Down syndrome)	pediatrician
skin wheals	dermatologist
skinny needle or Chiba needle	surgeon
sky suture	surgeon
sleep (inspissated mucus about the eyes)	a general term
smile or smiling incision	surgeon
smoker's face	a general term
snowball opacities	ophthalmologist
snowbanks	ophthalmologist
snuff box	orthopedist
SOAP note	chart note in following format: (S)ubjective (O)bjective (A)ssessment (P)lan of management
spoon nails	—
steeple sign (on chest x-ray)	radiologist
stick-tie	refers to suture ligature, transfixion suture, or a long strand of suture clamped on a hemostat
stonebasket	urologist
stoved (of a finger) means stubbed	orthopedist
strawberrry gallbladder	—
strawberry hemangioma	gynecologist, pediatrician
strawberry tongue	—
string sign	radiologist
sugar-tong plaster splint	orthopedist
sugar-tongs (instrument)	orthopedist
"surf" test (surfactant test of amniotic fluid)	pathologist
tailor's seat	orthopedist
tennis elbow	orthopedist
trick (of a joint) means unstable	orthopedist
trigger finger	orthopedist
tumor plot	cardiologist
two-flight dyspnea	respiratory system
two-pillow orthopnea	respiratory system
walking pneumonia	respiratory system
weaver's bottom	orthopedist
wet mount	pathologist
wing suture	surgeon
witches milk	neonatologist
yoga foot drop	orthopedist
ZEEP (zero end respiratory pressure)	pulmonologist
zit (comedo)	dermatologist

B

Index

Note: Page numbers in *italics* refer to figures; page numbers followed by t refer to tables.